A **NA**OMI SCHNEIDER BOOK

Highlighting the lives and experiences of marginalized communities, the select titles of this imprint draw from sociology, anthropology, law, and history, as well as from the traditions of journalism and advocacy, to reassess mainstream history and promote unconventional thinking about contemporary social and political issues. Their authors share the passion, commitment, and creativity of Executive Editor Naomi Schneider.

Partner to the Poor

CALIFORNIA SERIES IN PUBLIC ANTHROPOLOGY

The California Series in Public Anthropology emphasizes the anthropologist's role as an engaged intellectual. It continues anthropology's commitment to being an ethnographic witness, to describing, in human terms, how life is lived beyond the borders of many readers' experiences. But it also adds a commitment, through ethnography, to reframing the terms of public debate—transforming received, accepted understandings of social issues with new insights, new framings.

Series Editor: Robert Borofsky (Hawaii Pacific University)

Contributing Editors: Philippe Bourgois (University of Pennsylvania), Paul Farmer (Partners in Health), Alex Hinton (Rutgers University), Carolyn Nordstrom (University of Notre Dame), and Nancy Scheper-Hughes (UC Berkeley)

University of California Press Editor: Naomi Schneider

PAUL FARMER

Partner to the Poor

A Paul Farmer Reader

———

Edited by

Haun Saussy

Foreword by

Tracy Kidder

UNIVERSITY OF CALIFORNIA PRESS

Berkeley   Los Angeles   London

For Didi,
Catherine, Elisabeth, and Sebastien

University of California Press, one of the most distinguished
university presses in the United States, enriches lives around the
world by advancing scholarship in the humanities, social sciences,
and natural sciences. Its activities are supported by the UC Press
Foundation and by philanthropic contributions from individuals
and institutions. For more information, visit www.ucpress.edu.

University of California Press
Berkeley and Los Angeles, California

University of California Press, Ltd.
London, England

Library of Congress Cataloging-in-Publication Data

Farmer, Paul, 1959–
   Partner to the poor : a Paul Farmer reader / Paul Farmer ;
edited by Haun Saussy.
      p. ; cm.
   Includes bibliographical references and index.
   ISBN 978-0-520-25711-5 (cloth : alk. paper)
   ISBN 978-0-520-25713-9 (pbk. : alk. paper)
   1. Poor—Medical care.   2. Medical anthropology.   3. Social
medicine.   4. Epidemiology.   5. Public Health.   I. Saussy,
Haun, 1960–   II. Title.
   [DNLM: 1. Poverty—Personal Narratives.   2. Social Medicine—
Personal Narratives.   3. Internationality—Personal Narratives.
4. Physician's Role—Personal Narratives.   5. Social Justice—
Personal Narratives.   WA 31 F234p 2009]
   RA418.5.P6F375   2010
   362.1086'942—dc22   2009038154

Manufactured in the United States of America

19   18   17   16   15   14   13   12   11   10
10   9   8   7   6   5   4   3   2   1

This book is printed on Cascades Enviro 100, a 100% post consumer waste, recycled, de-inked fiber. FSC recycled certified
and processed chlorine free. It is acid free, Ecologo certified,
and manufactured by BioGas energy.

CONTENTS

Foreword

Seeing the Proof

Tracy Kidder

A few years back I wrote a book called *Mountains Beyond Mountains*. It has a subtitle: "The Quest of Dr. Paul Farmer, a Man Who Would Cure the World." I don't much like subtitles and I didn't add this one willingly, but I suppose it's accurate enough. My book is mostly about one person, Paul Farmer, and, as we all know, the old saw that one person can make a difference in this world really isn't the whole truth. Paul Farmer never wanted me to imagine that he alone was responsible for the early work of Partners In Health. In fact, I think that if he'd been the writer, he would have given equal time to all the people involved in the early days—to Tom White, and Jim Yong Kim, and Fritz Lafontant, and Ophelia Dahl, and Loune Viaud, and Todd McCormack, and Haun Saussy, and the rest of a cast of at least dozens. But I have to add that I couldn't have written a book like that, and I'm glad I didn't try.

I traveled quite a lot with Paul Farmer, and some of those trips were, collectively, like a harrowing of hell for me—to the famished, deforested Central Plateau of Haiti; to a periurban slum outside Lima, Peru, which, as the residents say, looks like the surface of the moon; to Moscow's Central Prison, where what the doctors described as an "uncrowded cell" contained fifty patients coughing up drug-resistant TB bacilli. In those places, particularly, Paul Farmer showed me more reasons for despair than I've ever seen before, or indeed imagined. And yet it was the most exhilarating experience of my life. PIH was still pretty small then, back in 2000, and yet they were creating vivid proof that diseases which could be treated successfully in the developed world could also be treated successfully and economically in some of the poorest, most difficult settings imaginable. That was the moving thing for me. Seeing the proof.

We also went to less difficult places. Havana, Cuba, for instance. We spent most of our week there in the company of a world-class infectious-disease doctor named Jorge Pérez Ávila, who all by himself—by example, as it were—corrected some of the prejudices I brought with me to Cuba. Years of bad publicity had left me imagining the place as gray and rather colorless, puritanically Stalinist. One night we ended up in the bar of a fancy hotel, renovated with European money. There we were fed dinner by the manager, a Cuban woman named Ninfa, a patient of Jorge's. At some point, Jorge turned to her and said, in words like these, "Ninfa. That is such a lovely name. But how did your parents know when you were born that you would be so beautiful?" Ninfa smiled, and turned to me. "Jorge has a very special way with all his female patients," she said. "We all want to sleep with him."

I began to sense that Cuba was a place where one might be able to have a pretty good time. I already knew that Paul Farmer's idea of a really good time was to visit patients. In Cuba, he did what he often did in other places where he had no patients of his own: he borrowed some from other doctors. Anyway, visiting patients also was Jorge's idea of rip-roaring fun, so that's what they did, while I tagged along. They visited Jorge's patients, mostly women, most of whom were pregnant. And after a while I would say to Jorge, "Is this patient pregnant, too?" just to hear his answer, which was, invariably, "Yes, but it is not my pregnancy."

I remember going on rounds with Paul and his students at the Brigham and Women's Hospital in Boston many times—evenings that would stretch late into the night, nights that were always the oddest mix of the comical and serious, yet always a cheerful experience somehow, rounds at the Brigham with Dr. Farmer, maybe because every tool ever invented for repairing patients was right at hand.

I remember a fashion show that the TB patients at Zanmi Lasante in Haiti put on, to celebrate Paul's birthday—I was sure that party would find its way into the book I was going to write, but it didn't, perhaps because I was laughing so hard at one moment and felt so enchanted the next that I couldn't take adequate notes. I remember Mamito, the matriarch of Zanmi Lasante, scolding me for something Paul had done about fifteen years before—scolding *me* because Paul had asked me, really almost begged me, to intercede on his behalf and explain to her why we had gone on an eleven-hour hike. I remember long treks and conversations with the wonderful, hot-headed Ti Jean, who built God knows how many houses for the poorest of Zanmi Lasante's patients. Ti Jean once carried me across a river. Another time he fed me and Paul a dinner of guinea fowl and Barbancourt rum. I miss him. He had a habit of telling Paul to shut up when Paul dared to interrupt one of his discourses—and the interesting thing about those moments was that Paul actually would shut up.

Then there were the christenings of patients' newborn babies—in Peru, for instance—with Paul in the role of godfather. This summer in Rwanda, I learned that this happens in Africa, too. And I found myself thinking, This is pretty cool, the guy has godchildren all over the world, more godchildren than a mafia don.

I remember quite vividly watching Paul testify in a grubby little courtroom in New York City—the INS was trying to deport a Haitian man with AIDS, and Paul was testifying to the effect that sending this man back to prisons in Haiti was tantamount to torture. The district attorney seemed like a pretty tough cookie, but after listening to Paul describe conditions in Haiti, she stopped putting up any fight at all and started asking him questions that seemed calculated to injure her case. Periodically, as I recall, this prosecutor would exclaim, "Good God! I had no idea it was that bad!" And I also recall that, on the way to the courtroom, Paul started worrying that his necktie was too flamboyant to wear before a judge. He insisted I give him my much more conservative tie. I still have the fiery red one that he gave me in return, though I do not wear it.

Finally, there was a night in Moscow. A congenial dinner with a famous personage in public health. By day Paul had been arguing with him. The fight had to do with milk: Paul wanted Russian prisoners with TB to get a glass of milk each day, and the public health expert didn't think this was necessary. I drank a therapeutic amount of Côtes du Rhône at dinner. Afterward, walking down a snowy Moscow street in the dark, I needled Paul a little. I may have recited a line I heard many times from people in the business of international health, which goes like this: "Doctors are very nice. They think the patient in front of them is the most important thing. But we care about something more important, which is the health of populations." I repeated something like that and then said of our dinner companion, "He's interested in public health."

"I'm interested in public health, too!" said Paul. "But what is the public? Is it a family, a village, a city, a country? Who are these people to say what the public is?" He was smiling. I think he'd had a therapeutic dose of Côtes du Rhône, too. His tone was jocular, but by then I knew that jocularity was often the tone in which he disguised statements of great importance to him. And I've been turning that statement over in my mind ever since, The Moscow Statement, as it were.

Partners In Health doesn't have all the answers as to how to go about fixing the dreadful poverty and disease that afflict billions of people today. I don't think anyone in the organization ever said they did. And even if they did have all the answers, they couldn't bring the terrifying pandemics of AIDS and TB and malaria under control all by themselves, any more than Paul Farmer could have created and nurtured Partners In Health all by himself. But they have shown the world that it is possible to control those diseases and to redress some of the underlying causes that have turned those diseases into pandemics. In some cases, with multidrug-resistant TB, for instance, they have given the world precise prescriptions, and they have made it possible for poor countries to use those prescriptions—largely thanks to Jim Kim, who figured out how to drive down the prices of the necessary drugs by about 90 percent.

But what they have done above all, I think, is to present both a rebuke and a challenge to the United States and the other wealthy countries and to offer all of us a real kind of hope, hope backed up by fact. They have done this, I believe, by paying attention to the needs of individual patients, in Haiti, Peru, Russia, Boston, and now Africa. It has been individual patients, people just like you and me, who have taught them how to treat a family, a village, a city, a country, maybe the world.

Introduction

The Right to Claim Rights

Haun Saussy

"BAGAY KI PA SENP / STUFF THAT IS NOT SIMPLE"

People sometimes refer to Paul Edward Farmer, MD, born in 1959, as a hero, saint, madman, or genius. Any or all of these descriptions may hold—but the essential thing about him is that he listens to his patients.

In the earliest piece of writing collected here ("Bad Blood, Spoiled Milk," from 1988), the young Paul Farmer, anthropologist, epidemiologist, doctor to the poor, gives an informant the last word:

> I consulted [Madame Gracia] regarding the ingredients of the herbal remedy for *move san/lèt gate*. Her response, and the tone in which it was delivered, brought me up short: "Surely you are collecting these leaves in order to better understand their power and improve their efficacy?" Had she added, "If you think we'll be satisfied with a symbolic analysis of *move san/lèt gate*, you're quite mistaken," I would not have been more surprised.[1]

As if Madame Gracia were telling Paul: "Here's the information you requested; do not file under 'Folklore.'"

A similar scene of instruction occurs early in Tracy Kidder's *Mountains Beyond Mountains*. A research project in rural Haiti had begun with the assumption that patients' beliefs about how they contracted tuberculosis—did they think it was caused by microbes or by sorcery?—made a difference for compliance and outcomes. The results of the study, however, showed no relation between belief and the results of treatment; the main factor influencing cure rates was the availability of food and social support. This might have meant that culture was irrelevant to practicing medicine in the Third World, a conclusion that this anthropologist-in-training was loath to adopt. Thinking that perhaps his own skills in eliciting tacit attitudes about sorcery were to blame for the discordant conclusions, Farmer began reinterviewing patients. Kidder describes him speaking to "a sweet, rather elderly woman":

> When he had first interviewed her, about a year before, she'd taken mild offense at his questions about sorcery. She'd been one of the few to deny she believed in it. "Polo, *chéri*," she had said, "I'm not stupid. I know tuberculosis comes from people coughing germs." She'd taken all her medicines. She'd been cured.
>
> But now, a year later, when he asked her again about sorcery, she said that of course she believed in it. "I know who sent me my sickness, and I'm going to get her back," she told him.
>
> "But if you believe that," he cried, "why did you take your medicines?"
>
> She looked at him. He remembered a small sympathetic smile. The smile, he thought, of an elder explaining something to a child—in fact, he was only twenty-nine. "*Chéri*," she said, "*èske-w pa konprann bagay ki pa senp?*" The Creole phrase *pa senp* means "not simple," and implies that a thing is freighted with complexity, usually of a magical sort. So, in free translation, she said to Farmer, "Honey, are you incapable of complexity?"[2]

Both of these tales end with an abrupt change of focus, an epiphany. Part of the change is evidenced by a stylistic shift in which the remarks of the Haitian informant are translated into language that we are more likely to attribute to a graduate seminar than to dwellers in palm-frond huts with dirt floors. The shift in linguistic register mirrors a change in the tacit rules of the conversation between doctor and patient or between anthropologist and informant: the person conventionally assumed to be tongue-tied—the patient, the layperson, the primitive—seizes authority over the discussion, redefining its subject and purpose.

At such moments, the reader has the sense of a new narrative opening. The future—like the futures to which the last pages of *Old Goriot, Great Expectations,* or *Crime and Punishment* deliver their characters—will be different. Dr. Farmer learns from his patients. Their stories change the story he tells and the way he tells it.[3]

Medicine is both a formidably walled fortress of specializations and a standing rebuke to specialization. It is perhaps the one true humanistic discipline. Everything that impinges on the human species, from chemistry to psychology, from particle physics to marital discord, falls under its survey. When your case becomes serious, the general practitioner gives way to the cardiologist or the oncologist, who may send you to see a further, even more minutely focused, specialist; but an adequate explanation of what has gone wrong with you, as opposed to the remedies to be applied to its effects, may demand the talents of the geographer, the economist, the historian, the hydroelectric engineer, the novelist.

Your feelings of despair may interest both the researcher of neuronal networks, armed with sensors and magnetic-resonance imaging machines, and the chronicler of the fading American auto industry, whose local subsidiary recently folded and left you with a mortgage to pay and only so many months of unemployment compensation. Case studies are never one-dimensional. The inherent multiplicity of medicine declares that things are "not simple," while also showing that they are never without reason.

Complexity—the ability to negotiate among widely variant frames and scales of explanation—is a necessity in Paul Farmer's chosen terrain. A given person's disease is both a biological event with microscopic agents and a social event with human determinants, some of them (for example, trans-Atlantic slavery) reaching back hundreds of years and involving millions of strangers in related patterns of action. Rudolf Virchow had in mind housing, diet, working conditions, and birthrates when, even in the pre-microbial era, he designated doctors "the natural attorneys of the poor."[4] In recent years, medical training has been broadened to include reflection on social and cultural factors of illness, not just clinical ones. Attention to such causes makes for better doctors and more perspicuous diagnoses. But the essential thing is to clarify the relations among biological, economic, social, cultural, and other determinants of disease, not to use one of these dimensions as a cover for impotence in another. Much of Dr. Farmer's effort has gone into a polite, persistent struggle against the "immodest claims of causality" that doom certain sick people to an epidemiological dungeon whose outlines precisely match their cultural dungeon.

We have a striking example from early analysis of the AIDS epidemic. Reporting, on June 24, 1983, on the basis of 1,641 HIV cases verified in the United States and Puerto Rico, the U.S. Centers for Disease Control observed: "Groups at highest risk of acquiring AIDS continue to be homosexual and bisexual men (71% of cases), intravenous drug users (17%), persons born in Haiti and now living in the United States (5%), and patients with hemophilia (1%). Six percent of the cases cannot be placed in one of the above risk groups."[5] Four risk groups and one "undetermined" group adding up, with suspicious neatness, to precisely 100 percent, as if it were impossible for a person to be, for example, a bisexual intravenous drug user of Haitian origin: the CDC's statistics show the usual flaws of rough-cut data gathering and do not begin to frame an explanation. Of the categories, one is definable genetically (absence of a clotting factor in the blood), two are definable by behavior (a history of engaging in certain sex acts or taking drugs in a certain way), and one is a matter of nationality. It makes no sense for the total of five such categories to amount to 100 percent, except as an artifact of the process by which the data were gathered. A more cynical and accurate description would have read: "In 71% of cases, the examining physician chose to check off the box marked 'homosexual man'; in 17%, the doctor marked 'drug injector,'" and so forth.

But despite these obvious flaws, the CDC's report on an as yet little-understood disease could be—and was—read as an epistemological riddle. *What do gay men, heroin addicts, Haitians, and hemophiliacs have in common? The answer might explain AIDS!* And so, with biomedicine slow to deliver its suspect (the responsible "agent"), the sciences of behavior leapt in to answer a poorly posed question with the tools of ethnography, rumor, and prejudice. Leaving hemophiliacs aside, and picking up the hint in the CDC report that the unknown agent was most likely transmitted through the blood, journalists, abetted by anthropologists, connected the dots in a fantastic shower of clichés: blood sacrifice, pederasty, barbarism, black magic. The *Journal of the American Medical Association* lent its professional majesty to the question, "Do necromantic zombiists transmit HTLV-III/LAV during voodooistic rituals?"[6] If this is medical anthropology, neither the medical personnel nor the social scientists did much honor to their professions by joining forces. To be sure, the disease was poorly understood, and a range of divergent hypotheses about its origin and transmission were, quite legitimately, being explored. And the gamut from blood to behavior to passports testifies once more to the inherent multidimensionality of medicine. But one would not have to be a Haitian to have felt at that moment that less interdisciplinarity, rather than more of it, would have been a good thing.

In those early years of the AIDS epidemic, Paul Farmer was a medical student at Harvard who spent most of his time helping out at a clinic in rural Haiti while also doing research for his doctorate in anthropology. He was in a good position, therefore, to replace bad interdisciplinarity with good. A sense for complexity ought to enlarge medicine by prompting investigators to trace the effects of behavior, culture, and economy on disease sufferers. The interdisciplinary task of these investigators would be to account for the inputs of these factors to the organism, not to guess wildly at the implications of category labels. (The hapless speculators would have made less of a foolish impression, besides, if the connotations of their categories—for example, that of "Haitian"—had been backed up with actual experience on the terrain: what does it *imply*, in terms of behavior and social networks, to be a Haitian immigrant in the United States?)

Farmer's essay "The Exotic and the Mundane: Human Immunodeficiency Virus in Haiti" (1990) and his book *AIDS and Accusation: Haiti and the Geography of Blame* (1992) showed the reasons for the association between Haitians and HIV. It had nothing to do with voodoo rites, African bloodlines, or other excuses for projecting impurity onto a tiny Caribbean nation, and a great deal to do with poverty and the desperation that drove country people to the city and reduced them to selling their bodies to tourists and their blood to commercial agencies. The wish to blame AIDS on Haitian immigrants appeared to be the latest rationalization for a longstanding prejudice, and the explanation for those "immodest claims" was to be found in "the North American folk model of Haitians."

The reversal implicit in the phrase "folk model"—for once, the Haitian version of world history being able to frame the other as a mere ethnographic curiosity—must have given Farmer a bitter satisfaction. At issue, however, was not denouncing sloppy scholarship or staring down stereotypes, but demonstrating the ease with which statistics, history, and pathology could be overwhelmed by an account of disease that was both wrong and utterly "simple." Of all the points of view recorded in *AIDS and Accusation,* the ones least often in accord with the findings of epidemiology are those of popular journalists, those amateur social scientists whose "knowledge base" often cannot tell rumor from well-established fact, yet who have tremendous powers of influence precisely because they tend to confirm what their public already believes.

Haitian villagers, on the other hand, gave accounts of disease history and transmission that seconded the conclusions of the virology labs. HIV crept along channels of inequality in the body politic. It took advantage of the many situations of sexual contact where one party had the edge and the other party had no choice: where one party was, typically, a U.S. tourist, a Haitian soldier or paramilitary, a truck driver, or a local bigwig; and the other was, typically, a handsome young man or woman who had left the poverty of the countryside to seek a better life doing menial labor in town. Haitians, especially poor rural Haitians, were not to blame for HIV; if anything, it was another curse among many visited on them from outside. So said the virology; so said the country people. The nonsense shouted about AIDS and Haiti gave Paul Farmer early lessons in how to think, and how not to think, about the diseases of the poor. It wasn't that rural Haitians' theories of disease transmission were superior or that the witnesses were monotonously truthful. One had to know how to listen.

THE OUTCOME GAP

"Blaming the victim"—in this instance, casting the sufferer as the source of the disease—is a crude version of a strategy of despair that Farmer has repeatedly challenged in his career. Many of the essays included in this volume document and counter the temptation to make social science the cover for ineffective or nonexistent medical treatment. Sometimes the excuses for which slapdash ethnography substitutes are comically transparent. For example, before the President's Emergency Plan for AIDS Relief, initiated in 2003, reversed standing priorities, officials of the U.S. Agency for International Development and the Department of the Treasury occasionally contended that distributing antiretroviral remedies to Africa and Asia would be irresponsible and futile because people in these regions lacked "the Western sense of time" and could not be taught to take their medications at regular intervals; the lack of paved roads and the absence of refrigeration (neither essential to delivering first-rate HIV care) were brought up as well.[7] Past experiences of failure in tuberculosis control were mustered up, too, bolstered by reductive, anecdotal accounts of culture that blamed "noncompliance" with the prescribed regimen on the patients' irrational beliefs or general fecklessness.[8] Good medicine was not to be wasted on undeserving people—and rather than adapting to poverty and decrepit infrastructure, or addressing as yet unknown beliefs that might drive patients away from clinics that offered antiretroviral therapy, critics preferred to exile the sufferers to a forest of dubious sociological constructs.

Social medicine, according to Paul Farmer and the medical charity he founded in 1986, Partners In Health, does not consist of ordering up social science research that justifies medical inaction. Rather, it is directed at identifying the obstacles to care and removing them. Often, the most obvious obstacle is the price of drugs, and it is usually sufficient to prevent the topic of effective treatment for poor people with maladies like HIV, cancer, or multidrug-resistant tuberculosis from ever coming up. To account for instances where drugs are within reach but beyond many sufferers' budgets, a considerable literature exists on the problem of patient "compliance." In the experience of PIH, the problem usually resides with the services offered, not the patients. When tuberculosis or HIV patients have to choose between buying pills and feeding their families, the result, more often than not, is missed appointments. When patients enrolled in a TB or AIDS program receive medicines along with food that can help to replace their lost incomes, compliance is no longer a problem, and cure rates rival those in the wealthiest, best-equipped settings. To this way of thinking, social medicine does not just analyze the social factors that contribute to populations' susceptibility to disease; it seizes on certain organizing principles of society (here, the market model for distribution of goods and services) and reworks them for the sake of medical efficacy.

In a series of medical journal articles in 2001 and 2002, Farmer and colleagues presented their model for treating HIV in settings of extreme poverty.[9] The model—including free voluntary testing and counseling; provision of antiretroviral medications, food, and social services; and daily accompaniment by community health workers, all free to the patient—was patterned on programs that the same group had used in treating multidrug-resistant tuberculosis in Peru, Haiti, and Siberia.[10] Writing in the *Bulletin of the World Health Organization*, Farmer's group reported on Haitian HIV sufferers who were being treated with antiretroviral medications:

> The clinical response to therapy was favorable in 59 of the first 60 patients (over 40 more were enrolled in 2001). We estimate that 48 of these patients were able to resume working and caring for their children. The weights of all but two patients

increased by more than 2 kg within the first 3 months of therapy. In a subset of 21 DOT-HAART [directly observed therapy with highly active antiretroviral therapy] patients whose viral loads were tested, 18 (86%) had no detectable virus in peripheral blood. This suggests that therapy was quite effective. Most studies based in the USA demonstrate viral suppression in only about 50% of patients after one year of treatment. . . .

The provision of life-saving care through the HIV Equity Initiative has had a favorable impact on staff morale. It is our belief that the stigma associated with AIDS has diminished as a result of dramatic responses to therapy. . . . A related consequence of introducing DOT-HAART is an increased use of the clinic's free HIV testing and counseling services. . . . Thus the provision of AIDS treatment has strengthened AIDS prevention.[11]

Beyond the immediate public of specialists in medicine and public health, the articles were addressed to the various factions implicated in one way or another in the AIDS crisis—governments, nongovernmental organizations, international bodies, charitable foundations, activist groups—and in not too roundabout a way sought their support. As the authors pointed out, "the DOT-HAART project described above is so small [1,350 patients diagnosed, approximately 150 of whom received antiretroviral therapy] that it would not merit attention in the public health literature if we could point to larger and better studies that respond aggressively to the growing challenge of HIV. Because we cannot, we hope that our experience might be instructive in other settings where HIV and poverty are the top-ranking threats to health." That is a quiet way of stating that PIH's efforts in the Central Plateau of Haiti were unique and ought to be emulated elsewhere.[12]

But how? And who would pay? Although no price tag was given (the authors acknowledged support from Partners In Health donors, hospitals, and foundations), at several points the article referred to "objections to the treatment of AIDS with HAART, including those of unfeasibility and patients' non-compliance."

> Our own attempts to obtain funding were often met with resistance on the grounds that the project would be unsustainable in a country as poor as Haiti. . . . We estimate that 75%–80% of project expenditures have been for medications. . . . Most regimens cost more than US$ 10,000 per year per person. . . . At such prices . . . the implementation of HAART in a poor country, even with the DOT-HAART approach to assure compliance, is considered in international medical and public health circles as neither sustainable nor cost-effective.[13]

The concluding section sharpened the ironies and all but implicated the very concept of "sustainability" wielded in those "international medical and public health circles" as a co-factor in the ongoing epidemic:

If HIV reveals a lack of basic primary care services for the poor, an aggressive response to this comparatively new disease may help to solve a host of old problems. High drug costs and the need for sustained monitoring have led many observers to conclude that aggressive treatment of chronic disease is neither feasible nor sustainable in those communities where the demand for treatment is greatest. The result is a growing "outcome gap" between rich and poor even as diseases become treatable by means of new medical technologies among people who have access to them.[14]

That sounds like a challenge. Responses by fellow experts in the same issue of the journal mainly sidestepped it. They chose not to address the objection to the criterion of "sustainability," or they simply repeated the words "neither feasible nor sustainable"; and some, in their recommendations, loaded the potential programs that might follow the model of PIH's pilot study with even greater financial and technological burdens. Anthony Mbewu was reluctant to generalize from the PIH study:

> Farmer et al. provide a starting point, but many more clinical trials are needed to investigate the efficacy of antiretrovirals in prolonging life and improving the quality of life lived with AIDS in developing countries. . . . Initial diagnosis should include a CD4 count, as accurate diagnosis and appropriate selection of patients for treatment [are] crucial. Treatment of newly infected patients requires more research. . . . Even with the drastic reductions in price of ARVs, to US$ 350 per annum, they remain unaffordable for most developing countries. Even in an "upper middle" income country such as South Africa, per capita health care expenditure in the public sector is only US$ 88 per annum.[15]

Richard Feachem struck a note of pathos:

> My dilemma is that the world is still a long way from being able to make antiretroviral drugs, even if they were free, effectively available to the majority of the people who are infected with HIV. I wish that the world was different. I wish that poor countries were not so poor. I wish that the health systems of poor countries were not so dysfunctional. I wish that rich countries were far more generous in their support for health sector activities in poor countries. Regrettably, none of this is the case in the real world in which we live. . . .
>
> [The position that access to HAART is a human right] may be right in a moral sense, but it is not practical. To advocate the impossible is to put at risk the achievement of more limited objectives. . . . An international effort focused on establishing and sustaining a number of islands of learning and good practice is likely to make a greater contribution to the reduction of suffering and unnecessary death than spreading limited resources thinly across the low-income countries.
>
> The approach that I recommend is very difficult for international agencies to adopt, for obvious political reasons. It is, however, an approach that the major foundations can take. . . . Let us make sure that the best is not seen as the enemy of the good.[16]

Charles Gilks, Carla AbouZahr, and Tomris Türmen suggested that the outcomes reported by PIH were the epidemiological equivalent of bonsai and should be viewed with clinical skepticism:

> Farmer et al. present a remarkable achievement: the establishment of a care service for people with HIV/AIDS in a community of poor displaced people living in a remote rural area of Haiti. . . . If the claims of the authors are substantiated, such a model would have enormous potential for replication in other resource-poor settings. If, on the other hand, the authors' claims are exaggerated, the potential for doing more harm than good would be great. . . .
>
> The authors' main contention is that the concerns voiced about treating HIV-positive people with HAART—namely high cost of drugs, lack of health system capacity to deliver them effectively, possibility of non-compliance, and risk of drug resistance—are ill-founded. If we are to be convinced that this is so, we need better evidence than that provided in this paper. . . .
>
> By any evaluation criteria—whether cost-effectiveness, sustainability, feasibility, or absence of unintended negative consequences—this success story must be classified as non-proven. Yes, we know with exceptional circumstances, motivation, resources and generous research funding positive outcomes can be achieved, but replication is something else entirely. Yes, it is true that with huge inputs the miracle of anti-retroviral therapy will produce stunning successes. And certainly, acting when others have failed to do so is noble. However, for lack of appropriate design and scientific evaluation, important lessons that might have been applied in other settings simply cannot be drawn from this study.[17]

The discussion around providing antiretroviral therapy to penniless Haitians suggested that the Partners In Health initiative was, however "noble," potentially capable of "doing more harm than good." From the point of view of international aid institutions, the PIH model of treatment had many drawbacks. It would involve spending large amounts of money outside existing budgets and breaking down distinctions between medical, economic, and social forms of intervention. Moreover, it reversed the usual pattern of action in medical assistance programs. It sought, as the PIH doctors proudly put it, to "remove the onus of adherence from vulnerable patients and place it squarely on the providers."[18] Rather than waiting in their clinics for patients to come in and ask for treatment (and get the best treatment commensurate with their ability to pay), the doctors and their colleagues were being told to go out into the villages, find the people suffering from contagious diseases, and give them medication, food, and social support.

In addition, far from aiming at some "sustainable" future in which Haiti or Peru would carry the costs of epidemic illness, this plan recognized that the only way to make modern medicine happen in the poorest countries of the world was for the wealthy countries to pay for it. Without a doubt, the PIH clinicians and researchers were addressing the "outcome gap": whether substantially or symbolically remained to be seen. For the time being, Richard Feachem's predictions were borne out: PIH continued to depend on foundations for the greater part of its funding. Nonetheless, in 2002 the people of PIH had the satisfaction of seeing the World Health Organization adopt guidelines similar to theirs for treatment of multidrug-resistant tuberculosis in settings of poverty, and then of observing the creation of the Global Fund to Fight AIDS, Tuberculosis, and Malaria. In 2003, the WHO declared the HIV epidemic a worldwide public health emergency and announced its intention to see three million people who were living in poverty begin to receive antiretroviral therapies by 2005 (a goal reached sometime in 2008 and amounting to 31 percent of the estimated need).[19]

But none of this amounted to a general recognition of HAART (or whatever approach sets the highest contemporary standard of care) as a human right. Only that position makes health care for the poor sustainable, as PIH understands "sustainable." Foundations, like wealthy individuals with a hobby, can change their minds; religious or political groups can distort the medical agenda; indispensable local allies can drop out of the picture; the epidemics can and will go on growing.[20] What can argument, or even an excellent example, do in the face of the thesis (self-confirming by merely being pronounced) that "resources are limited" and "the world is like that"?

To put into context the faint praise ("acting when others have failed to do so is noble") bestowed on Partners In Health by a trio of WHO analysts, it is useful to point out that in 2000, AIDS had already killed more people than any epidemic since the worldwide bubonic plague of the fourteenth century, and yet "the quasi-totality of AIDS assistance to the [most] heavily-burdened countries ... consisted of the promotion of education and condom distribution."[21] So ineffectual a response requires explanation. The reason cannot be medical, because the effectiveness of antiretroviral therapy was uncontroversial in the First World: thousands of men and women got up every day and went about their business thanks to the combination regimens devised in 1996, which turned AIDS into a manageable chronic disease. The justification for the "different standards of care—treatment for the affluent, no treatment for the poor"[22] and the consequent "outcome gap"—was presented in the language of economics: resources were scarce; it was not "cost-effective" to allocate drugs purely on the basis of need; the rationing of AIDS care had to be planned for guaranteed success.

But for Farmer and his associates, the issues could not be left in that language: they had to be translated into a logically and politically more powerful idiom. That was the only way to break out of the self-confirming loop described in a 2001 *Lancet* paper: "Funding for expansion of this pilot project [in central Haiti] was sought from a number of international agencies charged with responding to AIDS; all declined to support this effort on the grounds that the drug costs were too high to meet so-called sustainability criteria. Pharmaceutical companies were approached for contributions or concessional prices but referred us back to the same international agencies that had already termed the project unsustainable."[23]

The language that came naturally to Partners In Health in describing this predicament was philosophical and moral. Abandoning the vast majority of AIDS sufferers to their fate had to be presented and constantly re-presented as a moral and political decision that inscribed in the flesh of millions of people the differential valuation of human lives that had currency "in the halls of power" (to use the customary Farmer shorthand). The horrible irony of tuberculosis—that "the advent of effective therapy seems only to have further entrenched [the] striking variation in disease distribution and outcomes" between rich and poor—had recurred for these new plagues. The fact that the poor were condemned to die of treatable diseases like AIDS and TB symptomatized the condition of "structural violence" (another piece of Farmer shorthand); it emanated from decisions that had to be framed as political and moral, not technological, arithmetic, or biological.[24] In the compound noun "social medicine," the social analysis once more had to lead the medical application.

"A CERTAIN PERCENTAGE"

Early in *Crime and Punishment*, Raskolnikov, who has not yet advanced to ax murder, is wandering the boulevards of St. Petersburg and comes across a sixteen-year-old girl in a torn dress, drunk to the point of blacking out and already attracting the interest of a predatory-looking older man. Raskolnikov calls a policeman and attempts to send the girl home in a cab. His rescue plan fails, and as the girl, her would-be admirer, and the policeman move down the street, Raskolnikov consoles himself with the then-new science of statistics:

> "Poor girl! . . . ," he said, having looked at the now empty end of the bench. "She'll come to her senses, cry a little, and then her mother will find out. . . . First she'll hit her, then she'll give her a whipping, badly and shamefully, and maybe even throw her out. . . . Then right away the hospital . . . well, and then . . . then the hospital again . . . wine . . . pot-houses . . . back to the hospital. . . . in two or three years she'll be a wreck, so altogether she'll have lived to be nineteen, or only eighteen years old. . . . Haven't I seen the likes of her? And how did they come to it? Just the same way . . . that's how. . . . Pah! And so what! They say that's just how it ought to be. Every year, they say, a certain percentage has to go . . . somewhere . . . to the devil, it must be, so as to freshen up the rest and not interfere with them. A percentage! Nice little words they have, really: so reassuring, so scientific. A certain percentage, they say, meaning there's nothing to worry about. Now, if it was some other word . . . well, then maybe it would be more worrisome. . . . And what if [Raskolnikov's sister] Dunechka somehow gets into the percentage! . . . If not that one, then some other?"[25]

A few pages further on, an overheard conversation in a tavern sets Raskolnikov to thinking of the elimination of one aged money-lending woman as the spark to a vast operation of moral accounting: "Hundreds, maybe thousands of lives put right; dozens of families saved from destitution, from decay, from ruin, from depravity, from the venereal hospitals—all on her money. Kill her and take her money, so that afterwards with its help you can devote yourself to the service of all mankind and the common cause: what do you think, wouldn't thousands of good deeds make up for one tiny little crime?"[26]

If not that one, then some other, Raskolnikov thinks about the girl on the way to a life of trouble; *let that one bear the cost for many others,* he thinks in the first intuition of what will become his own defining crime. In both cases, his thinking about the lives and fates of others is "simple": a person is a data point, the consequences of his or her elimination are calculable in terms of benefit and loss.[27] Only the thought of a particular person—his sister Dunechka—arrests (momentarily) his calculation.

The framers of health care budgets, especially in the age of AIDS, are in Raskolnikov's world, although it must be said, to their credit, that they are not comfortable there. In what are known as "resource-poor settings," the market—that is, patients' ability to pay—will supply neither prevention nor cure. In the experts' jargon, prevention is "cost-effective" and treatment is considered not to be so, absent the ability to pay for it. If the goal is "to save the most years of life with the funding available," prevention may look like a rational choice—supposing that it works.[28] But measures of the success of prevention will become available only in the long run and only in the aggregate (when that population's rate of infection is observed to shrink in proportion to the progress of the disease elsewhere), and prevention does nothing for the people who have already been infected. To give priority to prevention is to sentence them to death—almost to urge them to get out of the way so that the serious business of prevention can start. And as Farmer has often observed, no one is suggesting that prevention be the dominant or only approach to AIDS in the wealthy countries of the world; the rationale of "cost-effectiveness" is applied selectively in keeping with political and economic inequalities that are no secret to the people who suffer from them.

If availability of resources is the problem, the history of modern epidemics suggests another interpretation of the slogan "cost-effectiveness." Multidrug-resistant tuberculosis emerged because drugs were rationed improperly, ensuring not that patients were cured but rather that the bacilli invading them were vaccinated against first-line therapies. The history of the Ebola outbreak gives a more vivid illustration. The nuns in charge of a charity hospital in Sudan evaluated the funding available to them and determined that five hypodermic syringes were the maximum that could be supplied to their clinic each day. Rinsed occasionally in a pan of warm water, those syringes passed through the skin of hundreds of patients. In short order, an unanticipated virus felled first the patients who had received injections, then their family members and others who had come into contact with them, and finally the medical personnel themselves. Similar causes were involved in the second outbreak of the epidemic in Zaïre.[29] No one could deny that the staff of the charity hospital recognized the limitations placed on their resources—in this instance, syringes. They were responsible to their budget, but not to their patients, perhaps thinking that when medical care is provided as an act of charity, the relevant standard is that it be "better than nothing." In this case, however, what they provided was a great deal worse. One would not have to be a visionary to see that it would have been better to ask for more syringes, even if the budget suffered.

The problem with the Sudanese incident is that it too easily becomes an example of bad nursing rather than of bad priorities. And yet the nurses' blunder is of the same cloth as the "prevention versus cure" debate and the reluctance of drug companies and international bureaucracies to expand access to a First World standard of care. All these arise from resource stinginess, which aggravates a public health shortfall, turning it from a problem into an emergency. Before 2002, the World Health Organization and numerous governments were ready to spend money to show that they were concerned about tuberculosis, but they were not ready to spend enough money to cure the drug-resistant TB that was killing the patients and thereby rein in the epidemic in Russian prisons.[30] "Managerial successes, clinical failures": the title of one of Farmer's short commentaries neatly frames, by symmetrical antithesis, his personal policy.[31]

One form of complexity with which Paul Farmer constantly has to grapple is that introduced by differences of scale. The doctor does everything possible for the patient; the administrator does everything possible for the program; and a sense for complexity is needed where one might conflict with the other. (The term "sustainable" marks very precisely one such area of conflict: it was because Farmer was intent on sustaining his patients that potential donors judged his program "unsustainable.") Raskolnikov's logic always threatens and must be kept at bay.

Readers of Tracy Kidder's *Mountains Beyond Mountains* will remember the chapter about the medical evacuation of John, a small Haitian boy with a rare form of nasopharyngeal cancer. Serena Koenig, a Boston physician and Partners In Health volunteer, took an interest in John on one of her visits to Haiti and persuaded colleagues at Massachusetts General Hospital to waive the fees (some $100,000) for his treatment. But getting John to Boston was difficult: well over $20,000 had to be disbursed for John's preliminary biopsy, an ambulance to take him down the mountain to the Port-au-Prince airport, and a Lear jet to get him to the States. To top it all off, the surgeons at Mass General found that his cancer had spread to so many parts of his body that nothing could be done to save him. He died a few weeks later.

Could this be deemed both a managerial and a clinical failure? Administrators at the PIH clinic in Haiti worried about the consequences before deciding to go ahead:

> "What are we going to do if another kid like this comes to us? It's not a one-time thing. We're not going to close the hospital after this. It's really tricky. The staff will be asking why did they spend this money. . . ."
>
> "I'm looking at only one child," Serena said.
>
> "That's the thing," said Ti Fifi. "There are so many kids waiting for heart surgery, and the staff is asking for more money. A medevac flight is not something you do in Haiti. . . . I am sure that people will say, If your child is sick go to Cange and they will fly him to Boston. In the central plateau, this is going to be an event."[32]

The doctor's focus on the "one child" collides with the program manager's anxiety about the infinite number of possible patients and the impossibility of treating them all equally. The group's efforts to remedy inequalities in health care between Haiti and the United States, pursued uncompromisingly in this particular instance, might create in the minds of Haitians a feeling that John had been singled out for inequitably favorable treatment, while other people's children had not. (In the end, these fears proved groundless, but Kidder does not explore the reasons: do they come down to good luck or to the extraordinary forbearance of the residents of Haiti's Central Plateau?) The review committees that had turned down PIH's requests for funding for the HIV Equity Project, had they been asked, would never have authorized John's flight, even with free medical care awaiting him in Boston. Kidder writes: "A feeling lingered with me that the whole episode was like an object lesson in the difficulty of Farmer's enterprise, perhaps in its ultimate futility."[33]

Kidder's narration of the episode brings out the awkward choices that PIH faced. A lot could have been done with $20,000. Raskolnikov might have found it expedient to delay the ambulance and use the money originally earmarked for John toward the good of the greater number. But that would be adopting the manager's position rather than that of the doctor, who quite rightly has the primary duty of advocating for her patient so long as the patient has a chance of being cured. And vetoing the child's evacuation would certainly not be adopting the patient's position. Raskolnikov might also have argued that, given the "percentage" of children that die from various causes every year in Haiti, withholding care from one more child would not add perceptibly to the catastrophe. If not this small boy, it would surely be another one; why single out this boy for a comfortable death? In Kidder's account, the doctor's perspective is the one that starts and ends with the plain bump-on-a-log of indelible fact: "'What will I say if I'm asked why we're doing this?' 'That his mother brought him to us,' said Farmer. 'And we're doing everything we can to help him.'"[34]

Complexity consists of maintaining the chance for the doctor to act as a doctor, proceeding as if there were only this one patient in the world. You don't "scale up" from the individual patient to the program, any more than you apply precisely the same feelings to the love of another person and to the love of humanity.[35] Pressures familiar in the world of medical insurers and "managed care"—pressures to contain costs, to maneuver the patient's ration of care toward the statistical mean—operate a thousand times more stringently in the realm of grants and assistance programs among the poor. Ingenuity, an irrational degree of effort, and the kindness of strangers have so far kept the budget of Partners In Health from being a restraint on the doctor's sense of priorities. The far goal is to transform institutions to the point that "because his mother brought him to us" is an explanation that evokes no protest.

VIABILITY

Skepticism about Paul Farmer and Partners In Health is often expressed with two related words, "sustainability" and "viability." Often while expressing admiration for the work of PIH, critics contend that the work is not sustainable, that it relies on the efforts of a small band of unreasonably decent people, that it cannot survive its founder, that it would evaporate were it not for an ever-increasing stream of charitable donations, that it creates an undesirable dependency of the Third World on the kindness of the First. The objection to dependency expresses itself in a curious variant of the metaphor of vitality. If maintaining PIH's patients in a state of viability comes at the price of making its programs appear nonviable, the very viability of PIH, its ability to sustain itself and grow, relies, in these critics' reading, on a kind of artificial life support doomed to collapse one day.

"Sustainability," "viability"—words redolent of good intentions, of careful planning, of stewardship and long-term forethought. Their very modesty makes them attractive. Rather than promising immediate utopia, they point to means of carrying on somehow, with limited expectations. The violence they contain is, if anywhere, well under the surface. But philology can bring it out.

The term "viability," originating in French, moved into English in the middle nineteenth century. The *Oxford English Dictionary* summarizes: "VIABILITY. The quality or state of being viable; capacity for living; the ability to live under certain conditions. Also *transf.*: now *esp.* feasibility; ability to continue or be continued; the state of being financially sustainable. In common use from c. 1860."[36] A little narrative, familiar in its outlines, inhabits the sequence of meanings given here: the word is said to depart from a core meaning that is human in connotation (what could be more intimately associated with humanness than "living"?) to extend its anthropomorphism to new and alien objects, such as defense policies, business plans, political programs.[37] Just as the human infant emerges from its initial life-support system, the mother's body, and begins to take air and nourishment from outside, eventually to stand autonomously on the ground of adulthood, so enterprises, policies, and so forth begin as uncertain projects needing investment or other inputs and eventually come to a self-sustaining maturity, or don't. As the *OED* observes, the standard uses of the term today are those referring to the nonbiological contexts; there has been not just an extension but a migration of sense. Thus the *OED* inserts the tag "*transf.*," indicating metaphorical transfer, between the biological and nonbiological contexts of use.

The word "sustainable" (a near-synonym of "viable") is a migrant from the sphere of engineering and environmentalism to that of business, and thence to that of political economy. Buckminster Fuller is responsible for the major shift in the word's meaning, through his speeches and activism on behalf of long-range planning and management of "Spaceship Earth."[38] With finite resources, how long could consumer societies prevail before consuming the very basis of their existence (air, water, food, raw materials)? Fuller's vision of a future economy would maximize the utility of the minimal resources extracted from the environment. A business is termed sustainable when its sources of income are expected to durably exceed its outlays. When used by specialists in international economics, the term refers to a fantasy in which the costs of development (say, the building of a health care infrastructure) are borne by the beneficiaries, something that was certainly not the case for Europe during the Industrial Revolution and is unlikely to occur elsewhere.

"Viability" and its predecessor, the adjective "viable," are words invented at a particular moment, having particular contexts of use and particular dimensions along which they extend themselves. The word *viable* first appears in the anonymous French translation of Castiglione's *Il Cortegiano* (The Courtier) published at Lyons in 1537.[39] At the textual juncture in question, Castiglione's assembly of learned and courtly persons is debating whether women are suited for public office, and one speaker contends that women, being better equipped for natural survival than men, ought to have at least the equivalent privileges in social life. The reason, couched in the "four humors" medical language of the time, is that "temperate bodies are most perfect . . . woman, taken in herself, is temperate, or at least more nearly temperate than man, because the moisture she has in her is proportionate to her natural warmth, which in man more readily evaporates and is consumed because of excessive dryness. . . . And thus, since men dry out more than women in the act of procreation, it frequently happens that they are not as *viable* as women."[40] Reckless expenditure contrasted with reserve and internal balance: the "viability" here ascribed to women exhibits the properties that would later, in a world with a different physics and a different economics, be designated by the word "self-sustaining."

The French translator added a discrimination of meaning to Castiglione's Italian, and a new word to the French language, for here the Italian text says *"spesso interviene che sono meno vivaci che esse."* *Vivace* is a correctly formed word in Italian, and the cognate *vivace* already existed in French (it is found in Rabelais and Montaigne); but French *vivace* did not specify how "endowed with life" should be taken, whether it indicated a degree of intensity or a degree of duration.[41] The context emphasizes longevity, not just liveliness; *viable,* it turns out, is the adjective that conveys a prediction of duration on the basis of preexisting qualities.

The main distinction introduced into French by the word *viable,* the asserted distinction between mere life and durable, self-sustaining life, gives opportunity for a further distinction on the border between medicine and law—two bodies of knowledge that perch nervously over the definition of life. For certain French legal purposes, such as assigning paternity or assigning guilt in cases of infanticide or abortion (turning out differently according to whether the child *would have* been expected to live), it is not enough that a child be born alive; it must be born both *alive and viable,* and the one condition does not entail the other.[42]

But the full meaning of the distinction between the French terms *en vie* (alive) and *viable* emerges in court cases centering, as if written by Balzac, around multiple deaths and disputed rights of succession to property. Here the Roman law, always touchy about family matters, provided guidance. "The child who comes dead into the world is not considered a child; it is not even a person," writes Alexandre Duranton in 1844, backing himself up with Justinian in the *Digests:* "Those who are born dead are deemed neither born, nor procreated." They can be forgotten as far as property rights go. But what about the child that is born in a state between life and death? As Duranton argues: "The law requires not only that, in order to have the capacity to be someone's successor, a child not be stillborn; the law demands that the child be born viable, that is, with the necessary conditions for living, with the aptitude for life; that its conformation be such that, on seeing it, no one will say: He was born for nothing but to die at the instant, and not for life." Imagine two children, both of whom live for only an hour. The law will treat them differently according to whether or not they were suited and equipped for life, that is, "viable."[43]

At this historical stage of French law, then, a judgment of "viability" constitutes the child as a juridical person, not life per se.[44] The decision is a legal one, but judges cannot make it; only a doctor is entitled to assign viability. In an 1871 case judged by the civil tribunal of Narbonne, a father was required to prove "that the child was born, that it lived outside its mother's body, however short its existence may have been, and that it therefore constituted a legal person capable of receiving goods by way of inheritance and of transmitting goods in the same manner." The testimony supplied by the father in this case, said the court, was inadequate because "he did not offer to prove that the child cried out, or even that it took a complete breath; he did not offer to prove that anyone's hand felt a heartbeat through the child's chest; he did not offer to prove that a mirror had been put before its mouth and been fogged by its breath"—all traditional means of ascertaining life. Against the father's claim that the child was born viable, though admittedly not alive, the court contended that the only signs of life it had given were "convulsive movements" and an accidental influx of air into its nonfunctioning lungs during the doctor's attempt at resuscitation.[45] "Convulsive," "accidental": the magistrate's language makes the nonviable child out to be a machine or other arrangement of movable matter, not yet an animal, much less a member of our species.

The law is concerned with the doctor's opinion of whether the child *would have* survived, not with his report on whether it *did* survive. The question is whether it had everything that was necessary for an autonomous existence outside its mother's body, the touchstone of viability. The opinion that the child was "viable," that is, "organized for life" and capable of living without external help, whether or not it actually goes on to live, pulls the switch that makes the child a possessor of legal rights and, in the cases just cited, an inheritor. Without this medical blessing, the child has bumped against the limits of the social world but has not been admitted to any role within it. Any social role, even the minimal one of inheritor, must be claimed; it does not follow from the nature of things, as Duranton says with emphasis.

Not just a matter of marking the alternative of life or death, the term "viability" opens a place of judgment about what is and is not to be considered human. With the constellation of meanings it implies, it takes up from the Roman legal doctrine that excludes nonviable children from the status of humanity.[46] One of the possibilities it opens is eugenics.

The uncertain status of the premature or incomplete child between viability and nonviability—particularly uncertain now that the means of prolonging life and substituting for vital functions are so much more advanced than they were in the 1870s—is a link between those scenarios in which a claim to property hinges on a judgment of viable personhood and the contemporary contexts in which the word "viability" is most often pronounced, namely, ecological predictions. For although the need to reverse damage done to the environment is well documented, and such actions are plainly in the interest of future generations, those future generations have no legal forum at which to present their case. Before he or she can inherit, as Duranton points out, a person must have judicial standing, and judicial standing goes only to those who exist at the time that a right is conferred—exist, that is, in the full sense of being both alive and viable.

The distinction between *vie* and *viabilité* comes up for the purpose of resolving an uncertainty—Was the product of the birth a human child? Was it therefore eligible to inherit and transmit property?—and always under counterfactual conditions. *Had the infant in question lived, would it have succumbed to external causes or to a consequence of its own malformation?* No question of viability arises in the case of a child who lives. The word's power derives not from the defined expertise of the doctor or the lawyer, but from the interchange of their two disciplines. The doctor answers a question of no medical relevance just because the law needs it answered. The question to which the term "viability" corresponds is not really about life and death but about transmission, inheriting, bequeathing. The people for whom such judgments make a difference are never the persons about whom the judgments are made. Those inheritors and experts appear in the story of viability or nonviability as specters with the power to shape a narrative in which they have an interest, but of which they are not the objects. And, mirror-fashion, current predictions of the viability of the present forms of human culture, made by us, will have consequences not particularly for us, but for people who are not able to sit in on our discussions. The medical "viability" judgments come too late; the ecological ones come too early.

These scenes in which something not quite yet existent, or not quite up to the definition of living, knocks on the door and desires to be admitted can be recognized as well in the articulation among medicine, the economics of aid, and human rights that forms the complex, contradictory object of Paul Farmer's efforts. In its medico-legal usage, as when an inheritance hangs on the status attributed to the dead child, the term "viable" stakes out the uneasy frontier between ways of life and "mere life,"[47] between social and biological existence. That is, it describes its own hybrid field of meaning in performing the work it does. When the word moves into political vocabulary, it serves to predict an outcome and at the same time to assert the reality of the object of its predictions, to make something viable or nonviable. Chateaubriand, in 1833, wrote to the Dauphine about the July Monarchy: "Although the present monarchy does not seem viable, I fear that it will live beyond the limits one might predict for it." Victor Hugo, in 1848: "It is because I long for the Republic that I long for it to be viable, that I desire it to be definitive." George Sand, in 1870: "Be well advised that the Republic will be born again, and that nothing can forestall it; viable or not, it occupies every mind."[48]

When we assess the viability of an animal species, an economic program, or a political entity, we are, as part of the implication of the word, imagining it as already dead or moribund and of retroactively questionable legal standing (recall that the child deemed not viable is considered not to have lost the status of a person or inheritor, but *never* to have had it). Thus the word carries a certain verbal magic, reinforced by its association with the language of experts, the power to say *what would have been* or *what was going to be all along.* "Viable" is never entirely in the present tense, or entirely in any one moment. Because it links two moments, it tells a story and creates a potential subject: the child, the patient, the Republic, all figures of frustrated possibility in need of something they cannot supply themselves. One such thing that must be supplied from outside, a necessary but certainly insufficient condition, is a narrator willing to identify them as protagonists of a story, like Dr. Farmer defending his patients against the narrative in which they were only features of a different protagonist, the unhealthy budget. (For that matter, he also defended his unhealthy budget, on the grounds not that bankruptcy was admirable but that in this situation a balanced exchange between Haitian sick people and international development agencies was both impossible and immoral.) It is a matter of asserting their lives against a model of viability from which they were peremptorily excluded.

SUBSTANTIVE RIGHTS AND UNIVERSAL OBLIGATIONS

The assignment of viability is the precondition for human status: those not yet in being, or no longer in being, lack a forum in which to be heard. That condition of being outside the reach of rights is one they share with many people currently in existence. Before he or she can possess any legal rights, a human being must have ongoing biological existence: this lesson, implicit in the legal history of the term "viable," forms the basis of Paul Farmer's uneasiness with the usual language of human rights as spoken in this country. A longstanding dispute, alluded to in "Rethinking Health and Human Rights" and "Making Human Rights Substantial" (chapters 21 and 25 in this volume), divides those who see the core human rights issue as protecting individual autonomy from the encroachment of the state and those who see it as securing economic and social rights. This division follows old Cold War precedent, with the socialist bureaucracies claiming to derive their authority from their provision of subsistence to the people, and the capitalist forms of organization claiming to derive it from the consent of the governed.

For Farmer, the culture of human rights harbors a disastrous tendency to forget the fact that human bodies need sustenance and medical care before they can claim the freedoms enshrined in the Bill of Rights or similar documents. The right to claim rights, it seems, is what "structural violence" denies the poor, and it does this by threatening to take away that indispensable infrastructure that is a body or to take away the food, clean water, and appropriate medication that underwrite the body's survival. "It is when people are able to eat and be well that they have the chance to build democratic institutions," Farmer notes. Substantive rights form the basis of legal rights; the human body is the indispensable infrastructure supporting any legal or political claim. Not to get the sequence backward: that is how to restore the meaning of the misused term "viability."

Conversely, it makes a great difference for Dr. Farmer's patients and potential patients to maintain, as a medical expert might, that the right to claim rights, however moribund in the greater part of the world today, was not stillborn but has at least drawn enough breath in the course of human history to be registered as viable and thus to have legal heirs. What those heirs inherit is a claim on certain substantive rights, rights entailing a share in goods. A business, a church, or a charity may extend the same goods to people—food, first-rate medicine, housing, and even that much-trumpeted commodity hope—but it will be as an exchange or as a gift. Rights belong to the traffic that people have with states. The privatization of social services has notoriously created obstacles to medical care by subjecting patients to user fees and by withdrawing services once provided as a public good, but the primary harm done is to the contact between citizen and state, which is no longer based on a mutual claim of rights. Of course, in much of the world, and especially where the poor are at home, the state operates more commonly to take rights away from the people than to grant rights; but no other actor is under a universal obligation, however frequently breached, to provide for the common good. It is astonishing that Paul Farmer has seen the worst effects of predatory states both strong and weak—not to mention bandits, structural-adjustment programs, and drug lords—yet considers the protection of primordial rights to be the business of the state. Has the twentieth century, with its lynchings, pogroms, camps, gulags, exterminations, and bombings, passed him by?

Under the withering-away of the welfare state and the privatization of police power, little stands between "unaccommodated man" and brutal economic, environmental, judicial, and viral conditions. Russia, Haiti, and Rwanda, three of the countries where PIH is most active, can illustrate the point. Kidder captures the ambiguous relation between Partners In Health initiatives and their political context in a bold simile:

> In daylight, in an all but treeless, baked brown landscape, Zanmi Lasante [PIH's Haitian sister organization] makes a dramatic appearance, like a *fortress* on its mountainside, a large complex of concrete buildings, half covered with tropical greenery. Inside the walls, the world turns leafy. Tall trees stand beside courtyards and walkways and walls, artful constructions of concrete and stone, which mount the forested hillside. . . . There is running water, and you can hear a big generator churning out electricity. The buildings have tiled floors and clean white walls and ceilings. [emphasis added][49]

A fortress: in other words, a place where people can band together for protection; an enclave holding out against erosion, lawlessness, and disease. Zanmi Lasante appears as a rebuilding of the mission of government, an act of resistance to the abdication of state responsibility imposed on Haiti by external powers—in sum, a replacement for the missing state. (By extending rights and imposing peace, the "fortress" could be said to pass two minimal tests of statehood.) There is something paradoxical—or "not simple"—about this quasi-fortress, this model for a welfare state, built with private donations. The ambition that directs it—to persuade states to get back into the business of guaranteeing substantive rights, central among them the right to health care—will, if successful, resolve that paradox in time. Perhaps the leafy fortress on the hill is analogous to the pinprick of immunization, a particle of privatization meant to enable the body to overcome the disease.

NOTES

1. Farmer, "Bad Blood, Spoiled Milk," pp. 80–81. Also see chapter 1 in this volume.

2. Kidder, *Mountains Beyond Mountains*, p. 35. Kidder tells in anecdotal form the story Farmer presents in social science terms in the 1999 essay "Optimism and Pessimism in Tuberculosis Control" (which appears in Farmer, *Infections and Inequalities*, pp. 211–27, and is also included in this volume as chapter 8). Farmer mentions this dialogue later in Kidder's book: "The woman who said to me years ago, Are you incapable of complexity? That was an epiphany for me. Are you going to punish people for thinking TB comes from sorcery?" (p. 293).

3. For another study in which the format of patients' narratives serves as a diagnostic of social and biological change, see Farmer, "Sending Sickness" (chapter 2 in this volume).

4. Virchow, "Was die 'medizinische Reform' will," cited in Ackerknecht, *Rudolf Virchow*, p. 46; see also pp. 130–32 of Ackerknecht's book.

5. Centers for Disease Control and Prevention, "Current Trends: Acquired Immunodeficiency Syndrome (AIDS) Update—United States."

6. Greenfield, "Night of the Living Dead II." For a fuller account of these baroque scenarios, see Farmer, "The Exotic and the Mundane" (chapter 3 in this volume).

7. See Herbert, "Refusing to Save Africans."

8. See Farmer, "Social Scientists and the New Tuberculosis" (chapter 7 in this volume).

9. Farmer, Léandre, Mukherjee, Gupta, et al., "Community-Based Treatment of Advanced HIV Disease"; Farmer, Léandre, Mukherjee, Claude, et al., "Community-Based Approaches to HIV Treatment in Resource-Poor Settings"; Farmer, "The Major Infectious Diseases in the World—To Treat or Not to Treat?" (chapter 12 in this volume); Singler and Farmer, "Treating HIV in Resource-Poor Settings."

10. Farmer and Kim, "Community-Based Approaches to the Control of Multidrug-Resistant Tuberculosis"; Farmer, "Managerial Successes, Clinical Failures"; Furin et al., "Effect of Administering Short-Course, Standard Regimens in Individuals Infected with Drug-Resistant Mycobacterium Tuberculosis Strains."

11. Farmer, Léandre, Mukherjee, Gupta, et al., "Community-Based Treatment of Advanced HIV Disease," pp. 1147–48.

12. Ibid., pp. 1149–50. Cf. Kidder, *Mountains Beyond Mountains*, p. 257.

13. Farmer, Léandre, Mukherjee, Gupta, et al., "Community-Based Treatment of Advanced HIV Disease," pp. 1146, 1148.

14. Ibid., p. 1149.

15. Mbewu, "Antiretroviral Therapy Is Only Part of It," p. 1152. Lacking lab equipment to per-

form CD4 counts and viral load tests in 2001, PIH's Haitian clinics had substituted a decision algo-rithm; hence Mbewu's recommendation.

16. Feachem, "HAART—The Need for Strategically Focused Investments," pp. 1152–53.

17. Gilks, AbouZahr, and Türmen, "HAART in Haiti—Evidence Needed," pp. 1154–55. One is reminded of Feachem's concern that "the best not be made the enemy of the good."

18. Farmer, Nizeye, et al., "Structural Violence and Clinical Medicine" (chapter 18 in this volume).

19. See World Health Organization, *Scaling Up Antiretroviral Therapy in Resource-Limited Settings;* World Health Organization, *Towards Universal Access,* pp. 16–18; Benkimoun, "Contre le sida, 'on peut soulever des montagnes.'"

20. In Haiti, Jean-Bertrand Aristide's presidency was abruptly terminated by U.S. intervention in February 2004, and membership in his Lavalas party became grounds for suspicion in the eyes of the new government and the occupying United Nations forces. Many PIH associates with a Lavalas background were killed, driven into hiding, or exiled. In Uganda, money for AIDS "prevention" was sidetracked into abstinence campaigns, which had predictably low efficacy.

21. Farmer, Léandre, Mukherjee, Claude, et al., "Community-Based Approaches to HIV Treatment in Resource-Poor Settings," p. 404.

22. Ibid., p. 408.

23. Ibid., p. 407; cf. Kidder, *Mountains Beyond Mountains,* pp. 242–43.

24. Farmer's lecture "An Anthropology of Structural Violence" (chapter 17 in this volume) was followed in the original publication by comments calling for a more precise and less unwieldy definition of the concept; see Bourgois et al., "Commentary on Farmer, Paul, 'An Anthropology of Structural Violence.'" Loïc Wacquant's critique is the most pointed of the lot: for him, the term "structural violence" "diffuses responsibility in order to expand its ambit," "conflates full-fledged domination with mere social disparity and then collapses forms of violence that need to be differentiated," and finally "is saturated with moral judgments that invite anachronism" (p. 322).

25. Dostoevsky, *Crime and Punishment,* p. 50. The translators (p. 555) suggest Adolphe Quételet as the source of the character's ideas about statistical regularity in human behavior. On incidental characters in fiction, see Woloch, *The One vs. the Many.*

26. Dostoevsky, *Crime and Punishment,* p. 65. The speaker is "a student [Raskolnikov] did not know or remember at all," but his words express "*exactly the same thoughts* [that] had just been conceived in [Raskolnikov's] own head" (pp. 63, 66). Even thoughts and words, it seems, occur with statistical regularity.

27. For another rumination about the uselessness of "simplicity" and "the straight-line approach" in contemplating matters of life and death, see Dostoevsky, *A Writer's Diary,* vol. 1, pp. 641–56, 721–29.

28. See Farmer, "Never Again? Reflections on Human Values and Human Rights" (chapter 23 in this volume) for a discussion of the costs of prevention versus care.

29. This example is taken from Farmer, "Rethinking 'Emerging Infectious Diseases,'" in Farmer, *Infections and Inequalities,* pp. 37–58 (also included in this volume as chapter 6). Once more, note the pattern in which a disease for which subpar hospital care—an effect of international inequality—is partially to blame nonetheless is characterized in the press as emerging from, and poetically belonging to, the Third World population it devours.

30. See Farmer, "The Major Infectious Diseases of the World—To Treat or Not to Treat?" (chapter 12 in this volume).

31. Farmer, "Managerial Successes, Clinical Failures."

32. Kidder, *Mountains Beyond Mountains,* p. 270.

33. Ibid., p. 279. For Farmer's response to Kidder's questions about the "futility" of the episode, see pp. 287–91.

34. Ibid., p. 264.

35. See Dostoevsky, *A Writer's Diary*, vol. 1, p. 735: "The awareness of one's own utter inability to assist or bring any aid or relief at all to suffering humanity, coupled with one's complete conviction of the existence of that suffering, can even transform the love for humanity in your heart to hatred for humanity." In *Pathologies of Power* (pp. 196–212, esp. pp. 204–5), Farmer elaborates on the divide between the medical ethics usually taught in hospitals, centered around end-of-life care and the "quandary ethics of individual patients," and the often unaddressed ethical problem of massive denial of care.

36. *Oxford English Dictionary (OED)*, s.v. "viability."

37. To quote the examples given by the *OED*: "Such narrowing or deformity of the female pelvis . . . as will absolutely preclude the birth of a *viable* child"; "I have repeatedly been astonished at the *viability* of the infant after traction had been applied to it"; "He also had some doubts about the *viability* of the work financially"; "They are a main factor in giving [the country] such economic *viability* as it possesses"; "The Russian nuclear capacity appears to be not capable of destroying anything like enough of the American potential for a Russian first strike to be a *viable* proposition"; "[Jordan] was not in economic terms a *viable* state without British support."

38. See Fuller, *Operating Manual for Spaceship Earth*. The word "sustainability" seems to have come into widespread use following the 1987 United Nations report *Our Common Future*, from the World Commission on Environment and Development, a document that is rife with Fullerisms.

39. *Trésor de la langue française (TLF)*, 1994, s.vv. "*viable*," "*viabilité*"; *Grand Larousse*, 1978, s.vv.

40. Castiglione, *The Book of the Courtier*, p. 219 (slightly modified).

41. See *TLF*, s.v. "*vivace*" (1).

42. For an application to paternity, see Frain, *Arrests du Parlement de Bretagne*, pp. 229–30. On the criteria for considering a child "*vitalis*" (equivalent to French *viable*), see Zacchia, *Quaestiones medico-legales*, pp. 47–49. For a discussion, see Fischer-Homberger, *Medezin vor Gericht*, p. 246.

43. Duranton, *Cours de droit français*, vol. 6, p. 92, citing Justinian, "De verborum significatione," *Digests* 50.16.129.

44. In U.S. law, the "threshold of viability" at twenty weeks is held to mark the beginning of the state's interest in protecting the child as a person; for the perhaps least controversial part of a controversial case, see *Roe v. Wade*, 410 US 113, at 163 (1973).

45. Dubrac, *Traité de jurisprudence médicale et pharmaceutique*, pp. 38–39.

46. "Those are not considered 'children' who are procreated contrary to the form of the human race, as when a woman gives birth to something monstrous or prodigious. But a birth that accomplishes the purposes of the human body shall in other respects be considered effective and thus be numbered among the children [of a man]" (Justinian, "De statu hominum," *Digests* 1.5.14; cited as well by Duranton, *Cours de droit français*, vol. 6, p. 95).

47. On "bare life," see Agamben, *Homo Sacer*.

48. Citations from *TLF* and *Grand Larousse*, s.v. "*viable*."

49. Kidder, *Mountains Beyond Mountains*, p. 19.

Ethnography, History, Political Economy

Introduction to Part 1

Paul Farmer

In rereading the studies and essays collected in this book—some of them published while I was still in graduate school, some of them quite recent and published here for the first time, the majority from the years in between—I discern trends different from the ones I had expected, even hoped for. After more than two decades of writing for peers in anthropology and medicine, one hopes to be impressed by (or at least to note) a steady improvement in the quality of writing, or by ever more thorough exploration of the implications of findings, or by the depths of one's insights. Do these chapters confirm progress? I hope any reader can observe, beyond the shifts of genre, discipline, and audience, the accretion of knowledge and experience that comes with simply sticking with certain topics for many years. I've tried to do that as both a physician and an anthropologist. When speaking to students, I can extol the advantages conferred by identifying important topics early on and sticking with them for a decade or two. I was lucky enough to happen on medical anthropology as an undergraduate biochemistry major bound for medical school, and this discovery has shaped my views on all the key topics reviewed in this book. At least, nearly a quarter-century of attention to a single set of topics should make one more credible as a student of (or spokesperson for) them.

It's less obvious that the results of academic inquiry, when not linked to substantive programs, have much impact on the topics explored. I prefaced the second edition of another book, *Infections and Inequalities*, with an essay finished on July 11, 2000. One of the topics discussed in that book, and this one, was the overweening role of "cost-effectiveness analyses" in determining what constitutes a worthy investment in health and what does not. In that essay, I was not seeking to impugn the logics that underpin cost-effectiveness analyses, but was rather seeking to offer a positivist critique of them by underlining, as a physician-anthropologist might, all the considerations (whether framed in monetary terms or not) that might make such analyses more sound. Writing on the way to attend an international AIDS conference in Durban, South Africa, I conveyed my hope that the book "might serve a pragmatic end by calling into question these and other logics that promise a future in which health equity will play a shrinking role. Only by struggling for higher standards for the destitute sick will we avoid another unappealing role—that of academic Cassandras who prophesy the coming plagues, but do little to avert them."[1]

Looking back now over two decades of writing, I am forced to wonder whether I have succeeded in avoiding the unappealing role of academic Cassandra. Students who find this reader helpful can trace the roots of these essays and studies and decide for themselves. Writing these brief introductions between Rwanda and Haiti and Harvard, I am not sure I can pin down my role, but I am happy to report some improvements since the somewhat discouraged preface to *Infections and Inequalities*. Since that time, we've seen an enormous boom in programs to promote global health equity. New funding mechanisms have arisen to support AIDS treatment programs, flourishing in the very settings in which they were so recently deemed not cost-effective. These new resources and programs have strengthened health systems broadly and allowed us to expand our work from Haiti and Peru and other places mentioned in these chapters to Africa, which has been a great privilege.

We'd like to think that documenting some early work in Haiti has been helpful in this expansion of life-saving medical care. But there are other reasons to write. Biosocially complex phenomena such as the epidemics and the human rights debates discussed here are hard to understand, and descriptions of them sometimes meet with resistance. In order to demystify the process of comprehension, I have encouraged students to try to write about complexity, in the hope (often rewarded) that illumination will follow. "I think with my hands" is the way I've tried to convey my own enthusiasm for writing to my students, most of them physicians-in-training.

George Orwell once wrote an essay called "Why I Write," and it's been helpful to me in contemplating this reader. Orwell enumerates four motives for writing: "sheer egoism," "aesthetic enthusiasm," "historical impulse" ("desire to see things as they are, to find out true facts and store them up for the use of posterity"), and "political impulse" ("desire to push the world in a certain direction, to alter other people's idea of the kind of society they should strive after").[2] I hope that the material published here is seen as falling under the latter two rubrics—that, and simply trying to figure things out. Physicians spend more time taking care of patients than writing, but anthropologists spend much of their time writing;

and for practitioners of the latter field, there's no shortage of angst about *how* we write. Clifford Geertz has examined anthropologists' obsession with "being there" and has argued that many of the conventions of anthropological writing—from the created tense, "the ethnographic present," to frequent recourse to local terminology, explained or translated parenthetically—are to be understood as efforts to show what might be termed, in modern parlance, the ethnographer's street cred.[3] Or, to use a Haitian expression, which will not appear here in the original, "you have to know there to go there."

I bought into this way of seeing the world as I devoured everything ever written about Haiti. It's a wonderful privilege to be awarded a doctoral degree for learning a language, obsessing about a culture, and reading anything one can find about the people and place in question. When I say "bought into," I am not suggesting that I now reject this rite of passage (ethnographic fieldwork followed by writing for one's peers). What I do hope is that my writings about other places I know less intimately—Russian prisons, Peruvian shantytowns, Rwandan settlements, or Guatemalan villages haunted by violence—are also illuminated by the instruction I received both from my professors (at Duke and Harvard) and from my first informants (in rural Haiti). Certainly, the many people cited in these pages have been my teachers in the best sense of the word, and I am grateful to them all. Classroom and clinic and fieldwork have taught me about social process and theory. If there is any unifying thesis here, it's that poverty, gender inequality, and racism—products of the heavy hand of history—powerfully constrain human agency. A decade ago I wrote, somewhat defensively perhaps, that "striving to understand a commonality of constraint is hardly tantamount to denying the salience of personal experience."[4]

Another thing I notice in this reader, which moves from research on epidemic diseases in poor places to essays about poverty and rights more generally, is the heightened affective tone of the later essays. The reason for this is not some temporal evolution in my writing or in the subjects that move me to conduct research and write; my subjects have remained constant since even before my first trip to Haiti, prior to medical school. What has changed is an ability to work more of these sentiments into my published work in journals and edited volumes. The strictures on such writing can be tight and reflect the priorities of the journals or volume editors as much as or more than the topic at hand. (I've been lucky enough to publish my own books, including three others with the University of California Press, in more or less the register I sought.)

For example, one study reprinted here was first published in *American Ethnologist* in 1988. Two years shy of either an MD or a PhD, I was proud of this piece, which I edited several times (along with Haun Saussy), trying to emulate the tone of that journal, prestigious among the few who read it. The research was based on fairly straightforward participant-observation, informed by many interviews, all duly recorded and transcribed and translated. It took two years to research and write just this one paper about a fairly obscure "culture-bound disorder" that afflicted certain nursing mothers in rural Haiti, and the text, as published and in keeping with conventions in anthropology, was replete with words in Haitian and their glosses. I was at the stage of having to prove my seriousness, and so I did, with documentation, methodology, and rewriting.

But early in the course of my youthful enthusiasm for research in rural Haiti, I was brought up short a number of times by my informants, as the jargon goes. Some of them wanted to know why I was spending so much time interviewing young women and herbalists and other local practitioners, rather than spending all my time improving the small clinic we had just built in the squatter settlement where I lived and worked (and where, almost twenty-five years later, I am writing these words). But how to insert the informants' reproach into a scholarly journal without offending the sensibilities of its potential readers, who at the time loomed large in my imagination as a pool of scholarly judges who desperately needed to read my work, whether they knew it or not? (The pool, it turned out, was rather smaller than I believed.) In the end, I decided to include at least one of the sharper rebukes, from a woman I called Mme. Gracia. Along with thousands of others, she had been flooded out of a fertile valley by a hydroelectric dam and was now living in a dusty squatter settlement. I must have recorded her remarks in 1986 and written them up in 1987 for publication in 1988. Hers was the final word:

> Mme. Gracia, a woman in her late sixties, insisted that I not forget recent history. She reminded me to attend to the larger context in which "malignant emotions" arose: "*Move san* is not something that was regularly seen before [the valley was flooded]. Some people died from it after the dam was finished. Now we are up here and we are poor. We have no livestock, no [sugarcane] mills. We suffer too many shocks (*sezisman*), too many problems. We are poor and we are weak, and that is why you see *move san*."

Mme. Gracia was among those who chided me gently for paying attention to issues that were less pressing than the need for water, health care, and education. That was it for me. I knew Mme. Gracia was right.

Thanks to undergraduate studies, to graduate school, and to Haiti, I had a good sense for what sort of anthropology I wanted to pursue. Shortly before I began my first year as an official MD-PhD student, I read a book by George Marcus and Michael Fischer about the state of anthropology: they noted that "an interpretive anthropology fully accountable to its historical and political-economy implications thus remains to be written."[5] That was precisely what I wanted to do and write, and the name of part 1 of this reader reflects this ambition. I wanted to link "experience-near" writing to an understanding of the larger structural underpinnings of lived experience in the places where I work. Haitians, after all, told me again and again that it was their poverty that led or pushed them into this or that catastrophe. I could see that they were right—but what, as my teachers often asked, was the theoretical underpinning of such work?

The obsession with "contributing to theory" saturated not only seminars but also discussions among graduate students. (Such discussions did not occur over at the medical school, where the task at hand was cramming what was termed "factual information" into one's head as fast as possible.) In graduate studies, it was all about theory—the more recondite, the better. There was, in the books we were reading at unsafe speeds, a good deal of distance, not to say a divorce, between what passed for empirical data, the fruit of ethnographic fieldwork, and the theoretical scaffolding on which this data, frequently in light doses, was hung. Also common, in the social sciences in general, was the feat of linking ethnographic information to one theory about society when the same information might as well have been advanced as support for another, completely discrepant theory. That was not the sort of anthropology I wanted to write.

The Haitians were training me to be skeptical about claims of causality (even as they advanced their own claims with great assurance), and I knew, before I embarked on graduate studies, that I wanted to be a practicing physician and—to the initial disappointment of some of my teachers—an activist. But an excellent course in social theory, reaching back to Comte, Weber, and Marx, while paying respect to Frantz Fanon (this respect moved me deeply) en route to Habermas and other luminaries, convinced me that there was more than enough social theory to go around. In addition to being influenced by my Harvard mentors, I was drawn to the work of Sidney Mintz, for he had built up an interpretive anthropology accountable to history and political economy—even if a lot of the interpretive stuff was buried in obscure papers about Haitian market women or in riveting life histories. At the same time that I was writing "Bad Blood, Spoiled Milk," which was based on ethnography, I was trying to write another paper about Haiti's history and political economy. The two papers were published simultaneously, the latter in a Marxist anthropology journal. (Perhaps the words of one of my mentors still reverberate in my memory—"Sure, they'll publish it, as long as you follow the party line"—since I did not object when Haun Saussy left the essay out of this reader.)[6]

Thanks to medical school and, especially, to Haiti, I also had a good sense of the kind of medicine I wanted to practice: infectious disease. The plagues I was seeing were both preventable and curable, I thought, as I turned reluctantly away from general surgery, another field that tempted me when I witnessed what the Haitians called "stupid deaths" from obstructed labor, gunshot wounds, injuries from falling rocks or machetes, and peritonitis. By 1988, Haiti and Haitians had steered me in certain directions within both anthropology and medicine. I was and am grateful for it. Surrounded by epidemic disease, I decided that I would both study epidemics and do my best, working with others, to stop them or at least lessen the suffering caused by them.

NOTES

1. Farmer, *Infections and Inequalities*, p. xxviii.
2. Orwell, "Why I Write," in Orwell, *The Collected Essays, Journalism, and Letters of George Orwell*, vol. 4, p. 2.
3. See Clifford Geertz's essay "Being There," in Geertz, *Works and Lives*, pp. 1–24.
4. Farmer, *Infections and Inequalities*, p. xli.
5. Marcus and Fischer, *Anthropology as Cultural Critique*, p. 86.
6. Farmer, "Blood, Sweat, and Baseballs." The argument of this essay is further developed in Farmer, *The Uses of Haiti*.

Bad Blood, Spoiled Milk

Bodily Fluids as Moral Barometers in Rural Haiti

(1988)

Current discourse in medical anthropology is marked by an increasing appreciation of the body as physical, social, and political artifact. Concepts such as somatization, which implies the making corporeal of nonbodily experience, are by now common coin, and there is considerable enthusiasm for the increasingly fine-grained analyses that appear in several new specialty journals. But others discern an overweening analytic urge that yields fragmentary knowledge resistant to synthesis. Illness experiences are picked apart under the dissecting gaze not only of biomedicine but of anthropology as well, a discipline long parsed into such officially sanctioned subfields as "psychological" and "biological" anthropologies. Appreciating the full weight of centuries of what has come to be called Cartesian dualism, Nancy Scheper-Hughes and Margaret Lock write forcefully of our "failure to conceptualize a 'mindful' causation of somatic states."[1] How might we gather up our fragmentary knowledge? Several of those seeking to reconcile the three bodies have turned, in the past few years, to emotion.

An illness widespread in rural Haiti speaks to this and several other dilemmas central to contemporary medical anthropology. To use the tropes now common in our field, *move san* is somatically experienced and caused by emotional distress. *Move san*—for which a literal English equivalent is "bad blood"—begins, report my informants, as a disorder of the blood. But it may rapidly spread throughout the body, so that the head, limbs, eyes, skin, and uterus may all be affected. It most frequently strikes adult women; some assert that only women are afflicted. Although considered pathological, *move san* is not an uncommon response to emotional upsets. The disorder is seen as requiring treatment, and this is commonly effected by locally prepared herbal medicines.

The course and outcome of this illness, if it is untreated or unsuccessfully treated, are reported to be dismal: several of my informants speak of friends and relatives who have succumbed to *move san*. Those most vulnerable are pregnant women or nursing mothers; in such cases, chances are good that the malady will affect the quality of breast milk. *Move san* is the chief—and some say the only—cause of the *lèt gate,* or spoiled milk, syndrome: "bad blood" is held to make it impossible for a lactating mother to afford her infant "good milk." It is thus a frequently cited motive for early weaning, which, in rural Haiti, often has disastrous effects on the infant's health. The chief effects of *move san,* however, are judged to be manifest in the mother.

Although I first encountered the *move san/lèt gate* complex in 1984 while doing research on childrearing in peasant families, its significance as a perceived threat to health was not clear until research conducted during a 1985 census revealed a 77 percent lifetime prevalence rate of *move san* (with or without *lèt gate*) in Do Kay, a small village in central Haiti and the site of most of the research reported here.

Move san has not been systematically studied, nor have thorough case studies been presented in the anthropological literature on Haiti.[2] The disorder is of interest to medical (and psychological) anthropology for several reasons, many of them obvious. Those who suffer from *move san/lèt gate* cite it as a danger to the health of women already beset with intractable and unrelenting difficulties. Child health specialists from several traditions would maintain that *move san,* like all other motives for early weaning, constitutes a threat to the health of infants. The disorder joins a long and varied list of conditions in which women question their ability to breastfeed.[3] But *move san* and *lèt gate* are more than ethnographic exotica or public health nuisances. The significance of the syndrome lies in the fact that social problems and their psychological sequelae usually are designated as the causes of the somatically experienced disorder. For this reason, the Haitian syndrome poses a challenge to overly simplistic interpretations of "folk illnesses."

Following the suggestion of others who advise that indigenous illness categories first be studied "emically," from within their cultural context, I will consider the *move san/lèt gate* complex to be an illness caused by malignant emotions—anger born of interpersonal strife, shock, grief, chronic worry, and other affects perceived as potentially harmful. It is thus not possible to relegate *move san* to such categories as "psychological" or "somatic." This stance, which avoids the strictures of a dogmatically "medicalized" anthropology, is reconsidered in the conclusions offered at the end of the paper.

THE RESEARCH SETTING

The Republic of Haiti occupies the western third of the island of Hispaniola. After the Dominican Republic, which borders it to the east, its nearest neighbors are Jamaica to the southwest and Cuba to the north and west. Haiti, born of a slave revolt that ended in 1804, is the hemisphere's second-oldest independent nation. Its inhabitants are largely the descendants of the African slaves that made western Hispaniola France's most lucrative colony. During the nineteenth century, the nascent peasantry, left to its own devices, developed richly syncretic linguistic, religious, and ethnomedical institutions. In 1982, Haiti's population was conservatively estimated to be 5.1 million, or 345 persons per exploitable square kilometer. Despite the alarming density, 57 percent of the labor force is involved in small-scale agriculture. Some 74 percent of the country's inhabitants are rural; many live in villages similar to the one described in this study. Estimates of per capita income usually put Haiti last among the countries of the Western Hemisphere, and this poverty is reflected in the health status of the nation: a life expectancy of forty-eight years and an infant mortality rate of 124 per 1,000.[4]

Do Kay stretches along an unpaved road that cuts through Haiti's Central Plateau. A small village in great flux, it has been the locus of almost all "development" efforts in the area. Consisting of 123 households in 1985, Do Kay had a total population of 677. Exactly one year later, a census by the same team revealed 11 new households, bringing the number of inhabitants to 772. Some of the increase in population is due, it seems, to the construction, since 1980, of a church, a school, a clinic, and a community bakery and the initiation of a project to make pigs available to the rural poor.

The area has a curious and ironic history. Before 1956, there was no Do Kay; the village of Kay was situated in the fertile valley of the nation's largest river. A great many of the persons now living in Do Kay then lived in an area adjacent to Kay called Petit Fond. When the valley was flooded to build a hydroelectric dam, the majority of villagers were forced to move up into the hills on either side of the valley. Kay became divided into "Do" (those that resettled on the stony backs of the hills) and "Ba" (those that remained down near the new waterline). Most villagers received no compensation for their land, nor were they provided with water or electricity. For many, the years following the inundation of their lands were bitter. As deforestation and erosion whittled away at the hills, it became more and more difficult to wrest sustenance from them. And yet Do Kay is typical of many small Haitian villages in which the great majority make a living by tending small gardens and selling much of their produce. Marketing is largely the province of young to middle-aged women, many of whom are also responsible for growing their merchandise.

The majority of the houses comprise two rooms: a *sal* with chairs, and a *cham* with straw mats or, occasionally, a bed. Although average household size in Do Kay is between five and six persons, it is not unusual to find more than ten sharing these two rooms. Typically, dwellings are constructed of stones covered with a cement-like mud, although wattle daubed with mud is not uncommon. There is still no electricity in the area, and none of the houses has running water.

Until recently, for their water supply, residents of Do Kay were forced to scramble down a steep hillside to a large spring 800 vertical feet below the level of the road. Although villagers seemed to know the dangers of drinking impure water, the temptation was to store water in large pots or calabash gourds. Infant deaths due to diarrheal disease were commonplace. A hydraulic pump now moves springwater up to three public fountains placed along the road and also to the school and other buildings run by the church.

There is no village center or "square," although the school-church-clinic complex may be beginning to take on this function. The clinic was inaugurated in 1985 and began offering consultations with a Haitian doctor two days per week. Until March of that year, when the bakery opened, there were no retail shops or businesses, though a few commodities (canned milk, local colas, small quantities of grain) could be obtained from the handful of families known to "resell."

Excluding the doctor, all the informants cited in this research were born and grew up in rural and agrarian Haiti. They are all, by their own criteria, extremely poor. This brief introduction is intended to situate the *move san/lèt gate* syndrome, primarily an affliction of women, against the background of the daily struggles of the remarkable women of Do Kay.

INTERVIEWING METHODS, CASE-FINDING, AND SURVEY RESULTS

The research on which this paper is based was conducted as part of a larger study of childrearing and nutrition in rural Haiti. When the study was initiated in 1985, I restricted in-depth interviewing to Do Kay. I had already lived in the village for over a year and knew many of its inhabitants. Other researchers working in Haiti have found familiarity with informants to be crucial to obtaining reliable data.[5] Initial interviews indicated the modal weaning age to be eighteen months, and so I decided to interview the mothers or primary caretakers of all children eighteen months and younger. By September 1985, there were forty-seven such infants in Do Kay. Interviews with mothers were preceded by three lengthy "pre-test" interviews with tried-and-true informants (such as Mme. Kado,[6] introduced later) who had helped me in the past. Most mothers (or primary caretakers) were interviewed, in their homes, more than once in 1985.

Although the interviews were open-ended and followed no rigid format, several issues were always addressed. Among these were *move san* and its relation to breastfeeding. As the significance of the disorder became manifest, I devoted more interview time to its characterization. Among my informants were three women who claimed to be experiencing *move san* at the time of the initial interview. These were considered "active cases." Two of the three were attempting to breastfeed infants; these women were interviewed several times over twenty months.

For purposes of this preliminary discussion, it is necessary to indicate that a startlingly high percentage (thirty-six mothers, or 77 percent) of those interviewed had experienced at least one identifiable episode of *move san*.[7] Thirty-two of the thirty-six, or 89 percent, sought treatment in the professional or popular health sectors: three went to a biomedical practitioner; thirteen consulted only a *dokte fey* or other herbalist; sixteen sought treatment from more than one source (although recourse to an herbalist was almost always included in the quest for therapy). In the majority of cases, professional care was preceded and then supplemented by home health care.

The central problematic of this paper is not, however, *move san* as an isolated disorder, but rather the *move san/lèt gate* complex. Of the thirty-six women who had experienced at least one episode of *move san*, seventeen, or 47 percent, stated that they had been breastfeeding an infant during an episode. (Of the three women who remarked that they felt that their lives had been in danger, two were among this group.) Of the seventeen, fifteen sought treatment outside the home for (or, in two cases, to prevent) *lèt gate*. One woman who had not sought treatment outside the home was one of the three respondents who had *move san/ lèt gate* at the time of the 1985 survey; she was gathering the funds necessary to defray her treatment expenses. The other respondent was treated effectively at home, by her mother's sister. Ten of the treatment regimens for *move san/lèt gate* met with success; these women declared that they had been "cured" by the remedies. The remaining six all weaned their children, citing *lèt gate* as the motive; only two of these six children were normal weight for age by the Gomez scale, a widely used measure of childhood malnutrition.

In all cases, the etiology of the *lèt gate* was held to be *move san;* in other words, their association, which was guaranteed by the methodology, was never labeled as chance by an informant.[8] The etiology of *move san* itself was invariably seen to be a malignant emotion, most commonly caused by interpersonal strife. Of the thirty-six informants with a history of *move san*, twenty-four cited such strife as the cause of the disorder. Seventeen of these conflicts involved a spouse, partner, or family member (in descending order of importance: husband or mate, brothers and sisters, parents and children); five involved *vwasinay*, or neighbors; and two involved near or total strangers. Of the remaining twelve informants with a history of *move san*, there were five related cases of shock (*sezisman*), and the other seven adduced a mixed bag of stressors, most related to chronic financial problems (for example, shame at being unable to feed children), all of which had led to "too much bad emotion." Distinctions between personal and social stress-ors seem significant, but I have not yet discerned any clear pattern of course or outcome that might be related to such differentiation. No clear symptomatology for *move san* emerged from the preliminary readings of the interviews.

CASE HISTORIES

Given that *move san* is a common problem among the mothers of children under eighteen months of age in Do Kay, what is the natural history of the illness? What are the psychological concomitants of "bad blood"? Who is at risk? How long does it last? What are its symptoms? How is it treated? Why do some women find successful therapy, while others do not? These were among the questions that led me to elicit more psychologically detailed case histories from the three women afflicted with *move san* at the time this study was initiated. Because I knew little about the perceived course of the illness, it seemed imperative to follow the cases over long periods of time. Two of these histories are presented here, the first in detail because it is a good example of the common scenario in which the label *move san* is invoked. It is also prototypical[9] in that it illustrates what appears to be the classical course of the disorder. The second case is one in which the *move san/lèt gate* syndrome was caused by "shock" (*sezisman*) or fright; though far less frequently invoked as precipitating the disorder, it was the second most common etiology given by my informants.

Case 1

Ti Malou Joseph, thirty years old, has had recurrent episodes of *move san;* each has been precipitated, she readily avers, by discord with the father of her children. She and her living children brought to a total of thirteen the number of persons sharing her parents' two-room house. Although I have only indirect indicators of socioeconomic status, the Joseph family is considered one of the poorest in the village. The house is roofed with tin, but the floor is tamped dirt. Both of her parents are frequently ill, and Ti Malou and a younger sister are usually the major breadwinners for the family. To generate income, they engage in small-scale gardening and the buying and reselling of produce and staples such as raw sugar. Often, Ti Malou lacks the (very small amount of) capital necessary to participate in the rural marketing network. Currently estranged from the father of her children, she is emblematic of the uncounted Haitian women who labor against increasingly dismal odds.

Ti Malou was interviewed several times. The first session took place late in the sixth month of her fourth pregnancy. When asked if she had ever suffered from *move san,* she replied that she had, asserting that she was experiencing it at that very moment. (Another informant, Mme. Kado, had hinted that I would find an active case in Ti Malou.) When asked to describe "the problem," she explained, "I think the problem is the result of fighting with the father of my children. He hit me, a pregnant woman, and made life very difficult for me." Several months after the birth of her child, and two months after being cured, Ti Malou had not significantly changed her ideas about etiology:

> If you're having troubles (*nan kont*) with someone, and they yell at you or strike you, you can become ill. My illness is the result of fighting with the father of my children. He struck me while I was pregnant and rendered my life very difficult. He struck me in the face. That's what makes the blood rise up to my head and spoil the milk; this happened during my fifth month, and by five and a half months, my *move san* had already erupted [in *bouton*, small, raised blemishes] all over my body. The blood mixes with the milk; if it reaches the uterus, it will kill you rapidly.

As her pregnancy progressed, Ti Malou became more and more uncomfortable. She complained of severe lower-back pains (*doulè senti*), muscle cramps, headaches, dizziness, light-headedness (*soulay*), diarrhea, and crampy stomach pain. She endured a month or so of these symptoms, seeking no care outside the home or family friends. By the end of her seventh month, she was "unable to get out of bed." In early July, she began experiencing tingling and then "numbness" in her legs. She fell one day "because I had no sensation in my left leg." In mid-July, a full month before her expected date of confinement, she began experiencing what she described as "labor pains":

> It wasn't my time, but something was happening. I thought they were labor pains (*tranche*). I began to worry about the fall (*sò*) I had taken. Madame Kado told me that I was carrying twins, and that one of them had been damaged when I fell. I suspect now that it was not the fall that was responsible for the death of one of them. That might have left a mark on the child, but it wasn't severe enough to kill her. I went to see the doctor [in Mirebalais, a nearby town], but he said that there was nothing wrong, and that the baby wasn't due yet. He didn't think there were twins.

Mme. Kado, an influential friend, had informed Ti Malou that her symptoms were "in large measure" due to *move san;* by the end of the pregnancy, her mother and other family members agreed. Herbal remedies, the therapy of choice, were interdicted during the pregnancy, because "the medicine is too strong for the baby." During her final month of pregnancy, Ti Malou was in bed more often than not. Everyone agreed that she looked ill; more than one member of her family remarked that she was "as white as a person with tuberculosis."

When labor pains did begin, it was decided that she should go to the hospital to deliver rather than having the usual home birth attended by a midwife. There were bound to be complications, according to Mme. Kado. Late one evening, about a week after her "date," Ti Malou and her mother left for the hospital in Hinche, about an hour away. They paid for a space on one of the trucks that carries produce and its vendors from the Central Plateau to Port-au-Prince and back again.

Rumors drifted back to Do Kay throughout the next day, with many versions of the story of her labor and delivery. All agreed, however, that the process was bedeviled from the start. One of Ti Malou's younger brothers followed them the next morning; he returned that evening, bearing bad news. His sister was "bleeding," he said, and needed a transfusion. This she would not receive without prepayment. The news was greeted by Mme. Kado and other friends (myself included) with horror. The requisite fifteen dollars (more than a month's income for many rural families) was collected in short order and dispatched with a kins-woman of Ti Malou. The next day we heard nothing. Mme. Kado feared the worst and suggested that *move san* was also to blame for Ti Malou's complications. On the third day of her hospitalization, Ti Malou gave birth to twins: one, Jules, was alive and well; the other was stillborn.

Her subsequent case of *lèt gate* was seen both as a confirmation of the *move san* diagnosis, if anyone doubted it, and as a further indication of the severity of the episode. Most of her symptoms persisted, but she delayed a trip to the *dokte fey*, or herbalist, citing financial worries. Ti Malou's father prepared a root-and-leaf concoction, but her relief was short-lived. The family became concerned that her breast milk would "pass" into her head and make her "crazy" or kill her. (No one in the Joseph family other than Ti Malou mentioned the uterus.) Three weeks after Jules's birth, he too broke out in *bouton*. He grew listless and stopped gaining weight.

Mme. Kado and others indicated that it was "scandalous" that Ti Malou had not yet attended to "their" illness properly. Mme. Kado recommended a midwife about an hour's donkey ride from Do Kay; she was reputed to be adept at cur-ing *move san/lèt gate*. Her rates were more reasonable than those of a *dokte fey*, but her results were as good. Finally, Ti Malou did go in search of the indicated root-and-leaf remedy. (Such an interaction is depicted by the midwife later in this study; see "The Healer's EM.") Ti Malou also made a second visit to the doc-tor while she was a *ti nouris*, as a mother is known for the first several weeks of nursing. Although the visit was only a few days before her trip to see the midwife, she again did not mention her disorder to the doctor. Her chief complaint, he reported, was a fungal infection in the infant's throat.

Case 2

Alourdes Surpris is the twenty-three-year-old mother of one of the most mal-nourished children in the village. At eleven months, her daughter Acephie weighed 5.7 kilograms; by the Gomez scale, she suffered from third-degree mal-nutrition. Although at the time of this writing Acephie is less malnourished, developmental delays are evident. Surprisingly, the child would seem to be one of those least at risk of nutritional disease: she lives with both parents in a three-room house directly across the street from the school. Her father is a schoolteacher and nets a small, but regular salary; Alourdes works in the new day care center and has received several years of formal education. Although the couple was not married when the child, their first, was conceived, both reported wanting a child very much.

How did this unlikely candidate become malnourished? The cause was probably early weaning: "I weaned her at five months. When she was born, I breastfed her, but my milk dried up; I had to wean her right away." Alourdes's notion of why her milk "dried up" is quite specific:

> I have had *move san* ever since a bolt of lightning struck my house and narrowly missed killing my husband and child. . . . It knocked us right out of bed. I was shocked (*sezi*) so much that I could never breastfeed again. I couldn't concentrate, I couldn't fall asleep. Whenever the baby cried, I'd jump. My heart was skipping. Even though I took a great deal of [herbal] medicine, my milk was never restored.

As noted earlier, five of the seventeen cases of *lèt gate* due to *move san* were caused by *sezisman*. Although further study is clearly necessary, it seems as if the course of *move san* is similar regardless of the source of the malignant emotion perceived to have caused it (for example, interpersonal strife, economic pressures, natural cataclysms). The healer I interviewed remarked that minor changes in the remedy are called for if the *move san* is caused by shock, though not all informants made such fine distinctions.

MOVE SAN/LÈT GATE AS "INTERPRETED DISORDER"

In a critique of methodologies grounded in an "empiricist theory of language," Byron Good and Mary-Jo DelVecchio Good suggest that an analysis of indigenous illness categories should include both an investigation of the sociocultural construction of illness realities and the analysis of the "semantic networks" that link "key public symbols both to primary social values and to powerful personal affects."[10] To put it somewhat differently, a symptom may be thought of as a vehicle of meaning that connects two different kinds of referents—the traditionally expected ones and the unexpected, "private" ones. As the first of several steps in the analysis of the *move san/lèt gate* complex, I will adopt a meaning-centered approach that encompasses both the more psychological as well as the more somatic components of a disorder that defies facile Cartesian classification. My task is not only to describe both shared and idiosyncratic meanings but also to answer some of the key questions listed at the outset: What is the natural history of the illness? How long does it last? What are its symptoms? How is it treated? Why do some women find successful therapy, while others do not? What sorts of emotional upset are most frequently associated with the illness? What triggers these emotions? Who is at risk?

One means by which semantic networks may be evoked—and an understanding of the construction of an illness experience approached—is through eliciting informants' explanatory models, or "EMs," to use the accepted shorthand.[11] Because such an approach takes informants' discourse seriously, it entails literal and liberal quotation. It attaches narrators to narratives and recognizes discourse as context-dependent. Space restrictions limit our discussion to one case, that of Ti Malou. (As a matter of convenience, I often refer to her as "the patient.") Although her case history, presented earlier, pointed out many facets of her EM, we have not examined in detail, much less contrasted, the discourses of the patient, her friends and family, and her healers. Those engaged in the clinical process include at least a confidante (Mme. Kado), the patient's mother, a midwife/healer, and a physician. Each was interviewed at length at least twice during the illness episode.

My analysis is also meant to be mindful of three fundamental charges that have been leveled at interpretive medical anthropology. Much of the material published to date has been narrowly focused on "the doctor/patient relationship." I thank my informants for making it clear that the doctor's EM was far less relevant to their own constructions than were the other EMs presented here. Further, slighting the individual psychological nature of the illness begs the entire question of intracultural variation. Finally, study of EMs too often ignores the fact that they change over time. Not only are explanatory models reformulated and even re-created during the same illness episode; they also may be reshaped in different contexts at the same point in the episode. The cases presented here have been followed over twenty months. Interviews with older women added a greater time depth than my own recent involvement could afford. The concluding section examines in more detail the correctives that a multiply-situated discourse and its inferred connections can bring to interpretive exercises.

The Patient's EM

Ti Malou's EM might be described as "somatosocial." Although she gave the *move san/lèt gate* complex a social etiology, Ti Malou tended to focus discussion of her illness on her shifting symptoms and on the pathophysiology and course of the illness. To cite an interview following her successful cure:

> I've had it before; my life has been full of problems like this. The first thing I noticed was a bumpy rash [*bouton*] that erupted all over my body. After that, I felt terrible; I couldn't sleep, I had no appetite, and I had diarrhea. I tried treating the diarrhea with clinic medicine, but it wasn't until I took the herbal remedy [over three months later] that I was really free of it. I also had a terrible headache, and my jaw was stiff and difficult to move and my mouth was always full of water.

Her selectivity is not to be mistaken for "lack of insight" or reluctance to confront "interpersonal" difficulties: when questioned, she unhesitatingly cited the social and psychological origins of her distress. But in her more unprompted discourse, she tended to dwell on her discomfort and her quest for treatment.

Another aspect of the treatment described most fully by Ti Malou was the necessity of separating blood from milk before therapy could be successfully initiated:

> As soon as the child was born, I knew that the milk was no good. My father went in search of a medicine for me to drink. I did indeed drink it, but it had no effect, because my father did not know to separate the blood from the milk . . . before making me take the remedy. It was the midwife who began by separating blood and milk. Only when this was achieved did she start me on the remedy.

When asked what was wrong with her milk, Ti Malou responded that it had become "weak, watery" and had been "invaded by bad blood." When asked quite pointedly what had caused her blood to go bad, she readily replied, "Emotion" (*emansyon*). *Move san* and *lèt gate*, it is clear, are embedded in social interactions. As noted, interpersonal strife is designated as the cause of most cases of *move san*. The household (*menaj*) is the context in which the majority of these cases occur. In Do Kay, at least, a woman's husband or lover is not infrequently regarded as a potential agent of discord. So it was with Ti Malou. One striking aspect of the nature of the interaction between Ti Malou (and her friends and family) and the man who is held to have caused "all her problems" is the considerable comity that marks their every public exchange. This important point will be considered more fully later.

The Mother's EM

In 1985, Jesula Joseph thought that she was approaching her fiftieth year, "but I don't pay much attention to things like that." Indeed, more pressing dilemmas crowd her life: thirteen people to feed, more than half of them children; her own considerable health problems, which include deteriorating vision and chronic back pain; her sickly husband's inability to work; a leaky roof and a rainy season; and two sick grandchildren. Ti Malou's illness arose against a backdrop of unremitting struggle. In our first session, conducted a week before I first interviewed her daughter, I thought I detected a resignation that bordered on lack of interest: "I don't know. Sometimes when you're pregnant it's like that. Some women have a harder time bearing children. It's God's will. I don't know. Maybe it is weakness (*feblès*)." Later in the same interview, when asked if she thought her daughter might have *move san*, she expressed doubt: "I think it is a difficult pregnancy, not *move san*." A month later, she stated that a third-trimester fall had caused many of Ti Malou's problems.

A few days before Ti Malou's confinement, however, her mother was confident that *move san* was at the root of her daughter's symptoms. Mme. Joseph's "lack of interest" dissipated as the family came to perceive Ti Malou's problem as their greatest worry. Mme. Joseph's comments remind us of the need to adopt a more process-oriented approach to the study of illness meanings. Five months and three interviews later, it had become clear to me that her central etiologic interpretations had been revised at least three times during that period. What was at first a difficult pregnancy (later exacerbated by a fall) came to be redefined as *move san,* and finally as the full diapason of *move san/lèt gate* triggered by a malevolent lover. Close attention to the temporal sequence of the revisions, as well as the changes in Ti Malou's EM, led me to believe that the persuasive force of Mme. Joseph's conceptions had been overshadowed by those of Mme. Kado's EM, examined next.

A Confidante's EM

Madame Anita Kado, a fifty-one-year-old widow, is the mother of nine children, seven of whom are living. She is a cook and an aide-de-camp to the priest who runs the school in Do Kay. She considers herself a resident of Mirebalais but has long spent most of her time in Kay. A presence there for over a decade, Mme. Kado now wields considerable influence. As the daughter of a midwife, she has a longstanding interest in health issues. She is clearly a member of what might be described as Ti Malou's health management group.[12] As far as I know, Mme. Kado was the first to suggest that Ti Malou's difficulties were due to *move san.* By the end of the pregnancy, everyone agreed that Ti Malou was suffering from the disorder and that it had to be treated as such.

Mme. Kado, always an excellent informant, had a good deal to say about *move san.* These quotations are from an interview that took place shortly after Ti Malou's effective treatment:

> If you have an argument or a fight with someone, and if [that person] yells at you while you're pregnant, when the child is born, it will have problems. If he doesn't have diarrhea, the sickness will cause *bouton* to erupt all over him. This indicates that the milk is spoiled. The baby will continue to nurse, but the milk isn't good for him and will give him diarrhea. It's necessary to wean the baby temporarily. If nothing is done about it, even the next child will be affected. A remedy is necessary. You must find a person who knows how to make the medicine, and get two or three doses—enough for about four days. The baby needs to start nursing again for the remedy to work properly. You don't have to give the baby any medicine; he'll take it from his mother's breast, it will reach his blood and take away the bad milk he's already consumed. When the diarrhea starts to go away, you know that the milk is starting to get back to normal. If the diarrhea persists, the milk is still spoiled.

I asked her if babies ever died from *lèt gate.*

> No, never. It's the mother who can die. Ti Malou is a good case. If you're not getting along with someone—perhaps you've said something bad to her, and she becomes angry with you or upset and starts to cry, she can have *move san.* With someone like Ti Malou, it was clear that she began to have *move san* after Luc hit her. But for some people, the first sign is after the baby is born, when you see the milk is no good. If the spoiled milk mixes with the mother's blood and then reaches her uterus, she can die. The milk can go to her head and make her crazy; it can even give her diarrhea as it does the child. It begins to dominate her until it gives her a very serious illness. If that happens, she will surely die.

How can one be sure that a baby's *bouton* and diarrhea are caused by *move san?* Mme. Kado's response was characteristically confident and empiric:

> Well, we knew the milk was no good: it was as clear as water. But to make sure, express some of the milk into a large spoon; if it's thick and white, it's probably not spoiled. Take the spoon and hold it over a flame. As it begins to boil, put a small twig in it. If the cream climbs up the stick, the milk is good. If it doesn't make cream, it's no good. But it's usually not necessary to do this.

The worthlessness of "thin" or "watery" milk is a theme that recurs not only in Mme. Kado's discourse but in that of most of my informants. Two women expressed breast milk into a cupped hand to demonstrate the patently inferior quality, in their eyes, of their milk. These adjectives were held in contradistinction to their antonyms: thick versus thin or watery, opaque white versus clear, strong versus weak, healthy versus unhealthy. The oppositions became a leitmotiv that ran through many of the interviews; as the healer's explanations make clear in the following section, they extend analogically from the body physical to the body social.

Opinion was split as to the cause of the stillbirth in Ti Malou's case, but the disorder was widely held to have complicated labor and delivery. Mme. Kado suggested that *move san* had been at the root of the problem:

> The milk begins to build up early in the pregnancy; it is spread throughout the body, like the blood, but must never mix with blood. In the girl's case, not only did the blood and milk mix, which made the milk turn (*tounen*), but I think it may have started to infiltrate the uterus (*lanmè*). This is very dangerous; she's lucky to have escaped. The guy probably did this on purpose.

Although Ti Malou and her mother were willing to state that the problem was *move san* and that *move san* is caused by emotion, they were less willing to discuss in detail the nature of the discord that engendered the malignant sentiment. Mme. Kado, on the other hand, was full of theories:

Certainly, it may have been only the emotion that turned the milk, and made it leave its place. But when the illness is so bad (*rèd*) that a baby dies, you begin to think that the bad person did more than yell at the woman. It's usually the *woman* who is sick with simple *move san*.

When asked what she intended by her comment, Mme. Kado hinted that Ti Malou's former consort may have tried to "poison" her. Further, Mme. Kado confided that Ti Malou's mother had similar suspicions. (On a subsequent interview of the patient's mother, I found that she had indeed come to believe that her daughter was the victim of maleficence.) When Mme. Kado was asked to fully explain what she meant by "poison," it became clear that she was not speaking of a toxin. She illustrated with a personal scenario:

> I had nine children, and I lost two. With the one who died when she was eleven days old, it seems as if it was a bad person (*move moun*) who did the damage [lit. "tempted it" (the fetus)] while I was still carrying the baby. This person gave me something, but I had no idea: I thought she was my close friend! She cooked for me, I cooked for her . . . she was always over at the house. And then she gives me a bit of *joumon* [a Haitian squash] during the very week that I gave birth. . . . On the seventh day [postpartum], things started going wrong. . . . I thought the baby was uninterested in nursing. She was not yet sick, but she was about to be. When I got up very early the next morning, her jaw was locked shut (*machwa-l te sere*). . . . When she reached the eleventh day, at four o'clock in the morning—the same time that she fell ill—she died. And when she died, out came the bit of *joumon*, exactly as I had eaten it.

Mme. Kado reports that the "bad person" is still living in Mirebalais. When I asked whether she still spoke to the perpetrator of the crime, she expressed surprise at the question: "Do I still speak with her? Of course! With people like that, you never let on that you know they're no good. If you do reveal that you know how bad they are, you'll never have children."

Mme. Kado's anecdote raises more questions than it answers. Did Mme. Kado have *move san* after this event? "Not really," she replied, "although I did take a leaf-and-root medicine to prevent my illness. I'm not very susceptible." Why not? What factors render Ti Malou more susceptible to the disorder (or Mme. Kado less susceptible), or does the difference reside in the precipitating events? How often does *move san* involve malevolent poisoning or magic poisoning? Mme. Kado felt that "you don't have to have a bad person trying to do something to you to have *move san*, but it happens like that sometimes." Some of these questions will be addressed later in this study.

The Healer's EM

Mme. Victor is known as a midwife who is knowledgeable about herbal remedies; she is not, however, a *dokte fey*. She does not know her age but looks to be at least sixty. She lives several miles from Kay in a very modest two-room house. When I interviewed her there, slightly more than two months after she had seen Ti Malou and cured her, she had just returned from delivering a baby. She remembered Ti Malou's case vividly, although she had met her client only once before the therapy. I did not ask how much she charged to cure Ti Malou, but Mme. Kado had estimated that her fee was about five dollars.

Her notion of etiology was not too different from those detailed earlier, although she contended that *move san* is not exclusively a woman's disorder:

> Anyone can fall ill with *move san;* it happens mostly to women, but it can also happen to men. If you are deceived, cheated, cuckolded, ostracized, or frightened, you must beware of *move san.* It can happen in a short amount of time; within a week you're very ill. The first thing you notice is an eruption of itchy bumps all over your body. Then you might have a headache, fever . . . your mouth becomes dry, you're very jumpy . . . your blood turns into water, and you feel weak or stiff. . . . A person with *move san* can sleep all day long. If you press on your nails, you note that there's no blood under there, and you know then that it's turned. Your eyes also turn white. If you're poor enough, you'll feel that you still have to go work in your garden, but if you let the sun cook your already watery blood, it will make it all worse. You become like a leaf: more and more withered. Soon you don't even look human. . . . If the victim is a nursing mother, the milk's as good as lost; it goes bad. You need the [herbal] remedy to make new milk. As soon as you've finished the first day or so of medicine, you can expect the milk to start coming down beautifully, then the headache will go away, as will the body stiffness.

Mme. Victor's discourse was rich in details, which is not surprising given her professional interest in the disorder. The theme of weak or watery blood is again linked to poverty, which is widely held to exacerbate *move san.* Botanical metaphors pepper her descriptions, which are also rich in herbal lore. Mme. Victor was quite willing to share her knowledge and even expressed a willingness to cull some of the scarcer ingredients. Her recipe was presented as a precise and somewhat ritualized regimen:

> To make the remedy, you soak the roots of *bwa lèt,* the roots of *kayimit, bwa jon,* and coconut, and the leaves of *sorosi* and *fey sezi.* If the person with *move san* is a woman with a nursing baby and her milk has gone bad, you need to add the leaves and roots of *bwa let* and also to add one small spoonful of the spoiled milk to the bottle [that contains the remedy]. This is for the person to drink, and will separate the blood from the milk. . . . But there's more to it than that: you must buy a piece of white soap and a coconut, a bit of coffee, a measure of black beans, and then you bring down the blood (*fe lèt la desann*). You grill the coffee together with the black beans and seven grains of salt. When you've finished grilling, you grind it up in a mortar and put it in a pan, add water, and mix it up. From this you make a compress for both the brow and the back of the head, and keep it moist with the

concoction all day long. . . . You can also place an empty shallow basket on the person's head and pour the medicine in the basket; it will run down over the head and body. Each time you dampen the compress, also rub down her arms and legs with the medicine. Do this for a week or so. Also put a grain of virgin salt [from a box that has not been used for cooking] in the palm of each hand. Place a grain of salt under each of [the patient's] feet and stand on a palm leaf. She must stand still. This will make the milk return to its rightful place.

Mme. Victor mentioned that there were several variations on this theme, but that these were the "principal ingredients." Some of these versions are designed to alleviate particular symptoms. (If swollen feet are part of the symptom cluster, Mme. Victor adds avocado-tree bark to the mixture.) A slightly different formula was indicated if the *move san* (or *lèt gate*) was caused by *sezisman*. Further, it is perfectly acceptable for someone suffering from *move san* to seek medical care from other practitioners, with the following caveat:

> The medicine I'm telling you about is the best one for *move san*, and you'd better take it before you spend your money to go to the hospital, because hospital medicines can't make the milk go down. After this remedy has made the milk go down, then you can go to the doctor.

Although such herbal remedies are clearly the therapy of choice, there are attendant risks:

> Don't put in too much of the ingredients. . . . If it's too strong, or you give her too much of the medicine, it can make the person go crazy. But if she doesn't take the medicine, the milk mixes with the blood, it rises to the head and that makes her crazy anyway. That's why nursing mothers are more susceptible, and when you don't see any milk, you'd better hurry and take the [herbal] medicine because you can be sure that the milk is going to her head and will kill her.

Further, the family of the sufferer must ensure that no repeated emotional shocks "interrupt the treatment. . . . The weak has to become strong." Unlike Ti Malou and Mme. Kado, Mme. Victor said nothing about the "infiltration of the uterus." When asked about the case of Alourdes (our second case study), who followed a similar regimen without results, Mme. Victor's disapproval was evident:

> If she weaned her baby, she has narrowly missed killing herself; it's the baby who makes the medicine work correctly. The infant sucks out the bad milk and can then be given a purgative (*lók*). Then both mother and child get well together. But if she has *move san* and doesn't take the right medicine, and the milk dries up within her and the child is weaned, she might look healed today, but she'll be sick again tomorrow.

After interviewing two *dokte fey* and several women with a history of successfully treated *move san/lèt gate,* it became clear that the most constant ingredient in the remedy for spoiled milk was *bwa lèt*. Literally "milk tree," *Sapium jamai-cense* exudes an opaque white sap when nicked or broken. Since Haitian ethno-botany so strikingly recalls a more famous "milk tree," I turn to Victor Turner's analysis of Ndembu ritual. He reminds us to seek three classes of data when attempting to analyze the structure and properties of ritual symbols: "(1) exter-nal form and observable characteristics; (2) interpretations offered by specialists and laymen; (3) significant contexts largely worked out by the anthropologist."[13] Observable characteristics as described by Mme. Victor seemed to typify those of other healers. The interpretations of "laymen," who were all women, tended to be rather thin when compared to the explications offered by Mme. Victor. A typical lay response: "The *bwa lèt* separates the milk from the blood; it makes the milk come back to its place. It strengthens the milk, too, and makes it thick again. The nursing child draws the new milk down into the breast."

The "significant contexts" slowly emerge with repeated interviewing. I attempted to answer basic enough questions: Why might two of our most vital constituents, blood and breast milk, be perceived as potential contaminants? Why would blood become a poison that can mix with breast milk and "climb" into the head or "descend" to the uterus with mortal effect? But before considering this illness in its symbolic register, let us explore the empirical meaning it holds for an "outside authority"—the village's visiting doctor.

The Doctor's EM

Dr. Jean Pierre is a thirty-five-year-old graduate of his country's only medical school. He has been practicing in rural Haiti for almost five years, since the completion of his year-long residency in a small city in the south of Haiti. After moving to the Central Plateau, Jean worked exclusively in the nearby town of Mirebalais; more recently, he has been spending two days each week in the new clinic in Do Kay. I have worked with him for over four years and know that he is from a middle-class family from the country's southern peninsula. Although he was raised by strict Catholic parents, attended parochial schools, and considered becoming a priest, he avows an interest in voodoo. His grand-uncle was a well-known *houngan,* or voodoo priest, in the area where Jean was raised. Despite professed interest in the local religion, Jean more often seems bemused by his patients' health beliefs.

Dr. Pierre saw Ti Malou twice: once in Mirebalais during her "false labor," and again a month or so after her hospitalization. During both visits he spent no more than five minutes per session with Ti Malou. Although I did not tape-record our discussions of her case, I did make the following note at her first consultation:

Jean states that Ti Malou is in "false labor," but that otherwise her pregnancy is progressing normally. He attributes most of her problems to folate deficiency, although I informed him that she was receiving 1 mg/day of folate supplement. The backache is due, he says, to the normal loosening of pelvic ligaments; the leg problems are sciatica from the same cause. When asked about *move san,* he laughed and said, "Everyone has *move san!* Her blood is 'bad' because she needs more folate and iron. Besides, there's nothing I can do about such disorders." He said that she did not bring up the issue with him, but spoke only of her back pain, diarrhea, a numbness in her legs, and of course the "labor pains."

Worth noting throughout these exchanges are, first, the degree to which the EMs of the patient, the mother, the confidante, and the local healer converge, and second, how little these have in common with the EM held by the doctor. Ti Malou knew very well that, in the clinic, complaints of *move san* were more likely to elicit scorn than sympathy. Again we are reminded that discourse depends on a setting for much of its meaning; rather than being neutrally descriptive, it always interacts performatively with a setting of expectations and admitted interpretations. The patient later insisted that her own etiologies were "too private" to discuss in front of the doctor. When I countered mildly that her disorder did not seem too private in Do Kay, she responded much as Jean had done: "There's really nothing he can do, anyway."

That the EMs of all those who accepted the reality of *move san* disorder should have so much in common ought not to surprise us. *Move san* is a "public health problem" in an unaccustomed sense: an illness with a public meaning. When a whole village knows the participants and follows the course of treatment, a case of *move san/lèt gate* serves as a stage on which social and psychological problems (mistreatment of pregnant or lactating women, for example) can be aired. The doctor refused to admit *move san* into the range of his competence, and the patient tacitly agreed to act as if the disorder had never occurred. Doctor and patient were not, therefore, speaking the same language.

Momentarily putting aside the doctor's opinion of the disorder's etiology and cure, we might sum up the villagers' shared understanding of the *move san/lèt gate* complex as including the following points:

A "malignant" emotion can cause sickness. Such emotions include anger, fright, and shock. Women who contract the illness are more often perceived as victims than as offenders.

Pregnant and lactating women are particularly susceptible to *move san.* They should therefore be protected from these malignant emotions.

If *move san* does occur in a pregnant or lactating mother, one common outcome is "spoiled milk."

With or without *lèt gate, move san* is appropriately but not always successfully treated with an herbal remedy.

> Body fluids like milk and blood are perceived as especially sensitive to
> "malignant" emotions; disorders involving them can therefore be seen
> as "barometers" of disturbances in the social field.

This last point, bringing physiological, pharmacological, psychological, interpersonal, and moral forces to bear on the etiology of *move san,* ought to be singled out as just the sort of emphatically loaded cultural *donnée* that an anthropology of suffering needs to examine. In this context, it is significant that Hazel Weidman wrote of a "blood paradigm" that seemed to underlie many of the health-related beliefs of her Haitian American informants.[14]

While a socially recognized disorder like *move san* in some regards resembles a code by which private messages are made public, this should not make us forget that a code can contain personal or regional "dialects," "styles," or "idioms." In Ti Malou's case, we can see personal meaning at work: her illness seems to chart the history of her relationship with Luc, the father of her children. An uninformed observer might not notice the tension that exists between the former mates. But in Do Kay there are plenty of open secrets and forbidden subjects. I recall Mme. Kado's response when I asked her if she still spoke to the woman she held responsible for the death of one of her children: "Do I still speak with her? Of course! With people like that, you never let on that you know they're no good. If you do reveal that you know how bad they are, you'll never have children." Illnesses, therefore, might speak louder than words in contexts such as those from which the *move san* disorder takes its meaning.

One hypothesis comes to mind for certain cases in which *move san* is intractable or difficult to treat: the "illness" might in fact be "illness behavior," a form of chronic somatization that is related to strong social pressures (as, for example, the pressure to avoid confronting those who wrong you). Somatization of distress is, in such cases, a form of metaphoric retaliation or resistance. Although somatization is clearly an important component of *move san,* there are substantial differences between the somatization depicted here and that described by Arthur Kleinman among the Chinese and Margaret Lock among Japanese women.[15] Among Kleinman's Hunanese patients, depression and psychosocial problems were either denied or taken to be the result, and not the cause, of pain. Etiologies were predominantly biologic, these being the culturally sanctioned causes of illness. My informants, in contrast, almost always designated social problems and their psychological sequelae as the cause of their illness but thereafter focused on their abundant somatic symptoms. Among Lock's Japanese informants, also women, we can see more similarities: somatization of distress is a form of women's protest, but the social dynamics of distress, however obvious, are often treated as a forbidden subject. More research should show how similar these patterns are.

Nonetheless, the model of "illness behavior" is inappropriate to many of the cases described by my informants. For a few, *move san* may be more of a coping style, an idiom of distress. For others, it recalls a more acute form of somatization similar to an acute stress syndrome. But if *move san* is in some way adaptive, "the work of culture," why is the outcome occasionally so dismal? As Gananath Obeyesekere writes, "Work also implies failure; if mourning is successful work, melancholia is failure."[16] Where people are under severe nutritional, political, and interpersonal stress, attempts to replace direct confrontation with some "safer" alternative are bound to fail sometimes. Seen as "work," acute *move san* may be successful, while the *move san/lèt gate* complex is frequently a failure.

Should *move san* and *lèt gate* be considered two different syndromes? If so, *move san* seems to be an "etiological category," one that suggests much about the origins of the problem, with wide variation in presenting symptoms. Spoiled milk, on the other hand, is virtually pathognomonic for the *move san/lèt gate* syndrome when it is seen in a previously healthy woman who is not pregnant. Is spoiled milk merely the symptom of bad blood in a pregnant or nursing mother? I believe that *lèt gate* is more than just a symptom of *move san*. Instead, let us suppose, as do my informants, that the two "run together"; it is widely believed that the added factor of milk complicates the course of the malady. It indicates, I suspect, the gravity of the initial offense, the malignancy of the emotion. It recalibrates the barometer.

Further, this barometer gives readings on the larger atmosphere. Everyone in Do Kay shares a background of great material and political stress. Social interrelations and psychological equilibrium are rendered more fragile under these conditions. In much of rural Haiti, women are frequently called upon to perform the Herculean task of providing for children and other dependents. Too often, like Ti Malou Joseph, they must do this alone. During pregnancy, and while a woman is a *ti nouris,* several strict rules are observed, all seeming to reflect a single concern: the protection of the woman. One must avoid, at all costs, startling or upsetting a pregnant or nursing mother. When this "taboo" is broken, *move san* as illness behavior is one means of articulating distress. Obeyesekere asserts that the "work of culture is the process whereby painful motives and affects such as those occurring in depression are transformed into publicly accepted sets of meanings and symbols."[17] In his work in Sri Lanka, Obeyesekere sees the work of culture in the ample Buddhist lexicon of suffering and despair. But the work of culture is found not only in well-articulated ideology or flashy ritual. It is also present in a more subtle illness syndrome that may afford beleaguered women, and especially mothers, a culturally sanctioned and relatively safe means of articulating displeasure with the behavior of consociates. It becomes, quite literally, an idiom in which many forms of misfortune—whether designated by outside observers as social, economic, psychological, or physical—are obliquely presented.

Whether or not an organic basis is ever found for the *move san/lèt gate* complex, it is clearly an illness rich in cultural and individual meaning. It is for this reason, too, that a more broadly conceived approach is now appropriate.

DISCUSSION: MODELS OF AN ILLNESS

A next step in the preliminary assessment of a heretofore undescribed indigenous illness category might be to apply to it several different varieties of cultural analysis, one after another, in an attempt to clarify the nature of the illness, and then compare the results. We shall bring three possible and complementary methods of explaining to bear on *move san/lèt gate*. The first is the meaning-centered psychological and ethnomedical analysis outlined earlier. A number of the questions posed at the outset remain unanswered, suggesting, perhaps, the limitations of an interpretive approach. If it hopes to answer questions of relative risk and changing incidence, an interpretive approach not only must be based on a painstaking phenomenology of illness and grounded in epidemiology but also must incorporate the lessons of history and political economy. Further, a comparative exercise might yield insights not apparent if an "emic" stance alone is adopted. What follows is a pair of methodological sketches, the sole purpose of which is heuristic.

Move San/Lèt Gate as a Product of Economic Forces

Is the *lèt gate* syndrome the product of an economy that forces women away from breastfeeding? In 1975, an estimated 46.2 percent of Haitian women participated in the labor force, making them far more economically active than any of their Latin American counterparts. In the entire Third World, only Lesotho boasts a formal economy more dependent upon women.[18]

In their detailed study of infant feeding practices in a Haitian village they call "Kinanbwa," Maria Alvarez and Gerald Murray note an alarming increase in the "spoiled milk syndrome." Their rural informants "believed that it is possible for the milk of a lactating mother to *gate*, to spoil and turn it into a poisonous substance that may, instead of nourishing the child, harm or even kill it." For this reason, women with *lèt gate* wean their children. As in Do Kay, "the most frequent cause for this is the onset of violent negative emotional state in the female." The authors attribute the "epidemic" to the gradually deteriorating economy of the village in which they worked: "It takes little imagination to perceive the manner in which this 'illness' provides precisely the cognitive rationale for turning to the increasingly early weaning that the worsening economic conditions in the village make practically desirable. The belief complex itself makes possible a behaviorally convenient symbolic metamorphosis of the meaning of early weaning. Traditionally, early weaning was seen as an injustice to the child. But when a woman has *lèt gate,* her early weaning is interpreted as a service to the child." Although Alvarez and Murray do not suggest a monistic economic model, favoring instead one that draws upon intimate familiarity with their informants, they do insist that "the epidemic of *lèt gate* which appears to have come over the village cannot be understood apart from the economic pressures which make early weaning desirable."[19]

It is unlikely, however, that the model they propose will fully illuminate the Do Kay data. First, although the prevalence of *move san/lèt gate* would seem to be as high among my informants as among the Kinanbwa mothers, the lactating women of Do Kay, unlike those who spoke with Alvarez and Murray, do not wean their children when their milk spoils; rather, they seek to treat it. Ten out of sixteen did so effectively. Second, in Do Kay, the threat is seen as chiefly to the mother, not the infant. One of the chief differences between the two groups of women is the Kinanbwa women's almost universal involvement in marketing, an activity that takes them to Port-au-Prince for much of the year. The women in Do Kay do far less marketing but still have a high incidence of *lèt gate.* More work is necessary to determine possible psychological and secondary "gains" derived from the *move san/lèt gate* label. Perhaps the course, rather than the incidence, of the illness is to some extent determined by the mother's occupation. No pattern was discernible among my informants: the six women who weaned their infants were no more involved in marketing than were the ten who continued breastfeeding after successful treatment.

During the past few years, a "critical medical anthropology" has taken shape. Although it seems to have no one agenda, a central criticism leveled against medical anthropology has been its failure to link local ills to the larger systems of domination that often influence or even generate them. Much psychological anthropology is vulnerable to the same critique. My own refresher course in political economy was taught by a more convincing teacher—one of my local informants. Mme. Gracia, a woman in her late sixties, insisted that I not forget recent history. She reminded me to attend to the larger context in which "malignant emotions" arose:

> *Move san* is not something that was regularly seen before [the valley was flooded]. Some people died from it after the dam was finished. Now we are up here and we are poor. We have no livestock, no [sugarcane] mills. We suffer too many shocks (*sezisman*), too many problems. We are poor and we are weak, and that is why you see *move san.*

For Mme. Gracia, as for many of my younger informants, *move san* was a channel through which broader experiences of suffering could be transmitted. That suffering is explicitly related to the humiliating frustrations of poverty, the ineffaceable pain of displacement. Mme. Gracia jogged my memory: seven of the thirty-six mothers with a history of *move san* cited financial difficulties as the prime etiologic factor. Poverty was mentioned in most talk about suffering and misfortune. I do not believe that *move san/lèt gate* is a direct product of economic forces. But I do believe that the weight of material deprivation may change the incidence and course of the illness, and even serve as a causal factor in some instances. In many of the Do Kay cases, then, a modified version of Alvarez and Murray's dictum holds true: the high incidence of *lèt gate* in Do Kay cannot be understood apart from the economic pressures that make emotional stability so elusive.

Move San as a Mental Disorder, American Style

One of the most consistently applied methods of examining a "new" disorder is to attempt to map it onto existing illness categories. This has become especially true if the disorder is labeled "psychological." For example, Ari Kiev has declared that culture-bound disorders "are not new diagnostic entities; they are in fact similar to those already known in the West." Each of the well-described culture-bound disorders, Kiev asserts, is actually an American psychiatric diagnosis in exotic clothing: *latah* is a hysterical disorder, *susto* and *koro* are anxiety disorders, *shinkeishitsu* is really obsessive-compulsive disorder, and so on.[20] As much recent work by anthropologists has shown, there is good reason to believe such transpositions inaccurate.

False starts do not excuse us, however, from seeking a genuine dialogue with other, related disciplines. In referring to the American Psychiatric Association's *Diagnostic and Statistical Manual of Mental Disorders* (DSM-III), we need not surrender our relativism, nor our attempts at autonomous theorizing. We can consider the textbook classifications as offering a comparative perspective, not an authoritative answer. In several circumstances, diagnoses from one nosology have served to illuminate diagnoses from another. In the spirit of such comparison, we will suspend skepticism and consider *move san* as a Haitian version of one of our own official labels. Further, the exercise is best conducted by clinically informed anthropologists with an understanding of indigenous categories, if only as a preemptive strike against those less aware of the slippery nature of categories and labels. With the growing hegemony of North American medicine in Haiti, it will not be long before DSM-III is aimed at *move san* with "therapeutic" intent.

For example, can *move san* be construed as a depressive disorder? Given the primacy of the "psychological" that is manifest in DSM-III criteria for Major Depressive Disorder (MDD), it is unlikely that any of my informants would be diagnosed as clinically depressed. If some of their somatic complaints were judged to be metaphoric expressions of sadness, however, several of them would meet MDD criteria. I am not sure that would be an appropriate or useful diagnosis; in those who are currently afflicted with *move san,* the affective component is more suggestive of anxiety than depression. Of the several anxiety disorders listed in DSM-III, only Generalized Anxiety Disorder (GAD) would be a candidate diagnosis for *move san.* DSM-III stipulates that the essential feature of the new category GAD is "persistént anxiety of at least one month's duration." Certainly, anxiety of one brand or another was present among the vast majority of those women suffering from *move san,* but it did not have the overwhelming character of an "essential feature" and was often of short duration. Further, anxiety is almost as prevalent among those women with no history of *move san.* Raising children in rural Haiti has become an anxiety-generating venture.

Taking the somatization of depression among the Chinese for a model, can a case be made for the somatization of anxiety disorder among rural Haitian women? DSM-III certainly makes it easier to arrive at a diagnosis of GAD than one of MDD. To diagnose the former, "generalized, persistent anxiety" must be continuously present for at least one month. Unlike the criteria for MDD, however, which are imbued with a marked primacy of the mental, the anxious mood may be manifested in symptoms from any three of the following four categories: motor tension, autonomic hyperactivity, apprehensive expectation, and vigilance and scanning.[21] Although a patient such as Ti Malou could be squeezed into a modified, "somatized" MDD category, a diagnosis of GAD might fit her more comfortably. At present, these diagnoses may not be entertained concurrently: DSM-III stipulates that a diagnosis of GAD may not be made when the criteria for MDD or any other Affective Disorder can be met. Since the publication of DSM-III, the hierarchical organization giving precedence to Affective Disorders has come under attack; Robert Spitzer and Janet Williams have reviewed the issues and propose a revision in which a "symptomatically more pervasive disorder preempts the diagnosis of a less pervasive disorder."[22]

One problem with such a "lenient" approach to diagnosis might be that, although criteria can be met using the somatic symptoms, the resulting clinical picture is not strikingly anxious. This leads, of course, to a conundrum and underlines a major source of anthropology's chronic vexation with psychiatry: none of the reported symptoms is specific to anxiety, and none of them allows us to distinguish "normal" from "pathologic" anxiety.

The APA classification holds that the essential feature of Adjustment Disorder is "a maladaptive reaction to an identifiable psychosocial stressor." The maladaptive nature of the response is manifested by "impairment in social or occupational functioning or symptoms that are in excess of a normal and expected reaction to the stressor."[23] If it falls to outsiders to decide what constitutes normal and abnormal reactions, these criteria are more easily met. Because appropriate social functioning for a *ti nouris* includes breastfeeding, and because bottle-feeding so often has adverse effects in settings such as rural Haiti, *move san* as a response to a stressor might very well be considered maladaptive.[24] Yet this diagnosis, even if embellished by tags such as "with Anxious Mood" or "with Mixed Emotional Features," would have no real utility and would offer little in the way of improving our understanding of the disorder.

Just as it would be premature to exclude an organic basis, so too is it unrealistic to consider as psychogenic in origin any illness "for which there is positive evidence, or a strong presumption, that the symptoms are linked to psychological factors or conflicts."[25] *All* symptoms, once perceived, are linked to "psychological factors or conflicts," even those symptoms that are positively valued. More useful in a preliminary examination of *move san* is the term "somatization" as used by Wayne Katon, Arthur Kleinman, and Gary Rosen;[26] they include under that label not only physical symptoms that occur in the absence of organic findings but also the amplification of complaints caused by established pathology, such as a chronic illness. The definition eschews an unrealistic faith in the ability of clinicians to detect "underlying" organic findings or pathophysiologic mechanisms on a case-by-case basis. In over four years of intermittent clinical experience in Haiti, I have never seen anything resembling a complete diagnostic workup.

Psychological reductionism would have us miss the possibility of significant biological disruption; in addition to the medicalization of social problems (for example, neurasthenia in China, "heart distress" in Iran), can we afford to miss or misinterpret the *physiologization* of social and psychological problems? An elegant psychoneuroendocrinologic model could be advanced to explain *lèt gate* (for example, neuromodulatory inhibition of oxytocin letdown or prolactin rise), as well as the more obvious symptoms of autonomic nervous system hyperarousal. And is our own relativism not called into question by our failure to entertain the possibility that *move san* might be just what it is said to be: a blood disorder caused by malignant emotions? Among my informants, the most common explanatory model seems to go *beyond* a somatosocial model—*move san/lèt gate* becomes a disorder of experience, without a great deal of Cartesian anguish as to whether it is more somatic than psychological. The disorder, and their view of it, calls into question the tenaciously dissecting gaze not only of psychiatry but of much medical anthropology as well.

CONCLUSION: MADAME GRACIA AND
THE ANTHROPOLOGY OF SUFFERING

Move san is an illness that has not yet been fully described in anthropological, medical, or psychiatric literature. How to begin? Anthony Marsella's suggestion that research start from an emic determination of popular categories[27] is accomplished by eliciting explanatory models from informants in order to clarify how the illness (often not neatly labeled "psychological" or "somatic" by the persons who suffer from it) is culturally constructed. After this preliminary description, how should the illness be examined? I have presented several different ways of interpreting the data—some of them reductionist and functionalist, but all heuristically useful. The mapping of "exotic" disorders onto North American psychiatric-diagnostic frameworks instructs mainly through its inadequacies; it neither helps us understand the "folk" nosology nor gives any assurance that the familiar categories are being applied correctly. In the attempt to formalize imaginary correspondences, an "unreal" illness is reinterpreted to fit the authoritative terms of a "real" one.

Considering *move san/lèt gate* as an interpreted disorder affords a privileged view not only of the disorder but of broader categories of affliction. Viewed as a cultural artifact, the most striking thing about *move san* disorder is the lurid extremity of its symbolism: two of the body's most vital constituents, blood and milk, are turned to poisons. The powerful metaphors serve, it may be inferred, as a warning against the abuse of women, especially pregnant or nursing ones. Transgressions are discouraged by their publicly visible, and potentially dire, results. As somatic indices, "bad blood" and "spoiled milk" submit private problems to public scrutiny. The opposition of vital and lethal body fluids serves as a moral barometer.

Up to this point, the nonbodily factors appealed to by our analysis of the disorder have been largely interpersonal and village-scale. The investigation remains shallow, however, if the "moral barometers" are viewed in a controlled and limited context. A village is not a bell jar, and, as Mme. Gracia attests, the syndrome is related to the historical and economic changes affecting women's increasingly difficult struggle for survival in rural Haiti. In their incisive evaluation of contemporary anthropology, George Marcus and Michael Fischer reach a similar conclusion: "An interpretive anthropology fully accountable to its historical and political-economy implications thus remains to be written."[28] This is no less true of medical and psychological anthropology. It is inexcusable to limit our horizons to the ideally circumscribed village, culture, or case history and ignore the social origins of much—if not most—illness and distress. An interpretive anthropology of affliction, attuned to the ways in which history and its calculus of economic and symbolic power impinge on the local and the personal, might yield new understandings of culturally evolved responses to illness, fear, pain, hunger, and brutality.

It is often remarked that contemporary academic approaches attempt to understand by dissection. We have this attitude to thank for much of our present-day rigor, and also for the specialization that renders accurate characterization of disorders like *move san* elusive. To diagnose such an affliction as somatic, psychological, or even psychosomatic is still somewhat different from and, it may be contended, something far less than examining it as it is experienced and interpreted. Perhaps what is necessary is a concerted and integrated effort, an anthropology that would seek underlying *forms* of suffering common to its many *aspects* (bodily, mental, economic, and so on). An anthropology of suffering would not stray far from the standard concerns of the ethnographer, for suffering strains cultural norms and brings them into sharp relief, as the Haitian material illustrates. Anthropologists are also in a position to discern epistemological and ontological differences (and similarities) between medicalized suffering and suffering that is understood in religious terms.

This is not to be mistaken for yet another call for holism. Rather, it is a reminder of the need to connect personal illness meanings with larger political and social systems. One way to approach such a project is simply to attend more closely to the way in which illness (and other misfortune) is worked into the narrative renderings of broader experience. In a 1986 study of urban, working-class France, we found that concepts such as "coping mechanisms" or "illness behaviors" were useful but inadequate to explore illness as experienced and discussed by our informants, who were mostly Iberian immigrants.[29] Pointed questions about specific episodes frequently elicited long and nonspecific narratives that seemed to address far larger, more existential questions of suffering. These narratives were typically couched in a sweeping "rhetoric of complaint," highly context-dependent and markedly performative. Illness episodes were commonly worked into this rhetoric in an attempt to make meaning out of a broader set of physical and social afflictions less easily classed as "psychological" or "physical" or "social" or "economic." That illness was often conceived in broad terms of misfortune meant that our subsequent analysis was reduced to a struggle, not entirely successful, for parsimony without reductionism.

Last come the moral dilemmas an anthropology of affliction must face. These are not new in our discipline, but they become particularly sharp when suffering forms both the subject and topic of research. Mme. Gracia made this painfully clear when I consulted her regarding the ingredients of the herbal remedy for *move san/lèt gate*. Her response, and the tone in which it was delivered, brought me up short: "Surely you are collecting these leaves in order to better understand their power and improve their efficacy?" Had she added, "If you think we'll be satisfied with a symbolic analysis of *move san/lèt gate,* you're quite mistaken," I would not have been more surprised.

NOTES

1. Scheper-Hughes and Lock, "The Mindful Body," p. 9.

2. Some of the most important research on Haitian "health beliefs" has been conducted, paradoxically, in the United States. Hazel Weidman (*Miami Health Ecology Project Report*) provides the most extended consideration of blood-related beliefs. She and her collaborators encountered *mau-*

vais sang (as interviews were conducted in Haitian Creole, the label may be considered a Galliciza-tion of *move san*) among their Haitian American informants; this and other disorders are considered as parts of a "blood paradigm" central to informants' perceptions of bodily functioning. Also on this topic, see "Haitian Blood Beliefs and Practices in Miami, Florida," by Clarissa Scott, a member of the research team led by Weidman. In research conducted in Haiti, the disorder is also mentioned en passant by Alfred Métraux in "Médecine et vodou en Haïti." It is discussed by Emmanuel Paul ("La première enfance") and considered at greater length in an excellent unpublished report by Maria Alvarez and Gerald Murray ("Socialization for Scarcity"). In his comments on a report by Jeanne Philippe and Jean Baptiste Romain ("Indisposition in Haiti"), Claude Charles, also a member of the Miami team, examines *indisposition* in relation to the blood paradigm prevalent among his infor-mants ("Brief Comments on the Occurrence, Etiology, and Treatment of Indisposition").

3. Interesting cross-cultural comparisons, beyond the scope of this paper, are to be made with the large literature treating disorders caused by emotional shocks, especially illnesses affecting breast milk. Unni Wikan ("Illness from Fright or Soul Loss") describes a group of illnesses called *kesambet* in northern Bali, which are very similar to the *move san/lèt gate* complex. Nancy Scheper-Hughes, working in urban Brazil, has recently described infant "death by neglect," one feature of which was perceived spoiling of breast milk. The discourse of her informants (the women of the community) recalls, I believe, that of many of the Haitian women who speak of *move san* in broad, "existential" terms (see Scheper-Hughes, "Culture, Scarcity, and Maternal Thinking"). There is also a large literature documenting the widespread belief that one's milk is insufficient, but milk insuf-ficiency is not necessarily the same as spoiled milk, nor do we have reason to believe that perceived insufficiency is often caused by malignant emotion. For a review, see Tully and Dewey, "Private Fears, Global Loss."

4. For an overview of the country, see Prince, *Haiti*.

5. Chen and Murray, "Truths and Untruths in Village Haiti."

6. All personal names are pseudonyms, as are "Do Kay" and "Ba Kay." Other geographical designations are as cited.

7. A follow-up survey was conducted at the time of the 1986 census, revealing even higher preva-lence (and thus increasing incidence) of *move san* as well as a new case of *move san/lèt gate*. It should be noted, however, that by then my interest in the disorder was well known; perhaps "questionable" cases were politely brought to my attention. Further longitudinal study is necessary to determine the chronicity of the complex and to elucidate patterns of recurrence or relapse.

8. There are, however, other causes of *lèt tounen*, or "turned milk," which often seemed to be synonymous with *lèt gate*. *Lèt tounen* was usually caused by the conception of another child, in which case the milk was described as "spoiled" or "turned." Many informants used the verb "to steal." One informant explained, "As soon as you become pregnant, any milk in your body must be for the baby in the womb. If the other [the nursing child] steals it, he can become sick."

9. Eleanor Rosch and others have questioned the validity of the prevailing "digital" model of categories, which assumes that "caseness" is determined by the absence or presence of discrete, criterial attributes. Instead, they propose an "analog" method that "represents natural categories as characterized by 'internal structure'; that is, composed of a 'core meaning' (the prototype, the clearest cases, the best examples) of the category, 'surrounded' by other members of increasing similarity and decreasing 'degree of membership'" (Rosch cited in Good and Good, "Towards a Meaning-Centered Analysis of Popular Illness Categories," p. 146). I present here two uncontested cases of *move san;* in some situations, *move san* is suspected to be the cause of certain symptoms, but there is not universal agreement.

10. Good and Good, "Towards a Meaning-Centered Analysis of Popular Illness Categories," p. 148.

11. Following Arthur Kleinman, explanatory models are "notions about an episode of sickness and its treatment that are employed by all those engaged in the clinical process" (*Patients and Healers in the Context of Culture*, p. 205). Formulated for each illness episode, EMs attempt to answer questions of etiology, type of symptoms and their onset, pathophysiology, the course of the sickness, and treatment. The methodology, when used in an open-ended way, has proven no less useful when the disorder is perceived as social or psychological in origin. Many of my rural Haitian informants were reluctant to be steered in any direction, however, and I am very tempted to refer to my transcripts as "ENs" (Elicited Narratives), rather than EMs.

12. For an evaluation of this concept, see Janzen, "Therapy Management."

13. Turner, *The Forest of Symbols*, p. 20.

14. Weidman, *Miami Health Ecology Project Report*.

15. Kleinman, "Neurasthenia and Depression"; Lock, "Protests of a Good Wife and Wise Mother." See also Kleinman, *Social Origins of Distress and Disease*.

16. Obeyesekere, "Depression, Buddhism, and the Work of Culture in Sri Lanka," p. 148.

17. Ibid.

18. Lundahl, *The Haitian Economy*. See also Neptune-Anglade, *L'autre moitié du développement*.

19. Alvarez and Murray, "Socialization for Scarcity," pp. 70–74.

20. Kiev, *Transcultural Psychiatry*, p. 66.

21. American Psychiatric Association, *Diagnostic and Statistical Manual of Mental Disorders*, s.v.

22. Spitzer and Williams, "Proposed Revisions in the DSM-III Classification of Anxiety Disorders Based on Research and Clinical Experience."

23. American Psychiatric Association, *Diagnostic and Statistical Manual of Mental Disorders*, p. 299.

24. Note, however, that Alvarez and Murray ("Socialization for Scarcity") discern the adaptive nature of "the spoiled milk syndrome" among their informants.

25. American Psychiatric Association, *Diagnostic and Statistical Manual of Mental Disorders*, p. 241.

26. Katon, Kleinman, and Rosen, "Depression and Somatization: A Review. Part I," and "Depression and Somatization: A Review. Part II."

27. Marsella, "Thoughts on Cross-Cultural Studies on the Epidemiology of Depression."

28. Marcus and Fischer, *Anthropology as Cultural Critique*, p. 86.

29. Gaines and Farmer, "Visible Saints."

2

Sending Sickness

Sorcery, Politics, and Changing Concepts
of AIDS in Rural Haiti

(1990)

AIDS presents new challenges to medical anthropology. Some are theoretical and not substantially different from the challenges faced by other ethnographers who seek to study, comprehend, and describe new phenomena. Others involve the ethical dilemmas inherent both in the study of a terrible new affliction for which (at the time of this writing) we have only limited therapeutic recourse and in the deeply vexed question of how anthropologists might best contribute to the effort to prevent transmission of HIV. What follows is a processual ethnography of the advent of AIDS in Do Kay, a small village in Haiti's Central Plateau. It is primarily descriptive, and the theoretical questions posed relate to the description of a new illness. Its chief goal is to call attention to the problems inherent in studying cultural meaning while meaning is taking shape.

The need for a more processual approach to the study of illness representations is most dramatically illustrated when one is witness to the advent of a new disorder or one previously unknown to one's host community. Some of the steps in this process of growing awareness are easily intuited. Before the arrival of the new malady, there exists no collective representation of the disorder; then comes a period of exposure, either to the illness or to rumor of it. With time and experience, disagreement and uncertainty about the nature of the disease may give way to a cultural model shared by the majority of a community.[1]

What determines whether or not consensus is reached? In studies of illness representations, medical anthropologists have usually asked, "To what degree is the model shared?" But when studying a truly novel disorder, a new set of questions pertains. How does cultural consensus emerge? How do illness representations, and the realities they organize and constitute, come into being? How are new representations related to existing structures? How does the suffering of particular human beings contribute to collective understandings, and how much of individual experience is not captured in cultural meaning?

My recent fieldwork in rural Haiti addresses these questions. Though primarily a study of a cultural model, the following account is also the story of three individuals with AIDS, for their experience is what made AIDS matter in Do Kay. This account is distilled from a series of interviews dating from 1983–84 to 1990, which reveal not just the role of culture in structuring illness narratives—we already know a great deal about that—but also the ways in which those narratives are elaborated, how they change over time, how representations (also changing) are embedded in narratives, and the significance of these narratives to the experience of illness.

THE CHANGING SIGNIFICANCE OF AIDS

The Republic of Haiti's role in the AIDS pandemic has been unique and unenviable. Like many other countries in the Caribbean, it has been gravely affected by HIV. Based on the number of AIDS cases per 100,000 in the population, Haiti is among the twenty most affected nations. Many more Haitians have been exposed to the virus. Although no large, random surveys have been conducted, a series of epidemiological studies conducted between 1985 and 1987 indicate that fully 9 percent of 2,152 "healthy urban adults" were seropositive for HIV.[2] Haitian radio has recently reported that AIDS is the leading cause of death among Haitian adults between the ages of twenty and forty-nine. While some contest this assessment, it is clear that HIV disease will mean great suffering in a nation that can ill afford yet another health burden.

For the inhabitants of Do Kay, the village in which most of the ethnographic material presented here was collected, the advent of a new and fatal disorder was, in the words of one person who lives there, "the last straw."[3] Early in 1987, the first case of AIDS was registered in Do Kay. Because we had already begun to investigate local understandings of AIDS four years earlier, it was possible to document the subsequent elaboration of a fairly detailed and widely shared cultural model of AIDS. By conducting serial interviews with the same people, it was possible to document the rate at which consensus was achieved and the events that led to it.[4]

An important national event also occurred during the course of this study. In 1986, Haiti's longstanding family dictatorship collapsed, which led to changes that were keenly felt in village Haiti. These changes also had a profound effect on the process of illness representation, for they altered substantially the ways in which illness and other kinds of misfortune were discussed. The following account attempts to illustrate the forces that were significant in defining a collective representation of AIDS and also to suggest how these forces were revealed to the ethnographer.

1983–84: "A CITY SICKNESS"

In 1983, when my research began, the word *"sida,"*[5] from the French acronym for *syndrome d'immunodéficience acquise,* was often heard in Port-au-Prince. The term had gained currency following speculation in the North American press about the association of this syndrome with Haiti. By early 1982, a number of Haitian immigrants had been seen in Florida and New York hospitals with infections characteristic of a new syndrome. Unlike other patients meeting diagnostic criteria for AIDS, the Haitians stated that they had not engaged in either homosexual activity or intravenous drug use; most had never had a blood transfusion. The U.S. Centers for Disease Control (CDC) inferred that Haitians as a group were in some way at risk for AIDS. The popular press drew upon readily available images of squalor, voodoo, and boatloads of "disease-ridden" or "economic" refugees and began to paint Haitians as the principal cause of the American epidemic.[6] As Dr. Robert Auguste of the Haitian Coalition on AIDS remarked in a *Miami Times* article in 1983, "In the annals of medicine, this categorization of a nationality as a 'risk group' is unique."

The effects on Haiti of this association with AIDS were quickly felt and far-reaching.[7] Throughout the 1970s, as international memories of "Papa Doc" Duvalier began to fade, tourism had assumed increasing importance in Haiti's economy. By 1980, it had become the country's second largest source of foreign currency, generating employment for thousands living in and around Port-au-Prince. The effects of the AIDS scare were dramatic and prompt: the Haitian Bureau of Tourism estimated a decline from seventy-five thousand visitors in the winter of 1981–82 to fewer than ten thousand the following year. Six hotels folded, and as many more declared themselves on the edge of bankruptcy. Several hotel owners were rumored to be planning a lawsuit against the CDC. Haitian government officials reacted in a manner reflecting the deep contradictions of the Haitian ruling class. Within months, one was hearing the classic mixture: antiracist nationalism, followed by local repression of those held responsible for "spreading AIDS." These measures did nothing to counter the collapse of the nation's tourist industry. As Elizabeth Abbott observed, "AIDS stamped Haiti's international image as political repression and intense poverty never had."[8]

As thousands of urban Haitians were left without jobs, the word *"sida"* took on specific connotations. Few city dwellers were unaware of the syndrome, though the majority of them could not have known individuals with AIDS. But the word *"sida"* was not yet well established in the rural Haitian lexicon. In interviews conducted in early 1984, only one of seventeen villagers mentioned *sida* as a possible cause of diarrhea. The term did not come up in unprompted discourse about tuberculosis, the most common infection among Haitians with AIDS, nor did it figure in talk about diarrhea or other disorders. When questioned, fifteen out of twenty villagers said that they had heard of *sida,* and a dozen of them associated certain symptoms or stigmata with this label, although many of these attributes were not, in fact, commonly seen in Haitians with AIDS.

Most of the villagers who spoke of *sida* noted that they had heard of the disorder on the radio or during trips to the capital.[9] There was considerable disagreement as to what the chief characteristics of *sida* might be. In the 1983–84 interviews, seven out of twenty mentioned at least one or two of these three aspects of *sida*: the novelty of the disorder, its relation to diarrhea, and its association with homosexuality. Only five remarked that *sida* was lethal. Three thought that it was originally a disease of pigs; three were also of the opinion that, despite claims to the contrary made by the foreign press, *sida* had been brought to Haiti by North Americans. Two others asserted that "*sida* is the same thing as tuberculosis."

In early 1984, Mme. Sylvain, a thirty-six-year-old market woman, offered the following commentary, which was similar to that of several of her neighbors:

> *Sida* is a sickness they have in Port-au-Prince and in the United States. It gives you a diarrhea that starts very slowly but never stops until you're completely dry. There's no water left in your body.... *Sida* is a sickness that you see in men who sleep with other men.

She had little else to say about the syndrome, although Mme. Sylvain was seldom at a loss for words when sickness was the topic.[10]

These preliminary interviews demonstrated that in Do Kay, where illnesses were usually the topic of much discussion, *sida* was not. When one villager was asked if he and his associates were reluctant to speak about *sida,* he responded, "Why should that be? There is no one who says we can't talk about *sida.* But it is nothing that we have seen here. It's a city sickness (*maladi lavil*)." In the first year of my research, all talk about the disorder was prompted by questioning; no one offered illness stories or "therapeutic narratives" about *sida.* For the people of Do Kay, already bent under the unremitting burdens of poverty and sickness, there was little at stake regarding AIDS.

Before 1985, then, one would have been hard-pressed to delineate a collective representation of AIDS in this part of rural Haiti. Despite several individuals' elaborate explanatory models, despite the savvy of market women like Mme. Sylvain, the lack of natural discourse about *sida* and the lack of agreement among informants about its core characteristics suggest that no cultural model of AIDS existed in the area around Do Kay during the 1983–84 period.

1985–86: *MÉLANGE ADULTÈRE DE TOUT*

During the course of 1985–86, relative silence concerning *sida* gave way to discussion of the new illness in the area surrounding Kay, and a more widely held representation slowly began to emerge. Villagers began to recount illness stories, but they were invariably the tales of someone else, somewhere else—people who had died in Mirebalais, the nearest large market town, or in Port-au-Prince. There was rumor, too, of mistreatment of Haitians in far-off North America; one villager often spoke of a cousin in New York who had lost her job "because they said she was a Haitian and an AIDS carrier."

Fully eighteen of twenty informants interviewed during this period referred directly to "blood" in our discussions of *sida,* and for many other residents of Do Kay as well, *sida* was a sickness of the blood. Perhaps the most commonly heard observation was that *sida* "dirties your blood" (*li sal san ou*). Villagers frequently alluded to "poor blood," usually a gloss for anemia, as a prodrome of *sida,* and some referred to the dangers of blood transfusion. For example, when Ti Malou Joseph needed a unit of blood during an obstetrical intervention, several villagers observed that, given the "sickness going around" (*maladi deyo a*), a transfusion was tempting fate.[11] For some, it was a question of exposing the transfusion recipient to a microbe (*mikwob*); for others, one of "mixing bloods that don't go together," causing reactions that eventually "degenerate into *sida.*" Several informants began to speak of *sida* as a slow but irreversible process that was invariably fatal.

Others interviewed in the summer of 1985 stated that "bad blood" (*move san*), a somatosocial disorder widespread among Haitian women, put one at risk for *sida.* As Mme. Mathieu put it, "You're very weak when you have *move san,* and you can more easily catch *sida.*" Although two of the twenty villagers interviewed in 1985 felt that the new illness was a "very severe form of *move san,*" the rest of those who mentioned *move san* underlined distinctions between it and *sida.* The observations of Mme. Kado, a fifty-one-year-old woman who worked with the priest who had founded the school in Do Kay, were typical of the opinions garnered in late 1985:

> [*Sida*] spoils your blood, makes you have so little blood that you become pale and dry. It first causes little blemishes (*bouton*) that rise all over your arms and legs. That tells you that the blood is bad and makes you think of a simple case of *move san.* But *sida* has no treatment; it's not like *move san.* Anyone can get this, but it is most common in the city.

In much of Haiti, disvalued experiences—shocks, disappointments, anger, fright—may be embodied as disorders of the blood. The significance of this conceptual framework led Hazel Weidman and her coworkers to speak of the "blood paradigm" underlying the health-related beliefs of their Haitian informants in Miami.[12] Within this paradigm are found the causal links between the social field and alterations in the quality, consistency, and nature of blood. During much of the 1985–86 period, preexisting beliefs about blood lent form to vague

understandings of *sida*, which was coming to represent an irreversible pollution caused, depending on whom you asked, by blood transfusions, same-sex
relations, weakness from overwork in the city, or travel to the United States. As
will be clear, however, the contributions of this paradigm to the emerging representation waned with direct experience of the disorder, and the "tuberculosis
paradigm" emerged as the more important of preexisting models.

The year 1985 also marked the debut of a preventive campaign conducted by
the nation's health authorities. There were songs about *sida* and numerous radio
programs, all in Creole and targeted toward the peasantry. Less important were
the many articles in the print media and the posters and billboards declaring
sida to be a public menace to which all were vulnerable. Although villagers may
have known more about the syndrome as a result of these public health efforts, it
was not yet a compelling subject of everyday discourse, which was increasingly, if
somewhat clandestinely, dedicated to discussion of national-level political events.
The Duvalier dictatorship, in place for almost thirty years, was beginning to
totter, and more and more rural Haitians joined the chorus calling for Duvalier's
removal.

After years of silence, the people of Do Kay joined in this chorus. Because
peasants had long been excluded from direct participation in politics, the shift
was a significant one and had an impact on the way that illness was discussed in
rural Haiti. At first, talk of *sida* was simply submerged in all-important discussions of national politics. When the syndrome was addressed, it seemed that it
was often invoked to malign the regime or the United States. On New Year's Day
in 1986, several of my friends from Mirebalais joked that Duvalier was a *masisi*
(homosexual) who had contracted the syndrome from one of his *masisi* min-
isters. Shortly after Duvalier's departure, one market woman in her mid-fifties
angrily denounced AIDS as part of "the American plan to enslave Haiti. . . . The
United States has a traffic in Haitian blood. Duvalier used to sell them our blood
for transfusions and experiments. One of these experiments was to make a new
sickness."[13]

Later it became clear that the fall of the Duvalier dictatorship had given a boost
to stories about *sida*. To judge from trends observed in Do Kay and surrounding
villages, rural Haitians began to feel that they could speak more candidly about
misfortunes in general, and this alteration in the "rhetoric of complaint" may
have had a determinant effect on what would prove to be enduring understandings of *sida*.[14]

One of the first slogans to become popular shortly after Duvalier's fall was
babouket la tonbe. A literal English equivalent would be "the bridle has fallen off,"
but the phrase would be better rendered as "the muzzle is off." Although few in
Do Kay began openly talking about politics until March, and a full year elapsed
before the adventurous were wholeheartedly joined by a majority of the villagers,

the transformation seemed complete by the spring of 1987. In the villages of the area, transistor radios suddenly began to proliferate, or at least to surface. Some persons, men especially, spent entire days cradling their radios, switching from one news program to another. Community councils, drastically overhauled in other villages, were strengthened in the area around Do Kay; meetings that once drew a score or so now frequently drew well over a hundred people. New groups were formed and set to civic activities such as repairing roads and planting trees. All this was worked into the daily round of gardening and marketing, but the changes stood out nonetheless.

The subject of *sida*, however, was only temporarily submerged. In Port-au-Prince, many knew people who had died or were ill with the syndrome. Hospitals and sanatoriums were faced with large numbers of *moun sida*, as persons with AIDS were labeled. Haitian researchers continued to document a large and growing epidemic. Government health officials conceded that *sida* was not a public relations issue but rather a major public health problem.

In Do Kay, *sida* was once again a regular topic of conversation. In the summer of 1986, questions I posed about the sickness triggered long and elaborate responses. Yet respondents expressed many discrepant ideas.

In natural discourse about *sida*, the number of references to blood declined. In interviews conducted late in 1986, only eleven of nineteen informants used the term when speaking at length about the new sickness. Public health campaigns may have contributed to this shift. The more one heard about it on the radio, the less it seemed to resemble other well-known disorders of the blood. The declining significance of the blood paradigm is suggested by a comment from a 1986 interview with Tonton Sanon, a *dokte fey* (herbalist): "I'm wondering if it is really a sickness of the blood, because we know how to put blood in its place. There's a part of it that is in the blood, yes, but it is not only in the blood, and it's not blood that is the principal problem. The problem is in other systems."

He was seconded by others who spoke as if the blood paradigm had been used to assess the nature of *sida* and found wanting. Interviews with other healers revealed a similar lack of accord about the new illness, although many allowed that *sida* was beyond their competence. "Truly it's a sickness that is slippery (*enpwenab*)," observed Mme. Victor, a midwife known for her efficacious herbal remedies. "To this day, they're struggling with it, but they haven't yet found an herbal treatment for it." A *dokte fey* predicted that "the herbal remedy that will heal *sida* has not yet reached us, but when it does, we'll learn how to use it."[15]

In summary, it seemed that during 1985 and 1986, when mention of *sida* began to stimulate more interest, villagers attempted to compare the disorder to other illnesses, especially those involving the blood. But *sida* failed to fit neatly into the existing blood paradigm. Lack of a perfect fit between the new disorder and the old framework posed no real problems, however, as clear and defensible understandings of *sida* were not yet a necessity: no one from Do Kay had fallen ill with the syndrome.

1987: PROTOTYPES AND PROTOMODELS

In many ways, 1987 was the decisive year in the process leading to a shared understanding of AIDS. During the course of that year, a protomodel of illness causation rose to prominence, a model that proved influential in the elaboration of a more stable collective representation of *sida*. By the fall of that year, narratives about *sida* were easily triggered, and it was clear that a consensus, albeit tenuous, had emerged.

Interviews conducted in 1987 and afterward revealed that the semantic network in which *sida* was embedded had changed substantially since 1983–84. In 1987, the syndrome was mentioned by over half of those asked to cite possible causes of diarrhea in an adult. The majority also associated *sida* with tuberculosis. Furthermore, ideas about how the new disorder became manifest in the afflicted were more widely shared. Equally striking was the increasing frequency with which the social and political origins of illness, including *sida,* were mentioned. There are perhaps two primary reasons for this: first, the unmuzzling of the rural poor had led to a new rhetoric of complaint; and second, and most important, the syndrome had come to matter locally. Someone in Do Kay had fallen ill with *sida.*

Comparing early interviews to these later ones reveals the increasing importance of the shift in styles of complaining, which was triggered by the large-scale political changes that were occurring. Although interviewing style and methods were not altered, the narratives, whether relating a case of diarrhea or some other misfortune, became increasingly tinged with a new political sensibility. Yet "politicization of discourse" is an altogether unsatisfactory description of a far more complicated process. The stories told were superficially similar to those heard earlier, but how tellers gave shape and sense to their stories had changed. For example, in speaking of misfortune, informants' attributions of blame seemed to be changing subtly. Narrative shifts similar to those in the following interview with Mme. Jolibois abound.

Mme. Jolibois, a young woman who supports her family by working a small patch of land, had traveled from the Kay area to a clinic in a nearby town in February 1984 because her infant son had a bad case of diarrhea. When she was asked in an interview that year what had caused the diarrhea, she answered, "I don't know what causes it. Microbes, perhaps, or gas from milk. Microbes, especially—they're little bugs that can make children sick. Or it could be my milk. I think he must be getting too old for milk."

In May 1987, over three years after the first interview, she again went to the clinic, a new one in Do Kay. This time, a nine-month-old daughter had severe diarrhea. When asked the same question, "What caused the diarrhea?" she responded, "It's the bad water we have in [my village]. We have to drink it even when it's muddy and full of microbes. It gives the babies diarrhea, and they die, and the government does nothing about it. It's always promises without action (*promet san bay*)."

The methodologically minded reader might ask a series of important questions. Were the differences related to the severity of the episode? The sex of the child? Are contextual or performative factors important? Did the ethnographer have a closer rapport with the informant years later? Perhaps Mme. Jolibois was simply in a bad or accusatory mood? Such questions were slowly revealed to be secondary, however, as I began to note similar trends in the discourse of other villagers.

The collapse of the Duvalier regime also had a palpable effect on the way in which AIDS-related accusations were marshaled and used. Conspiracy theories abounded: the Duvalier regime had caused *sida,* asserted some. Others thought that, no, the Duvaliers were too stupid to create a sickness, despite a talent for creating zombies, but that they had allowed the people of their nation to be used as guinea pigs in an American plan to stem migration. Referring to the North American speculation that AIDS originated in Haiti, more than one villager was heard to remark, "Of course they say it's from Haiti: whites say all bad diseases are from Haiti."[16] Indeed, accusations against the accusers were perhaps the most prevalent of these commentaries.

The illness of Manno Surpris was the second reason that the same villagers who were aware of but generally uninterested in *sida* in 1984 were universally interested in the syndrome less than three years later. In 1987, *sida* came to be a social drama that left few adults in Do Kay untouched.[17] The impact of this change is suggested by the observations of a young schoolteacher, himself a native of the village in which we worked. He was interviewed several times between 1983 and 1990. In a 1984 interview, he told us, "Yes, of course I've heard of [*sida*]. It's caused by living in the city. It gives you diarrhea and can kill you. . . . We've never had any *sida* here. It's a city sickness." A long exchange recorded late in 1987 clearly revealed that the man's understanding of *sida* had changed substantially. He could now hold forth at great length about the disorder, especially since he could now refer to the death of Manno Surpris, his fellow schoolteacher: "It was *sida* that killed him; that's what I'm trying to tell you. But they say it was a death sent to him. They sent a *sida* death to him . . . *sida* is caused by a tiny microbe. But not just anybody will catch the microbe that can cause *sida*." Manno's illness and death made a lasting contribution to the cultural model of *sida* that took shape in these years, and this contribution was not substantially lessened by the subsequent deaths from AIDS of two other villagers.

Born in a small village in another part of the Central Plateau, Manno was the son of peasant farmers. After passing his primary school exams, he moved to Mirebalais, a large market town not far from his home village, and there he began his secondary school education. Several months thereafter, he left to complete his secondary education in the capital. As is often the case for rural children with such expectations, Manno did odd jobs in order to pay tuition at one of what many urban Haitians label "lottery schools" (so called because, as far as learning is concerned, "you take your chances"). In five years, Manno completed only two more grades. Concluding that he would never finish his high school degree, he moved back to Mirebalais and began searching for a job.

Manno moved to Do Kay in 1982, when he became a teacher at a large new school established there by a Haitian priest. He was then twenty-five years old, and his eighth-grade education was no impediment. An enthusiastic and hard-working man, Manno came to be held in high esteem by the school administrators. He was entrusted with a number of public tasks, including taking care of the village's new water pump and the community pig project, both of which were administered by the priest who ran the school. Père Jacques later recalled: "I felt that he was good-natured and dependable. But most of all, he didn't seem to be in much of a hurry to get back to Mirebalais on Friday afternoon. He really seemed to like working in the village." Alourdes Monestime, also a teacher, was one reason that Manno enjoyed staying in Do Kay. In 1984, their daughter was born; a year later, they began building their own house not far from the school. A second child was on the way.

I knew that Manno was not universally popular. He was a salaried teacher, and some of his other duties were remunerated, so he was sometimes confronted with the envy of the less fortunate. This jealousy was compounded because the villagers considered him *moun vini*, a "newcomer" or "outsider." It was obvious that at least one person resented Manno's status: shortly after Baby Doc Duvalier's departure in February 1986, Manno's half-finished house was knocked down. Although these kinds of events were common throughout Haiti, this was the only such incident in the Kay area.

The significance of the sentiment against Manno was not clear to me until August, when he beat an adolescent schoolboy for some transgression in the pigsty. I was surprised by the intensity of the community's reaction to the beating. The "facts" were quickly circulated by word of mouth. The schoolboy had inadvertently let several pigs escape. Upon discovering this, Manno attacked him with a length of rubber hose. The elderly man who had unofficially adopted the orphaned boy was not in the village, and a couple of local men were heard muttering about settling the score with Manno themselves. Someone sent word to the boy's grandmother, who lived a couple of hours' walk from Do Kay. A few schoolboys began carrying their own lengths of hose "for self-defense." The crisis was defused by Mme. Alexis, Père Jacques's wife, who called for a meeting of the adults concerned (Manno, the boy's grandmother, and the foster father at Do Kay). During this meeting, Manno apologized to the boy. With the apology, I thought that the whole affair was closed.

After a day or two, I heard no more grumbling against Manno. Perhaps the grumbling ended because he had fallen ill. Beginning in early 1986, he had been bothered by intermittent diarrhea. Superficial skin infections recrudesced throughout the summer; the patches would clear up with treatment, only to appear again, usually on the scalp, neck, or face. By December, his decline was drastic, and he began to cough. In January 1987, Manno's physician in Port-au-Prince referred him to the public clinic for the test necessary to diagnose HIV infection.

In the first week of February, while awaiting the results of an HIV antibody test, Manno revealed his fears about the disorder. "Most of all, I hope it's not tuberculosis. But I'm afraid that's what it is. I'm coughing. I've lost weight. . . . I'm afraid I have tuberculosis, and I'll never get better, never be able to work again. . . . People don't want to be near you if you have tuberculosis."

Manno did indeed have tuberculosis and initially responded well to the appropriate treatment; by March he no longer looked ill at all. However, the test had revealed that he also had antibodies to HIV, which suggested immune deficiency caused by the virus as the root of his health problems. On his next visit to the doctor, Alourdes went with him. She tested seronegative, and the doctor advised her to avoid unprotected sexual contact with Manno.

Although other villagers were not privy to the results of Manno's test, they had other reasons for believing that his tuberculosis was "not simple," as was often remarked. A rumor circulated around Do Kay, which was not dampened by Manno's clinical improvement: he was the victim, it was whispered, of sorcery. Some angry or jealous rival had consulted a voodoo priest in order to have a *mo*, or dead person, "sent" against Manno.[18] One of Manno's former students told me of gossip to this effect: "I don't believe it myself, but that's what some people say," the young man commented. "Some people can do it by themselves; others go to a *bokor* [a voodoo practitioner adept in the skills necessary to heal and to harm]." Having been exposed to dramatic descriptions in the ethnographic literature of "voodoo death" in Haiti and elsewhere, I was concerned about the possible effects of the rumor on Manno's health.

In conversations during his first period of convalescence after the diagnosis, Manno shared with me the history of his sexual activity. For a thirty-year-old man carrying antibodies to HIV, his sexual history was strikingly sparse, especially when compared to those elicited from North Americans with AIDS or their HIV-seronegative, age-matched controls. Manno reported sexual contact with only four persons, all of them women. None of them was involved in prostitution. Two of these women he met in Port-au-Prince, the third in Mirebalais, and the fourth was Alourdes, whom he had met in Do Kay in 1982. Since the beginning of his involvement with Alourdes, about four years before, he said, he had slept with no one else. He denied ever having had sexual contact with a man or boy; he denied use of any narcotics (indeed, he had heard of neither heroin nor marijuana, although he was familiar with the Haitian word for "illicit drug"). He had received, however, "at least a dozen" intramuscular injections, usually of penicillin or injectable vitamins. Although many of these had been administered in the preceding months, several injections had been given years before. He had never received a transfusion; the intravenous fluids he had received in the past month had been administered with sterile needles.

Although disheartened by the lab results and fully aware of the usual course of the disease, Père Jacques spared no expense in treating Manno. Prescriptions were filled promptly, well-balanced meals were prepared and delivered, staff members of the clinic at Do Kay were encouraged to visit Manno regularly. His mother came from their home village; Alourdes's sister came from a village near Do Kay. No one seemed afraid to touch him, although family members had been warned that Manno's illness was "caused by a microbe." By late February, Manno was going for walks and had put on twenty pounds. He had stopped coughing completely and looked well. Père Jacques wondered whether Manno might return to teaching by the fall semester. Mme. Alexis was sure that he had been misdiagnosed, despite warnings from the staff doctor that his apparent recovery was in keeping with the course of the disease.

Manno did so well, in fact, that his neighbors and coworkers soon began to wonder why he had not returned to Do Kay. If no one seemed particularly leery of Manno, the same could not be said of Manno himself. He was frightened of something, or someone. His wife, when she returned to her teaching post, chose to stay at her mother's house, almost an hour's dusty walk from the school. When I asked Père Jacques why Manno was reluctant to return to Do Kay, he responded candidly:

> I have heard that Manno believes that he is the victim of someone's ill will. I hope you can at least see why this sort of accusation is dangerous. It doesn't hurt anyone if you blame a microbe, but blaming someone else for your misfortunes leads to division and hatred. That's why I'm so unhappy that Manno believes he's been the victim of evil.

Père Jacques's unhappiness may have resulted in a confrontation between him and Manno. In any case, when Manno left Mirebalais, his departure was surreptitious. "He should at least have come by before leaving Mirebalais," Père Jacques complained, "but I haven't seen him at all."

Manno was indeed difficult to track down. In March, I traveled to Alourdes's mother's house at least three times. Her son-in-law was never there: he was "in his own region, at his mother's," or he was "in Mirebalais for a couple of days." These responses seemed fine to me, and I would have kept on believing them if one of my coworkers had not lived next door to Alourdes's mother. Community health worker Christian Guerrier was also related to Alourdes: his father and her father were brothers. The day after my third futile visit, Christian explained to me what I had failed to understand:

> There's something you need to understand about Haitians, at least some of them. They believe that there are different kinds of medications for different kinds of illnesses. Some illnesses require several different kinds of medication. . . . Manno is not at his mother's house. He is in Vieux-Fonds [a small village about two hours' walk from Do Kay] being treated by a *houngan* [voodoo priest]. He believes that, because someone sent him the illness, it must be taken away.

Christian observed that Manno's treatment might take a long time—"many days or weeks." I would not see him until the *houngan* had finished treating him. Finally, Christian intimated that I might wish to confront Alourdes about her husband's whereabouts, taking care not to let her know who had revealed the reason for his absences.

In a subsequent interview, Alourdes did not seem reluctant to impart more detailed information about Manno's treatment. Alourdes had been among those interviewed about AIDS in 1984. At the time, she had opined that *sida* was "a form of diarrhea seen in homosexuals." In 1987, again, she had no difficulty accepting a physiological origin for *sida*. But she also attributed her husband's illness to sorcery:

> Manno believes that they did this to him because they were jealous that he had three jobs—teaching, the pigsty, and the water pump. . . . The people who did this to him already know what they've done; they know what kind of illness they've sent. He won't survive. There are people who know how to send a TB death (*voye yon mo tebe*) on someone; that person gets TB.

At first Alourdes was reluctant to name a perpetrator, but at last she told me:

> Yes, you know the people who did this. One comes from my husband's hometown; another comes from here; the third is even related to me, although he pretends that he is not. Two of them work inside the school complex. The one who comes from my husband's region is at the head of it . . . he's the master of the affair, he arranged it.

I knew that one of the schoolteachers, Fritz, was from the same town as Manno, so I asked if he was one of those who had bewitched her husband. Alourdes nodded and then quickly added that another teacher was the second member of the group. She adamantly refused to name the third. I discovered only later that the triad was completed by her cousin, Christian's sister—and Fritz's fiancée.

Knowledge of the family's suspicion of sorcery seemed to be widespread. Mme. Alexis brought up the subject on several occasions and continued to express her exasperation over "their persistent superstition": "I know people believe that someone can send a tuberculous death, but how can they think such a thing when they know the diagnosis? I was sure that when the family received the [HIV antibody] tests they would abandon the notion that a person was responsible."

A full month elapsed before I saw Manno again. In early May, I stopped by his wife's mother's house. The family owned two small houses, built side by side with a granary between them. One of them had been emptied for Manno and his family. When I reached the yard, I saw Manno lying inside the house in bed, but he jumped to his feet when I greeted him. "Manno, I never seem to see you." His handshake was firm; he had put on at least another fifteen pounds. "Oh, you know, I just don't seem to get down to Do Kay," he responded.

If Manno's medical condition had temporarily improved, his social dilemma had not. He and his family blamed close friends and relations for what they feared to be an inevitably fatal illness. He had abandoned his house and become estranged from Père Jacques, his and his wife's employer. In late June, when Manno began to develop diarrhea and fever, I learned from Christian that the sick man and his family were increasingly obsessed not with the course of the disease but with its ultimate origin. But he was not yet willing to speak more candidly with me about his suspicions, and the course of the disease remained the chief focus of our discussions.

The subject was finally broached on a day during which Manno had an appointment with his physician in Port-au-Prince. I found Manno waiting for a jitney, and I offered to drive him to Mirebalais, where he could more easily catch a ride to Port-au-Prince. While on the road, I asked, "Tell me more about your illness—the sort of things we haven't been able to talk about for lack of privacy."

His response was direct: "I know that I am very sick, even though I don't look it. They tell me there's no cure. But I'm not sure of that. If you can find a cause, you can find a cure."

When I asked, "What is the cause of your illness?" he unhesitatingly replied, "A microbe." Silence followed this response.

I asked, "Why aren't you staying in your house?"

"Well, my mother-in-law suggested that we move in with her until I was feeling better."

"But you've been feeling better for months now."

"Yes," he said after a pause. "That's true."

We had been through this already more than once, and I decided to press him.

"It has been suggested," I remarked, "that you moved out of your house because you thought someone from Do Kay was trying to harm you."

Manno weighed my question. I began to wonder if he might be short of breath, but he answered in a steady voice: "Perhaps that's what they say, but that doesn't mean it's true. . . . Well, I don't know if someone is trying to harm me, but I don't know that someone isn't. Maybe, maybe not." Manno was clearly not in a mood to divulge more, but we agreed to continue the "frank discussion" the following week.

The summer of 1987 was a difficult period for keeping appointments. On several occasions, political unrest paralyzed the major cities. Our meeting was canceled by a strike that shut down most roads. Manno missed at least two more appointments at the AIDS clinic, one because gunfire in the streets scared away the staff and patients. By late July, he had begun complaining again of diarrhea. And his neighbor, Christian, informed me that Manno was coughing again. Political problems prevented Manno from refilling his supply of one of the antituberculous drugs. By early August, he was vomiting and complained of "terrible headaches."

By the third week in August, Manno was once more gravely ill. A group of young men from Do Kay, most of them my coworkers, asked me to drive them to Manno's house "for a prayer meeting." "We have heard," one of them said, "that he and his wife are in spiritual danger." We reached the house by 9 P.M. and found the family in bed. The children were asleep on their little mat on the floor, and their mother appeared to be sleeping there with them. Manno was in his bed, and he seemed somewhat embarrassed by our visit. When I asked him about his headaches, he described them as "no better, no worse." One visitor initiated a couple of songs; a few Bible verses were recited. Another person prayed, asking the Almighty to send down his "spiritual medication."

By the end of the month, Manno's breathing had become labored. The painkillers no longer helped, and he had not been sleeping. He vomited after most meals and had lost a great deal of weight. In mid-September, Christian informed me that Manno was worse than ever.

We reached the house late in the afternoon. His mother was there, which I took to be a bad sign. Also present were his brother and a cousin, neither of whom I had met before. When I arrived in the yard, I could hear Manno's short, labored breathing. Christian and the others remained outside during the half-hour I was in the house. Manno had great difficulty speaking but seemed to be lucid. His eyes rolled a bit when he spoke, and he was as thin as he had been in January. I realized that Manno was dying, and my subsequent request seemed hollow. "Allow us to take Manno to the hospital," I said to his wife's father. "No, no—I'm in the middle of treating him with herbs," he answered evenly but forcefully. "I'll give him to you, but only after twenty-one or so days."

Manno died the next morning. I heard the news just before midday and went immediately to the house. A dozen or so friends and family were sitting quietly under the granary. Alourdes's mother was wailing in the doorway of her house. I found Alourdes inside her mother's front room, sitting on the bed. She looked more tired than grief-stricken. Her little boy was nursing. Manno had not slept the last night, said Alourdes, nor had she. He had asked for some cola and milk early in the morning but vomited it almost immediately. At about 10:30 or so, Manno had complained that he was almost out of breath. This must be due, he felt, to his short rations. So he asked his wife to prepare him a plantain. He was groaning. "A few minutes later, when I noticed he wasn't groaning, I went back in. He had died while I was cooking the plantain."

I sat in the room for a while, on the floor. Someone brought us chairs, and we continued to sit in silence. Finally I decided to leave in order to bring news of the death to Père Jacques, who was visiting a mission station on the far side of the reservoir. When I returned, Alourdes had commissioned a coffin to be made, and her father had gone off to make arrangements for the grave and the funeral, to be held the following day.

That evening, I went to the wake. There was a good deal of crying and little attempt at the sort of humor I had seen at the wakes of older rural Haitians. Alourdes wrote a note to Père Jacques concerning the funeral, but the priest had departed for Mirebalais. It was left to Gerard, the lay leader of the Do Kay mission and the principal of the school that had employed Manno, to conduct the sacraments. By the time Gerard and I returned the next morning, Manno had already been buried. There were no more than a dozen people milling about the yard. Gerard announced that he would offer his "ministrations at the time of death," which meant, I soon discovered, that he would read from the Creole version of the *Book of Common Prayer* and hold forth on any lessons to be learned from the brief life of Manno Surpris. When Gerard stepped into the room in which Manno had died, he was followed only by Alourdes, carrying her son, and Manno's mother.

I was very uncomfortable when Gerard called me into the house, where he was lecturing to his polite but distracted audience. Like Père Jacques, Gerard sought to enlist both moral and medical authority against the theory of baleful enchantment:

> Man cannot hurt man. Manno never hurt anyone; on the contrary, one thing he was known for was his ready smile. So why would anyone wish to harm him? It is a very bad thing to accuse someone else of trying to harm him, a very heavy load. No, we all know what illness he had. He had *sida*.

He turned to me and added, "Didn't he?" It was the first time I had heard Manno's family publicly confronted with the word *sida*, though everyone in the family knew of the diagnosis. Naming the illness did not disturb me, but I was afraid that Alourdes would think I had betrayed her confidence by discussing the subject with Gerard. At about this time, Alourdes's father entered the room. Gerard might as well have spoken to a mahogany tree, for the man began whispering unabashedly about the latest signs of Fritz's malevolence. It was never clear if Gerard understood that the family might agree that Manno had died of *sida* but simultaneously hold that someone—and Fritz's name kept surfacing—had "sent the illness on him." In any case, Gerard was not to be allowed to have the last word.

The Haitians I interviewed are not ignorant of the modes of transmission of infectious disease. On the contrary, their ideas of etiology and epidemiology reflect the incursion of the "North American ideology" of AIDS—that the disease is caused by a virus and is somehow related to homosexuality. These ideas were later subsumed, however, in uniquely Haitian beliefs about illness causation. Sorcery accusations did not surprise Père Jacques and Mme. Alexis, although the latter expressed dismay that such a "false idea" could be held concurrently with knowledge of "the real cause." Although Père Jacques cast his analysis in terms of the familiar dichotomy of voodoo versus Christianity, my coworkers from Do Kay or surrounding villages spoke in less clear-cut terms. A series of oppositions, rather than one, came to guide many of our conversations: an illness might be caused by a "microbe" or by sorcery or by both. An intended victim might be "powerful" or "susceptible." For example, some spoke of the night, years ago, when Manno had been knocked out of bed by a bolt of lightning. The shock, they said, had left him susceptible to a disease caused by a microbe and "sent by someone." An illness as serious as *sida* might be treated by doctors, or voodoo priests, or herbalists, or prayer, or any combination of these. The extent to which Manno believed in each of these treatment modalities remains unclear. I believe he was glad to receive all of them.

The first case of *sida* to affect our village summoned up, as happened elsewhere, the powers of explanation and prediction latent in shared models of disease. It seems that wherever AIDS strikes, accusation is never far behind.[19] In the United States, blame and counter-blame played large roles in public discourse on AIDS risk groups. In at least one Haitian village, however, the calculus of blame was strikingly different from that seen in North America. Blame was directed not at the sick person, but at the person or persons seen as having caused, through envy or resentment, the victim to fall ill of a fatal disease.

Noticeably absent was the revulsion confronting AIDS patients in North America, in both clinical settings and home communities. In the United States, we read of employers summarily firing workers with AIDS; in rural Haiti, we encounter an employer angry because his employee with AIDS is avoiding him. In North America, AIDS becomes a reason for marking and excluding members of groups associated with the virus (Haitians, intravenous drug users, male homosexuals); in Do Kay, the sick man's self-exile from social networks reflects his fear of further persecution, and his outsider status is seen as having triggered the "sent sickness," not as resulting from it. North Americans with AIDS have left eloquent testimony to the meaning of the syndrome there: "You get fired, you get evicted from your apartment. You're a leper. You die alone."[20] This summary is far from describing Manno's experience, nor would it describe that of a young woman from Do Kay who died of AIDS several months after him.

Anita Joseph was the second villager to fall ill with *sida*. Anita once referred to herself as "a genuine resident of Kay," but her name did not surface in the census of 1984. The following year, however, a study of villagers' ties to Port-au-Prince and the United States revealed that Luc Joseph had a daughter in "the city." She was, he reported, "married to a man who works in the airport."

Less than two years later, Anita, gravely ill, was brought back to Do Kay by her father. Her husband had died some months previously, of a slow, wasting illness. Shortly after Anita's return to Do Kay, I heard that she might have *sida*. The rumor was not surprising, as there was at that time a great deal of talk about Manno's illness. Anita, people remarked, looked the way Manno had earlier that year. She had been in the city, and was *sida* not a city sickness?

More than one villager opined that Anita did not have *sida,* as she was "too innocent." The logic behind this statement was radically different, however, from that underpinning similar statements made in North America. "Innocence" had nothing to do with such things as sexual practices (though some villagers believed that Anita had led a "free life"); rather, it underlined the assertion that a string of bad luck typically signifies that one is the victim of *maji*, sorcery. Sorcery is never random; it is sent by enemies. Most people make enemies by inspiring jealousy (often through inordinate accumulation) or by their own malevolent magic. Dogged by bad luck, Anita had never inspired the envy of anyone, and she was widely regarded as unwise in the ways of *maji*. Two persons who had earlier explained the role of sorcery in Manno's illness queried rhetorically, "Who would send a *sida* death on this poor unfortunate child?" Since many believed that the sole case of *sida* known in the Kay area had been caused by sorcery, and since Anita was an unlikely victim of this form of malice, it stood to reason, some thought, that Anita could not possibly have *sida*.

Perhaps equally important to this interpretation was the course of Anita's illness. She did not have skin infections or other dermatologic manifestations, as had Manno. Furthermore, as Manno began his final descent, Anita was recovering her strength under a treatment regimen for tuberculosis. When Manno died, Anita was hard at work in Mirebalais. That Manno had initially shown a striking response to antituberculous medications (or some other concurrent intervention) seemed irrelevant to the widely shared assessment of Anita's malady. To judge from the total absence of reference to Anita in interviews about *sida* conducted in the autumn of 1987, it was widely assumed that she was not in fact ill with the new disorder.

Six months after the initiation of the antituberculous regimen, however, Anita declined precipitously. Her employer in Mirebalais sent her back to Do Kay. Anita had bitter words for the woman, stating that "they just use you up, and when they're finished with you, they throw you in the garbage." She also felt that she had made an error in returning to "the same kind of work that got me sick in the first place." By early December, she could no longer walk to the Do Kay clinic; she weighed less than ninety pounds and suffered from intermittent diarrhea. Convinced that she was indeed taking her medications, her physicians were concerned about AIDS, especially when she recounted the story of her husband and his illness.[21]

Her deterioration clearly shook her father's faith in the clinic, as well as her own, and they began spending significant sums on herbal treatments. As her father later reported, "I had already sold a small piece of land in order to buy treatments. I was spending left and right, with no results." Since the treatment for tuberculosis was entirely free of charge, it was clear that Luc had spent his resources in the folk sector. He later informed me that he had consulted a voodoo priest but soon abandoned that tack, as he came to agree that his daughter was an unlikely victim of sorcery.

By the close of 1987, Anita was widely believed to be ill with *sida,* and this time the label stuck. The disorder was again a frequent topic of conversation, edged out of prominence only by national politics. The election-related violence of November 1987, in which Duvalierist thugs massacred people waiting in line to cast the first ballots of their lives, shocked villagers and led many to observe that "things simply can't continue like this." The unpleasant turn of national events was related in several ways to continued hard times for "the people." The advent of *sida* was simply one manifestation of these trials.

Another concern was the predicted return of the big *tonton makout,* the members of the Duvaliers' security forces, who had fled Haiti after February 1986. Several people whispered that some of the cruelest of the *makout,* even those rumored dead, were bringing back new weapons. One twenty-three-year-old high school student from Do Kay informed me that one of the Duvaliers' most notorious henchmen was returning from South America with "newly acquired knowledge." In a manner revealing not his own cynicism but rather that of Duvalierism, the student continued:

> They say he went [to South America] to study the science of bacteriology. He learned how to create microbes and then traveled to [North] America to study germ warfare. . . . They can now put microbes into the water of troublesome places. They can disappear all the militant young men and at the same time attract more [international] aid in order to stop the epidemic.

1988: NEW DISORDER, OLD PARADIGMS

In Do Kay, an increased concern with *sida* fit neatly into the almost apocalyptic winter of 1987–88. Manno was dead, and Anita was dying. Why was it, several villagers queried, that Do Kay alone of the villages in the area had people sick with *sida?* If the disorder was indeed novel, as most seemed to believe, why should it strike Do Kay first? Some cautioned that the mysterious deaths of two persons from nearby villages might not have been the result of "sent" tuberculosis, as had been suspected: perhaps they had died, undiagnosed, from *sida.* Other questions were asked in more hushed tones: Were others, such as Dieudonné and Celhomme, also ill with the disorder? Was it really caused by a simple microbe, or was someone at the bottom of it all?

Rumors flew. Some said that Acéphie had contracted the disorder by sharing clothes with Germaine, a kinswoman from another village on the plateau. A voodoo priest in a neighboring village was reported to have signed a contract with a North American manufacturing firm that would authorize him to "load tear-gas grenades with *mo sida.*" Demonstrators who found themselves in a cloud of this brand of tear gas would later fall ill with a bona fide case of *sida.* One person with tuberculosis was cautioned not to cross any major paths, stand in a crossroads, or walk under a chicken roost, lest his malady "degenerate into *sida.*"

At the same time, I noted the parallel activities of the village representatives of community medicine. At the January 1988 meeting of the village health committee, there was talk of initiating a much-needed antituberculosis project, one that would also include the task of HIV education. The community health workers from Do Kay and surrounding villages held a second conference on *sida,* but these attempts at activism seemed mired in a widely shared resignation that cast the new disorder as a ruthless killer against which "doctors' medication" could offer little comfort. The dispirited physicians seemed to feel that any assertions to the contrary were hollow, that there really was nothing they could do.

Anita's death in mid-February coincided with an obvious dampening of discussion about the disorder. What had once seemed a sort of struggle for preeminence between politics and *sida,* with the former eclipsing the latter whenever "the thing was hot," now appeared to be more like a symbiotic relationship between the two. When the muzzle was off, it was off for everything; when it was reapplied with new force, those with the most to lose simply spoke less. *Sida* was discussed less and less as villagers, increasingly cowed by "the climate of insecurity," stopped discussing national politics.

During the months following Anita's death, there seemed to be a new confidence and clarity in the commentaries offered by the villagers. It was widely agreed that she had died of *sida,* yet people remarked that her sickness was outwardly different from that of Manno. It was almost universally accepted that *sida* was a "sent sickness" (that is, the result of sorcery), and yet few believed that Anita had been the victim of sorcery. How did the nascent representation accommodate the disparities offered by her sickness? As one of Anita's aunts put it, "We don't know whether or not they sent a *sida* death to [her lover], but we know that she did not have a death sent to her. She had it in her blood; she caught it from him." Her father's lack of success in his quest for magical therapy was seen as an indication not of the power of her enemies but of the virulence of her "natural" illness.

Anita's aunt was reflecting the view of many in Do Kay who had come to understand that a person may contract *sida* in two ways:

> You catch it by sleeping with a person with *sida*. You might not see that the person is sick, but the person nonetheless has it in the blood. The other way is if someone sends a *mo sida*. When Manno died, he didn't have *sida* in the blood. They sent a *mo sida* to him, but it wasn't in his blood.

The proof that Manno's *sida* was "not simple" was that his wife did not have the disorder. "If it was in his blood, his wife would have it, and she did not," observed one of Anita's aunts. "She had a test, and she did not have it."

By the end of Anita's illness, these distinctions between causal mechanisms operating in Manno's case and in hers became sharper and had a great influence on a rapidly evolving collective representation of *sida*. In the eyes of a majority of those interviewed in early 1988, Manno's sickness had been sent to him by a jealous rival or a group of rivals. Anita had contracted *sida* through sexual contact with a person who had the syndrome. She was not the victim of sorcery. Indeed, this would have been a very unlikely fate for Anita Joseph. As villagers repeated many times, Anita had lost her mother, run away at fourteen, and been forced into a sexual union by poverty. Several people, including Anita's uncle, added that they were all victims of the dam at Péligre, whose construction in 1956 had displaced and impoverished them.

Dieudonné Gracia was the third villager to fall ill with *sida,* and once again many features of the case were found to be compatible with the nascent model. He had spent two years in Port-au-Prince. Through a relative from Do Kay, he had found a position as "yard boy" for a well-to-do family. He worked opening gates, fetching heavy things from the car, and tending flowers in the cool heights of one of the city's ostentatious suburbs. Dieudonné's subsequent illness was seen by most as the result of an argument with a rival domestic, which led him to return to Do Kay in 1985. Two informants felt that his *sida* was the result of poison, an invisible "powder" laid in his path. But most villagers, including his family, came to agree that Dieudonné's was another "sent sickness," a suspicion later confirmed by a voodoo priest consulted by Boss Yonel, the young man's father.

Although Dieudonné had visited the clinic for recurrent diarrhea and weight loss in 1986 and early 1987, his cousin, a community health worker, felt that his illness had begun in August of 1987:

> His gums began to hurt him, to bleed easily. He was coughing, and he had diarrhea that went on and on, and fever and vomiting. This was when he was first ill, when he was working in Savanette [a neighboring village]. It was on the way home from Savanette; he got to [another community health worker's] house, and he thought it was a cold. He gave him cold medications, and I took care of him when he came home. He got better.

Dieudonné did seem to improve, which may explain why his illness was not attributed to sent *sida* until about the time of Anita's death, when he was again coughing and complaining of shortness of breath *(retoufman)*. By April, his night sweats led the physicians in Do Kay to suspect tuberculosis, but Boss Yoncl was reluctant to believe that diagnosis. Physicians from another clinic offered the same opinion.

During the last week of September 1988, Boss Yonel took his son to see Tonton Meme, a well-known voodoo priest who lived in a neighboring village. Meme diagnosed *sida* and stated that it had been sent by "a man living in Port-au-Prince, but from somewhere else." This was seen as confirmation of the original reading of the illness. Tonton Meme explained that *sida* "is both natural and supernatural, because they know how to send it, and you can also catch it from a person who already has *sida*." He spoke, too, of the protections he could offer against the sickness, of charms *(gad* and *aret)* that could "protect you against any kind of sickness that a person would send to you."

In an interview shortly before his death, Dieudonné observed that "*sida* is a jealousy sickness." When asked to explain more fully what he intended by his observation, he replied:

> What I see is that poor people catch it more easily. They say the rich get *sida*; I don't see that. But what I do see is that one poor person sends it to another poor person. It's like the army, brothers shooting brothers. The little soldier *(ti solda)* is really one of us, one of the people. But he is made to do the bidding of the State, and so shoots his own brother when they yell, "Fire!" Perhaps they are at last coming to understand this.

Dieudonné was not calling for international peace and friendship across borders, but was alluding to the fact that since independence the Haitian army has been unleashed on no other enemy than the Haitian people. Brothers shooting brothers, indeed. Dieudonné's optimism about people "coming to understand this" was based on the September coup d'état, which was initially viewed as "deliverance" from the bloody and now universally detested rule of the most recent in a series of military governments.

Dieudonné's diarrhea and cough worsened, and villagers compared his open sores to Manno's dermatological problems. He died in October. His mother told me that she had been alerted well in advance: "A woman I know came to the clinic. . . . She was sitting with me and said, 'Oh! Look how death is near you!' (*gadejan lamo a pre ou!*) So I knew the week before."

Although one dissenting opinion had it that "tuberculosis killed him because it circulated too long in his blood," most agreed with Dieudonné's cousin, who explained the relationship between tuberculosis and sent *sida:*

> Tuberculosis and *sida* resemble each other greatly. They say that "TB is *sida's* little brother," because you can see them together. But if it's a sent *sida*, then it's really [*sida*] that leaves you weak and susceptible to TB. You can treat it, but you'll die nonetheless. *Sida* is TB's older brother, and it's not easy to find treatment for it.

At this writing, villagers continue to talk about *sida*, although they still greatly fear it—as they do many other misfortunes.[22] Based on statements like that of Dieudonné's cousin and also on more structured interviews, the following points summarize the shared understanding of AIDS in a Haitian village in 1989:

Sida is a "new disease."

Sida is strongly associated with skin infections, "drying up," diarrhea, and especially tuberculosis.

Sida may occur both naturally (*maladi bondje*, "God's illness") and unnaturally. Natural *sida* is caused by sexual contact with someone who "carries the germ." Unnatural *sida* is "sent" by someone who willfully inflicts death upon the afflicted. The mechanism of malice is through *expédition* of a "dead [person]," in the same manner that tuberculosis may be sent.

Whether "God's illness" or "sent," *sida* may be held to be caused by a "microbe."

Sida may be transmitted by contact with contaminated or "dirty" blood (but earlier associations with homosexuality and transfusion are rarely cited).

The term *"sida"* reverberates with associations drawn from the larger political-economic context, associations with North American imperialism, a lack of class solidarity among the poor, and the corruption of the ruling elite.

For many living in Do Kay, there exist two related but distinguishable entities—"*sida* the infectious disease" and "*sida* caused by magic." One may take preventive measures against each. Condoms are helpful against the former, useless against the latter. Certain charms (*gad* and *aret*) are widely believed to offer some protection against *sida*-caused-by-magic, but there is uncertainty about whether the charms will work in the event of exposure to *sida*-the-infectious-disease.

Whether this uncertainty is supplanted by consensus remains to be seen, but the rapid rate of change in local understandings of *sida* appears to be a thing of the past. Although the current meanings will be contested and will change, the *cultural* model described here reflects the evolution of a high level of agreement among informants regarding the nature of the illness. And although significant "surface variation" in models may be elicited from individuals, even these discrepant versions seem to be generated by a schema that includes the points just listed.[23] In the absence of dramatic group experience, collective accord tends to be more stable and to shift more slowly than individual models, which are often more vulnerable to disputation and subject to rapid revision.

DISCUSSION

Tracing the emergence of *sida* as a collective representation illuminates our understanding of AIDS in rural Haiti. Recall that in 1984, when *sida* was a "city sickness," the most frequent comments about it concerned the novelty of the disorder, its relation to diarrhea, and its association with homosexuality. The absence of illness stories regarding the malady calls into question the very notion of a cultural model of *sida* at that time. As of October 1988, however, there were many stories to tell. Manno's remained the prototypical case, the standard against which other illnesses could be judged. When two other villagers succumbed to *sida,* their illnesses, though quite different in several ways from Manno's, confirmed many of the tentatively held understandings that were elaborated in 1987.

While many of the ideas and associations were indeed new, the term *"sida"* and the syndrome with which it is associated came to be embedded in a series of distinctly Haitian ideas about illness. This "adoption" of a new illness category into an older interpretive framework is well documented. "As new medical terms become known in a society," Byron Good has noted, "they find their way into existing semantic networks. Thus while new explanatory models may be introduced, it is clear that changes in medical rationality seldom follow quickly."[24]

The causal language used in reference to *sida* is in many respects similar to that employed when speaking of tuberculosis. For example, the new illness became linked to other diseases that are believed to be caused by malign magic. Just as it is possible to "send a chest death" *(voye yon mo pwatrinè),* so, too, it is possible to send an AIDS death to someone. The relation of these ideas to voodoo is unclear. Certainly, some of my informants readily ascribed both the ideas and the practice of sorcery to the realm of voodoo. But most of those interviewed made no such Manichean distinctions. Instead of adherence to a neatly defined "belief system," we found almost universal acceptance of the possibility of "sending sickness." This was as true of virulently antivoodoo Protestants as it was of regulars of Tonton Meme's temple.

The scholarly literature on voodoo documents this form of illness causation. Alfred Métraux refers to the "sending of the dead" as "the most fearful practice in the black arts" and describes Haitian understandings of *expédition:* "Whoever has become the prey of one or more dead people sent against him begins to grow thin, spit blood and is soon dead. The laying on of this spell is always attended by fatal results unless it is diagnosed in time and a capable *hun-gan* succeeds in making the dead let go."[25]

In Haiti, a fatal disease that causes one to "grow thin, spit blood" is tuberculosis until proven otherwise. Once referred to as "little house illness," in reference to the tuberculous person's separate sleeping quarters, tuberculosis remains a leading cause of death among adults and is still greatly feared. Although some say that virtually any death can be sent, the people of Do Kay and surrounding villages agree that a *mo pwatrinè* (a tuberculous death) is the one most commonly "expedited." In research concerning tuberculosis that was conducted before the advent of AIDS, a few informants asserted that only a *mo pwatrinè* can be sent. These same informants, when interviewed in 1988, all agreed that now there was a new "expeditable" death to be feared.

These two major causal schemes—magic and germ theory—are elaborately intertwined and subject to revision. For example, one person who was widely believed to have been the victim of a *mo pwatrinè* was considered to have "simple TB" after antituberculosis therapy led to her dramatic recovery. As another person with tuberculosis put it, "If they had sent a *mo pwatrinè* to me, your medicines wouldn't be able to touch it." For *sida,* conversely, some consider the sent version to be the less virulent form of the disease, since at least magical intervention is possible. As of 1989, the "natural" form was universally and rapidly fatal.

The cultural discourse that emerged around *sida* developed largely through a shrinking set of intracultural variations in representations of the new disorder. Yet important variation remained even after a genuine cultural model of the illness had come into being. The relation of representation to illness stories was paramount in Do Kay, as stories were the matrix in which such representations took form. The fact that representations were necessarily embedded in narratives meant that rhetorical exigencies and performative factors could be shown to have determinant effects on shaping the cultural models.

The term *"sida"* has become a prominent part of everyday Haitian discourse about misfortune. It has been the topic of several nationally popular songs, all of which tend to affirm associations that are important to the Haitian cultural model of AIDS. This discourse reveals the semantic network in which the term is embedded, a network that has come to include such diverse associations as the endless suffering of the Haitian people, divine punishment, the corruption of the ruling class, and the ills of North American imperialism.

These shifts in the rhetoric of complaint were brought into relief by the political turmoil of the late 1980s. The collapse of the Duvalier dictatorship had a palpable effect on the way AIDS-related accusations were marshaled and used, further emphasizing the effects of performative factors on illness representations. One noted a shift in the target of recrimination, from a focus on racist North America—a rhetoric encouraged by the regime—to one suggesting the ill will of the Haitian rulers. For example, when the military government organized a carefully policed forum on the mechanics of army-run elections, the gathering was widely referred to as a "forum *sida*," a play on the official term "forum CEDHA" (the acronym designating the army's proposed electoral machinery). The significance of conspiracy theories, some of which point to powerful *makout* and their allies, has yet to decline. Although such expressions emanated from Port-au-Prince, it is possible that they have had a greater effect on the elaboration of rural illness realities than has the virus itself. Many areas of rural Haiti had registered no local cases of *sida* as of 1990; travel in northern and southern Haiti during that period nonetheless suggested to me that inhabitants of these regions were familiar with many of these expressions.

When framed as an illness caused by sorcery, *sida* stands for local, rather than large-scale, dissatisfaction. Several villagers referred to *sida* as a "jealousy sickness," an illness visited on one poor person by another, even poorer person. As such, the disorder has come to connote an inability of poor Haitians to develop enduring class solidarity. Such observations often served as codas in the illness stories recounted in Do Kay, as when Dieudonné concluded a conversation with a deep sigh and the prediction that "Haiti will never change as long as poor people keep sending sickness on other poor people." These associations are also important in other parts of Haiti. The most recent pre-Lenten carnival was marred by a widespread rumor of a group of people who planned to spread *sida* by injecting revelers with HIV-infected serum. Some urban Haitians described the alleged planners as "poor people hurting their own brothers and sisters."

It is possible to delineate several factors important to the crafting of this illness representation. Most significant, of course, has been the advent of the illness itself, with the suffering and pain it has introduced into the lives of particular individuals and their families. *Sida*'s debut in Do Kay prompted its residents to care about AIDS and created an urgent need to find a means of talking about the new affliction with one another. Thereafter, Manno's illness served as a prototypical case, and, though the presentation and course of subsequent cases were much different, they did not quickly alter ideas about the etiology, symptomatology, and experience of *sida*.

When Manno's affliction made *sida* matter to the people of Do Kay, what organizing principles did they use to make sense of a new kind of suffering? The flurry of information that followed the arrival of AIDS in Haiti was important. Billboards, posters, and t-shirts all proclaimed AIDS to be a menace. But it was the radio that offered a largely nonliterate population a certain exposure to biomedical understandings of the syndrome, shaping at least the contours of a cultural model of AIDS. Although the radio did not immediately stimulate strong interest in the disease in rural Haiti, it seems to have provided a vague grid— associations with homosexuality, blood transfusions, "America"—upon which genuinely interested villagers would later evaluate their neighbors' illnesses. In this respect, the efforts of a local clinic to disseminate information about AIDS in church, at community council meetings, and at conferences for health workers, injectionists, and midwives supplemented the national media.

These sources of information seem far less significant, however, than the preexisting meaning structures into which *sida* so neatly fit. The blood paradigm, which posits causal links between the social field and alterations in the quality, consistency, and nature of blood, was invoked early on, before the virulence of *sida* became clear. Disorders of the blood are all considered dangerous and require intervention, but they are rarely refractory to treatment, unlike the new disorder. *Sida* also recalled tuberculosis in many ways. All three of the villagers who fell ill with *sida* eventually developed active tuberculosis. In addition, the new disorder is far more serious than "bad blood" and evokes significant fear. It is not only disfiguring but also chronic, sapping the body's strength over months or years. Given certain similarities in presentation, it is not surprising that the tuberculosis paradigm has been invoked in reference to *sida*. This longstanding conceptual framework includes elaborate understandings of causality, most notably through sorcery, divination, and treatment. Finally, the microbe paradigm, which has the official blessing of the local representatives of cosmopolitan medicine, has long endured alongside the other explanatory frameworks. It is widely accepted, with provisos, in rural Haiti.

These three frameworks—in which are embedded understandings of blood, tuberculosis, and microbes—have been worked into a "master paradigm" that links sickness to moral concerns and social relations. Writing of North America, Michael Taussig has observed that "behind every reified disease theory in our society lurks an organizing realm of moral concerns."[26] This is no less true in the Kay area, where *sida* has come to represent a "jealousy sickness" and a disease of the poor—victims' moral readings of the sources of their suffering.

AIDS AND THE STUDY OF ILLNESS REPRESENTATIONS

Medical anthropology has by and large followed its parent discipline in studying illness representations in cultural, political, and historical contexts. When the illness under consideration is a new one, it is clear that our ethnography must be not only alive to the importance of change but also accountable to history and political economy.[27] AIDS, an illness that "moves along the fault lines of society," demands nothing less.[28]

Such a mandate is no license to give short shrift to the lived experience of the afflicted, however. Indeed, by attending closely to the understandings of the ill and their families, we are led to precisely this conclusion. I think of the words of Manno, who said of his disorder, "They tell me there's no cure. But I'm not sure of that. If you can find a cause, you can find a cure." Manno's search for a cause was the search for the enemies who had ensorcelled him, and it was guided by an assessment of his relations with those around him. Who was jealous of his relative success in the village?

Anita, even younger than Manno and a native of Do Kay, was not a victim of sorcery. In contrast to the etiologic theories advanced by Manno and his family, Anita felt that she had "caught it from a man in the city." The rest of her analysis was much more sociological, however, as she added that the reason she had a lover at a young age was "because I had no mother." She continued:

> When she died, it was bad. My father was just sitting there. And when I saw how poor I was, and how hungry, and saw that it would never get any better, I had to go to the city. Back then I was so skinny. I was saving my life, I thought, by getting out of here.

Anita was equally clear about the cause of her family's poverty: "My parents lost their land to the water," she said, "and that is what makes us poor." If there had been no dam, insisted Anita, her mother would not have sickened and died; if her mother had lived, Anita would never have gone to the city; had she not gone to Port-au-Prince, she would not have "caught it from a man in the city."

Neither the dam nor the AIDS epidemic would have been as they are if Haiti had not been caught up in a network of relations that are political and economic as well as sexual. Dieudonné underlined this point on several occasions. Like Manno, he was a self-described victim of sorcery; but, like Anita, he tended to cast things in sociological terms. Dieudonné voiced what have been deemed "conspiracy theories" regarding the origins of AIDS. On more than one occasion, he wondered whether *sida* might not have been "sent to Haiti by the United States. That's why they were so quick to say that Haitians gave [the world] *sida*." When asked why the United States would wish such a pestilence on Haitians, Dieudonné had a ready answer: "They say there are too many Haitians over there now. They needed us to work for them, but now there are too many over there." A history of Haiti's entanglement in this international network should inform any understanding of *sida* as "sent sickness." The spread of HIV across national borders seems to have taken place within our lifetimes, but the conditions favoring the rapid, international spread of a predominantly sexually transmitted disorder were established long ago and further heighten the need to historicize any understanding of this pandemic.

The path from dissensus to consensus has many forks, and also dead-ends: not all forks lead to high rates of interindividual agreement. Some steps in this process are intuitively obvious; others are not. There are two main reasons for a failure to reach consensus in representation. First, some disorders are "epidemiologically excluded" from the list of illnesses that people can care about: Is there a contemporary North American cultural model of yaws, for example, as there is in Haiti? Is there a Haitian model of anorexia nervosa? The second reason relates to the perceived severity of the disorder: some illnesses are banal and, though widely recognized, never generate enough collective concern to trigger illness stories. But a life-threatening illness quickly stimulated a critical mass of both local interest and interested parties, and the formation of illness stories seemed to follow naturally.

As time passed, these narratives became much more similarly structured. As Manno's illness triggered a great deal of natural discourse about the new sickness, people began to recount the "same story," and the illness of which they spoke came to have characteristics and features that varied less and less from informant to informant. This consensus was cobbled together toward the end of 1987, and subsequent events tended to inflect the nascent model of *sida* rather than remake it. Anita's symptoms, though strikingly different from Manno's, served largely to reinforce features of a model put into circulation by stories relating the details of Manno's illness. It was for this reason that his experience may be termed "prototypical."

We may conclude that a certain critical mass of community engagement is necessary before a new affliction engenders illness stories with moral bite. That effective illness stories have a moral, moving component has been observed by many who have studied them. Indeed, Laurie Price has argued that "affective propositions are so central to most of these illness narratives that it can be said that if cultural models of social roles drive the narratives, emotional propositions are the fuel that empower them."[29] These affectively laden commentaries, over the years, were the web in which were enmeshed new ideas, tentative suggestions, timid conclusions, and, finally, growing consensus about a new sickness.

This account has underlined the central role of illness stories in the emergence of a new cultural model. But one cannot easily fashion something out of nothing, at least not in the unforgiving harshness of rural Haiti. It was the intrusion of *sida*—and not of the ethnographer asking questions about *sida*—that triggered genuine illness stories. By offering a plot and characters, Manno's illness served as a model for the etiology, symptomatology, and experience of *sida*. Perhaps the final tie to time was offered by the fact that this new illness was, clearly, mortal.

Each of these components—a critical mass of fearful concern, a prototypical case, employment in moving narratives—was a necessary part of the process described here. Paul Ricoeur puts it well: "time becomes human to the extent that it is articulated through a narrative mode, and narrative attains its full meaning when it becomes a condition of temporal existence."[30]

NOTES

1. Several of the concepts in this article—cultural model, prototypical model, semantic network, social construction, and so on—have been used in different ways in medical anthropology. This study is informed by the critique of an "empiricist theory of language" offered in Good and Good, "Towards a Meaning-Centered Analysis of Popular Illness Categories," and by work in cognitive anthropology, which has begun shifting its attention from the formal properties of illness models to their relation to natural discourse and thus to context and performance characteristics of illness representations (see Price, "Ecuadorian Illness Stories"). A focus on *lived experience* is crucial to this view, even in a study of the emergence of a collective representation. (For a forceful statement of such a position, see Kleinman and Kleinman, "Suffering and Its Professional Transformation.") We can now make headway by merging these groups of concerns. One important "bridge concept" might be the cultural model, an idea formalized by cognitive anthropologists seeking to show how "cultural models frame experience, supplying interpretations of that experience and inferences about it, and goals for action" (Quinn and Holland, "Culture and Cognition," p. 6).

2. Pape and Johnson, "Epidemiology of AIDS in the Caribbean."

3. On the ecological and social history of Do Kay, see Farmer, "Bad Blood, Spoiled Milk" (included in this volume as chapter 1).

4. The processual ethnography of the changing understanding of AIDS in Do Kay is based on a large body of interviews, most of which are not cited here. As they all inform my understanding of the significance of the comments that are cited, it is necessary to detail here the methodology of the larger project, which was initiated in 1983. At least once during each of the subsequent six years, the same twenty villagers were interviewed regarding tuberculosis and AIDS; during three of those years, a third disorder *(move san)* was also discussed. The majority of these conversations were tape-recorded. In 1988, it was impossible for me to interview seven of the informants myself, but a research assistant was able to speak with them regarding tuberculosis and AIDS. All other taped exchanges were initiated by me and took place in a variety of settings, most often in the informants' houses. Of the twenty adults, two have now died, and one has left Do Kay.

The interviews were open-ended and usually focused on specific "illness stories," always including discussion of the following topics regarding each of the three illnesses: its key features (including typical presentation, causes, course, and understandings of pathogenesis when relevant), appropriate therapeutic interventions, its relation to other sicknesses common in the area, and questions of risk and vulnerability. In addition to these interviews, the research involved lengthy conversations with all villagers afflicted with tuberculosis and AIDS and the majority of those with *move san*. Members of victims' families were also interviewed, as were other key actors in the events described here. These qualitative data were complemented by information from several structured surveys and an annual census, conducted by myself and other members of Proje Veye Sante, a locally directed public health initiative based in Do Kay. Since May 1983, I have spent an average of six months per year in Do Kay and have therefore witnessed the changes described here.

5. The French acronym is commonly rendered as S.I.D.A., SIDA, or Sida; *sida* is the Creole

orthography. I have adopted the latter here in order to reflect the substantial difference between the terms as used in different national and cultural settings.

6. See Centers for Disease Control and Prevention, "Opportunistic Infections and Kaposi's Sarcoma among Haitians in the United States"; also Nachman and Dreyfuss, "Haitians and AIDS in South Florida."

7. The anti-Haitian backlash may have been felt as keenly in New York, Miami, Boston, Montreal, and other North American cities in which large numbers of Haitians reside; see Farmer, "AIDS and Accusation." For a review of AIDS-related discrimination against Haitians, see Sabatier, *Blaming Others.*

8. Abbott, *Haiti,* p. 255.

9. Three of the five who had never heard the term were men who "never traveled to Port-au-Prince." Such homebodies are rare in the Central Plateau, where most inhabitants are highly involved in the marketing of produce.

10. In Haiti, market women are known for their up-to-date information. Their "frequent trips to neighboring cities and to Port-au-Prince make [them] aware of everything—not just the rise and fall of prices, but also national events, not only the genuine ones, but the false rumors that spread through the marketplaces" (Bastien, *Le paysan haïtien et sa famille,* p. 128).

11. It should be noted, however, that Ti Malou was widely believed to have *move san,* a common disorder that is treated by herbal medications and not transfusion; see Farmer, "Bad Blood, Spoiled Milk" (included in this volume as chapter 1). Some observed that when one is ill with *move san,* any intravenous solution can be dangerous.

12. Weidman, *Miami Health Ecology Project Report;* see also Laguerre, *Afro-Caribbean Folk Medicine.*

13. James Ferguson documents the role of the *duvaliériste* Luckner Cambronne in a trade in Haitian blood, which was used for medical experiments and for its antibody-rich serum (see *Papa Doc, Baby Doc*).

14. For a discussion of rhetorics of complaint and their relevance to illness representations, see Gaines and Farmer, "Visible Saints." It has long been recognized that Haitians have complicated, multifactorial ideas about illness causation. A large body of ethnographic literature shows that rural Haitians often entertain explanatory frameworks that make room for "naturalistic" causation as well as lines of causality dominated by human agency. Particularly relevant is Coreil, "Traditional and Western Responses to an Anthrax Epidemic in Rural Haiti."

15. For discussion of health care practitioners in rural Haiti, see Coreil, "Parallel Structures in Professional and Folk Health Care"; as well as Laguerre, *Afro-Caribbean Folk Medicine.*

16. As Renée Sabatier notes, "Syphilis was referred to by the Spanish as 'the sickness of Hispaniola,' believing it to have come from what is now Haiti when Columbus returned from his voyage to the Americas" (*Blaming Others,* p. 42).

17. The advent of AIDS to this village is more fully described in Farmer, "AIDS and Accusation."

18. The term *"expedition"* is also used to describe this process, which requires the services of a *houngan,* or voodoo priest. In translating the term *"voye yon mo sida,"* I have used the less accurate "send a *sida* death" rather than the more cumbersome "send a dead person who has died from *sida.*"

19. For a discussion of folk representations invoked in the popular press and even by specialists, see Farmer, "The Exotic and the Mundane" (included in this volume as chapter 3).

20. Whitmore, *Someone Was Here,* p. 26.

21. Anita's story has been told more fully in Farmer and Kleinman, "AIDS as Human Suffering."

22. Things do not appear to have changed altogether. Ethnographic research conducted decades ago led Alfred Métraux to observe that "in everyday life the threat of charms, sorcery and spells makes it but one more care to be listed with drought and the price of coffee and bananas. Magic is at

least an evil against which man is not entirely powerless" (*Voodoo in Haiti*, p. 269). Laënnec Hurbon offers a similar insight when he notes that "spells are part of the daily struggle in a world already littered with traps" (*Le barbare imaginaire*, p. 260).

23. See Garro, "Explaining High Blood Pressure."

24. Good, "The Heart of What's the Matter," p. 54.

25. Métraux, *Voodoo in Haiti*, p. 274.

26. Taussig, "Reification and the Consciousness of the Patient," p. 7.

27. Moore, "Explaining the Present."

28. This expression is borrowed from Bateson and Goldsby, *Thinking AIDS*. Shirley Lindenbaum used a similar image in her classic study of sorcery and the advent of *kuru,* another novel infectious disease, in rural Papua New Guinea: "A geography of fear tracks unequal relations" (*Kuru Sorcery,* p. 146).

29. Price, "Ecuadorian Illness Stories," p. 319.

30. Ricoeur, *Time and Narrative,* vol. 1, p. 52.

The Exotic and the Mundane

Human Immunodeficiency Virus in Haiti

(1990)

Early in the pandemic of the acquired immune deficiency syndrome (AIDS), a number of Haitians fell ill with opportunistic infections characteristic of the new syndrome. Some of the ill Haitians lived in urban Haiti; others had emigrated to the United States or Canada. Unlike other patients who met the diagnostic criteria for AIDS, the Haitians diagnosed in the United States denied having participated in homosexual activity or intravenous drug use. Most had never had a blood transfusion. AIDS among Haitians was, in the words of many researchers, "a complete mystery." Public health officials therefore inferred that Haitians per se were in some way at risk for AIDS, and it was suggested that unraveling "the Haiti connection" would lead researchers to the culprit. In the colorful prose that came to typify commentary on Haitians with AIDS, one reporter termed the incidence of AIDS in Haitians "a clue from the grave, as though a zombie, leaving a trail of unwinding gauze bandages and rotting flesh, had come to the hospital's Grand Rounds to pronounce a curse."[1]

The Haitian cases spurred the publication of a wide range of theories purporting to explain the epidemiology and origins of AIDS. In December 1982, for example, a physician with the National Cancer Institute was widely quoted as follows: "We suspect that this may be an epidemic Haitian virus that was brought back to the homosexual population in the United States."[2] This theory, echoed by other scientists and in the popular press, had a considerable impact on Haiti itself, which once counted tourism as an important source of foreign currency. But it also affected Haitians everywhere, especially those living in the United States and Canada. Sander Gilman might not have been exaggerating when he wrote that "to be a Haitian and living in New York City meant that you were perceived as an AIDS 'carrier.'"[3] Many of the million or so Haitians living in North America argued that speculation about a Haitian origin of AIDS led to a wave of anti-Haitian discrimination, which in turn led to loss of jobs and housing.[4]

The link between AIDS and Haiti, strengthened in innumerable articles in the popular press, seemed to resonate with what might be termed a North American folk model of Haitians.[5] One of the most persistently invoked associations related the occurrence of AIDS in Haitians to voodoo. Something that happened at these ritual fires, it was speculated, triggered AIDS in cult adherents, presumed to be the quasi-totality of Haitians. In the October 1983 issue of the *Annals of Internal Medicine,* Peter Moses and John Moses, two physicians affiliated with the Massachusetts Institute of Technology, related the details of a visit to Haiti and wrote, "It seems reasonable to consider voodoo practices a cause of the syndrome."[6] Why, precisely, would it be "reasonable" to consider voodoo practices a cause of the syndrome? Did existing knowledge of AIDS in Haiti make this hypothesis reasonable?

In 1986, the official organ of the American Medical Association published a consideration of these theories under the fey title "Night of the Living Dead II." In it, the author asks, "Do necromantic zombiists transmit HTLV-III/LAV during voodooistic rituals?" Tellingly, he cites not the scientific literature on AIDS in Haiti, which by that time was substantial, but the popular press:

> Even now, many Haitians are voodoo *serviteurs* and partake in its rituals *(New York Times,* 15 May 1985, pp. 1, 6). (Some are also members of secret societies such as Bizango or "impure" sects, called "cabrit thomazo," which are suspected to use human blood itself in sacrificial worship.) As the HTLV-III/LAV virus is known to be stable in aqueous solution at room temperature for at least a week, lay Haitian voodooists may be unsuspectingly infected with AIDS by ingestion, inhalation, or dermal contact with contaminated ritual substances, as well as by sexual activity.[7]

In a heroic effort to accommodate all of the exotic furbelows available in the North American folk model of Haitians, another essay, written by two social scientists, depicts the following scene: "In frenzied trance, the priest lets blood: mammal's [sic] throats are cut; typically, chicken's [sic] heads are torn off their necks. The priest bites out the chicken's tongue with his teeth and may suck on the bloody stump of the neck." These sacrificial offerings, "infected with one of the Type C oncogenic retroviruses, which is closely related to HTLV," are "repeatedly [sic] sacrificed in voodoo ceremonies, and their blood is directly ingested by priests and their assistants." The authors complete the model with the assertion that "many voodoo priests are homosexual men" who are "certainly in a position to satisfy their sexual desires, especially in urban areas."[8]

The following essay will review the epidemiology of AIDS and HIV in Haiti. What is known about transmission of HIV in Haiti? Does it remain a "mystery"?

That such questions remain critical is apparent from a February 1990 ruling from the Food and Drug Administration (FDA), which banned all Haitians from donating blood. In response to this ruling, thousands of Haitians brought Miami traffic to a standstill as they protested in front of the local FDA headquarters, with shouts of "Racists!" The demonstrations culminated in a mammoth rally in New York City, where so many marchers—fifty thousand according to the police, more than twice that according to organizers—crossed the Brooklyn Bridge that it was closed to traffic: "The number of protesters—college students, factory workers and families with picnic baskets—surprised the Police Department, which had expected several thousand people."[9]

What, exactly, had prompted the FDA ruling? The *New York Times* explained that the decision was based on what was known about HIV transmission in Haiti: "The Centers for Disease Control have stopped publicly specifying that Haitians are at risk for contracting AIDS, but the agency's statistics still carry a category of 'pattern II countries,' where heterosexual transmission is the primary mode of infection. And these are defined by the World Health Organization as Haiti and sub-Saharan Africa."[10]

In overviews of the world epidemiology of HIV/AIDS, it is usually remarked that three general types of epidemiological "patterns" currently exist. Pattern I, to use the terminology of the World Health Organization (WHO) Global Program on AIDS, is seen in North America and Europe. It is characterized by a preponderance of cases among gay and bisexual men, with variable attack rates among intravenous drug users. Haiti (and sometimes the entire Caribbean) is characterized, along with much of Africa, as reflecting Pattern II: "Pattern II is seen in the Caribbean and in large areas of sub-Saharan Africa, and differs [from Pattern I] in that heterosexual intercourse has been the dominant mode of HIV transmission from the start. Blood transfusion, the reuse of contaminated needles, and intravenous drug use contribute to a variable degree, but homosexuality generally plays a minor role in this pattern."[11] Pattern III countries are considered areas of low incidence of AIDS.

This essay suggests that the terminology used by the World Health Organization and many other agencies may not reflect the reality of the epidemic, especially with regard to Haiti and much of the rest of the Caribbean. In fact, careful epidemiological research has cast doubt on many early assumptions about the Haitian epidemic and its role in the larger epidemic to the north. I will further argue that the course of the American pandemic, including the epidemic in Haiti, has been determined to no small extent by structures long in place.

A CHRONOLOGY OF THE AIDS/HIV EPIDEMIC IN HAITI

Most chroniclers of the AIDS pandemic agree that awareness of the new syndrome began in 1980 in California. Several physicians in Los Angeles observed that *Pneumocystis carinii,* a harmless parasite to those with intact immune defenses, had caused pneumonia (P.C.P.) in several young men who did not exhibit recognized states of immunodeficiency. The only epidemiological clue linking the cases was the sexual preference of the men. By June of 1981, the U.S. Centers for Disease Control (CDC), monitoring the distribution of drugs used to treat P.C.P., reported that "in the period October 1980–May 1981, 5 young men, all active homosexuals, were treated for biopsy-confirmed *Pneumocystis carinii* pneumonia at 3 different hospitals in Los Angeles."[12] By the end of the summer, 108 cases of Kaposi's sarcoma and unexplained opportunistic infections had been reported to the CDC. The vast majority of cases were from California and New York. Of those afflicted, 107 were men; more than 90 percent of these men stated that they were gay and sexually active.

Alerted to the possibility of an epidemic, North American public health specialists reviewed available documentation and observed that unexpected clusterings of Kaposi's sarcoma and opportunistic infections had begun early in 1977. Haitian physicians began to see similarly puzzling cases of immunosuppression shortly thereafter. The first Haitian case of Kaposi's sarcoma was detected in June 1979, when dermatologist Bernard Liautaud diagnosed the disorder in a twenty-eight-year-old woman from a city in western Haiti. She had been referred to the university hospital for worsening lower-extremity edema and nodular and papular lesions on her face, trunk, and extremities. Neither her demographic variables nor clinical presentation fit the standard description of patients with the sarcoma: before the AIDS pandemic, Kaposi's had been described as a rare and slow-growing malignancy seen largely in elderly men of Eastern European and Mediterranean descent. The tumor behaved quite differently in Dr. Liautaud's patient—it was aggressive and fatal.

When the presence of the cancer in a young Haitian man was confirmed later that year, Liautaud posed the following question: was Kaposi's sarcoma of longstanding and unappreciated importance in Haiti, or was the cancer new to the country? A survey of colleagues led him to conclude that Kaposi's sarcoma was virtually unknown in Haiti. Liautaud and his coworkers reported their findings to an international medical conference held in Haiti in April 1982.[13] Concurrent "outbreaks" of Kaposi's reported in California and New York lent force to the idea that the tumor might be in some way related to an epidemic triggered by an infectious agent.[14]

Several cases of inexplicable opportunistic infection, first noted in February 1980, were also described at the 1982 conference. These suggestions of immunosuppression were strikingly similar to those termed "AIDS" in the North American medical literature. The conviction that something new and significant was afoot led to the formation, in May 1982, of the Haitian Study Group on Kaposi's Sarcoma and Opportunistic Infections (GHESKIO). The study group comprised thirteen physicians and scientists who would eventually treat hundreds of patients with AIDS and conduct important clinical and epidemiological research.

In May 1983, the Association Médicale Haïtienne sponsored a medical conference in Port-au-Prince. Research presented there left little doubt that in urban Haiti, at least, a new state of immunodeficiency was striking increasing numbers of young adults, especially men. In the Haitian medical community, few doubted that the patients were ill with AIDS as defined by the CDC. By the time of the conference, twenty cases of Kaposi's sarcoma and more than sixty otherwise unexplained opportunistic infections had been recorded, as shown in table 3.1. Using CDC criteria, Haitian researchers diagnosed a total of sixty-one cases of AIDS between June 1979 and October 1982.

Despite the obvious parallel—in both Haiti and the United States, the suggestion of a new, acquired, and epidemic immunosuppression—there were important disparities between the two epidemics. When compared to cases in the United States, a smaller proportion of the Haitians with AIDS had P.C.P., the most common opportunistic infection in North Americans with AIDS. Although the Haitian patients did have mycobacterial infections, their infection was almost exclusively tuberculosis; *M. avium-intracellulare,* an infection often found in North Americans with AIDS, was rare in Haiti. But oroesophageal candidiasis was extremely common in Haitians with AIDS, so much so that some have seen it as an early marker for AIDS.[15] Data also showed disparities in time of survival after diagnosis: whereas mean survival after diagnosis was usually greater than a year in the United States, survival was less than six months in the majority of Haitian patients, and none survived more than twenty-four months. Despite these differences, most researchers were confident that the Haitian and North American epidemics were caused by the same organism.

The research presented in 1983 offered important epidemiologic clues to Haiti's "role" in the larger pandemic. Although the Haitian researchers initially concluded that "no segment of Haitian society appears to be free of opportunistic infections or Kaposi's sarcoma,"[16] AIDS did not strike randomly. Jean W. Pape and his coworkers found that 74 percent of all men with opportunistic infections lived in Port-au-Prince, home to approximately 17 percent of all Haitians. Curiously, 33 percent of all AIDS patients lived in a single suburb, Carrefour. This finding was underlined because several of the patients interviewed by Pape and other researchers reported that they had been remunerated for sex: "The prevalence rate of men with opportunistic infections in Carrefour was significantly higher than that of men in Port-au-Prince (p < 0.001 by the chi-square test). This is of interest since Carrefour, a suburb of Port-au-Prince, is recognized as the principal center of male and female prostitution in Haiti."[17]

The investigations also revealed that only 13 percent of the remaining men

Table 3.1 AIDS Cases Diagnosed by the Haitian Study Group on
Kaposi's Sarcoma and Opportunistic Infections (GHESKIO), 1979–83

	Number of Cases	
	Kaposi's Sarcoma	Opportunistic Infection
1979	2	0
1980	2	5
1981	7	9
1982	5	35
1983 (January to May)	4	12

SOURCE: Pape et al., "Characteristics of the Acquired Immunodeficiency Syndrome (AIDS) in Haiti."

with opportunistic infections were from elsewhere in the country. An equal number had been living outside Haiti: two patients had resided in New York, one in Miami, one in Belgium, and one in the Bahamas. Five of twenty-one men interviewed by one of the GHESKIO clinicians stated that they were bisexual, as did two patients referred by other Haitian physicians. These seven men had all lived in Carrefour (four) or the United States (three). Three of them reported sexual contact with North American men in both Haiti and the United States, and two others had had sexual contact with Haitian men known to have opportunistic infections.[18] Furthermore, fully half of the allegedly heterosexual men had either lived or traveled outside Haiti.

Research presented at the 1983 meetings made it clear that none of the Haitians ill with the new syndrome had ever been to Africa.[19] All denied sexual contact with persons from that continent; most, in fact, had never met an African. But 10 to 15 percent of these patients had traveled to North America or Europe in the five years preceding the onset of their illness, and several more admitted to sexual contact with tourists.[20] Other important demographic data offered by the GHESKIO team included high prevalence of venereal disease (71 percent) and histories of blood transfusion (20 percent) in these patients.

Also in 1983, members of the GHESKIO team surveyed the twenty-one dermatologists and pathologists known to be practicing in Haiti and asked them to provide information regarding their experience with diagnosis and treatment of Kaposi's sarcoma. More than a thousand biopsy specimens from the Hôpital Albert Schweitzer were also reviewed. The survey revealed that before June 1979 only one case had been diagnosed in Haiti, in 1972, and it had afflicted a man in his sixth decade. The course of his illness was not known, but it had not aroused suspicions of immunodeficiency. GHESKIO concluded, as had Liautaud, that the new cases of Kaposi's sarcoma represented an epidemic of recent onset.

In summary, those who attended the conference could draw several important conclusions based on the data presented at the meetings:

Haitians with AIDS were then largely men, although increasing numbers of women were reporting to the GHESKIO clinic.

The epicenter of the Haitian epidemic was the city of Carrefour, a center of prostitution bordering the south side of Port-au-Prince.

A large percentage of the early cases had been linked to homosexual contact, some of it with non-Haitians.

The rate of transfusion-associated transmission was higher in Haiti than in the United States.

Although the opportunistic infections often differed from those seen in North Americans with AIDS, the Haitian epidemic was manifestly related to that in the United States.

The microbial agent that led to AIDS was probably new to Haiti, since no one could report cases predating the North American epidemic.

Subsequent research, based on the development of assays for antibodies to the newly discovered HIV, also suggests that the virus was new to Haiti. Blood samples drawn from adults during the course of a 1977–79 outbreak of dengue fever were later tested for antibodies to HIV. The enzyme-linked immunosorbent assay (ELISA, whole virus) and radioimmunoprecipitation assay (RIPA) for antibody to the p25 and gpl20 antigens revealed that none of the 191 samples tested had antibodies to HIV.[21] The sole indication that AIDS existed in Haiti before 1979, when Dr. Liautaud had noted two cases of Kaposi's sarcoma, was the autopsy record of a previously healthy twenty-year-old man who had died in 1978, two weeks after the sudden onset of generalized seizures. Postmortem studies at the Hôpital Albert Schweitzer revealed cerebral toxoplasmosis, an opportunistic infection common in persons with AIDS. "These data and studies from Africa," conclude Warren Johnson and Jean Pape, "are consistent with the hypothesis that HIV most likely originated in that continent, came to the United States and Europe, and subsequently was introduced into Haiti by either tourists or returning Haitians."[22]

The research conducted in the first years of the Haitian epidemic also addressed many of the questions raised by the speculations of North American researchers. Was AIDS caused by "an epidemic Haitian virus," as some had postulated? Had overworked or undertrained Haitian physicians merely overlooked the disease, as others seemed to imply?[23] Was AIDS caused by an African virus brought to the United States by Haitians?[24] Was AIDS caused by an organism endemic among isolated, superstitious peasants who transmitted it through some bizarre voodoo practice? Some of the Haitian researchers felt that these questions had been answered by their research, which had been published in refereed, international journals. Yet their contributions did little to dampen the apparently self-sustaining "exotic theories" that continued to influence popular opinion in the United States and elsewhere.

HIV IN HAITI: THE DIMENSIONS OF THE PROBLEM

How far has HIV spread in Haiti? Given the natural history of HIV infection, this question is best answered not by the epidemiology of AIDS but through the study of HIV seroprevalence in asymptomatic populations. Researchers in Haiti have studied seroprevalence of HIV using both ELISA and RIPA (p25, gpl20). During 1986 and 1987, blood samples from several cohorts of healthy adults were analyzed for antibodies to HIV; table 3.2 summarizes the results. In a group of individuals working in hotels catering to tourists, HIV seroprevalence was 12 percent. Among urban factory workers, 5 percent were found to have antibodies to HIV. In both series, *rates were comparable for men and women,* which suggested to many that the high attack rate in Haitian men would slowly give way to a pattern like that seen in parts of Central Africa, where men and women are equally affected.

In a group of 502 mothers of children hospitalized with diarrhea, and in a group of 190 urban adults with low socioeconomic status, the seroprevalence rates were 12 percent and 13 percent, respectively (table 3.2). All of the 57 medical workers involved in the care of AIDS patients were seronegative, which corroborates data indicating that HIV is not easily spread by nonsexual contact. Overall, GHESKIO researchers found that approximately 9 percent of 912 healthy urban adults (in the urban categories listed in table 3.2, excluding pregnant women) were seropositive for HIV.

Additionally, a group of researchers based in Cité Soleil, a slum on the northern fringes of Port-au-Prince, reported that 8.4 percent of 1,240 healthy women receiving prenatal care in 1986 were seropositive for HIV.[25] In 1987, 9.9 percent of 2,009 sexually active women in Cité Soleil were HIV-positive; in 1989, 10.5 percent of 1,074 similar women were found to have been exposed to HIV (seropositivity in Cité Soleil was confirmed by Western blot).[26] In Gonaïves, the third-largest Haitian city, 9 percent of 1,795 patients reporting to a clinic that serves a predominantly low-income clientele tested seropositive in 1988.[27] The highest rates were found in female Haitian prostitutes (53 percent),[28] underlining for some their role in the transmission of HIV. Few observed that high rates of seroprevalence among prostitutes might simply reflect "occupational risk"—an increased likelihood of coming into contact with a seropositive man—proving nothing about their role in spreading the virus.

Other investigations confirmed the high rates of seroprevalence among people living in or near the capital. Pape and coworkers also tested sera that had been

Table 3.2 HIV Seroprevalence among Healthy Adults in Haiti, 1986–87

	N	Mean Age (Years)	% HIV+
Urban Haiti (Port-au-Prince area)			
Hotel workers	25	45	12.0
Factory workers	84	30	5.0
Pregnant women (1986)	1,240	29	8.4
Mothers of sick infants	502	29	12.0
Other adults:			
High socioeconomic status	54	35	0.0
Low socioeconomic status	190	33	13.0
Medical workers	57	40	0.0
Total	2,152	27	9.0
Rural Haiti (outside Port-au-Prince)			
Mothers of sick infants	97	25	3.0
Pregnant women	117	27	3.0
Blood donors	245	32	4.0
Other adults (rural village)	191	29	1.0
Total	650	30	3.0

SOURCE: Pape and Johnson, "Epidemiology of AIDS in the Caribbean," p. 35.

collected for other diagnostic procedures and reported that, of 1,037 adults phlebotomized during the first six months of 1986 by three commercial laboratories in Port-au-Prince, 8 percent were seropositive for HIV antibodies.[29] The health status of these persons is not known, but since none of the three laboratories performed HIV serology at the time of phlebotomy, the sera had not been collected to diagnose HIV infection. These samples represent 10 percent of the total number of persons bled by the three laboratories during that period.

When all available data from seroprevalence studies of healthy urban adults are compiled, one is led to conclude that a substantial number of urban Haitians have been exposed to HIV. In contrast, in 1986–1987, the seroprevalence rate averaged 3 percent in rural areas. The seroprevalence rate was 3 percent among 97 mothers of children hospitalized with dehydration; 4 percent of 245 unscreened rural blood donors had antibodies to HIV. In an area even more distant from urban centers, only 1 percent of 191 adults who came for immunizations were seropositive (see table 3.2).

What of seroprevalence among children? The GHESKIO team studied three groups of children: the offspring of a parent with AIDS; children hospitalized in Port-au-Prince with diarrheal disease; and healthy, age-matched controls from the same neighborhoods as the hospitalized children. Their findings, summa-

Table 3.3 Prevalence of HIV Antibodies among Haitian Children, 1985–86

Age in Years	Children of a Parent with AIDS		Children Hospitalized with Diarrhea		Controls	
	N	% HIV+	N	% HIV+	N	% HIV+
Younger than 1	96	28.0	260	8.0	119	3.0
1–4	252	3.0	52	2.0	41	2.0
4–10	218	2.0	5	0	7	0
Older than 10	43	0	0	—	0	—
Total	609	6.5	317	6.5	167	2.0

SOURCE: Pape and Johnson, "Epidemiology of AIDS in the Caribbean."

rized in table 3.3, suggest that pediatric infection with HIV is perinatal: rates are highest in the children of parents with AIDS, especially among those less than one year old, when maternal antibodies may give false-positive antibody tests. Further, the children of a seropositive father and a seronegative mother were all seronegative, also strongly suggesting vertical (mother-to-infant) transmission.

It is especially disturbing that the rates of seropositivity were identical for the children of parents with AIDS and the children hospitalized with diarrhea: 6.5 percent in both groups, three times greater than the rates documented in control samples. This finding implies that, in Port-au-Prince at least, pediatric infection with HIV may lead to significant morbidity (for example, diarrheal disease) even before pediatric AIDS can be diagnosed. The relative contribution of HIV compared to that of other pathogens is difficult to assess in Haiti, where infant death due to diarrheal disease has long been commonplace.

In summary, large numbers of Haitians have been exposed to HIV. The speed of spread has been great indeed: stored blood samples from 1977–79 were found to be free of HIV. Since then, most of the tested populations without a single seropositive adult have been small cohorts of rural Haitians. The only other completely seropositive results have been for a group of health care workers and a series of adults from relatively privileged backgrounds, which has led some observers to question the conclusion, advanced early in the epidemic, that Haitians from all economic backgrounds were equally vulnerable to AIDS. As Johnson and Pape concluded, "Collectively, these data indicate that HIV infection is widespread and more prevalent in urban areas and in lower socioeconomic groups."[30] It is precisely this group of people—poor city dwellers—who were most at risk during the early years of the epidemic. They remain more vulnerable than their wealthy counterparts both to HIV infection and to virtually every other infectious disease known in Haiti.

HAITI AND THE "ACCEPTED RISK FACTORS"

In Haiti, the epidemiological questions were the same as those posed in other nations that were the focus of the AIDS pandemic: Who is at risk for acquiring HIV infection? How is the virus transmitted? To what extent has it spread in groups engaging in "high-risk behaviors"? A good deal of evidence indicates that answers to these questions have changed through the years. The initial research had identified none of the "accepted risk factors"—homosexuality, bisexuality, intravenous drug use, a history of transfusion, and hemophilia—in the vast majority of Haitian Americans with AIDS.[31] In Haiti, however, risk factors often were identified, although the specific factors deemed important have changed over the years.

Spurred by calls for careful research that could answer the questions raised at the 1983 conference, the GHESKIO investigators began to gather much more information from each new patient in an effort to identify activities or events that could have led to HIV exposure. Unfortunately, questions pertaining to sexual history were not standardized, and little effort was made to gather ethnographic data that might have complemented information garnered in the clinic. However, when Pape developed a standardized questionnaire, which he and the GHESKIO physicians began to administer in July 1983, they discovered that they were able to identify "accepted risk factors" in the majority of cases. Data on the first thirty-four patients were presented at a conference in Washington the following summer (see table 3.4).

When comparing the GHESKIO data with reports concerning Haitian Americans with AIDS, the most striking revelation was that fully 50 percent of the men interviewed in Haiti had a history of sexual relations with men. None of them, however, were exclusively homosexual: "The fact that all the male AIDS patients who have had sex with men are bisexual would also provide greater opportunity for heterosexual transmission of AIDS in Haiti. This also may contribute to the finding that 21 percent of our Haitian AIDS patients are women, as compared with only 7 percent in the United States."[32] Pape and his team also reported that half of the women patients had received a blood transfusion in the five years before the onset of symptoms, and the researchers observed that Haitian women are more likely to receive blood—often in the course of an obstetrical intervention—than are Haitian men.

Do these data, which clearly demonstrate "accepted risk factors" in a majority of those studied, suggest that transmission in Haiti was occurring through the same mechanisms that had been elucidated in the United States? To determine the significance of presumed risk factors, the researchers initiated a control study with an ambitious design: "Each of the most recent 36 AIDS patients was asked to provide three "healthy" persons to serve as controls. The controls included a

Table 3.4 Risk Factors in Thirty-Four Patients, 1983–84

	Males (N = 26)		Females (N = 8)	
Bisexual contact	13	(50%)	0	
Blood transfusion	3	(11%)	4	(50%)
IV drug abuse	1	(4%)	0	
Spouse with AIDS	0		1	(12%)
None apparent	9	(35%)	3	(38%)

SOURCE: Pape et al., "Risk Factors Associated with AIDS in Haiti."

sibling of the same sex closest in age to the patient, a friend of the same sex who shared social activities, and a current or recent sexual partner."[33]

Despite the audacity of this request, Pape's patients complied by recruiting twenty siblings, twenty friends, and twenty sexual partners. It is interesting that all the patients—including the men who had histories of homosexual contact—provided "current or recent sexual partners" of the opposite sex. Among the risk factors studied were blood transfusions, the use of parenteral medications, and frequency of "heterosexual promiscuity" (arbitrarily defined as more than twelve different partners during the six months preceding onset of their illness).

Early in the epidemic, researchers had noted another potential mode of transmission of HIV: the use of contaminated needles. In Haiti, intramuscular injections may be given either by medical personnel or, in areas without access to medical facilities, by those known as "injectionists." Disposable needles and syringes, not readily available in Haiti, are frequently reused without sterilization. Pape and colleagues found that, during the five-year period before the onset of AIDS symptoms, 83 percent of male and 88 percent of female AIDS patients had received parenteral medications.[34] Although these figures are suggestive, more than 67 percent of the controls (seronegative siblings and friends) also reported having had injections in the preceding five years, implying that other factors were involved in HIV transmission.

Because homosexual contact was already a documented risk factor, researchers hypothesized that an additional factor might be the number of opposite-sex partners. The female siblings and friends had a mean of one sex partner per year during the five years preceding the study and an HIV seroprevalence rate of 9 percent. Male siblings and friends, in contrast, had six or seven opposite-sex partners annually and a seroprevalence of 22 percent. Although the numbers are small and the sample was not random, these figures corroborate the initial impressions of those studying the epidemic: urban Haitian men seemed to have significantly more sexual partners than urban women did, suggesting a greater role for men in the spread of HIV. The predominantly male role would be further

Table 3.5 AIDS Cases Diagnosed by the Haitian Study Group on
Kaposi's Sarcoma and Opportunistic Infections (GHESKIO), 1979–87

	Kaposi's Sarcoma	Opportunistic Infection	Total
1979	2	0	2
1980	2	5	7
1981	7	9	16
1982	5	35	40
1983	8	53	61
1984	11	103	114
1985	8	136	144
1986	10	160	170
1987	8	159	167
Total	61	660	721

SOURCES: Pape et al., "Characteristics of the Acquired Immunodeficiency
Syndrome (AIDS) in Haiti"; Pape et al., "The Acquired Immunodeficiency Syndrome in Haiti"; Johnson and Pape, "AIDS in Haiti."

amplified if the viral agent were more easily transmitted from male to female
than from female to male.[35]

Based on the control study initiated in 1983, the GHESKIO team initially concluded that "accepted risk factors" were present in more than two-thirds of the
Haitians diagnosed with AIDS. This figure was compared to those published in
reports from the United States, where only 6 percent of Haitian Americans with
AIDS "were bisexual" and only 1 percent used intravenous drugs. As Pape and
coworkers later observed, "the disparity in the data from the United States and
Haiti may be attributable, in part, to a greater willingness of Haitians to provide
reliable responses to personal questions in their native country and language."[36]

The patterns that had emerged in the first control-study cohort were soon
shown to be shifting. Indeed, the Haitian epidemic was changing. Most striking
was the changing incidence of opportunistic infections versus Kaposi's sarcoma
in Haitians with AIDS; this shift in clinical features is illustrated in table 3.5. The
percentage of AIDS patients with Kaposi's decreased from 15 percent of the cases
that occurred before and in 1984 to 5 percent of the cases in 1986–88.

Important shifts were also evident in the sex distribution of persons with
AIDS in Haiti. An overwhelming majority of the early patients had been men,
but the percentage of women among the GHESKIO patients was increasing with
each passing year, as indicated in table 3.6.

In addition to the diminished sex differences in the incidence of AIDS, more
and more patients were denying that their personal histories included "accepted
risk factors." Risk factors were noted in only 20 percent of the first Haitian cohort

Table 3.6 Sex Distribution of Patients with AIDS in Urban Haiti

	Female Patients (N)	Total Patients (N)	% Female Patients
1979–82	10	65	15
1983–85	86	319	27
1986–88	144	458	31

SOURCE: Marie-Marcelle Deschamps, personal communication to the author, 1989.

(before 1983) because, it was hypothesized, a standardized approach to these questions had not been applied. In a second cohort (1983–84), researchers identified risk factors in a majority of patients. Of the men, 50 percent had histories of sexual contact with both men and women. However, only 11 percent of the 170 male and female patients who were diagnosed with AIDS in or after 1986 reported bisexuality, blood transfusions, or intravenous drug use.

The changing significance of these risk factors was reflected in the control study, in which a total of 384 persons with AIDS (278 male and 106 female) have been evaluated, along with 174 of their heterosexual sex partners and 224 of their siblings and friends. Among the sex-matched siblings, none of whom had been transfused and all of whom denied bisexuality, 17 percent were seropositive. Sex differences in this group were not striking: 19 percent of the brothers were seropositive, as were 14 percent of the sisters. Among 108 of the patients' sex-matched friends, none of the women screened were seropositive, whereas 26 percent of the men were. All but 5 percent of the male friends screened denied homosexuality or bisexuality; all of those who had same-sex sexual relations were seropositive. Blood transfusion seemed to be a less important mode of transmission as the epidemic progressed: 2 percent of male and 3 percent of female respondents had received transfusions during the preceding five years, and none of them were seropositive.

Finally, 55 percent of 174 regular sexual partners or spouses of AIDS patients had antibodies to HIV: 61 percent of male partners and 54 percent of female partners. Only 3 percent and 6 percent of the male and female partners, respectively, had received a transfusion, and neither group reported bisexuality or intravenous drug use. Study of the regular sexual partners of Haitians with AIDS underlined the disturbing proposition that AIDS was becoming "just another" sexually transmitted disease, but still there were no data to suggest *efficient* female-to-male transmission of HIV.

In summary, then, the relative number of Haitians with AIDS reporting a history of transfusion or same-sex contact has decreased markedly.[37] The GHESKIO clinic has seen a marked increase in the percentage of patients who have a spouse

Table 3.7 Risk Factors in 559 Haitian AIDS Patients

	1983 ($N = 38$)	1984 ($N = 104$)	1985 ($N = 132$)	1986 ($N = 185$)	1987 ($N = 100$)	Total ($N = 559$)
Bisexual contact	50%	27%	8%	4%	1%	13%
Blood transfusion	23%	12%	8%	7%	10%	10%
Intravenous drug use	1%	1%	1%	0%	1%	1%
Heterosexual contact	5%	6%	14%	16%	15%	13%
Undetermined	21%	54%	69%	73%	73%	64%

SOURCE: Pape and Johnson, "Epidemiology of AIDS in the Caribbean," p. 37.

or regular sexual partner with AIDS, a history of prostitution, or none of the accepted "risk factors." When data from the various "phases" of the epidemic are considered together, it appears that "accepted risk factors" could be identified for only 20 percent of Haitians with AIDS at the outset of the epidemic. A couple of years later, risk factors were reported in a majority of Haitians with AIDS, but by 1986 the number of patients with these risk factors began to decrease. The shape of this curve, which hints at a rise and fall of the importance of bisexual contact, is in all probability an artifact of research design. It is far more likely that preliminary low rates of detection of bisexual contact (and perhaps transfusion) resulted from the stigmatization of homosexuality and from nonstandardized approaches to eliciting the data.[38]

A more probable curve would be one that reveals a high prevalence, among the first Haitians with AIDS, of "accepted risk factors"—that is, the "North American/European" risk factors identified by the CDC. Of all these factors, bisexual activity was by far the most significant in Haiti. With the passage of time, however, it has become increasingly clear that AIDS can be heterosexually transmitted, especially from men to women. By 1988, heterosexual transmission was presumed in 16 percent of patients who were female prostitutes or in those who had a spouse with AIDS; it is a probable source of infection in the patients who deny all other "accepted risk factors." By 1986, as table 3.7 indicates, these patients represented more than 70 percent of Haitian AIDS cases. Additional evidence for heterosexual transmission of HIV is the finding that more than half of 139 Haitian prostitutes in the Port-au-Prince area were seropositive: the rate of seropositivity increased from 49 percent in 1985 to 66 percent in 1986.[39]

The data from Haiti do not offer strong support for *efficient* female-to-male transmission, although this route is clearly not trivial: if bisexuality is decreasingly common and yet HIV seropositivity continues to increase among men, women are necessarily a source as well as a "sink" for infection. The conclusions we can draw from these studies are important: HIV is heterosexually transmitted, but it is much more efficiently transmitted from male to female than vice versa. At this writing, heterosexual transmission is thought to account for the majority of Haitian AIDS cases, and cases associated with perinatal transmission are increasing at a rate greater than that of the epidemic in general. In Haiti, AIDS is afflicting increasing numbers of women, and especially poor women.

AIDS IN THE CARIBBEAN:
THE "WEST ATLANTIC PANDEMIC"

The history of the Haitian AIDS epidemic is brief and devastating. Less than two decades ago, HIV may not have been present in the country. Now, complications of HIV infection are among the leading causes of death in urban Haiti. How are other Caribbean islands affected? Is Haiti, as some believe, an AIDS-ridden pocket in an otherwise low-prevalence region? Answering these questions is no mean task, as Pape and Johnson explain:

> First, in many countries there is no registry system for AIDS and it was only in 1984 that most nations started reporting cases to [the Pan American Health Organization]. Secondly, the widely used CDC case definition for AIDS is inappropriate for defining tropical AIDS and requires sophisticated laboratory support that is not readily available in most countries. In our experience in Haiti, the new CDC case definition for AIDS, which relies more on HIV testing and clinical presentation, should increase the actual number of reported cases by at least 30 percent.[40]

Given the extreme poverty of Haiti, it is ironic that Haitians with AIDS stand a better chance of an adequate medical workup than the citizens of several other Caribbean nations. Although Haiti has the weakest health infrastructure in the region, it has had the largest number of cases, received the greatest amount of international scrutiny as "the source of AIDS," and sustained the most substantial economic blows, relative to gross national product (GNP). Perhaps in part as a result of these negative forces, many Haitian physicians and researchers have been involved in the professional response to the epidemic. Haitians publish more HIV-related studies than researchers in other Caribbean countries, and the GHESKIO-run national laboratories are experienced in AIDS diagnosis.

With this in mind, what do we know about the contours of the Caribbean pandemic? All of what are termed "the Caribbean basin countries" have reported AIDS cases to the Pan American Health Organization (PAHO). Among the islands, Haiti, the Dominican Republic, Trinidad and Tobago, and the Bahamas account for 82 percent of all cases reported to PAHO between the recognized onset of the epidemic and September 1987. Haiti reported the largest number of cases in the Caribbean region, which at first appears to lend credence to the widely shared belief that citizens of the nation are somehow uniquely susceptible to AIDS. When the number of cases is standardized to reflect per capita caseload, however, the uniqueness of Haiti disappears: the attack rate is actually lower in Haiti than it is in several other countries in the region.[41]

During the twelve months preceding September 1987, the number of reported Caribbean cases doubled, with the largest rates of increase occurring in Barbados, Jamaica, Martinique, Guadeloupe, French Guiana, the U.S. Virgin Islands, and Grenada. The epidemic in the Dominican Republic continues to grow: although no cases were reported in 1983, 62 were reported in the subsequent two years. During 1986, the number of Dominican cases more than doubled, and as of the end of 1989, 856 cases had been reported to PAHO.

What has been the nature of HIV transmission in these countries? As noted earlier, many public health specialists speak of the entire Caribbean basin as an example of Pattern II, which differs from Pattern I "in that heterosexual intercourse has been the dominant mode of HIV transmission *from the start . . .* [and] homosexuality generally plays a minor role in this pattern" (emphasis added).[42] But the preceding review of the data from Haiti suggests that this WHO terminology obscures more than it illuminates. First, although "the start" was never accurately documented, it seems clear that same-sex relations between men played a crucial role in the Haitian epidemic. Second, the WHO scheme underlines similarities between Haiti and Africa, comparisons that unfortunately tend to draw attention away from the history of the Caribbean pandemic, which is in fact much more intimately related to the North American epidemic. Third, the WHO scheme is static, whereas the Haitian epidemic has been rapidly changing. Data from other Caribbean countries indicate that the WHO terminology is equally inappropriate there and that the patterns seen in Haiti are similar to those in other countries in the region.

The data provided in table 3.8 suggest that homosexual contact has also played an important role in other Caribbean islands. "For these homosexuals," Pape and Johnson write, in reference to gay men in Jamaica, the Dominican Republic, and Trinidad, "sexual contact with American homosexuals rather than promiscuity per se appeared to be associated with increased risk of infection."[43] An important study of Trinidad bolsters this conclusion. The first case of AIDS in the West Indies was reported in that country in February 1983. Since then, the number of cases has risen steadily, leaving Trinidad with one of the highest attack rates in the Americas. In a 1987 study, Courtenay Bartholomew and coworkers compared the epidemiological correlates of infection with two retroviruses: HTLV and HIV. Infection with the former virus, thought to be long endemic in the Caribbean, was significantly associated with age, African descent, number of lifetime sexual partners, and duration of homosexuality. In sharp contrast, "age and race were not associated with HIV seropositivity. The major risk factor for HIV seropositiv-

Table 3.8 HIV Seroprevalence among Caribbean Homosexuals and Bisexuals

	Jamaica 1986		Dominican Republic 1985		Trinidad[a]	
	N	% HIV+	N	% HIV+	N	% HIV+
Homosexual/bisexual	125	10.0	46	17.0	106	40.0
Controls	4,000	0	306	2.6	983	0.2

SOURCE: Pape and Johnson, "Epidemiology of AIDS in the Caribbean."

[a] For Trinidad, information about the control group was gathered in 1982; figures for the homosexual/bisexual group are from 1983–84.

ity was homosexual contact with a partner from a foreign country, primarily the United States. Duration of homosexuality and number of lifetime partners were not significantly associated with HIV seropositivity."[44] The Haitian experience would suggest that Trinidad can expect the relative significance of sexual contact with a North American gay man to decrease, as other risk factors—most notably, high numbers of partners—become preeminent.[45]

A similar risk factor was observed in the Dominican Republic, where Haitians, long despised in this neighboring country, have come under even heavier fire as "AIDS carriers." Yet studies reveal high seroprevalence among homosexual/bisexual male prostitutes living in the tourist areas of the country: 10 percent in Santiago and 19 percent in Puerto Plata. "Tourists, and not Haitians, were the most likely source of virus transmission to Dominicans, because contact occurs frequently between tourists (e.g., male homosexuals) and Dominicans but rarely between Haitians and Dominicans."[46] Further, the epidemiology of HIV in the Dominican Republic may resemble that in Haiti even more than the Trinidadian epidemiology does. R. Ellen Koenig and coworkers underline the role of economically driven prostitution among young Dominican men who consider themselves heterosexual: "Persons who engage in homosexual acts only to earn money usually consider themselves heterosexual. This situation, public health workers have indicated, is particularly prevalent in the tourist areas with young adolescents. It could explain our finding of three positive serum samples in schoolchildren from Santo Domingo."[47]

Together, these data suggest that many of the forces that have helped to shape the Haitian epidemic have been economic and historical: sufficient data now exist to support the assertion that economically motivated male prostitution, catering to a North American clientele, played a major role in the introduction of HIV to Haiti. Why might Haiti be particularly vulnerable to the commodification of sexuality? It is almost a cliché now to note that Haiti is the poorest country in the hemisphere, and one of the twenty-five poorest in the world. A per capita annual income of $315 in 1983 masks the fact that annual income hovered around $50 in the countryside. In a country as poor as Haiti, AIDS might be thought of as an occupational hazard for workers in the tourist industry. A similar observation could be made concerning several other Caribbean nations.

Tourists' attitudes toward Haiti throughout the first half of the twentieth century are nicely summarized by Frank Carpenter, whose guidebook to the Caribbean qualifies Haitian culture as "a deplorable and almost unbelievable mixture of barbaric customs and African traditions."[48] Later, in a slightly different atmosphere, Haiti's "exoticism" could be peddled as an attraction. Tourism began in 1949, when Port-au-Prince celebrated its bicentennial with the inauguration of the "Cité de l'Exposition," a long stretch of modern buildings built on the reclaimed swampy waterfront of the capital. The country had approximately 20,000 visitors that year, and slightly fewer in 1950 and 1951. During the first half of the 1950s, approximately 250,000 tourists spent an average of three days and $105 in Haiti—bringing in approximately 25 percent of Haiti's foreign currency.[49]

There was every sign that the gains in tourism would be steady, but political instability in 1957, followed by the tyrannical rule of François Duvalier, meant that North Americans avoided Haiti for several years.[50] Duvalier attempted to court tourists and their dollars later in the 1960s, after he had silenced domestic opposition. In the same speech in which he welcomed U.S. vice president Nelson Rockefeller to Haiti and promoted the country as an ideal site for U.S. assembly plants, Duvalier proposed that "Haiti could be a great land of relaxation for the American middle class—it is close, beautiful, and politically stable."[51]

By 1970, the annual number of visitors was close to 100,000; not counting brief layovers and "afternoon dockings," the annual tally had risen to 143,538 by 1979. Club Méditerranée opened its doors the following year.[52] It seemed as if tourism had arrived. Indeed, it was predicted that the industry would soon supplant coffee and the offshore assembly plants as the capital's chief source of foreign exchange. But the effects of the "AIDS scare" were dramatic and prompt: the Haitian Bureau of Tourism estimated a decline from 75,000 visitors in the winter of 1981–82 to fewer than 10,000 the following year. "Already suffering from an image problem, Haiti has been made an international pariah by AIDS," concluded one 1983 report. "Boycotted by tourists and investors, it has lost millions of dollars and hundreds of jobs at a time when half the work force is jobless. Even exports are being shunned by some."[53]

Tourism did bring something of lasting significance, however: institutionalized prostitution. And as Haiti became poorer, both men and women became cheaper. Although no quantitative studies of Haitian urban prostitution have been conducted, it is clear that a substantial sector of the trade catered to tourists, and especially to North Americans. As one physician-author put it, "this country had—as far as promiscuity was concerned—replaced Cuba."[54]

A portion of the tourist industry catered specifically to a gay clientele, and it was not long before interviews with Haitians suffering from AIDS revealed sexual contact with gay men from North America. In a key paper published in 1984, Jean-Michel Guérin and coworkers from Haiti, North America, and Canada state that "17 percent of our patients had sexual contact with [North] American tourists."[55] During the AMH-sponsored conference in 1983, one Haitian American researcher read aloud from the pages of the 1983 *Spartacus International Gay Guide,* in which Haiti was enthusiastically recommended to the gay tourist: handsome men with "a great ability to satisfy" are readily available, but "there is no free sex in Haiti, except with other gay tourists you may come across. Your partners will expect to be paid for their services but the charges are nominal." Another advertisement, which ran in *The Advocate* ("The National Gay News Magazine"), assured the prospective tourist that Haiti is "a place where all your fantasies come true."[56]

Of course, the existence of sexual tourism, some of it gay, does not prove that this commerce was in any way related to the Haitian AIDS epidemic. It does, however, symbolize the ties between Haiti and nearby North America—ties that did not find their way into early discussions of AIDS among Haitians. In fact, a review of even the scholarly literature on Haiti leaves one with the impression that the country is the most "isolated" or "insular" of Caribbean countries. In an assessment resonant with the AIDS-related speculations of the U.S. medical community, the author of one standard text remarks that "Haiti in 1950 was in general what it had been in 1900: a preindustrial society inhabited by ignorant, diseased peasants oblivious to the outside world."[57]

But a study of Haiti's economy reveals that the nation has long been closely tied to the United States. In fact, Haiti plays an interesting role in the "West Atlantic system," an economic network encompassing much of the Caribbean basin and centered in the United States. Haiti's position in this network was secured during the U.S. military occupation of the country, which began in 1915: "The Occupation also secured a niche for Haiti in the emerging West Atlantic system. As the amount of cultivatable land continued to drop, peasants began to swell the ranks of the reserve armies of Port-au-Prince, North America, and neighboring Caribbean countries. When a pliant dictator could assure a favorable economic setting . . . the United States began installing, or helping local entrepreneurs to install, offshore assembly plants in Port-au-Prince."[58]

By 1978, exports from offshore assembly operations had surpassed even coffee in importance. The World Bank and the U.S. Embassy estimate that as of 1980 there were approximately 220 assembly plants employing some sixty thousand persons. These factories were (and are) all located in the capital. "Assuming a dependency ratio of 4 to 1," add Joseph Grunwald, Leslie Delatour, and Karl Voltaire, "this means that assembly operations supported about one-quarter of the population of Port-au-Prince in 1980."[59] The population of Port-au-Prince, a city approximately ten times larger than the country's second-largest city, doubled in size between 1970 and 1984. Many of the newcomers had been lured by the false promise of jobs in the tourist industry or the assembly plants. Kenneth Boodhoo remarks that in 1978, "unemployment remained (almost unbelievably) in the 70–80 percent range."[60]

The Caribbean nations with high attack rates of AIDS are all part of the West Atlantic system. A relation between the degree of involvement in this network and the prevalence of AIDS is reflected in the following exercise. Excluding Puerto Rico, which is not an independent country, the five Caribbean basin nations with the largest numbers of cases by 1986 were the Dominican Republic, the Bahamas, Trinidad and Tobago, Mexico, and Haiti. In terms of trade, which five countries are the most dependent on the United States? Export indices offer a convenient marker of involvement in the West Atlantic system. In both 1983 and 1977, the years for which data are available, the five countries with the greatest economic ties to the United States were precisely those with the largest numbers of AIDS cases. The country with the largest number of AIDS cases, Haiti, was also the country most dependent on U.S. exports. In the entire Caribbean basin, only Puerto Rico is more economically dependent on the United States, and only Puerto Rico has reported more cases of AIDS to the Pan American Health Organization.

To understand the West Atlantic AIDS pandemic, a historical understanding of the worldwide spread of HIV is crucial. Jacques Leibowitch's fascinating sketch of the history of a related virus is suggestive: "The map of HTLV in the New World is that of the African diaspora."[61] Because he refers to the massive dislocations of Africans through the slave trade, another way of stating this relationship would be that the map of HTLV in the New World is the map of European expansionist imperialism. An analogous observation holds for the even more recently recognized virus: the map of HIV in the New World reflects to an important extent the geography of North American neocolonialism. That these considerations are lineaments of the American epidemics is suggested by comparing Haiti with a neighboring island. In Haiti, several epidemiological studies of asymptomatic city dwellers reveal HIV seroprevalence rates of approximately 9 percent. In 1986 in Cuba, only 0.01 percent of a million persons tested were found to have antibodies to HIV.[62] Had the pandemic begun a few decades earlier, the epidemiology of HIV infection in the Caribbean might well be different. Havana might have been as much an epicenter of the pandemic as Carrefour.

CONCLUSIONS

The occurrence of a "mysterious new disease" in Haitians resonated with an existing stock of imagery: haggard refugees, barbaric rituals, poverty, and hunger. In her study of Haiti after Duvalier, North American journalist Amy Wilentz highlights the power of these images and the place of AIDS among them:

> If Duvalier left it would be big news. Family in power for thirty years. Bloodthirsty dictatorship. Fall of the Tontons Macoutes. Beautiful wife flees with millions in jewels. Chaos in the streets. All this, added to the regular Haitian features, made the editors back in the world's capitals salivate: Plenty amid poverty. ("Great.") Voodoo's hold on the peasantry. Voodoo's hold on the elite? ("Maybe. How do we illustrate it, though? That's my problem. You see?") Voodoo and the Catholic Church. Just plain voodoo. ("Yeah, uh-huh. Good idea. Great pictures.") Deforestation. ("Can we get art? I mean, face it. Tree stumps. Do they read?") Drought? Boat People. ("Get me those bodies that washed up in Florida. Who took those pictures?") A refrigerated suite in the palace where wife and friends store their furs. ("Yeah, but has anyone ever *seen* it?") And now AIDS. The best.[63]

Whether for the popular press or for medical journals, AIDS in Haitians made great copy—but only when AIDS was linked to the exotic. Given the publication dates of the early reports on AIDS in Haiti, it is puzzling that "exotic theories" regarding Haitians have continued to receive so much play in the scientific and popular presses of North America. The persistence of these theories represents, in fact, a systematic misreading of existing epidemiological data. Careful study of the hypotheses surfacing in the scientific sector reveals that they are not very different from the popular semantic network that surrounds the label "Haitian." Historical regard points out the importance of racism and voodoo to this associative network. Even cannibalism, the most popular nineteenth-century smear, was resuscitated during discussions of Haiti's role in the AIDS pandemic.

That these referents continue to play important roles in determining the boundaries and content of a North American semantic network about Haiti is evident in a popular 1990 novel. In *Mile Zero,* set in Key West in the not-so-distant past, we learn that there is "some weird stuff going down in town," and that "ever since the last boatload of Haitian refugees came in it's been getting weirder."[64] The novel describes a boat full of Haitians who had perished in their efforts to escape the violent misery of their home country. In one scene, a policeman appears on television, fielding questions from reporters: "There's no proof of cannibalism on this boat. I don't know where that rumor got started. These people died of exposure, starvation and drinking seawater. There will be an investigation. Yes, one survivor. No, I already told you, no signs of cannibalism have been exhibited on any bodies."[65]

The one survivor is Voltaire Tincourette, a peasant who is taken off the boat, clutching an amulet, and is dispatched to an Immigration and Naturalization Service detention camp on the edge of the Everglades. Voltaire hails from the southern mountains of Haiti: "*Paysans* up there have really been isolated, more African than Haitian," announces the book's protagonist. "Very superstitious people," he adds, in response to his interlocutor's whistled "*Grande* voodoo."[66]

The Africa-Haiti connection is underlined by an omniscient narrator, who appears to be the Devil. He too is Haitian, and he offers the following warning: "Do you see the green monkey grinning in Africa, high in the tree? The green monkey has a secret he shares with me and withholds from you."[67] It seems that the reader is to infer that the monkey also shared, through unspecified routes, his secret with Voltaire.

Voltaire and another Haitian, Hippolyte, escape from the camp and flee on foot until Voltaire is struck by a car and killed. His autopsy is recalled in the context of other medical examinations of the inmates:

> They found some men had yaws, a flesh-rotting disease the United Nations claims had been wiped out. They found something else, a lingering pneumonia which wastes a person away. The pneumonia is linked to a virus in Africa, started as a green monkey or something, nobody knows for certain, so it doesn't have a name. Immigrant Haitians have the highest chance of developing it, except for homosexuals. The doctors had no idea how many men in camp were homosexuals, they know to a man how many were recent arrivals from Haiti. They asked permission to run tests on blood from Voltaire's body. He had the green monkey virus, they figured Hippolyte had it too.[68]

These excerpts offer a classic example of the network of meanings evoked, in the United States, at the mention of Haiti. The story of Voltaire is a more florid version of the pseudoscientific hypotheses of Alexander Moore and Ronald LeBaron,[69] cited earlier, as well as many others. All these speculations resemble one another; they do not resemble what is known about HIV and AIDS in Haiti and among Haitian Americans. It is precisely individuals like Voltaire Tincourette—"*Paysans* up there [who] have really been isolated"—who have *not* been exposed to HIV.

AIDS in Haiti is not so mysterious after all. It is, in some senses, rather mundane. Much is made in the public health literature of the similarities between the Haitian and the African AIDS epidemics, but the Haitian epidemic is representative of the Western Hemisphere. Indeed, the entire Caribbean pandemic is derivative of the North American and European pandemic, and it began in communities related to the "outside world," most notably gay and bisexual men and others related to the tourist industry. With the exception of intravenous drug users and hemophiliacs, the North American and European pandemic has thus far been, to some extent, contained in the gay/bisexual population. In Haiti, a host of forces conspired to decrease the efficacy of preventive programs, and HIV began to spread rapidly through the heterosexual population, especially to women and children.

The Haitian epidemic tells a changing story. The current chapters of this tale are about sexually active men, who transmit HIV to women far more efficiently than women can infect them. The chapters to come will be about their suffering, compounded by wretched poverty, and about the infected babies born to these women. But the ongoing story of AIDS in Haiti will always have a beginning. AIDS in Haiti is about proximity rather than distance. AIDS in Haiti is a tale of ties to the United States, rather than to Africa; it is a story of unemployment rates greater than 70 percent. AIDS in Haiti has more to do with tourism and trade in a dirt-poor country than with the bloody bodies of chickens sacrificed in voodoo rituals.

NOTES

1. Cited in Abbott, *Haiti*, pp. 254–55.

2. Bruce Chabner of the National Cancer Institute, cited in the *Miami News*, December 2, 1982, p. 8A.

3. Gilman, "AIDS and Syphilis," p. 102.

4. Farmer, "AIDS and Accusation."

5. See Lawless, *Haiti's Bad Press*.

6. Moses and Moses, "Haiti and the Acquired Immune Deficiency Syndrome." Peter Moses and John Moses also made the following, apparently offhand, comment: "If the syndrome originates in rural people, *and it seems likely that it does,* it occurs among those who have had little or no direct or indirect contact with Port-au-Prince or other urban areas" ("Haiti and the Acquired Immune Deficiency Syndrome"; emphasis added).

7. Greenfield, "Night of the Living Dead II," p. 2200.

8. Moore and LeBaron, "The Case for a Haitian Origin of the AIDS Epidemic," pp. 81, 84.

9. Lorch, "F.D.A. Policy to Limit Blood Is Protested."

10. Lambert, "Now, No Haitians Can Donate Blood."

11. Osborn, "Public Health and the Politics of AIDS Prevention," p. 126.

12. Centers for Disease Control and Prevention, "*Pneumocystis* Pneumonia—Los Angeles."

13. Liautaud et al., "Le sarcôme de Kaposi en Haïti."

14. Some oncologists suspect that Kaposi's sarcoma is somehow related to previous infection with cytomegalovirus. For a review of these data, see Groopman, "Viruses and Human Neoplasia." For a study revealing a lack of association between cytomegalovirus and endemic Kaposi's, see Ambinder et al., "Lack of Association of Cytomegalovirus with Endemic African Kaposi's Sarcoma."

15. Guérin et al., "Acquired Immune Deficiency Syndrome."

16. Pape et al., "Characteristics of the Acquired Immunodeficiency Syndrome (AIDS) in Haiti," p. 949.

17. Ibid., p. 948.

18. In another review, Jean Pape and Warren Johnson state that "in 1983, the majority of male patients with AIDS were bisexuals who had at least one sexual encounter with visiting North Americans or Haitians residing in North America" ("Epidemiology of AIDS in the Caribbean," p. 32).

19. The Collaborative Study Group of AIDS in Haitian-Americans ("Risk Factors for AIDS among Haitians Residing in the United States") was similarly unable to find a single Haitian with AIDS who had a history of residence or travel in Africa.

20. Guérin et al., "Acquired Immune Deficiency Syndrome." See also Johnson and Pape, "AIDS in Haiti."

21. Johnson and Pape, "AIDS in Haiti," p. 67. The advent of antibody tests put an end to suggestions that malnutrition or some other disorder was masquerading as AIDS: fully 96 percent of the clinically diagnosed AIDS patients were found to be seropositive for HIV (ibid.).

22. Ibid.

23. For example, in a letter responding to the 1983 article by Pape and coworkers in the *New England Journal of Medicine* (Pape et al., "Characteristics of the Acquired Immunodeficiency Syndrome [AIDS] in Haiti"), two researchers from Yale University suggested that "Pape et al. do not convincingly exclude malnutrition as a cause of immune deficiency and opportunistic infection in the patients described" (Mellors and Barry, "Malnutrition or AIDS in Haiti?" p. 1119). An earlier letter to the same journal suggested that "malnutrition is likely to be present in Haitians recently immigrated to Europe, Canada, or the United States," which might explain AIDS in Haitian infants (Goudsmit, "Malnutrition and Concomitant Herpesvirus Infection as a Possible Cause of Immunodeficiency Syndrome in Haitian Infants," p. 554). The theory was echoed in Beach and Laura, "Nutrition and the Acquired Immunodeficiency Syndrome." These letters, unaccompanied by new data, reflect not only a poor understanding of the sociology of Haitian malnutrition and of Haitian outmigration but also the willingness of medical journals to publish AIDS-related speculations.

24. This is the thesis argued by Jacques Leibowitch (*A Strange Virus of Unknown Origin*).

25. Halsey, Boulos, and Brutus, "HIV Antibody Prevalence in Pregnant Haitian Women."

26. Brutus, "Séroprevalence de HIV parmi les femmes enceintes à Cité Soleil, Haiti."

27. Brutus, "Problèmes d'éthique liés au dépistage du virus HIV-1."

28. Johnson and Pape, "AIDS in Haiti," p. 69.

29. Pape and Johnson, "Epidemiology of AIDS in the Caribbean."

30. Johnson and Pape, "AIDS in Haiti," p. 70.

31. The literature regarding Haitians residing in the United States is reviewed in Farmer, "AIDS and Accusation."

32. Pape et al., "Risk Factors Associated with AIDS in Haiti," p. 7.

33. Ibid.

34. Pape et al., "The Acquired Immunodeficiency Syndrome in Haiti."

35. An analogous mode of transmission has been described for HTLV-1, a retrovirus closely related to HIV, for which female-to-male transmission is thought to occur rarely, if at all (Kajiyama et al., "Intrafamilial Transmission of Adult T-Cell Leukemia Virus"; Murphy et al., "Sexual Transmission of Human T-Lymphotropic Virus Type I (HTLV-I)"). There are other reasons to believe that HIV is more efficiently transmitted from men to women. HIV is concentrated in seminal fluid, but it is often difficult to isolate in vaginal secretions. It is important to note that, when male ejaculate is compared to vaginal secretions, inoculum size is of course different by several orders of magnitude. In a 1990 colloquium, Dr. Andrew Moss, director of the Department of AIDS Epidemiology at San Francisco General Hospital, observed that women are ten times more likely than men to become infected upon sexual exposure to HIV: "It worries me that the number of sexual partners is a risk factor for transmission [even among those who use intravenous drugs], and it worries me that the rate is twice as high in women as in men because this indicates that heterosexual transmission, not needle sharing, is responsible for new infections" (cited in Harvard AIDS Institute, "HAI Forum Panelists Debate the True Numbers of the AIDS Epidemic," p. 5).

36. Pape et al., "Risk Factors Associated with AIDS in Haiti," p. 6.

37. In Haiti, the decreasing *relative* significance of same-sex contacts in the spread of HIV is the cause, it seems, for a decreasing incidence of Kaposi's sarcoma. Among North Americans with AIDS, Kaposi's sarcoma is seen most frequently among gay men (rather than among drug users, for example), especially those with histories of repeated exposure to cytomegalovirus.

38. It is not my intention to suggest that homosexuality is more stigmatized in Haiti than in other parts of Latin America. In fact, some ethnographic studies suggest the opposite; see Murray, "A Note on Haitian Tolerance of Homosexuality." It is nonetheless true that homosexuality remains stigmatized among Haitians, wherever they live.

39. Pape and Johnson, "Epidemiology of AIDS in the Caribbean," p. 36.

40. Ibid., p. 32.

41. Lange and Jaffe, "AIDS in Haiti," p. 1410.

42. Osborn, "Public Health and the Politics of AIDS Prevention," p. 126.

43. Pape and Johnson, "Epidemiology of AIDS in the Caribbean," p. 36.

44. Bartholomew et al., "Transmission of HTLV-I and HIV among Homosexual Men in Trinidad," p. 2606.

45. This has been the case in Denmark, where sexual contact with a North American gay man, rather than promiscuity per se, was an important risk factor in the first cases of AIDS (Gerstoft et al., "The Acquired Immunodeficiency Syndrome [AIDS] in Denmark"). A similar pattern was reported in Bogotá, Colombia, where Nhora Merino and colleagues observed that "significant behavioral risk factors for HIV-1 seropositivity among this sample of Colombian homosexual men included receptive anal intercourse and, for the subgroup reporting receptive roles, contact with foreign visitors" ("HIV-1, Sexual Practices, and Contact with Foreigners in Homosexual Men in Colombia, South America," pp. 333–34).

46. Koenig et al., "Prevalence of Antibodies to the Human Immunodeficiency Virus in Dominicans and Haitians in the Dominican Republic," p. 634.

47. Ibid.

48. Carpenter, *Lands of the Caribbean*, p. 236.

49. Francisque, *La structure économique et sociale de Haïti*, p. 139.

50. The protagonist of Graham Greene's *The Comedians* is a Port-au-Prince hotelier who in 1961 remembers fondly the days when tourists flocked to his bar and made love in the pool. "The drummer's fled to New York, and all the bikini girls stay in Miami now," he explains to two prospective clients. "You'll probably be the only guests I have" (p. 11).

51. Trouillot, *Haiti, State against Nation*, p. 200.

52. Barros, *Haïti, de 1804 à nos jours*, p. 750.

53. Chaze, "In Haiti, a View of Life at the Bottom."

54. Métellus, *Haïti*, p. 90.

55. Guérin et al., "Acquired Immune Deficiency Syndrome," p. 256.

56. Cited in Moore and LeBaron, "The Case for a Haitian Origin of the AIDS Epidemic," p. 82. Stephen Murray and Kenneth Payne question the relevance of gay tourism in the Haitian AIDS epidemic: "Insofar as gay travel can be estimated from gay guidebooks, Haiti was one of the least-favored destinations in the Caribbean for gay travelers during the 1970s and the less-favored half of the island of Hispaniola" ("Medical Policy without Scientific Evidence," pp. 25–26). But their assessment is based only on "frequency of listing in gay guidebooks," surely a less significant indicator of the relevance of this type of tourism than the cluster studies that revealed direct sexual contact between Haitian men and North American gay tourists.

It is important to note that the introduction of a sexually transmitted disease need not involve some "critical mass" of sexual contact; it requires only that the disorder be introduced into a sexually active population (in this case, Haitian men), which the study by Jean-Michel Guérin and colleagues documents (Guérin et al., "Acquired Immune Deficiency Syndrome," p. 256). Interestingly, Murray and Payne cite an American journalist's interview with Guérin and not his research published in the *Annals of the New York Academy of Science:* "At the Haitian end of the hypothesized transmission vector, Dr. Jean-Michel Guérin of GHESKIO told [journalist Anne-Christine] d'Adesky . . . that all his patients—without exception—had denied having sex with tourists" (pp. 25–26). In fact, Guérin's *Annals* article, which brought together the research of ten physicians representing research centers in Haiti, the United States, and Canada, clearly specifies which patients acknowledged sexual relations with gay tourists from North America. It is thus evident that Guérin meant that these patients *initially* denied such contacts. D'Adesky's later essay underlines the sex-for-money exchanges that took place between tourists and poor Haitian men ("Silence = Death, AIDS in Haiti").

57. Langley, *The United States and the Caribbean in the Twentieth Century,* p. 175.

58. Farmer, "Blood, Sweat, and Baseballs," p. 96.

59. Grunwald, Delatour, and Voltaire, "Offshore Assembly in Haiti," p. 232.

60. Boodhoo, "The Economic Dimension of U.S.-Caribbean Policy," p. 81.

61. Leibowitch, *A Strange Virus of Unknown Origin,* p. 57.

62. Liautaud, Pape, and Pamphile, "Le sida dans les Caraïbes," p. 690.

63. Wilentz, *The Rainy Season,* pp. 22–23.

64. Sanchez, *Mile Zero,* pp. 59–60.

65. Ibid., p. 24.

66. Ibid., p. 43.

67. Ibid., p. 252.

68. Ibid., p. 323.

69. Moore and LeBaron, "The Case for a Haitian Origin of the AIDS Epidemic."

Ethnography, Social Analysis, and the Prevention of Sexually Transmitted HIV Infection among Poor Women in Haiti

(1997)

Social scientists and physicians alike have long known that the socioeconomically disadvantaged have higher rates of disease than those not hampered by such constraints. But what are the mechanisms and processes that transform social factors into personal risk? How do forces as disparate as sexism, poverty, and political violence become embodied as individual pathology? These and related questions are key not only to medical anthropology but to social theory in general.

These questions are posed acutely in considering HIV infection, now that AIDS has become a leading cause of death among young adults throughout the world. As HIV advances, it is becoming clear that, in spite of a great deal of epidemiological and ethnographic research, we do not yet understand risk and how it is structured. Who is likely to become infected with HIV? A number of trends in the pandemic undermine the falsely reassuring—and inappropriately stigmatizing—notion of discrete "risk groups" that might be identified by epidemiologists.

The increasing incidence of HIV disease among women is a case in point. In a sobering 1992 report, the United Nations observed that "for most women, the major risk factor for HIV infection is being married. Each day a further three thousand women become infected, and five hundred infected women die. Most are between 15 and 35 years old."[1]

It is not marriage itself that places women at risk, however. Throughout the world, most women with HIV infection are living in poverty. The study of the dynamics of HIV infection among poor women affords a means of examining the complex relationships among power, gender, and sexuality. To focus the earlier questions: how, precisely, do social forces (such as poverty, sexism, and other forms of discrimination) translate into risk for infection with HIV?

Although many observers would agree that such social forces are the strongest enhancers of risk for infection, the subject has been neglected in both the biomedical and anthropological literature on HIV disease, to the benefit of a narrowly behavioral and individualistic conception of risk.[2] Take, for example, a 1992 investigation of heterosexually transmitted HIV infection in what is described as "rural" Florida. The study, by Tedd Ellerbrock and colleagues, revealed that fully 5.1 percent of 1,082 women attending a public prenatal clinic in rural Florida had antibodies to HIV. What risk factors might account for such a high rate of infection? The researchers reported a statistically significant association between HIV infection and a history of using crack cocaine, having more than five sexual partners in a lifetime, or having more than two sexual partners per year of sexual activity. Also associated with seropositivity to HIV were histories of exchanging sex for money or for drugs or having sexual intercourse with a "high-risk partner." The study concludes that "in communities with a high seroprevalence of HIV, like this Florida community, a sizeable proportion of all women of reproductive age are at risk for infection through heterosexual transmission."[3]

One might argue that these are not, in fact, the most significant conclusions to be drawn from such a study. In settings with an even higher seroprevalence of HIV, such as New York City, it is now clear that not all women of reproductive age are at increased risk for HIV infection: poor women, who are usually women of color, are the ones at high risk. But nowhere in Ellerbrock's article does the word "poverty" appear, though the authors mention that, of the women who knew their incomes, more than 90 percent belonged to households earning less than $10,000 per year. Nowhere in the article do we see the word "racism," though in Florida, as elsewhere, African American and Hispanic communities bear the brunt of the epidemic. The terms "sexism," "despair," and "powerlessness" are also absent from the discussion. And yet one might as easily argue that in the setting described here, Palm Beach County—a district more notable for its harsh juxtaposition of extreme wealth and poverty than for its "rurality"—women who are "at risk" of attending a public prenatal clinic are statistically at higher risk of acquiring HIV; they are mostly unemployed women of color who are more likely to have unstable sexual unions or to exchange sex for drugs or money.

How representative of the biomedical literature is this paper, which was published in the *New England Journal of Medicine?* "To date," note Nancy Krieger and coworkers in an important review of the epidemiological literature, "only a small fraction of epidemiological research in the United States has investigated the effects of racism on health." They report a similar dearth of attention to the effects of sexism and class differences; studies that examine the conjoint influence of these social forces are (as of 1997) nonexistent.[4] Vicente Navarro, noting growing class differentials in mortality rates in the United States, has deplored the "deafening silence on this topic." In a 1994 review of changes in mortality rates, Michael Marmot observes wryly that such trends are "of much interest to demographers but, judging by papers in the major medical journals, of little interest to doctors."[5]

Why might this be so? Granted, canonical issues are pertinent in explaining the silence: most epidemiological and biomedical journals do not consider racism, sexism, and class differentials to be subjects of professional discussion. But significant theoretical and methodological difficulties also impede investigation of these issues (as does, perhaps, a sense of helplessness about the practical implications of a careful examination). Some difficulties are perennial: how broadly must we cast the net in order to capture both the large-scale forces structuring risk and the precise mechanisms by which these forces affect the lives of individuals?

A nascent anthropology of infectious disease suggests that the net must be cast widely. In a 1997 review of this subject, Marcia Inhorn and Peter Brown argue that "any anthropological study that hopes to shed light on the etiology and transmission of infectious diseases must ultimately adopt both a macrosociological perspective . . . and a microsociological perspective."[6] A decade of research on AIDS among the Haitian poor leads me to agree, and to argue for a "responsible materialist" approach to a disease that has run along the fault lines of an international order linking "remote" Haitian villages to, say, cities in the United States.[7]

Many issues of individual agency are illuminated only by examining the gritty details of biography; life stories must be embedded in ethnography if their representative quality is to emerge.[8] We must embed these local understandings, in turn, in the larger-scale historical system of which the fieldwork site is a part.[9] This approach must thus be geographically broad and historically deep and must include critical rereadings of relevant data from epidemiology, history, and political economy. Only through such a broad approach will the role of "structural violence"—the degree to which a society (itself a problematic concept, as we shall see) is characterized by economic inequity, sexism, or racism—come into view.[10]

LINKING MICRO TO MACRO

After caring for dozens of poor Haitian women with HIV disease, I can testify to the deadly monotony in their stories: young women—or teenage girls—were drawn to Port-au-Prince by the lure of an escape from the harshest poverty; once in the city, each worked as a domestic; none managed to find the financial security that had proven so elusive in the countryside. The women I interviewed were straightforward about the nonvoluntary aspect of their sexual activity: in their opinions, poverty had forced them into unfavorable unions.

Over the past several years, the medical staff of the clinic in Do Kay has diagnosed dozens of cases of HIV infection in people who have presented to the clinic with a broad range of complaints. With surprisingly few exceptions, however, those so diagnosed shared a number of risk factors, as the small-scale case-control study summarized in table 4.1 suggests. We began the study by interviewing the first seventeen women diagnosed with symptomatic HIV infection (most had full-blown AIDS) who were residents of Do Kay or its two neighboring villages. Their responses to questions posed during a series of open-ended interviews were compared with those of seventeen age-matched, seronegative controls. In both groups, ages ranged from seventeen to thirty-seven, with a mean of about twenty-five years. None of these thirty-four women had a history of prostitution; none had used illicit drugs; only one, a member of the control group, had a history of transfusion. None of the women in either group had had more than six sexual partners. In fact, four of the afflicted women had had only one sexual partner. Although women in the study group had (on average) more sexual partners than those in the control group, the difference was not striking. Similarly, there was no clear difference between the two groups in education level or history of intramuscular injections.

The chief risk factors in this small study group seemed to involve not the number of partners in a lifetime, but rather the professions of these partners. Fourteen of the women with HIV disease had histories of sexual contact with soldiers or truck drivers. Two of these women each reported having only two sexual partners, one a soldier and one a truck driver. Of those women diagnosed with HIV disease, none had a history of sexual contact exclusively with peasants. Among the control group, only one woman had a truck driver as a regular partner; none reported contact with soldiers, and most had had sexual relations only with peasants from the region. Histories of extended residence in Port-au-Prince and work as a domestic were also strongly associated with a diagnosis of HIV disease.

Conjugal unions with nonpeasants—salaried soldiers and truck drivers, who are paid on a daily basis—reflect these women's quest for some measure of economic security. In this manner, truck drivers and soldiers have served as a "bridge" for transmitting HIV to the rural population, just as North American tourists seem to have served as a bridge to the urban Haitian population.[11] But just as North Americans are no longer important in the transmission of HIV in Haiti, truck drivers and soldiers will soon no longer be necessary components of the rural epidemic. Once introduced into a sexually active population, HIV will work its way into those with no history of residence in the city, no history of contact with soldiers or truck drivers, and no history of work as a domestic.

The research presented here underlines the importance of social inequalities

Table 4.1 Case-Control Study of HIV Infection
in Thirty-Four Rural Haitian Women

Patient Characteristics	Patients with HIV Disease ($N = 17$)	Control Group ($N = 17$)
Number of sexual partners	2.7	2.2
Partner of a truck driver	9.0	1.0
Partner of a soldier	7.0	0.0
Partner of a peasant only	0.0	15.0
Lived in Port-au-Prince	14.0	4.0
Worked as a servant	11.0	0.0
Years of education	4.8	4.0
Received a blood transfusion	0.0	1.0
Used illicit drugs	0.0	0.0
Received more than ten intramuscular injections	11.0	13.0

of the most casual, everyday sort in determining who is most at risk for HIV infection. In Haiti, HIV is sexually transmitted, and sexual unions are clearly made and unmade by economic pressures in a context of harsh poverty and steep inequality. Neither several years of participant-observation by the author nor a critical review of existing epidemiological data from urban Haiti and the rest of the Caribbean suggests that additional factors are involved in the transmission of HIV in Haiti. (Both popular and scientific literature in North America had hinted that "voodoo practices," including animal sacrifice and ritualized sex, were implicated.)[12]

When ethnographic and clinical-epidemiological research are linked to un-flinching social analysis, the contours of a rapidly changing epidemic—and the forces promoting HIV transmission—come into focus. Concluding that, in Haiti, "poverty and economic inequity serve as the most virulent co-factors in the spread of this disease,"[13] we can identify seven other socially conditioned forces increasing the rates of HIV transmission among Haitian women:

Gender inequality, especially concerning control of land and other resources

Traditional patterns of sexual union, such as stable concubinage, or *plasaj*, in which sexually transmitted pathogens are much more likely to be shared among three or more persons

Emerging patterns of sexual union, such as serial monogamy

Prevalence of sexually transmitted diseases and other genital-tract infections (such as trichomoniasis or infections causing mucosal lesions) and, perhaps more significant, lack of access to treatment for them

Lack of timely response by public health authorities, a delay related not
   merely to lack of resources but to the persistence of a political crisis

Lack of culturally appropriate prevention tools

Political violence, much of it state-sponsored and directed at poor people[14]

Each of these forces plays a part in the lives of our patients, according to their
own testimony. These are the "givens," the structural violence of their country
and, indeed, of the larger historical system in which it is ensnared.[15] Of all the
millions of persons on the losing end of the system, few are more trammeled by
punitive constraints than Haitian women living in poverty. For poor Haitian
women, often enough, the structures are more like strictures.

For reasons I explore in the remainder of this chapter, these are not factors regularly discussed in the medical journals that publish epidemiological studies of HIV
infection. Yet there is ample reason to believe that similar factors help to determine
the epidemiology of HIV infection in wealthier countries too, especially those
characterized by high indices of economic disparity, such as the United States.[16]

One reason the biomedical press does not candidly discuss social forces may
be related to the way AIDS research funds have been doled out. Quick to associate
anthropology with studies of exotic animal sacrifice, say, or ritual scarification,
those in control of funds ask anthropologists to perform "rapid ethnographic
assessments" of settings with high rates of HIV transmission. And medical
anthropologists have too often assented, restricting their inquiries to "delineating
the cultural component" of illness. Because culture is merely that, a component,
such research has been the object of legitimate critiques: "Medical anthropologists and sociologists have tended to elevate the cultural component into an omnibus explanation. The emphasis is on cultural determination. Even when social
relations receive more than reflexive recognition, medical social scientists restrict
the social relations to small "primary" group settings, such as the family, and factions at the micro unit. . . . Little or no attempt is made to encompass the totality
of the larger society's structure."[17]

In my view, obscuring "the totality of the larger society's structure" (including
its place in international systems) is all too frequently the mission of anthropological assessments whose goal is to assign origins or vectors for disease in such
"barbaric" practices as animal sacrifice and blood ritual. In the vast majority of
settings in which anthropologists work, HIV is transmitted through much more
mundane mechanisms.

Finally, such "exotic" practices are out of the ordinary, isolated, and to a large
extent voluntary. By associating them with AIDS, do we not silently reassure ourselves that the disease we study is equally voluntary, exceptional, and experience-
distant? If that is the profile of medical anthropology in the AIDS pandemic,
Haiti has a lesson to teach it.

ETHNOGRAPHY, SOCIAL THEORY, AND EPIDEMIOLOGY:
BRINGING IT ALL TOGETHER IN AIDS PREVENTION

If the chief forces promoting HIV transmission are powerful political and economic currents, what meaningful interventions might be made on the local level? If one of the chief reasons poor women engage in sexual relations is to conceive a child, what are the chances of promoting condom use? In a setting of political upheaval and violence against community organizers, what hope is there of seeing projects through to fruition?

Two community-based organizations, one Haitian and one North American, have attempted to incorporate insights gained from ethnographic, epidemiological, and clinical work in an AIDS prevention project in rural Haiti. In early 1992, Partners In Health and Zanmi Lasante received funds from the World AIDS Foundation to inaugurate "Une Chance à Prendre" (UCAP), a comprehensive, community-based response to a rapidly advancing epidemic. The project includes efforts to prevent the spread of HIV and other sexually transmitted pathogens, and it also introduces training programs for Haitian health workers. A significant component of UCAP attempts to improve clinical care for those already infected with HIV and to enhance providers' abilities to diagnose opportunistic infections (and other complications of HIV infection) in a timely fashion.

In spite of a very adverse political climate—a coup d'état took place months before the project was initiated, crippling the team's ability to work outside the Zanmi Lasante catchment area—each of these aspects of UCAP was inaugurated, and most of them were completed as planned. I will focus here on one small project within UCAP, as it demonstrates both the utility and the limits of culturally appropriate efforts to prevent HIV transmission among the poor.

Zanmi Lasante is the parent organization for a large and vibrant women's health project, one that sponsors interventions ranging from women's literacy to screening for cervical disease. A group of women involved in these efforts decided to create, in the context of UCAP, a series of AIDS prevention tools for women like themselves: poor, landless, and subject to discrimination at many levels. HIV-positive women also participated in the project, which has led, we believe, to the first prevention tools designed by and for poor Haitian women.

Because most rural Haitians do not read or write, and because UCAP had funds for a video recorder and portable generator, the women's group settled on making a video. Basing their script on the life story of the first woman from Do Kay to die of AIDS, the women created *Chache lavi, detwi lavi.* This expression (literally rendered as "looking for life, destroying life") is used whenever someone dies in the course of honest efforts to make a living—for example, when a market woman dies in a truck accident while transporting her produce to market. Many people in rural Haiti feel the expression is apposite to the stories of young women who are infected with HIV in the course of their struggle to survive.

The half-hour program tells the story of Jocelyne, a young woman who loses her family land to a hydroelectric dam—and, shortly thereafter, her mother to tuberculosis. Soon she is responding to the overtures of a truck driver. Jocelyne hopes that, through him, she can pull her family out of poverty. After she gives birth to a child, she finds herself alone and again penniless. Jocelyne sees work in the city as her only hope of surviving, and the only chance for a brighter future for her daughter.

What happens to Jocelyne in the city is typical of the lot of poor women in Haiti. Her next sexual union is with a second truck driver, who promises to help her find a job. Soon Jocelyne is working as a servant for a pittance and, unbeknownst to her employer, becomes pregnant. She is fired abruptly when her pregnancy becomes evident, but the truck driver is no longer around to help. Her next—and final—liaison is with a soldier, with whom she conceives twins. Sick and beaten down by her experience, she returns to Do Kay. There she is diagnosed with AIDS.

Marie, one of the seropositive actors who has since died of AIDS, offered the following observations in an interview conducted as the video was being edited:

> There are so many people who think that you get AIDS by being promiscuous (nan vilib), but through this story we are able to show what's really happening in Haiti. People like Jocelyne are everywhere—there's nothing for them, so they have to put themselves in peril to feed their children. Perhaps if she had known what was waiting for her, she could have taken precautions.

It is not clear, of course, that Jocelyne would have been able to alter her course had she been better informed, but the video has other merits as well. A Haitian nurse who directs a women's clinic in Port-au-Prince commented after viewing the video:

> The video really shakes you to your core, because it takes a hard look at the real culprits in this epidemic. It's so easy to say that poverty and oppression are to blame, and it's true. But when you see how Jocelyne's life is squashed at every turn by these forces. . . . It's so commonplace, it's banal—and yet why is this not part of our discussions of the disease? The video also helps to denounce a series of "myths"— that you can stop AIDS by merely circulating condoms, that you can stop AIDS by educating people, that AIDS is a result of promiscuity, et cetera.

In spite of the many forces conspiring to make a video irrelevant among the Haitian poor—who have no electricity, much less televisions with VCRs—*Chache lavi, detwi lavi* is proving to be more durable than might have been expected. The video's narrator has since become a skilled facilitator and has presented the group's work in many settings, sometimes with the help of a portable generator and projector. The video has twice been shown on national television (which has, admittedly, limited reach among those most at risk). Other community groups have petitioned Zanmi Lasante for help, as they would like to make AIDS prevention videos, too.

UCAP has also been instructive in its failures. These have included fallout from the coup d'état (from expulsion of two project coordinators to threats from soldiers who quite correctly saw our work as "anti-military"); problems among the professional staff (burnout as a result of high patient load, a problem dramatically worsened by the breakdown of the public health sector after the coup); and a lack of passion for some aspects of UCAP (for example, repetitive community meetings). There have also been worse-than-anticipated shortages of materials and unanticipated bureaucratic barriers that slowed down the training component of the project.

What effects might such a modest project have had in the face of such overwhelming odds? It is not possible to prove that *Chache lavi, detwi lavi* prevented a single case of HIV transmission. But it is possible to argue that tens of thousands of Haitians have encountered their first candid discussions of these issues in hearing the story of Jocelyne Gracia. It is possible to observe that the relationship between AIDS and gender inequality has become, as a result of UCAP, the subject of sustained community discussion. It is possible to speculate that "people who can name the source of their problems may be better off than those who are uncomprehending or silent."[18]

Although a realistic analysis should lead one to a more pessimistic assessment of the value of preventive efforts in a setting like Haiti, perhaps the last words should go to the women who made the video. Convinced that their efforts will not be in vain, members of the group repeatedly express the hope that women elsewhere can use the ideas presented in *Chache lavi, detwi lavi* to make their own AIDS prevention tools. To cite Marie again:

> We're telling this story to show how the circumstances of our lives have forced us to enter into bad situations like [Jocelyne's]. As poor women, we are committed to sharing what we've learned with other women like ourselves, especially those who don't have the means to create a video like this one.

CONCLUSION:
POVERTY AND POWERLESSNESS AS CO-FACTORS

Poverty and powerlessness can serve as powerful co-factors in the spread of HIV. An anthropology of infectious disease that is more than mere ethnography—one that plumbs social and political-economic analysis in an effort to discern the forces that structure risk—would certainly seem to buttress this assertion. Do these insights hold for infectious diseases other than HIV infection? Piecemeal evidence would suggest that poverty and inequality (including gender-based discrimination) are significant risk enhancers for most sexually transmitted diseases, including chlamydia, syphilis, gonorrhea, lymphogranuloma venereum, hepatitis, and syndromes such as pelvic inflammatory disease.[19] Because human papilloma virus is similarly influenced by social forces, perhaps even cervical cancer can be said to be a disease of poverty—in some developing countries, it is the leading neoplasm in women.[20] Surely a majority of parasitic diseases—including amebic dysentery, malaria, schistosomiasis, trypanosomiasis, and onchocerciasis—are similarly disproportionately distributed among the poor.

Studies spanning time, geographical space, and cultural diversity all point to an important thesis: poverty and inequality put people at risk for infectious diseases. With regard to certain diseases in specific settings, such as tuberculosis in the poor countries of the Southern Hemisphere, it may be that absolute poverty, with its attendant malnutrition and immunosuppression, is responsible for striking mortality differentials among those with reactivation disease.[21] Regarding other diseases, such as HIV infection, it seems that multiple inequities are to blame: steep grades of inequity (gender-based, economic, environmental) seem to put the disempowered at risk of AIDS as a sexually transmitted disease. Social discrimination and the violation of human rights have also been strongly implicated as risk factors for exposure to HIV.[22]

These tentative conclusions have a number of implications for further anthropological research on infectious disease. When behavior is strongly constrained by social forces, it is not illuminating to lump these forces under the catch-all category of "behavioral factors." As Jonathan Mann commented, "the study of the behavioral determinants of risk behavior, using standard concepts and classical methods, may have reached its limit."[23] A new research agenda would do more than stress the importance of socioeconomic status; surely this has been well enough established. It would also seek to explore the translation of large-scale forces—here I have focused on poverty and gender, but other factors may be equally important—into risk for populations and for individual patients.

In order to exploit fully the fruits of basic research, we now need large-scale investigations that would allow us to understand both the dynamics of infectious diseases within certain populations and the precise mechanisms by which social forces become embodied as risk for infection. The idea, here, would not be to "control" or "adjust" for socioeconomic status or race, but to study their effects on the distribution and course of infectious disease. Such research, based on prospective studies and sociocultural analysis, would attempt to ascribe relative weights to various social factors—a critical epidemiology that would link variations in incidence or prevalence (risk) to socioeconomic status and gender, including factors such as discrimination, sexism, and political upheaval.

These variables have always proven difficult to measure, and anthropologists could help bring important contextual considerations to the center of the large-scale epidemiological projects that will be necessary to bring these mechanisms into relief. Krieger and her coworkers—whose magisterial review of epidemiological studies of the health effects of racism, sexism, and social class should be read by all medical anthropologists—outline an alternative research agenda for an epidemiology that would address such questions, underlining four key elements and assumptions:[24]

> Patterns of disease, whether in individual bodies or in populations, are the result of "a dynamic interplay between exposure and susceptibility."
>
> The processes of both exposure and susceptibility are themselves structured over time and "conditioned by history."
>
> The social forces and relations manifest in racism, sexism, and social class will influence, one way or another, the exposure and susceptibility of those whose lives are defined by these relations.
>
> The mechanisms by which these social forces affect the health of populations include the shaping of exposure and susceptibility to both pathogens (and pathogenic processes) and protective factors, events, and processes; the degree of access to, and type of, health care; and the shaping of health research and health policies.[24]

Research would also examine the rate of disease progression in light of these and other factors, linking them to nutritional and immunological status. The explanatory power of models stemming from such research would be enhanced by their ability to account for variation over time and across geographical and cultural divides and would thus be informed by history and political economy. Although ethnography tends to bring life to the often arid studies of economists and historians, I am not convinced that maintaining disciplinary boundaries between economics, history, sociology, and anthropology is helpful. Immanuel Wallerstein pushes this line of thought even further: "The question before us today is whether there are any criteria which can be used to assert in a relatively clear and defensible way boundaries between the four presumed disciplines of anthropology, economics, political science, and sociology. World-systems analysis responds with an unequivocal 'no' to this question. All the presumed criteria—level of analysis, subject-matter, methods, theoretical assumptions— either are no longer true in practice or, if sustained, are barriers to further knowledge rather than stimuli to its creation."[25]

Such cross-disciplinary research has been inaugurated at times in the past, both in anthropology and in related fields. Indeed, exemplary studies were conducted in the earlier part of this century, when, for example, Joseph Goldberger, G. A. Wheeler, and Edgar Sydenstricker examined the occurrence of pellagra, whose etiology was then unknown, in seven cotton-mill villages in South Carolina.[26] Although the received wisdom was that high rates of this disorder among the poor were due to "poor hygiene" (or, among blacks, to innate "racial weakness"), these researchers disproved these notions with a careful study that analyzed not merely household diets and finances but also how foodstuffs and income were obtained and how seasonal variation affected access to both. Their research suggested that income alone did not determine rates of pellagra in these towns; instead, susceptibility to pellagra was related to the degree of dependency on cash cropping for cotton, thus linking the disorder to the larger political economy. Because Goldberger—who later discovered that niacin deficiency was the etiologic factor in pellagra—called for changes in the southern economy that he believed would lower rates of pellagra among these groups, he was vilified by many of his contemporaries in the medical field.

Today, Goldberger's work is regarded as exemplary public health research. But, as Krieger and coworkers write, "it is hard to imagine present U.S. epidemiologic studies explicitly testing detailed hypotheses about the social production and political economy of disease, as Goldberger and Sydenstricker once did." And why should that be so? The authors speculate that there exists within epidemiology a certain reluctance "to discuss uncomfortable subjects or to tackle issues whose remedies could lie outside the bounds of traditional public health interventions."[27]

While this is true, I doubt that this reluctance is in any way native to epidemiology. Nor is it the province of medicine, although it may be, as Sandra Gifford argues, that "greater control on the part of the medical profession over the diagnosis and treatment of risk . . . has diverted attention away from translating epidemiologic knowledge into population level interventions and has allowed the focus to be directed towards the medicalization of risk within individuals."[28]

In anthropology, similarly, Peter Brown's study of malaria control in Sardinia "emphasizes the need to understand the political economic variables which influence both the rates of disease and development."[29] Other researchers in the social sciences—including Brooke Grundfest Schoepf in anthropology, Meredeth Turshen in political science, and Randall Packard in history—have reached very similar conclusions in examining modern epidemics.[30] And yet all deplore a recurrent tendency, noted in each of these fields, to divert attention from the obvious conclusions of investigations into the patterning of disease, similar to my critique of epidemiology at the outset of this chapter.

The obvious conclusion is that risk for most diseases is structured in large part by social—political and economic—forces. If the distribution of these diseases is to be altered, it will be done by social—political and economic—responses. It is only appropriate to recall that sound anthropological research on infectious diseases is by no means among the most important task at hand for those seeking to diminish the suffering of the destitute sick. Nor is it being called for by the sick themselves. For the mechanisms of the uneven distribution of the world's resources—including the fruits of technology and science—are no longer obscure, if indeed they ever were. Sound research should be embedded in efforts to make available to the poor the resources and information already available to the more fortunate. If anything redeeming could have come from this latest plague, it might be that it has thrown into relief the vast disparity in resources available to people caught in the same web of social and economic relations.

Even the pessimists involved in the Haitian AIDS prevention efforts described earlier—those who doubt that educational efforts could have much of an effect on a rapidly advancing epidemic—share the women's group's hope that their example will inspire other women to organize their communities in order to promote a broader program of social justice. All the project participants agree that educational programs are not enough to prevent AIDS: poor women, no matter how dignified or well-informed, will remain at risk as long as they are not liberated from the myriad conditions, large-scale and local, that keep them dependent and vulnerable.

NOTES

This essay is offered in memory of Marie-Andrée Louihis.

1. United Nations Development Programme, *Young Women*, p. 3.

2. This emphasis is also obvious at the AIDS megaconferences held each year. Of the thousands of epidemiology-track posters and abstracts presented at the Eighth International Conference on AIDS, only three used "poverty" as a keyword.

3. Ellerbrock et al., "Heterosexually Transmitted Human Immunodeficiency Virus Infection among Pregnant Women in a Rural Florida Community," p. 1708.

4. Krieger et al., "Racism, Sexism, and Social Class," p. 86. Nancy Krieger and coworkers conclude their review with this reproach: "The minimal research that simultaneously studies the health effects of racism, sexism, and social class ultimately stands as a sharp indictment of the narrow vision limiting much of the epidemiological research conducted within the United States" (ibid., p. 99).

5. Navarro, "Race or Class versus Race and Class," p. 1240; Marmot, "Social Differentials in Health within and between Populations," p. 197.

6. Inhorn and Brown, "The Anthropology of Infectious Disease," pp. 98–99.

7. Farmer, *AIDS and Accusation*.

8. I have found that relating the narratives of individuals is the most effective way of making plain the effects of poverty and oppression on a population. Three such narratives of Haitian women are recounted in detail in chapter 15 of this volume.

9. The term "historical system" follows Immanuel Wallerstein, whose world-systems analysis "substitutes for the term 'society' the term 'historical system.' Of course, this is a mere semantic substitution. But it rids us of the central connotation that 'society' has acquired, its link to 'state,' and therefore of the presupposition about the 'where' and the 'when.' Furthermore, 'historical system' as a term underlines the unity of historical social science. The entity is simultaneously systemic and historical" (Wallerstein, "World-Systems Analysis," p. 317). I have made the argument for applying

a world-systems approach to a "responsible materialist" investigation of AIDS in Haiti in Farmer, *AIDS and Accusation,* pp. 13, 256–62.

10. What is intended by this use of the term "structure"? I would agree with Jonathan Turner, who reminds us that "structure is a process, not a thing" and that it "refers to the ordering of interactions across time and in space" ("Analytical Theorizing," pp. 169–70). By "structural violence," then, I refer to the processes, historically given and often economically driven, by which human agency may be constrained, whether through ritual, routine, or the hard surfaces of life. For some, including many of my informants and patients, life is structured by racism, sexism, *and* grinding poverty.

11. Farmer, *AIDS and Accusation.*

12. For both the research and the review, see ibid., chapters 7–14 and 19.

13. Farmer, "Culture, Society, and the Dynamics of HIV Transmission in Rural Haiti."

14. Indeed, the evacuation of several urban slums—such as Cité Soleil, with its alleged 10 percent seropositivity rate—meant that many with asymptomatic HIV infection returned to low-prevalence home villages to wait for the violence to subside. No research has addressed the means by which political violence thus changes the equations that might describe the rates of HIV transmission in Haiti.

15. As Wallerstein has noted, "by the late nineteenth century, for the first time ever, there existed only one historical system on the globe. We are still in that situation today" ("World-Systems Analysis," p. 318). I have examined Haiti's "fit" into this system in a recent study, which also examines how this "political economy of brutality" comes to have its effects in the lives of poor women; see Farmer, *The Uses of Haiti.*

16. In the United States, the fastest-growing subepidemic is among those who contract HIV heterosexually, a group consisting largely of poor African American and Hispanic populations. For example, Michael St. Louis and coworkers ("Human Immunodeficiency Virus Infection in Disadvantaged Adolescents") found that 3.6 percent of disadvantaged teenagers applying for work in the U.S. Job Corps were already seropositive for HIV. See also the special issue of *Culture, Medicine, and Psychiatry* (vol. 17, no. 4, 1993) titled "Women, Poverty, and AIDS."

17. Onoge, "Capitalism and Public Health," p. 221. As Peter Brown has noted, anthropology "is particularly well adapted to meet such a challenge because the holistic approach provides the 'big picture' of interacting cultural, demographic, economic and political variables which might evade other social scientists" ("Introduction," p. 6). Unfortunately, the big picture has all too often evaded anthropologists as well. In addition, see Sandra Gifford's discussion of the "medicalization" of the concept of risk, and also her warning: "we should be wary that social and cultural processes do not become reduced to factors which are translated *only* into individual health promotion" ("The Meaning of Lumps," p. 239). A critical discussion of the cooptation (theoretical, methodological, and moral) of anthropology by the AIDS establishment can be found in Farmer, "Culture, Society, and the Dynamics of HIV Transmission in Rural Haiti." See also Farmer, Robin, et al., "Tuberculosis, Poverty, and 'Compliance.'"

18. Krieger et al., "Racism, Sexism, and Social Class," p. 103. Krieger and coworkers are referring to a small literature examining hypertension among African Americans living in the United States. There are as yet no data suggesting that naming the sources of one's oppression (or dignity in the face of oppression) can alter the nature of risk in settings such as Haiti. Such research is certainly called for. I trace links between greater opportunities for political expression and the development of a rhetoric of illness causation in chapter 2 of this volume.

19. See Aral and Holmes, "Sexually Transmitted Diseases in the AIDS Era." See also Goeman, Meheus, and Piot, "Epidemiology of Sexually Transmissible Diseases in Developing Countries in the Era of AIDS"; Muir and Belsey, "Pelvic Inflammatory Disease and Its Consequences in the Developing World."

20. Paavonen, Koutsky, and Kiviat, "Cervical Neoplasia and Other STD-Related Genital and Anal Neoplasias"; Reeves, Rawls, and Brinton, "Epidemiology of Genital Papillomaviruses and Cervical Cancer"; Standaert and Meheus, "Le cancer du col utérin en Afrique."

21. See Farmer, Robin, et al., "Tuberculosis, Poverty, and 'Compliance.'"

22. Mann, "Global AIDS." It may be true that, in many instances, *setting*, and not type of infection, is the most important determinant of mortality. In a recent review of national trends in morbidity and mortality, Richard Wilkinson notes that the relationship between per capita GNP and mortality "peters out in the developed world. Apparently there is some minimum level of income (around $5,000 per capita in 1990) above which the absolute standard of living ceases to have much impact on health" ("The Epidemiological Transition," p. 63). It is important to add that any nation-based study has limitations in comparison to those adopting a broader systems approach.

23. Mann, "Global AIDS," p. 555.

24. Krieger et al., "Racism, Sexism, and Social Class," p. 100.

25. Wallerstein, "World-Systems Analysis," p. 312.

26. Goldberger, Wheeler, and Sydenstricker, "A Study of the Relation of Family Income and Other Economic Factors to Pellagra Incidence in Seven Cotton-Mill Villages of South Carolina in 1916."

27. Krieger et al., "Racism, Sexism, and Social Class," p. 99.

28. Gifford, "The Meaning of Lumps," p. 239.

29. Brown, "Introduction," p. 6.

30. Schoepf, "Women, AIDS, and Economic Crisis in Central Africa"; Turshen, *The Political Ecology of Disease in Tanzania*; Packard, *White Plague, Black Labor*.

5

From Haiti to Rwanda

AIDS and Accusations

(2006)

LEARNING LESSONS

AIDS and Accusation, published in 1992, summarized a number of lessons gleaned from my fieldwork, research, and clinical practice. First, I learned that AIDS, although a new disease, is deeply embedded in social and economic structures long in place—and that poverty and inequality are the fault lines along which HIV spreads. Even when I wrote the book, those of us working with the disease saw that AIDS was likely to become a major killer of people living in poverty.

I also learned how medical errors, bad diagnoses, and confidently expressed but incorrect claims of causality could themselves cause great suffering. Some claims came from the popular press, but many, as the book documents, came from officially accredited speakers: scientific and medical authorities as well as political figures. Some authorities claimed, for example, that HIV came to the United States from Haiti—"the little Africa off the coast of Florida," as the popular press calls it—despite the fact that data available at the time, which I review in the book, suggested the opposite. In *AIDS and Accusation*, I characterized the Haitian epidemic as a direct subepidemic, or offshoot, of the much larger U.S. pandemic—one that is quite unrelated to the epidemic in Africa. Technologies developed since that 1992 study have characterized the genetic subtypes, or clades, of HIV and corroborate the thesis laid out there: the Haitian epidemic is indeed caused by subtype B, the clade prevalent in the United States. AIDS did not come to Haiti from Africa, where other clades are prevalent; it came south with North American tourists. But the myth that AIDS came to the United States from Haiti persists in the popular press and, at times, in the popular imagination.

Similarly erroneous claims about the role of stigma, a traditional topic of anthropology and other social sciences, were also common. It's true that AIDS was entangled with stigma in many ways. In rural Haiti, social responses were often tied to accusations of sorcery, a system of attitudes with deep roots in Haiti's history as a slave colony. The modern-day accusations registered in rural Haiti were almost invariably embedded in local social inequalities. Accusing someone of sorcery is a way (maladaptive, perhaps) for the victim to transfer blame for misfortune to another person, the alleged perpetrator. But in the United States and other wealthy post-slavery societies of the Americas, the stigma of AIDS combined with inveterate racism to ensure that victims of the disease would always bear the blame for their own misfortune. Moreover, not only sufferers from HIV but all Haitians were branded as AIDS carriers. This variety of stigma cannot be reduced to a matter of personal concern, though I have heard hundreds of anecdotes of landlords and employers acting out of prejudice and fear, and I have no reason to doubt the veracity of these stories. Racism was central to the early international responses to AIDS, too, and remains a problem today, as AIDS takes its greatest toll on the continent of Africa, where the heritage of colonialism and racism weighs heavily.

In all these settings, however, accusation remained a constant, prompting the subtitle of the book: *Haiti and the Geography of Blame.* I learned that stigma, always socially constructed, works in different ways in different places and that the most important stigma in rural Haiti resulted from people's belief, correct at the time, that AIDS was an inevitably fatal disease. Stigma would later be a major barrier to the introduction of proper AIDS care when, once again, poverty and a lack of access to even the most rudimentary medical care were far more likely to determine the efficacy of AIDS screening and prevention efforts than were purely clinical issues. In rural Africa, as in rural Haiti, stigma is less a barrier to providing AIDS care than it is the reflection and result of a complete lack of decent health care for the poor. Stigma is a symptom of this grotesque failure but is commonly used as an excuse for further inaction. How often do we read in the popular press that stigma, rather than poor-quality services, slows HIV screening? Even today, a fundamental misunderstanding of stigma continues to hamper effective responses to the pandemic.

Among the other central lessons laid out in the book is that the mechanisms by which poverty and other social injustices, such as racism and gender inequality, hasten the advance of HIV and tuberculosis are knowable. The book thus closes with a call for an "anthropology of human suffering." Social conditions shape not only epidemics themselves but also social responses to them. I dared to make a few predictions at the end of the book, fairly obvious ones, as they seemed at the time, and I can say without triumph that they have come true. Near the end of *AIDS and Accusation,* I wrote:

If a disaster is to be averted in rural Haiti, vigorous and effective prevention campaigns must be initiated at once. And although such efforts must begin, the prospects of stopping the steady march of HIV are slim. AIDS is far more likely to join a host of other sexually transmitted diseases—including gonorrhea, syphilis, genital herpes, chlamydia, hepatitis B, lymphogranuloma venereum, and even cervical cancer—that have already become entrenched among the poor.

I take no pleasure in pointing out that a geographically broad and historically deep examination of the nascent pandemic in the 1980s showed that this disaster would occur unless vigorous and fundamentally structural interventions took place. Not until better treatment for these diseases was put in place and integrated with AIDS prevention did the Haitian epidemic begin to come under control. As I write this, the Haitian epidemic is at last shrinking, a major victory for public health in one of the most poverty-stricken countries on the planet.

I've spent much of the past two decades studying these infectious killers. To be frank, however, I was never asked, in Haiti or in any of the other places in which we work, to do much in the way of *studying* suffering. In fact, I cannot remember a single such invitation from patients or their families. Instead, we were inundated in Haiti and elsewhere with a different sort of request: to *do* something to allay the awful suffering associated with these infectious diseases and with the host of other problems—hunger, malaria, death during childbirth, mistreatment at the hands of the powerful or less impoverished—that people afflicted with the new disease, AIDS, had long faced.

Partners In Health, a nongovernmental organization seeking to put into practice the conviction that health care should be viewed as a human right, was born in the village of Do Kay and is rooted in the experiences and years of work described in *AIDS and Accusation*. To make a long story short—and these past two decades have felt very long—the years described in the processual ethnography in the book led me to contemplate some hard choices. On the one hand, a life of careful scholarship requires all one's attention, and no graduate student can afford to lose deep respect for careful scholarship; indeed, every graduate student has been the direct beneficiary of one or more mentors who have dedicated their lives to careful scholarship and teaching. On the other hand, one can choose a life of service and make common cause with people struggling under heavy burdens of poverty, AIDS, tuberculosis, malaria, and other causes of "stupid deaths," to use the Haitian term. At the time of the book's publication, this latter choice seemed both geographically and pragmatically remote from a research university like Harvard, an institution that had already afforded me an excellent education and was now prepared to offer the promise of a rewarding teaching career.

I've called these choices "hard." They do not have the gravity of those made each day by people living in poverty and facing the threat of disease and hunger and violence. But these decisions, mine and those of my coworkers, felt hard at the time and still do. Anyone who has spanned the worlds of the rich (any First World university qualifies as such) and the poor (of which Haiti and Rwanda are extreme examples) knows exactly what I mean. Many young scholars face similar dilemmas upon returning from fieldwork—especially medical anthropologists who, in their study, gaze down steep gradients of class and privilege. But not many scholars are also physicians, though other avenues of service are open to them.

WHAT IS TO BE DONE?

Partners In Health was, to some extent, born of the opportunity to study and reflect upon an emerging epidemic that collided with other catastrophes long in the making in central Haiti. My colleagues and I have worked there since the first months chronicled in *AIDS and Accusation;* we have also grown and had the privilege of caring for more than a million patients in places as far-flung as Peru, Siberia, Chiapas, Guatemala, inner-city Boston, and now rural Rwanda. Our choices about where to work were responses to a constant nagging voice, with a distinctly Haitian accent, as I hear it, that says, "Don't just study our suffering— do something to allay it."

But, as my students ask, do what, exactly? This question is difficult but not impossible to answer. At the end of the period I described in that 1992 book, no effective antiretroviral therapies existed to treat AIDS. But much could be done to prevent HIV transmission, so we launched "culturally appropriate prevention campaigns," which are described elsewhere.[1] In addition, each of the opportunistic infections that afflicted AIDS patients, often killing them, could be countered with therapies known to be effective. In Haiti, as in Africa, the main such infection is tuberculosis. So the response to the question "do what?" in that instance was to start an effective tuberculosis control program in rural Haiti. That's precisely what we did. As a result, we saw cure rates go from less than 50 percent to close to universal cure among those for whom all social barriers to care—from hunger to user fees, lack of water, and lack of transportation—were removed.

Scholarship also had work to do in this area, since we encountered no shortage of silliness—again, immodest claims of causality—among people attempting to explain, without alluding to the concept of neglect, why so many people died in places like Haiti from an eminently treatable disease such as tuberculosis.[2] The ranking explanation among Haitian and certain non-Haitian health professionals was that the peasants believed in sorcery and thus had no confidence in biomedicine. We learned, instead, that rural Haitians had no access to biomedicine and that they did just fine, regardless of their views on disease etiology, once we fixed the dysfunctional tuberculosis program. What needed to change was not the cultural beliefs of the patients but rather the quality of the tuberculosis program—and with it, perhaps, the cultural beliefs of part of the medical community.

Even as I was completing *AIDS and Accusation,* my colleagues and I were publishing, in medical journals, our experiences of setting up a community-based program to bring *all* tuberculosis patients to cure.[3] A significant number of these tuberculosis patients were also infected with HIV, but we found that they, too, did well once they received treatment for their tuberculosis, enjoying cure rates almost as high as those for patients not co-infected with HIV. But eventually, even after their tuberculosis was declared cured, patients infected with HIV would fall ill and die of other opportunistic infections or become ill again with tuberculosis. What could we do for them?

By 1995, ample evidence existed that antiretroviral "drug cocktails"—ARVs—could transform the formerly fatal affliction of AIDS into a manageable chronic disease. But although these drugs rapidly transformed the epidemic in the United States, cutting mortality dramatically and almost wiping out mother-to-child transmission and thus pediatric AIDS, the drugs were nonexistent in the world of the poor, where AIDS was having its greatest impact. People knew that treatment existed, but the drugs were unavailable to those who couldn't pay top dollar for them. Although we were never swayed much by arguments that prevention alone was the only "sustainable" intervention in settings riven by poverty, we were unable to acquire ARVs until 1998. Too little, too late, we thought, but we pressed on.

When our small organization decided to import these medications to treat the sickest AIDS patients in central Haiti, the cost of the drugs exceeded $1,500 per patient per year—even though we benefited from concessional prices and some donated medicines. This amount was and remains roughly six times the per capita income there. But while we, and many of our patients in Haiti, despaired about lagging behind, we soon discovered that Partners In Health was probably the first group working in the poorest parts of the world to introduce modern AIDS care as a public good—free of charge to the patient, as is tuberculosis care.[4] We based our policy on a simple premise: these people are sick, we're health care providers, and these medications are part of the same global economy that, after all, created Haiti as a slave colony to provide Europe with sugar, coffee, and other tropical produce. But we also reasoned that if AIDS had become the leading infectious cause of adult death in Haiti, it was also a public health challenge (to Haiti and to the rest of the world), and authorities needed to view prevention *and* treatment as a public good, not merely as commodities that only those with resources could purchase.

The introduction of antiretroviral therapy to a squatter settlement in rural Haiti—in a sense, the epilogue to the story told in *AIDS and Accusation*—provoked radically different responses in different quarters. Rural Haitians largely greeted our efforts with gratitude and even cheers, and the growing number of people within Partners In Health were confident that we were doing the right thing, even though paying for the drugs initially accounted for about 90 percent of all program costs. But in circles often mistakenly called "the international community," including some people with an avowed interest in the health of the poor, cheers were not forthcoming. These parties greeted the use of ARVs in places like rural Haiti or Africa with skepticism—deeming such projects wasteful and neither "sustainable" nor "cost-effective" in the paradigms of our day—and sometimes even derided the treatment programs as irresponsible. I am still struck, some twenty years after I learned to listen to patients and to people living in poverty, that such criticisms come not from the intended beneficiaries but rather from people with backgrounds more akin to mine. The critics at the time were professionals from North America or Europe or officials in poor countries who had been trained in the affluent world. They had accepted, as rural Haitians would not, the notion that the poor world would remain poor and that people so unfortunate as to be born there were out of luck when it came to receiving expensive but effective AIDS therapy.

This view changed as underfunded prevention strategies failed in much of the poor world, as new infections continued to multiply (in more or less the manner predicted in my book), and as AIDS mortality continued to climb. Many millions died unattended long after wealthy nations had shown that ARVs could suppress HIV in their patient populations; millions more are dying today wherever AIDS is prevalent but AIDS treatment is not. The need for urgent interventions is certainly evident to anyone who spends time in places like Haiti or Rwanda. Many others have tried to document "the race to treat AIDS," as one writer termed the phenomenon, and I won't try to do so here.[5] But I will say that Partners In Health continued to share its experiences in integrating AIDS prevention and care with the medical and health policy "community" in articles and in countless presentations and conferences—it would be impossible to tally the number of conferences held during those long years of inaction.

Moreover, by 2001, the "we" of Partners In Health was growing quickly, in part because so few other groups were pursuing a social justice agenda in introducing the highest possible standard of care for people living with both AIDS and poverty, and in part because the project was expanding rapidly—"scaling up"—in central Haiti. In every village we visited, we met people dying of AIDS, but we also met plenty of people anxious to serve as *accompagnateurs* who could help the afflicted by giving them their pills and social support each day.[6] When effective therapy became available, stigma, the topic of much of *AIDS and Accusation* and the factor that many policymakers believed was a barrier to effective care in Africa and Haiti, began to decline. Tens of thousands of people came to our clinics to be tested, knowing that they would receive care if we found them to be sick. In scaling up the effort we had launched in Do Kay, we learned that one can deliver high-quality health care in rural central Haiti, which lacks both paved roads and electricity and whose public health system long ago faltered and collapsed.

Indeed, Haiti and Haitians, who suffered greatly from social responses to the new and then untreatable disease with which they were initially identified, can also claim to have led the charge against AIDS. They have launched some of the poor world's first integrated prevention and care programs. Over the past few years, these efforts have not gone unnoticed. The policymakers who had earlier declared that prevention alone would have to suffice in settings as poor as Haiti had to modify their positions, not so much because the model developed in Haiti proved to be effective but because models that ignored treatment proved so utterly ineffective. In 2003, a new funding mechanism, the Global Fund to Fight AIDS, Tuberculosis, and Malaria, allowed Haiti to ramp up longstanding efforts to prevent new infections and to improve care for the sick; U.S. federal funds eventually followed. Even as some poor nations seemed ready to concede defeat in the struggle against AIDS, Haiti could point to real victories. Laurie Garrett, writing in the *New York Times* in July 2004, noted that "a new Global Fund report shows that of the 25 projects supported by the fund for more than a year, 80 percent have already either achieved or even surpassed their five-year goals. As chaotic as it is, Haiti surpassed its 2006 targets after only a year of Global Fund support."[7] A more detailed *New York Times* article, based on reporting from Do Kay, announced in its title "Rural Haitians Are Vanguard in AIDS Battle."[8]

Here in Rwanda, in the rural reaches of the world's poorest continent, some responses to the idea of integrating AIDS prevention and care were much the same as the global authorities' initial responses to the idea of treating AIDS in Haiti. Once again, we heard claims that stigma would prevent Rwandans from coming to clinics to be tested, but these claims were not supported by data. In Africa, as in Haiti, AIDS is stigmatized because it is a fatal wasting disease, but stigma did not prevent hundreds of Rwandans from seeking care once it was finally available. In Rwinkwavu, a town said to consist mostly of former exiles and people displaced by the 1994 genocide, hundreds have undergone screening for HIV infection in the past few months alone. Many of the people we found to be infected are now on proper therapy, again with the help of *accompagnateurs*. Indeed, veterans of the Haiti scale-up effort, which has long been led by a dynamic and experienced Haitian physician, came to rural Rwanda to help train *accompagnateurs* and nurses to build a similar project in the Rwandan countryside.

Haiti and Rwanda are about the same size, and both countries crowd more than eight million people into a mountainous area about the size of Maryland. Most inhabitants, in both places, are or have been peasant farmers. Haiti was colonized by France, Rwanda by Belgium. However, when we began work in Rwanda, I quickly realized the lack of cultural similarities between rural Rwanda and rural Haiti—indeed, my Haitian colleagues needed translators to speak with the rural Rwandans, who spoke Kinyarwanda and not French. The similarities of note were of the structural sort: deep poverty, a history of postcolonial violence, and a similar burden of disease (with AIDS, tuberculosis, malaria, and hunger heading the list).

Although the Haitian epidemic is unrelated to the African pandemic in the direct ways that the popular press asserted in the 1980s, the two epidemics do have striking parallels. The first AIDS case in Rwanda was detected in 1983, while the first cases were properly documented in Haiti in 1981, at the same time as the first cases in the United States. Rates of infection are roughly the same in both places. Tuberculosis is also the ranking opportunistic infection in Rwanda. And here, as in Haiti, great local enthusiasm exists for scaling up an integrated AIDS prevention and care program.

Given my training in anthropology, I know better than to claim that I have any knowledge of Rwandan culture until I'm conversant in the language and have spent at least a couple of years here. But I'm already convinced that a "geographically broad and historically deep" approach to learning will teach us about the relationship between AIDS (and other epidemics) and heavy-handed colonialism, poverty, violence, and genocide. I'm convinced, too, that the more we learn, the more we will see how Rwanda fits into a transnational web of meaning and social process, as does Haiti. Granted, Haiti's trials at the hands of the outside world have gone on nearly five times longer than those that Rwanda has endured; granted, too, Haiti's indigenous population was exterminated completely after the Europeans arrived in 1492, and almost all Haitians today are the descendants of kidnapped Africans. But I've little doubt that significant connivance from the great powers was required to arm Rwanda prior to the 1994 genocide; I'm confident that growing social inequality in a field of great social scarcity played a role in both the violence and the spread of HIV here. And in Rwanda, as in Haiti, poverty will constitute the most daunting barrier to the establishment of effective AIDS prevention and care.

GRAPPLING WITH THE NEW MYTHS AND
MYSTIFICATIONS ABOUT AIDS IN AFRICA

Here in rural Rwanda and in central Haiti, I still encounter little demand for book-length studies of AIDS or social responses to it. But that need is real, and I'm grateful to have had the chance, at least once, to spend several years working to unravel the complex skein of meaning and social process and epidemiology. Allow me to close these reflections by returning to the role of scholarship and by considering some of the analytic challenges now facing those who will confront the so-called new AIDS—new because, as noted in *AIDS and Accusation,* the epidemic changes rapidly, as do social responses to it, as does, we now know, the virus itself. Once again, we need processual studies, and these studies must be properly biosocial because one of the reasons the epidemic in Africa is changing is that ARVs are at last becoming available here, where the need is greatest. I still believe that perhaps only anthropology has the scope to understand this complex disease, but ethnographic studies will be accurate only if anthropologists work with others who are familiar with the pathophysiology and epidemiology of AIDS and of other infectious pathogens. Ethnographic studies will be accurate only if they rest on a sound knowledge of history and political economy.

Many studies similar to *AIDS and Accusation,* with AIDS in Africa as their topic, have been published recently, but much remains to be done. Surely, enterprising graduate students in medical anthropology would find a rich subject in the myths and mystifications swirling around Africa today, during this period that should be the post-antibiotic era but isn't yet. Across the continent, most of the people infected with HIV are not "living with AIDS," to use the American catchphrase. They are dying of AIDS.

Yet Africans everywhere know that medications exist to treat AIDS and tuberculosis (and, indeed, malaria and each of the pathologies mentioned in this book). So we see in Africa, as in Haiti, accusations and blame, myths and mystifications. If Haitians have any rivals in their degree of subjection to racist and ridiculous commentaries, or to immodest claims of causality from experts who should know better, they exist here on this continent.

We can identify some of the most pernicious myths and half-truths, especially those serving to explain inaction. People say that the medications are too expensive, which is true. But is this statement the beginning of a conversation or the end of one? In Haiti and elsewhere, the introduction of generic ARVs has lowered the price of a three-drug cocktail from about $10,000 per patient per year (the U.S. price tag for branded pharmaceuticals) or $1,500 per patient per year (the concessional price we paid in 1998) to less than $150 per patient per year. And the prices are still dropping. Surely such a welcome and vertiginous drop should make economists and public health specialists who claim treatment is not cost-effective a little more humble. How can we make confident claims about cost-effectiveness when both the cost and the "effectiveness" of our interventions change so rapidly?

Even if we agree that AIDS care is a right, there are significant challenges. We need to understand that as long as these medications remain commodities on the open market, they will be available only to those who can afford them. Regardless of how low the costs go, there will always be some who cannot pay. For those interested in health as a human right, the sale of ARVs will always pose problems.

Experts point out that the poorer parts of Africa lack the public health infra-structure needed to treat AIDS. This statement too is true. But, again, is it the end of a discussion of the disastrous impact of divesting from public health, or is it the beginning of one about building or rebuilding such infrastructures in the places that need them most? In Haiti, we've shown that investing in integrated AIDS prevention and care can strengthen faltering public health systems and improve women's health, tuberculosis and vaccination programs, and primary care.[9] If recent statements about the lack of health care infrastructure are the beginning of a long-overdue conversation, we will soon realize that one of the most important components of such infrastructure—personnel—is readily avail-able. Unemployment is high in the places that need AIDS treatment the most, and many people can be trained to be *accompagnateurs* or community health workers; their engagement will ensure that the quality of long-term care is sus-tained and improved. An honest discussion about the "brain drain" that sucks trained medical personnel out of Africa to more affluent settings in Europe and North America would also be welcome.[10]

Meanwhile, some people complain that AIDS-related stigma in Africa is over-whelming. This statement too is true. But, as we learned in Haiti, stigma is not often a barrier to actual AIDS treatment; rather, proper AIDS treatment, and indeed quality medical care for any affliction, is simply unavailable to the poor. Social barriers are, in truth, economic barriers, and these barriers will not be addressed by patient education or other attempts to change the patients rather than to change their social conditions. Empty clinics and testing centers sud-denly fill up when user fees are dropped and quality services become available to the poor.

Poverty is also at the heart of many of the problems facing those who seek to prevent mother-to-child transmission of HIV. We were assured, frequently by "experts," that the highest standard of care—ARVs during pregnancy and avoid-ance of breastfeeding after parturition—is impossible in Africa not only for the obvious reason (that children who do not breastfeed are at risk of gastroenteritis if clean water is unavailable) but also because bottle-feeding will stigmatize moth-ers. Our experience in rural Rwanda has already taught us that, as real as the challenges of clean water are, little evidence exists that stigma will undermine the success of ambitious programs that prevent babies from ingesting HIV-positive breast milk. In fact, we discovered quickly that some poor women borrowed their neighbors' children or claimed to be infected with HIV in order to receive the meager assistance—powdered milk, a kerosene stove to boil water, and a modest stipend for school fees—that our "AIDS program" offers in the Rwinkwavu area. So much for AIDS stigma. The challenges to efforts to prevent mother-to-child transmission of HIV are, rather, of a different order: avoiding stockouts of for-mula; reaching the poorest women; increasing access to reliably clean water.

Debates about what is to be done in Africa rage on. Some authorities continue to tell us to focus solely on prevention in the poorest countries, as if treatment and prevention somehow contradict each other. In fact, plenty of evidence is emerging that good treatment can strengthen prevention efforts.[11] Others have admonished us to focus solely on tuberculosis, which, unlike AIDS, is a curable disease. But these two chronic infectious diseases are tightly intertwined in Africa, and we focus on only one at the peril of our patients and the public at large. HIV-infected patients with tuberculosis will one day fall ill again, sometimes with a second case of tuberculosis (whether from relapse or from reinfection), and they will continue to expose those around them to this airborne disease, rendering tuberculosis control more and more difficult. This dynamic explains why rates of tuberculosis have skyrocketed across much of Africa during the past decade.

Other experts raise the specter of developing resistance to ARVs in Africa in order to slow down introduction of the medications. But any student of social behavior knows that this ploy is as wrongheaded as it is unethical. Throughout the world, people living with HIV want to stop dying of AIDS; their loved ones want them to survive. These families will sell their belongings to buy ARVs in a haphazard, off-and-on way. Intermittent access to these drugs is one of the quickest ways to fan an epidemic of drug-resistant HIV, as we have learned in the United States and elsewhere. Again, removing AIDS care from the market and putting it into the public domain—a public good for public health—is the smartest and most humane way to slow the emergence of acquired drug resistance, a problem seen with almost every infectious disease for which a treatment is available. And if AIDS is not the ranking public health threat in much of Africa, what is?

I have described just a few of the major analytic challenges now before us, and few of them have been addressed in a properly biosocial fashion. If today one cannot easily argue that ARVs cannot be used in the poorest parts of the world—a major victory for the afflicted and those who stand in solidarity with them—confused debates nonetheless continue to waste precious time. We should brace ourselves for the next great wave of debate, which will undoubtedly focus on what the modern world owes the destitute sick. If AIDS care becomes a right rather than a commodity, some people believe we will open a Pandora's box. Others, including me, believe that we have no more excuses for ignoring the growing inequality that has left hundreds of millions of people without any hope of surviving preventable and treatable illnesses. Those hundreds of millions are the same people who entered the new millennium without access to clean water, primary education, proper housing, and decent jobs. Taking on AIDS forcefully would allow us to start a "virtuous social cycle," long overdue, that might begin with one disease but end with a lot less inhumanity directed toward others with whom we share this fragile planet.

NOTES

1. We have described these programs in optimistic terms, probably in large part because obtaining financing was so hard in the early days. See, for example, Farmer, "Ethnography, Social Analysis, and the Prevention of Sexually Transmitted HIV Infection among Poor Women in Haiti" (included in this volume as chapter 4). For à more critical review of these programs, see Farmer and Walton, "Condoms, Coups, and Ideology of Prevention." Note that the latter essay, though published in 2000, was written just as we were beginning to scale up ARV therapy in central Haiti, an effort that quickly led to improved prevention outcomes.

2. These "immodest claims of causality" regarding tuberculosis and AIDS care are the chief topic of Farmer, *Infections and Inequalities.*

3. See Farmer, Robin, et al., "Tuberculosis, Poverty, and 'Compliance.'"

4. The concept of "public goods for public health" is explored in Kim, Shakow, Castro, et al., "Tuberculosis Control."

5. For an engaging account of the spread of HIV to the poorest parts of the world and a description of attempts, including ours, to introduce proper AIDS care as a human right, see d'Adesky, *Moving Mountains.*

6. *Accompagnateurs* are almost always neighbors of patients—some of them patients themselves—who accept responsibility for supervising daily care and support for people suffering from AIDS or tuberculosis; they are trained by Partners In Health staff and are the cornerstone of our projects in Haiti, Peru, Boston, Rwanda, and elsewhere. This strategy for treating AIDS in areas now termed "resource-poor settings" is described in a number of papers in the medical literature. See, for example, Farmer, Léandre, Mukherjee, Claude, et al., "Community-Based Approaches to HIV Treatment in Resource-Poor Settings"; Farmer, Léandre, Mukherjee, Gupta, et al., "Community-Based Treatment of Advanced HIV Disease"; Behforouz, Farmer, and Mukherjee, "From Directly Observed Therapy to *Accompagnateurs.*"

7. Garrett, "Bragging in Bangkok."

8. Dugger, "Rural Haitians Are Vanguard in AIDS Battle."

9. See Walton et al., "Integrated HIV Prevention and Care Strengthens Primary Health Care" (included in this volume as chapter 13).

10. We've also sought to address this issue in considering the social barriers to proper care for AIDS and other epidemic diseases; see Walton, Farmer, and Dillingham, "Social and Cultural Factors in Tropical Medicine." For more on burnout among African physicians in a Kenyan teaching hospital, which admits hundreds of patients dying of AIDS and tuberculosis but cannot care for them properly, see Raviola et al., "HIV, Disease Plague, Demoralization and 'Burnout.'"

11. See, for example, Blower and Farmer, "Predicting the Public Health Impact of Antiretrovirals."

Anthropology amid Epidemics

Introduction to Part 2

Paul Farmer

This part of the book groups a second set of (sometimes yeomanlike) studies and essays under the rubric "Anthropology amid Epidemics." The first of these essays builds on lessons learned: that large-scale social forces are what drive forward epidemic diseases, and that this is just as true of what have been called "social diseases" (tuberculosis, for example, and what were once termed "venereal diseases") as it is of, say, dengue or typhus or even Ebola. Sometimes these largely economic considerations are referred to as structural forces. That structural forces are the motive power behind contagious disease is obvious to historians of medicine, to social scientists who study epidemics, and to those epidemiologists not blinkered by what they consider ever more refined methodologies, which too commonly move such large-scale socioeconomic forces out of consideration altogether in favor of mathematical modeling or genetic fingerprinting (useful *components*, often, of biosocial analysis).

The failure to contemplate social and economic aspects of epidemics stunts our understanding of them. Thus can tuberculosis, for many decades the leading infectious killer of young adults around the globe, have been considered a "conquered" disease when it stopped killing people in the wealthy world (and in that world alone), and an "emerging" one only when a series of complex forces (again, largely social) led in recent decades to a series of rather spectacular nosocomial outbreaks in the United States.

So how does an anthropologist (who happens to be a physician) practice anthropology amid epidemics? I hope that it will be clear from these chapters that my intent has always been to link sound analyses to improved interventions, whether these interventions were designed to improve cure rates in tuberculosis programs in Haiti or to strengthen HIV prevention efforts there and elsewhere. The link between analysis and intervention is far and away the leading unexamined problem in public health. As analyses are desocialized, so too are interventions. Insofar as public health involves an educational component, analysis should be tightly allied with relevant interventions. But here is the conundrum: if structural forces, rather than cognitive considerations (patient knowledge of transmission, say), are what shape the broad outlines of epidemic disease, then why are so many of the interventions conceived by physicians and epidemiologists and public health specialists designed to instruct patients how to behave and even, at times, what to believe? The full weight of many old-school "hygiene programs," which sought to alter behavior and belief and even culture, is felt in modern public health and indeed in many attempts to advance programs for social change.

The tough question is, Whose culture are we seeking to change? Looking back to my undergraduate training, I think I'd been warned about easy answers to this question by books like *Tally's Corner,* which seemed to dissuade anyone from seeking to discern and then change the "unique culture" of urban black America: in this version of ethnography, culture was held to explain (to cause or account for) the creation and re-creation of an American underclass.[1] If culture re-creates class, then reformers seeking to improve the lot of unemployed men of color should seek to change their culture rather than to change the society in which subaltern classes and culture emerge. This "culture of poverty" argument hinged on a claim of causality that sidestepped the obvious pressure of economic and social structures on "culture"—and the result is the classic stratagem of "blaming the victim," as William Ryan noted in an important essay by the same name.[2]

One could discern the same tendency among those working in development assistance and international health: the causes of persistent or deepening poverty and growing inequality were structural and transregional, such as unfair trade agreements or poor labor conditions or unjust land tenure, whereas many of the proposed interventions were cognitive and local ("teach a man to fish," and so on). I've spent a lot of time underlining this mismatch. The startling thing, to me, was that even when social scientists agree on claims of causality, they too often end up participating in programs that focus only on one small part of the puzzle. Thus anthropologists become experts on "culture," as if the chief problem to be addressed were the locals' culture. This gap between analysis and interventions is the reason that the term "myths and mystifications" appears in more than one of the chapters in this book.

But the converse view—that because poverty is the root cause of these epidemics, poverty reduction should be our sole focus in public health—is not adequate either. I have termed this view the "Luddite trap." It amounts to throwing one's hands up in the face of an unbeatable (indeed, almost incomprehensible) "sea of troubles." If the cultural models are too narrow to lead to a solution, the Luddite problem is too big. Prescriptions exist for AIDS, tuberculosis, malaria, typhoid, and the other ills described in this section; but no one has yet discovered (even with double-blind, controlled studies) an effective prescription for poverty. To this day, leading macroeconomists cannot agree on the best remedy for poverty in Africa (or Haiti); by contrast, competent clinicians can usually agree on the proper treatment for every disease mentioned in this book and more.

Mindful of the skepticism with which my Haitian neighbors greeted ethnographic research, during my first years as a physician I spent most of my time working with Partners In Health and seeing patients, writing field notes and conducting interviews only in what little time was left. What struck me in considering—indeed, in combating—AIDS and tuberculosis and malaria was that success or failure in efforts to control these epidemics could be attributed, once again, to completely discrepant claims of causality on the part of the interveners. This was startling. Persistent tuberculosis could be attributed to persistent poverty (social limitations) or to ignorance about tuberculosis (cognitive limitations, which were curiously limited, in this view, to people living in poverty). But both hypotheses could not possibly be true, unless, by some miracle of predestination, poor people and only poor people suffered from the ignorance that caused tuberculosis. Yet too few seemed to be ready to address tuberculosis with more than a pedagogical solution.

The mismatch between the problem and the solutions proposed, even more striking as regards AIDS, was deeply troubling to me and to the growing number who worked with us in Partners In Health projects in Haiti and elsewhere. We were physicians and nurses and community health workers, primarily; none of us had been trained to deal with structural problems such as fair trade and labor markets (forget about undoing the legacy of slavery and colonialism). We were trained to take care of the sick and to focus our prevention efforts on vaccination campaigns—when we were lucky enough to have vaccines; there is none for AIDS, tuberculosis, or malaria—or on cognitive interventions designed to change what people understand or know about health and illness.

It's the hypothesis of these chapters that in each of the epidemics examined, causation is more social than cognitive; *it's the conditions* in which people live, rather than their cognitive limitations, that intensify risk. This is true whether examining an airborne pathogen, a sexually transmitted one, or a vector-borne disease such as malaria, though the dynamics of spread differ, as do the mechanisms by which these diseases come to be embodied in flesh and blood, even when the outcome is the same: very different pathogens move, through paths of least resistance, into the bodies of the poor. The chapters in this section set out my understanding of epidemic disease as a phenomenon that is fundamentally biosocial. By "biosocial," I mean that disease is a composite event-process involving some factors that can be identified and isolated in a laboratory, and some that are economic and social in nature: the disruption of stable families by migration in southern Africa, say, as well as brute forces such as food insecurity, landlessness, or the complex interplay between poverty and gender inequality.

Since the biosocial realm is a composite one, analysis will have to identify, among many possibilities, the best point at which intervention should take place. The "immodest claims of causality" I often critique here have the shared weakness of singling out one factor as the explanation, as if others can then be neglected. Our work with poor communities has taught us that neither medication, nor food support, nor accompaniment, nor prevention, nor public health education can provide a stand-alone answer to the problem of contagious disease. The good news: when comprehensive approaches to these epidemics are applied, they work. Pessimism regarding the design and outcomes of comprehensive programs then gives way to pessimism regarding our ability to muster resources, mobilize political will, and implement comprehensive programs. I've been working with Partners In Health long enough to see that, in certain times and places, optimism regarding these epidemics is warranted. Over the past two decades, in rural Haiti, overall HIV prevalence fell from 5 percent of the population to 2.2 percent in 2008. Although much debate will surround discrepant claims regarding this decline, the retreat of the epidemic is both welcome and gratifying to all who have sought to meet this goal.

NOTES

1. Liebow, *Tally's Corner.*
2. Ryan, *Blaming the Victim.*

6

Rethinking "Emerging Infectious Diseases"

(1996, 1999)

However secure and well-regulated civilized life may become, bacteria, Protozoa, viruses, infected fleas, lice, ticks, mosquitoes, and bedbugs will always lurk in the shadows ready to pounce when neglect, poverty, famine, or war lets down the defenses. And even in normal times they prey on the weak, the very young and the very old, living along with us, in mysterious obscurity waiting their opportunities.

HANS ZINSSER, *RATS, LICE, AND HISTORY*

The microbe is nothing; the terrain, everything.

LOUIS PASTEUR, 1822–95

AIDS. Ebola. Flesh-eating bacteria. One of the most significant events of the past ten or fifteen years is the explosion of "emerging infectious diseases." Some of these disorders—such as AIDS and Brazilian purpuric fever—can be regarded as genuinely new. Others were clinically identified some time ago but have newly identified etiologic agents or have again burst onto the scene in dramatic fashion. For example, the syndromes caused by Hantaan viruses have been known in Asia for centuries, but they now seem to be spreading beyond that continent as a result of ecological and economic transformations that increase contact between humans and rodents. The phenomenology of neuroborreliosis had been tackled long before the monikers "Lyme disease" and *Borrelia burgdorferi* were coined, and before suburban reforestation and golf courses complicated the equation by creating an environment agreeable to both ticks and affluent humans. Hemorrhagic fevers, including Ebola, were described long ago, and their etiologic agents were in many cases identified in previous decades. Still other diseases grouped under the "emerging" rubric are ancient and well-known foes that have changed, either in pathogenicity or distribution. Multidrug-resistant tuberculosis and invasive or necrotizing Group A streptococcal infection—the "flesh-eating bacteria" of the popular press—are cases in point.

Popularizing the concept of "emerging infectious diseases" has helped to marshal a sense of urgency, notoriously difficult to arouse in large bureaucracies. Funds have been channeled, conferences convened, articles written, and a dedicated journal founded. The research and action programs elaborated in response to the perceived emergence of new infections have, by and large, been sound.

But the concept also carries complex symbolic burdens—as do some of the diseases most commonly associated with it. Such burdens have certainly complicated and, in some instances, hampered the laying down of new knowledge. If certain populations have long been afflicted by these disorders, why are the diseases considered "new" or "emerging"? Is it simply because they have come to affect more visible—read, more "valuable"—persons? This would seem to be an obvious question from the perspective of the Haitian or African poor.

In the emerging literature on emerging infectious diseases, some questions are posed while others are not. A subtle and flexible understanding of emerging infections would be grounded in critical and reflexive study of how our knowledge develops. Units of analysis and key terms would be scrutinized and regularly redefined. These processes would include periodic rethinking not only of methodologies and study design but also of the validity of causal inference, and they would allow reflection on the limits of human knowledge.

The study of such processes, loosely known as epistemology, often happens in retrospect. To their credit, however, many of the chief contributors to the growing literature on emerging infectious diseases, accustomed to debate about microbial nomenclature, have shown exceptional self-awareness in examining the epistemological issues surrounding their work. Many are also thoroughly familiar with the multifactorial nature of disease emergence. In a 1995 review, one of the prime movers in the field (a virologist) noted that the emergence of a newly recognized or novel disease is rarely a purely virological event without identifiable causative co-factors: "Responsible factors include ecological changes, such as those due to agricultural or economic development or to anomalies in the climate; human demographic changes and behavior; travel and commerce; technology and industry; microbial adaptation and change; and breakdown of public health measures."[1] Similarly, the Institute of Medicine's influential report on emerging infections categorizes microbial threats not by type of agent, but rather according to major factors held to be related to their emergence: "human demographics and behavior; technology and industry; economic development and land use; international travel and commerce; microbial adaptation and change; and breakdown of public health measures."[2]

Many students of emerging diseases thus distinguish between a host of phenomena directly related to human actions—ranging from improved laboratory techniques and scientific discovery to economic development, global warming, and failures of public health—and another set of phenomena, much less common and deriving more directly from changes in the microbes themselves. Even in cases of microbial mutations, however, we commonly find signs that human actions have played a large role in enhancing pathogenicity or increasing resistance to antimicrobial agents. In one long list of emerging viral infections, for example, only the emergence of Rift Valley fever is attributed to a possible change in virulence or pathogenicity; and this cause is enumerated after social factors, for which better evidence exists.[3]

No need, then, to launch a campaign calling for a heightened awareness of sociogenesis, or "anthropogenesis," of disease emergence. Ironically, perhaps, some of the bench scientists involved in the field are both more likely to refer to a broad range of social factors and less likely to make immodest claims of causality about any one of them than are behavioral scientists who study infectious diseases.

Yet a *critical* epistemology of emerging infectious diseases is still in the early stages of development. A key task of this endeavor is to take our existing conceptual frameworks and ask, If we conceptualize disease in this way, what is obscured? What is brought into relief?

For example, a first step in understanding the epistemological dimension of disease emergence involves, as Irina Eckardt argues, developing "a certain sensitivity to the terms we are used to."[4] When we think of "tropical diseases," for instance, malaria comes quickly to mind. But not too long ago, malaria was a significant problem far from the tropics. Although there is imperfect overlap between malaria as currently defined and the malaria of the mid-nineteenth century, some medical historians agree with contemporary assessments that this illness "was the most important disease in the United States at the time." In the Ohio River Valley, according to Daniel Drake's 1850 study, thousands died in seasonal epidemics. A million-odd soldiers were afflicted with malaria during the U.S. Civil War. During the second decade of the twentieth century, when the population of the twelve southern states was about twenty-five million, the region saw an estimated one million cases of malaria per year. Malaria's decline in this country was "due only in small part to measures aimed directly against it, but more to agricultural development and to other factors some of which are still not clear."[5]

One responsible factor that is clear enough, if little discussed in the literature, is the reduction of poverty, including the development of improved housing, land drainage, mosquito repellents, nets, and electric fans—all of which have been (and remain) beyond the reach of those most at risk for malaria.[6] In fact, many "tropical" diseases predominantly afflict the poor; the groups at risk for these diseases are typically bounded more by socioeconomic status than by latitude. In Haiti, for example, my patients with malaria are almost exclusively those living in poverty.

None have electricity; none take prophylaxis; many have lost kin to malaria. This aspect of disease emergence is thus obscured by an uncritical use of the term "tropical medicine," which implies a geographic rather than a social topography.[7]

Any modern practitioner dealing with infectious disease knows this well, even if he or she sits in a travel clinic in New England. Those who come in for malaria prophylaxis and ask about appropriate vaccinations are students, professionals, and tourists. But when practitioners are called into the emergency room for an imported case of malaria, we usually see a very different patient shuddering on a damp gurney. In Boston, at least, the patient with malaria is likely to have been born in an endemic region—Haiti, say, or West Africa—and to be working as a laborer in the U.S. service economy. And that patient is also likely to tell us the diagnosis, for it will not be the first time that he or she has had malaria.

Similarly, the concept of "health transitions" is influential in what some have termed "the new public health" and also among sectors of the international financial institutions that typically control development efforts.[8] The health transitions model suggests that nation-states, as they develop, go through predictable epidemiological transformations. Death due to infectious causes is gradually supplanted by death due to malignancies and complications of coronary artery disease; the latter deaths occur at a more advanced age, reflecting progress. Although it describes broad patterns now apparent throughout the world, the concept of national health transitions masks other realities, including morbidity and mortality differentials *within* nationalities, which show that health conditions are often more tightly linked to local inequalities than to nationality.

For example, much was made of the fact that noncommunicable pathologies such as coronary artery disease and malignancies caused the majority of all world deaths in 1990. A very different picture emerges, however, when we compare causes of death among the wealthiest fifth of the world's population to the afflictions that kill the poorest fifth: although only 8 percent of deaths among the world's wealthiest were caused by infections or by maternal and perinatal mortality, fully 56 percent of all deaths among the poorest were caused by those pathologies, with infectious diseases at the head of the list.[9] How do the variables of class and race fit into such paradigms? In Harlem, where age-specific mortality in several groups is higher than in Bangladesh, leading causes of death are infectious disease and violence.[10]

The units of analysis are similarly up for grabs. When Surgeon General David Satcher, writing of emerging infectious diseases, reminds us that "the health of the individual is best ensured by maintaining or improving the health of the entire community,"[11] we should applaud his clear-sightedness. But we should also go on to ask, What constitutes "the entire community"? In a few instances—the 1994 outbreak of cryptosporidiosis in Milwaukee, say—the answer might be part of a city.[12] In other instances, "community" may mean a village or a group of passengers on an airplane. But the most common unit of analysis referred to in public health, the nation-state, is not all that meaningful to organisms such as dengue virus, *Vibrio cholera* O_{139}, HIV, penicillinase-producing *Neisseria gonorrhoeae,* multidrug-resistant tuberculosis, and hepatitis B virus. Such organisms proudly disregard political boundaries, even though a certain degree of "turbulence" in their dynamics may be introduced at national borders. The dynamics of disease emergence are not captured in nation-by-nation analyses any more than the diseases are contained by national boundaries, which are themselves emerging entities. (Most of the world's nations are, after all, twentieth-century creations, which might also give pause to those buying into the two-worlds myth.)

The limitations of these three important ways of viewing the health of populations—the concepts of tropical medicine, health transitions, and national health profiles—demonstrate that models and even assumptions about infectious diseases need to be *dynamic, systematic,* and *critical.* That is, models with explanatory power must be able to track rapidly changing clinical, even molecular, phenomena and link them to the large-scale (frequently transnational) social forces that shape the contours of disease emergence. I refer here to questions less on the order of how pig-duck agriculture might be related to the antigenic shifts central to influenza pandemics and more on the order of the following: Are World Bank policies related to the spread of HIV, as some have claimed?[13] What is the connection between international shipping practices and the spread of cholera from Asia to South America and elsewhere in the hemisphere?[14] How is genocide in Rwanda related to cholera in Zaïre?[15]

The study of anything said to be "emerging" tends to be *dynamic.* But the very notion of emergence in heterogeneous populations poses analytical questions that are rarely tackled, even in modern epidemiology, which, as Anthony McMichael argues, "assigns a primary importance to studying interindividual variations in risk. By concentrating on these specific and presumed free-range individual behaviors, we thereby pay less attention to the underlying social-historical influences on behavioral choices, patterns, and population health."[16]

Systematic analyses of disease emergence are not hemmed in by political or administrative borders. New tools based on DNA analysis allow us to rethink comfortable conclusions regarding treatment for some but not for others. The notorious "W strain" of multidrug-resistant tuberculosis, for example, spread quickly through New York City but then moved on to Atlanta, Miami, and Denver.[17] Later data suggest that the W strain's family tree has roots in Asia and Russia.[18] If these are transnational pandemics, spread through sharing air, then surely responses must be transnational—although, thus far, such responses have been hobbled by short-sighted parochialism. Genetic subtyping of HIV leads to the same conclusions.

A *critical* (and self-critical) approach would ask how existing frameworks might limit our ability to discern trends that are in fact related to the emergence of diseases. Not all social-production-of-disease theories are equally alive to the significance of how relative social and economic positioning—inequality— affects the risk of infection. For example, neither poverty nor inequality appears as a "cause of emergence" in the self-described "catalog" of emerging infections compiled by the Institute of Medicine.

Further, a critical approach would push the limits of existing academic politesse in order to ask more difficult and rarely raised questions, questions that still need to be answered if we are to better understand disease emergence. Examples might include issues such as these: By what mechanisms have international changes in agriculture shaped recent outbreaks of Argentine and Bolivian hemorrhagic fever, and how do these mechanisms derive from international trade agreements such as GATT and NAFTA? How might institutional racism be related to both urban crime and the epidemics of multidrug-resistant tuberculosis registered in New York prisons? Does privatization of health services buttress social inequalities, increasing risks for certain infections—and worsening outcomes— among the poor of sub-Saharan Africa and Latin America? How do the colonial histories of Belgium and Germany, and the neocolonial histories of France and the United States, tie into genocide in Rwanda—which was itself related to an epidemic of cholera? We can productively pose similar questions about many of the diseases now held to be emerging, as a few examples will suggest.

EMERGING HOW AND TO WHAT EXTENT? THE CASE OF EBOLA

Hemorrhagic fevers have been known in Africa since well before the continent was dubbed "the white man's grave" (an expression that, when used to refer to a region with such high rates of premature death, speaks volumes about the differential valuation of human lives). Ebola itself was isolated more than two decades ago.[19] Its appearance in human hosts has at times been insidious but more often takes the form of explosive eruptions. In accounting for recent outbreaks, it is unnecessary to postulate a change in filovirus virulence through mutation. For filoviruses, the Institute of Medicine catalog lists a single "factor facilitating emergence": "virus-infected monkeys shipped from developing countries via air."[20] Other factors can be easily identified, however. As with many infectious diseases, the distribution of Ebola outbreaks is tied to regional trade networks and other evolving social systems. And, as with many infectious diseases, Ebola explosions afflict—researchers aside—certain groups (people living in poverty, health care workers who serve the poor) while largely sparing others in close physical proximity.

Take, for example, the 1976 emergence of Ebola in Sudan. This epidemic was anything but random, for it was amplified by substandard medical practices in a mission hospital. Richard Preston recounts the story in his best-seller *The Hot Zone:* "It hit the hospital like a bomb. It savaged patients and snaked like chain lightning out from the hospital through patients' families. Apparently the medical staff had been giving patients injections with dirty needles."[21] Two months later, the better-known and more virulent outbreak in the region drained by Zaïre's Ebola River gave the disease its name and its fame.

The story was almost identical in both instances. The nuns who ran the Yambuku Mission Hospital started their busy day, notes Preston in his dramatic account of the Sudanese outbreak, by laying out five hypodermic syringes. These were used on the hundreds of patients who each day sought care there. "The nuns and staff occasionally rinsed the needles in a pan of warm water after injection, to get the blood off the needle." "The virus erupted simultaneously in fifty-five villages surrounding the hospital," Preston writes. "First it killed people who had received injections, and then it moved through families, killing family members, particularly women, who in Africa prepare the dead for burial. It swept through Yambuku Hospital's nursing staff, killing most of the nurses, and then it hit the Belgian nuns."[22]

The 1976 Zaïre outbreak afflicted 318 persons. Although much speculation about respiratory spread arose at the time, it has not been conclusively demonstrated as a cause of human cases. Most expert observers felt that the cases could be traced to failure to follow contact precautions, as well as improper sterilization of syringes and other paraphernalia—measures that, once taken, terminated the outbreak.[23]

It would be a grave error, however, to conclude that poor nursing practices were the *cause* of Ebola's emergence. Such simplifications desocialize our understanding by masking the contributions of social inequalities to the shape of these epidemics. On closer scrutiny, such an "explanation" suggests that Ebola does not emerge randomly: in Mobutu's Zaïre, one's likelihood of coming into contact with, say, unsterile syringes was inversely proportional to one's social status there. Local elites and sectors of the expatriate community with access to high-quality biomedical services (namely, the European and American communities and not the Rwandan refugees) were quite unlikely to contract such a disease.

The changes involved in the disease's *visibility* are equally embedded in social context. The "emergence" of Ebola has also been partly a question of our consciousness. Modern communications, including print and broadcast media, have been crucial in the casting of Ebola—a minor player, statistically speaking, in Zaïre's long list of fatal infections—as an emerging infectious disease.[24] Through CNN and other television networks, names such as "Kikwit" became, however briefly, household words in parts of Europe and North America. Journalists and novelists wrote best-selling books about small but horrific plagues, which in turn became profitable cinema. Thus, symbolically if not epidemiologically, Ebola spread like wildfire—as a danger potentially without limit. It emerged.

EMERGING FROM WHERE? THE CASE OF TUBERCULOSIS

Tuberculosis is considered another emerging disease, although in this case, "emerging" is synonymous with "reemerging." Some attribute its recrudescence to the advent of HIV—the Institute of Medicine's catalog lists "an increase in immunosuppressed populations" as the sole named factor facilitating the resurgence of tuberculosis[25]—and to the development of drug resistance. In a book subtitled *How the Battle against Tuberculosis Was Won—and Lost,* Frank Ryan states that "throughout the developed world, with the successful application of triple therapy and the enthusiastic promotion of prevention, the death rate from tuberculosis came tumbling down."[26] A 1998 piece in the *Washington Post* observes that "the invention of antibiotics quickly tamed the epidemic and most Americans put it out of mind."[27]

But can these claims of causality be taken seriously on the merits of the evidence? To be sure, the discovery of effective antituberculous therapies has saved hundreds of thousands afflicted with the disease, primarily in developed countries. But deaths from tuberculosis—once the leading cause of mortality among young adults in Europe and North America—were already declining there well before the 1943 discovery of streptomycin. In the rest of the world, and in small pockets of the United States and Europe, tuberculosis remains undaunted by ostensibly effective drugs, which are used too late, inappropriately, or not at all. From our clinic in central Haiti, it is impossible not to regard the notion of "tuberculosis resurgence" as something of a cruel joke—or yet another reminder of the invisibility of the poor.

Not all U.S. specialists are deaf to the persistent hack of patients far away. "It is sufficiently shameful," writes Michael Iseman, "that 30 years after recognition of the capacity of triple-therapy . . . to elicit 95%+ cure rates, tuberculosis prevalence rates for *many* nations remain unchanged."[28] Some estimate that over 1.7 billion persons are currently infected with quiescent but viable *Mycobacterium tuberculosis,* and, failing dramatic shifts in local epidemiology, a global analysis does not project major decreases in the importance of tuberculosis as a cause of death. Tuberculosis has retreated in certain populations, maintained a steady state in others, and surged forth in still others, remaining, at this writing, the world's leading infectious cause of preventable deaths.[29]

At mid-century, tuberculosis was still acknowledged as the great white plague. What explains this killer's invisibility by the 1970s and 1980s? Again, one must look to the study of disease *awareness*—that is, of consciousness and publicity—and its relation to power and wealth. "The neglect of tuberculosis as a major public health priority over the past two decades is simply extraordinary," wrote Christopher Murray in 1991. "Perhaps the most important contributor to this state of ignorance was the greatly reduced clinical and epidemiological importance of tuberculosis in the wealthy nations."[30]

Perhaps more telling was the lack of official concern evinced over persistently high, then rising, rates of tuberculosis among U.S. citizens living in poverty. TB's resurgence in the United States has occasioned more commentary than trends elsewhere, and it merits special scrutiny. The resurgence was initially signaled by an alteration in the trend of steady decline. Beginning in 1985, national data revealed a slowing of this downward trend: the decline was 0.2 percent in 1985, while 1986 saw a 2.6 percent increase in reported cases. In 1987, the decline was 1.1 percent. This failure to improve was described by the term "excess cases," but the true dimensions of the problem, concealed in national statistics, are revealed by breaking down the "excess cases" according to other variables.

For the Centers for Disease Control and Prevention (CDC), the salient variables are race, age, and geography. Basing an analysis on these variables reveals a much more disturbing pattern. During the years 1985–87, we find no mere "failure to decline," but rather a sharp increase in tuberculosis case rates among certain people in certain places. For example, nationwide the case rate increased 6.8 percent among blacks and 12.7 percent among Hispanics, although it *decreased* 4.8 percent among non-Hispanic whites. The increases were largest among young adults of color. Among blacks and Hispanics in the age group twenty-five to forty-four, increases in tuberculosis were reported at 17 and 27 percent, respectively.[31]

It is thus clear that some groups—ethnic minorities—account for the majority of excess cases in the United States. Dixie Snider, Louis Salinas, and Gloria Kelly estimate that 85 percent of cases among minorities can be defined as "excess," and in 1987 the absolute number of cases among blacks exceeded that among non-Hispanic whites for the first time. But we find striking geographic focus as well. Two-thirds of tuberculosis cases among blacks were reported from nine states. Between 1980 and 1987, New York City experienced a 45 percent increase in the number of persons with tuberculosis, with the burden again borne by people of color: "Increases have been most pronounced in blacks (79 percent) and in Hispanics (115 percent), especially in the 25- to 44-year age group where increases of 152 percent in blacks and 216 percent in Hispanics have been observed."[32]

In a sense, then, this "race-and-place" approach yields great insights. What at first appeared to be relatively insignificant changes in national data—a decline in the decline, as it were—were in fact significant focal outbreaks of a transmissible disease. But since race and place are largely proxies for poverty, a variable not recorded in national data on tuberculosis, there is still more to the story. For example, one study of welfare recipients in New York City found rates of tuberculosis that were seventy times the national average.[33] Clearly, the "resurgence" of tuberculosis has been felt largely by those who were already living with elevated tuberculosis risk. "Tuberculosis is not 'resurgent,'" writes Katherine Ott, "to those who have been contending with and marginalized by it all their lives."[34] In the communities most affected by tuberculosis, the disease in fact has never disappeared. Ott continues: "The story ends up as 'Tuberculosis is Back' rather than, more appropriately, 'Tuberculosis is Back in the News.' It is not its return that is extraordinary, but that its decline was to a great extent an artifact of socially constructed definitions."[35]

When complex push-pull forces move more poor people into the United States or reduce the standard of living of many people in the country, an increase in U.S. tuberculosis incidence is likely. A 1995 study of tuberculosis among foreign-born persons in the United States essentially credits immigration with the increased incidence of tuberculosis morbidity in this country. The authors observe that in some of the immigrants' countries of origin, the annual rate of infection is as great as two hundred times that registered in the United States; they further observe that those sampled included many living in homeless shelters, prisons, and camps for migrant workers. But the study contains no discussion of poverty or inequality, even though these are, along with war and political disruption, leading reasons for both high rates of tuberculosis *and* immigration to the United States. "The major determinants of risk in the foreign-born population," conclude the authors, "were the region of the world from which the person emigrated and the number of years in the United States."[36]

Mycobacteria do not respect national boundaries. The fact that endemic areas are settings from which will come many future North American tuberculosis cases argues for a more systemic approach to treatment and prevention as well as to our understanding of TB's reemergence. For this reason, at the very least, cooperation between industrialized nations and poor communities hard-hit by tuberculosis should be a new priority in tuberculosis control efforts in North America.

GOING WHERE? THE CASE OF HIV

To grasp the complexity of the issues—medical, social, and communicational— that surround the emergence of a disease into public view, consider AIDS. In the early 1980s, health officials informed the public that AIDS had probably emerged from Haiti. This speculation proved incorrect, but not before doing significant damage to Haiti's tourist industry and economy. The result: more desperate poverty, and an even steeper slope of inequality and vulnerability to disease, including AIDS. The label "AIDS vector" was also a heavy burden for the million or so Haitians living elsewhere in the Americas and certainly hampered public health efforts among them.[37]

HIV disease has since become the most spectacularly studied infection in human history. But some questions have been much better studied than others, and among those too well studied are a number of utter dead ends. Nonetheless, error is worth studying, too. Careful investigation of the mechanisms used to propagate immodest claims is an important part of a critical epistemology of emerging infectious diseases. As regards Haiti and AIDS, these mechanisms included the "exoticization" of Haiti, the existence of influential folk models about Haitians and Africans, and the conflation of poverty and cultural difference. Critical epidemiological studies might well reveal such folk models and half-baked cultural generalizations as unfortunate co-factors in the disease's spread.

HIV may not have come *from* Haiti, but it certainly went *to* Haiti. A critical reexamination of the Caribbean AIDS pandemic reveals that the distribution of HIV disease does not follow the outlines of nation-states but rather matches the contours of a transnational socioeconomic order. Much of the spread of HIV in the 1970s and 1980s moved along international "fault lines," tracking along steep gradients of inequality, which are also the paths of labor migration and sexual commerce.[38]

Also lacking, then, are considerations of the multiple dynamics of AIDS. In an important overview of the pandemic's first decade, Jonathan Mann, Daniel Tarantola, and Thomas Netter observe that its course "within and through global society is not being affected—in any serious manner—by the actions taken at the national or international level."[39] HIV has emerged, but where is it going? Why, how, and how fast? The Institute of Medicine catalog lists several factors facilitating the emergence of HIV: "urbanization; changes in lifestyles/mores; increased intravenous drug abuse; international travel; medical technology."[40] Much more could be said. HIV has spread across the globe, often wildly but never randomly. Like tuberculosis, HIV is entrenching itself in the ranks of the poor and marginalized.

Take, as an example, the rapid increase in AIDS incidence among women. In a 1992 report, the United Nations observed that "for most women, the major risk factor for HIV infection is being married."[41] It is not marriage per se, however, that places young women at risk. Throughout the world, most women with HIV infection, married or not, are living in poverty. The means by which confluent social forces—here, gender inequality and poverty—come to be embodied as risk for infection with this emerging pathogen have been neglected in biomedical, epidemiological, and even social science literature on AIDS. Fifteen years into an ever-emerging pandemic—in October 1994—editorialists writing in *Lancet* could comment concerning a new study: "We are not aware of other investigators who have considered the influence of socioeconomic status on mortality in HIV-infected individuals."[42] Thus AIDS follows the general rule that the effects of certain types of social forces on health outcomes are less likely to be studied.

Yet AIDS has always been a strikingly patterned pandemic. Despite the message of public health slogans—"AIDS Is for Everyone"—some groups are at high risk of HIV infection, whereas others clearly are shielded from risk. Furthermore, although the terminal events have been grimly similar across the board, the course of HIV disease has been highly variable. These disparities have sparked the search for hundreds of co-factors, from *Mycoplasma* and ulcerating genital lesions to voodoo rites and psychological predispositions. To date, not a single one of these associations has been convincingly shown to explain disparities in distribution or outcome of HIV disease. The best-demonstrated co-factors are *social inequalities,* which structure not only the contours of the AIDS pandemic but also the nature of the outcomes once an individual is sick with complications of HIV infection.[43] And a "cure," though eminently desirable, will not change the prognosis for the vast majority of AIDS sufferers. The advent of more effective antiviral agents promises to heighten those disparities even further: a three-drug regimen including a protease inhibitor costs $12,000 to $16,000 a year.[44] The formulators of health policy have already declared antiviral therapy to be "cost-ineffective" in the very regions in which HIV is most endemic.

TAKING A SECOND LOOK AT
EMERGING INFECTIOUS DISEASES

Writing in 1934 of typhoid fever, the emerging infectious disease of the previous century, Hans Zinsser observed that "the appraisal of the appearance of a so-called 'new' disease is fraught with many pitfalls."[45] Even a cursory reading of the literature on emerging diseases makes it clear that the examples cited here— Ebola, tuberculosis, HIV—are in no way unique in demanding contextualization through approaches offered by the social sciences. Ethnographic work can be a powerful corrective for tendencies to generate flimsy hypotheses and to rely on outmoded or inappropriate categories.[46] For example, an anthropologist working in Haiti in the early 1980s would have quickly questioned the hypothesis that voodoo was somehow related to the occurrence of the new disease known as AIDS. The "risk groups" identified by slipshod epidemiological research would have been called into question by an intimate acquaintance with the emerging epidemic in Haiti and the nearby United States.

Such approaches also include the grounding of case histories and local epidemics in the larger biosocial systems in which they take shape—which calls, most of the time, for the exploration of social inequalities. Why, for example, were there ten thousand cases of diphtheria in Russia from 1990 to 1993? It is easy enough to answer, as did the CDC, that the excess cases were due to a failure to vaccinate.[47] But only if we link this *distal* (and, in sum, technical) cause to the much more complex socioeconomic transformations altering the region's morbidity and mortality patterns will we discover compelling explanations.[48]

An epidemiology that is narrowly focused on individual risk and short on critical contextualization will not reveal these deep transformations, nor will it connect them to disease emergence. "Modern epidemiology," observes one of its leading contributors, is "oriented to explaining and quantifying the bobbing of corks on the surface waters, while largely disregarding the stronger undercurrents that determine where, on average, the cluster of corks ends up along the shoreline of risk."[49] Nor will standard journalism add much: "Amidst a flood of information," complains one of the chief chroniclers of disease emergence, "analysis and context are evaporating. . . . Outbreaks of flesh-eating bacteria may command headlines, but local failures to fully vaccinate preschool children garner little attention unless there is an epidemic."[50]

For understanding and eventually controlling emerging infectious diseases, the research questions identified by various blue-ribbon panels are incontestably important; they are, no doubt, the primary issues raised by the epidemics in question.[51] Yet there exists a series of corollary questions posed both by the diseases and by popular and scientific commentary about them. These questions pose, in turn, a series of research questions that are the exclusive province of neither social scientists nor bench scientists, neither clinicians nor epidemiologists. Indeed, we will need genuinely transdisciplinary collaboration to tackle the problems posed by emerging infectious diseases. As prolegomenon, four areas of corollary research, outlined in the following sections, are easily identified. In each is heard the recurrent leitmotiv of inequality.

Emerging Infectious Diseases and Social Inequalities

Study of the reticulated links between social inequalities and emerging disease would not construe the poor simply as "sentinel chickens" or mineshaft canaries. Instead it would ask, What are the precise mechanisms by which these diseases come to afflict some bodies but not others? What propagative effects might inequality per se contribute?[52] Similar queries were once major research questions for epidemiology and social medicine, but they have fallen out of favor, leaving a vacuum in which scholars and officials can easily stake immodest claims of causality.

Studies that examine the conjoint influence of social inequalities are virtually nonexistent; Nancy Krieger and colleagues, in a magisterial review, conclude that "the minimal research that simultaneously studies the health effects of racism, sexism, and social class ultimately stands as a sharp indictment of the narrow vision limiting much of the epidemiological research conducted within the United States."[53] And yet social inequalities shape not only the distribution of emerging diseases but also the health outcomes of those afflicted—a fact that is often downplayed: "Although there are many similarities between our vulnerability to infectious diseases and that of our ancestors, there is one distinct difference: we have the benefit of extensive scientific knowledge," wrote David Satcher in 1995.[54] True enough, if one is willing to gloss over the all-important question of who "we" are. The persons most at risk for emerging infectious diseases generally do not, in fact, have much of the benefit of scientific knowledge. We live in a world where infections pass easily across borders—social and geographic—while resources, including cumulative scientific knowledge, are blocked at customs.

Emerging Infectious Diseases in Transnational Perspective

"Travel is a potent force in disease emergence and spread," as Mary Wilson reminds us, and the "current volume, speed, and reach of travel are unprecedented."[55] Although the smallpox and measles epidemics accompanying the European colonization of the Americas were early and deadly reminders of the need for systemic understandings of microbial traffic, recent decades have seen a certain reification of the notion of the "catchment area." A useful means of delimiting a sphere of action—a district, a county, a country—has been erroneously elevated to the status of explanatory principle whenever the geographic unit of analysis is other than that defined by the disease itself.

Almost all diseases held to be emerging—from increasing drug resistance to the great pandemics of HIV and cholera—stand as modern rebukes to the parochialism of this and other public health constructs, as those who study such diseases are well aware.[56] Nevertheless, a critical sociology of liminality—of both the advancing, transnational edges of pandemics and the impress of human-made administrative and political boundaries on disease emergence—has yet to be attempted. But this sort of pragmatic solidarity, even if born of self-interest, seems unlikely to occur without new and aggressive advocacy. "Unless there is a clear and substantial immediate local need," noted a 1995 *Lancet* editorial, the "long-term implications of transnational disease spread are rarely addressed."[57]

The study of borders qua borders means, increasingly, the study of social inequalities. Many political borders serve as semipermeable membranes, quite open to diseases and yet closed to the free movement of cures. Thus inequalities of access can be created or buttressed at borders, even when pathogens cannot be so contained.

Research questions might include, for example, the following: How does the interface between two very different types of health care systems affect the rate of advance of an emerging disease? What turbulence is introduced when the border in question lies between rich and poor nations? Writing of health issues at the U.S.-Mexican border, for example, David C. Warner observes: "It is unlikely that any other binational border has such variety in health status, entitlements, and utilization."[58] Among the infectious diseases registered at this border are multidrug-resistant tuberculosis, rabies, dengue, and sexually transmitted diseases, including HIV (said to result, in part, from "cross-border use of red-light districts"). As Russia's epidemic of multidrug-resistant tuberculosis continues to grow, wealthy Scandinavia—and eventually other parts of Europe—will be hard-pressed to argue that treatment of the disease is not "cost-effective" in Russia.

As increased air and sea travel changes our notion of shared borders, steep grades of transnational inequality become more significant. Methodologies and theories relevant to the study of borders and emerging infections can come from disciplines ranging from the social sciences to molecular biology; mapping the emergence of diseases is now more feasible with the use of DNA fingerprinting and other new technologies.[59] Again, such investigations will pose difficult questions in a world where plasmids move freely but compassion is often grounded.

Emerging Infectious Diseases and the Dynamics of Change

As we elaborate lists of the factors that influence the careers of infectious diseases, we need conceptual tools that will perforce be historically deep, geographically broad, and at the same time *processual,* incorporating concepts of change. Above all, these tools must allow us to incorporate complexity rather than merely dissect or dismiss it. As Richard Levins argues, "effective analysis of emerging diseases must recognize the study of complexity as perhaps the central general scientific problem of our time."[60]

But the complexity of operators is convincing only when the variables on which it operates are well chosen. Can integrated mathematical modeling be linked to new ways of configuring systems, avoiding outmoded units of analysis such as the nation state in favor of the more fluid biosocial networks through which most pathogens clearly move? Can our embrace of complexity also encompass social complexities, including the unequal positioning of groups within larger populations? Such perspectives could be directed toward mapping the progress of diseases ranging from cholera to AIDS and would be suited to analysis of more unorthodox research subjects—for example, the effects of World Bank projects and policies on diseases ranging from onchocerciasis to plague.

Emerging Infectious Diseases and Critical Epistemology

I have argued that when we ask, What qualifies as an emerging infectious disease? we should understand that we are also asking, What is meant by "emerging"? This is no trivial shift of topic. It leads to other questions: Why do some persons constitute "risk groups," while others are "individuals at risk"? Why are some approaches and subjects considered appropriate for publication in influential journals, while others are dismissed out of hand? A critical nosology would explore the boundaries of polite and impolite discussion in science, interrogating the ways in which *perceptions* of a disease might contribute to its career. A trove of complex, affect-laden issues—the attribution of blame to perceived vectors of infection, the identification of scapegoats and victims, the role of stigma—though rarely discussed in academic medicine, are manifestly part and parcel of many of the epidemics in question.

Finally, why are some epidemics visible to those who fund research and services, while others are invisible? Certainly the degree to which multidrug-resistant tuberculosis is seen as a threat varies with the degree to which the powerful—or, at least, the nonpoor—are deemed to be "at risk." In its recent statements on tuberculosis and emerging infections, the World Health Organization manifestly attempts to use fear of contagion to goad wealthy nations into investing in disease surveillance and control out of self-interest—an age-old public health ploy acknowledged as such in the Institute of Medicine report on emerging infections: "Diseases that appear not to threaten the United States directly rarely elicit the political support necessary to maintain control efforts."[61]

The rhetoric of immediacy has been central to professional commentary on emerging infectious diseases, a strategy that is not without risk for those who have been silently suffering with these diseases, sometimes for generations. In fact, differential valuation of human life runs throughout this commentary and throughout much of the policy designed to address epidemic disease. Critical reexamination of the impact of such differential valuation and its effect on the allocation of resources must figure in discussion of emerging infections. That it does not is a marker more of analytic failures than of editorial standards.

More than ten years ago, the sociologist of science Bruno Latour reviewed hundreds of articles appearing in several Pasteur-era French scientific reviews in order to constitute what he called an "anthropology of the sciences" (he objected to the term "epistemology"). Latour cast his net widely. "There is no essential difference between the human and social sciences and the exact or natural sciences," he wrote, "because there is no more science than there is society. I have spoken of the Pasteurians as they spoke of their microbes."[62] Here, perhaps, is a reason to engage in a proactive effort to explore themes usually relegated to the margins of scientific inquiry: those of us who describe the comings and goings of microbes—feints, parries, emergences, retreats—may one day be subjected to the scrutiny of future students of the subject.

But there are more compelling reasons to seek a sounder analytic grasp of disease emergence. The Pasteurians' microbes remain the world's leading cause of death.[63] In an essay titled "The Conquest of Infectious Diseases: Who Are We Kidding?" two researchers from the CDC argue that "clinicians, microbiologists, and public health professionals must work together to prevent infectious diseases and to detect emerging diseases quickly."[64] Clearly such transdisciplinary work is necessary if we aspire to a sound analytic purchase on disease emergence—a prerequisite of effective control measures.

My intention is ecumenical and complementary. A critical framework would not aspire to supplant the methodologies of the many disciplines, from virology to molecular epidemiology, that now concern themselves with emerging diseases. "The key task for medicine," argued the pioneers Leon Eisenberg and Arthur Kleinman almost two decades ago, "is not to diminish the role of the biomedical sciences in the theory and practice of medicine but to supplement them with an equal application of the social sciences in order to provide both a more comprehensive understanding of disease and better care of the patient. The problem is not 'too much science,' but too narrow a view of the sciences relevant to medicine."[65]

NOTES

1. Morse, "Factors in the Emergence of Infectious Diseases," p. 9.

2. Lederberg, Shope, and Oaks, *Emerging Infections*, pp. 34–112. For a similar broad view of the emergence of viral hemorrhagic fevers, see Oldstone, *Viruses, Plagues, and History*.

3. Morse, "Factors in the Emergence of Infectious Diseases."

4. Eckardt, "Challenging Complexity," p. 409.

5. This history of malaria in the United States is detailed in Norman Levine's preface to Drake's study ("Editor's Preface," esp. p. 3). The estimate of malaria cases among the Civil War troops is drawn from Garrett, *The Coming Plague*, p. 47.

6. For a helpful look at malaria as a reemerging disease, see Olliaro, Cattani, and Wirth, "Malaria, the Submerged Disease." For a critical review of recent malaria control failures, see Garrett, *The Coming Plague*, chap. 2.

7. Note that mine is a fairly innocent rereading of the term "tropical medicine," which has well-known roots in the colonial enterprise. Sheldon Watts offers a more trenchant and informed reevaluation of tropical medicine: "From its very onset tropical medicine was thus an 'instrument of empire' intended to enable the white 'races' to live in, or at the very least to exploit, all areas of the globe" (*Epidemics and History*, p. xiii). See also Cueto, "Sanitation from Above"; and Solórzano, "Sowing the Seeds of Neo-Imperialism."

8. See Frenk and Chacon, "Bases conceptuales de la nueva salud internacional." See also Arthur Kleinman's excellent critique of "objectivity" in international health (*Writing at the Margin*, pp. 68–93).

9. See Gwatkin and Heuveline, "Improving the Health of the World's Poor."

10. McCord and Freeman, "Excess Mortality in Harlem."

11. Satcher, "Emerging Infections," p. 3.

12. MacKenzie et al., "A Massive Outbreak in Milwaukee of Cryptosporidium Infection Transmitted through the Public Water Supply."

13. Lurie, Hintzen, and Lowe, "Socioeconomic Obstacles to HIV Prevention and Treatment in Developing Countries."

14. World Health Organization, "Cholera in the Americas." See also McCarthy et al., "Toxigenic Vibrio Cholerae O1 and Cargo Ships Entering Gulf of Mexico."

15. Goma Epidemiology Group, "Public Health Impact of Rwandan Refugee Crisis."

16. McMichael, "The Health of Persons, Populations, and Planets," pp. 633–34.

17. Bifani et al., "Origin and Interstate Spread of a New York City Multidrug-Resistant Mycobacterium Tuberculosis Clone Family."

18. Barry Kreiswirth, personal communication to the author.

19. Johnson et al., "Isolation and Partial Characterisation of a New Virus Causing Acute Haemorrhagic Fever in Zaire."

20. Lederberg, Shope, and Oaks, *Emerging Infections*, p. 223.

21. Preston, *The Hot Zone*, p. 68.

22. Ibid., p. 71.

23. The 1978 report by the World Health Organization ("Ebola Haemorrhagic Fever in Zaïre, 1976"), though less eloquent than Richard Preston's account, also underlined the failure to follow contact precautions. "In some cases," observes Preston, "the medical system may intensify the outbreak like a lens that focuses sunlight on a heap of tinder" (*The Hot Zone*, p. 68).

24. Garrett, "Public Health and the Mass Media."

25. Lederberg, Shope, and Oaks, *Emerging Infections*, p. 213.

26. Ryan, *The Forgotten Plague*, p. 384.

27. DiBacco, "Tuberculosis on the Rebound—A Disease Thought Tamed Is Again Causing Concern."

28. Iseman, "Tailoring a Time-Bomb," p. 735.

29. Bloom and Murray, "Tuberculosis."

30. Murray, "Social, Economic, and Operational Research on Tuberculosis," p. 150.

31. Snider, Salinas, and Kelly, "Tuberculosis," p. 647.

32. Ibid.

33. Friedman et al., "Tuberculosis, AIDS, and Death among Substance Abusers on Welfare in New York City."

34. Ott, *Fevered Lives*, p. 158.

35. Ibid., p. 157.

36. McKenna, McCray, and Onorato, "The Epidemiology of Tuberculosis among Foreign-Born Persons in the United States, 1986 to 1993," p. 1073. Katherine Ott notes sharply, "It is not being foreign-born that puts a person at risk but the likelihood of repeated exposure to risk, compounded by poverty and ill health" (*Fevered Lives*, p. 163).

37. See Farmer, *AIDS and Accusation*.

38. Farmer, "The Exotic and the Mundane" (included in this volume as chapter 3).

39. Mann, Tarantola, and Netter, *AIDS in the World*, p. 1.

40. Lederberg, Shope, and Oaks, *Emerging Infections*, p. 39.

41. United Nations Development Programme, *Young Women*, p. 13.

42. Sampson and Neaton, "On Being Poor with HIV," p. 1100. They missed one study, however, as did my coauthors and I in our 1996 survey (Farmer, Connors, and Simmons, *Women, Poverty, and AIDS*). In a short communication published in 1990, Leigh Krueger and colleagues reported from Seattle "an independent effect of self-reported income on HIV-antibody status." They get to the point in their conclusion: "Since poverty spans the lines of age, ethnicity and sexual orientations, programs targeted specifically to the impoverished may be difficult to devise and implement" ("Poverty and HIV Seropositivity," p. 813).

43. Chaisson, Keruly, and Moore, "Race, Sex, Drug Use, and Progression of Human Immunodeficiency Virus Disease." See also Farmer, Connors, and Simmons, *Women, Poverty, and AIDS*; Fife and Mode, "AIDS Incidence and Income"; Wallace et al., "Will AIDS Be Contained within U.S. Minority Urban Populations?"

44. Waldholz, "Precious Pills." Some of the newer agents are even more costly.

45. Zinsser, *Rats, Lice and History*, p. 87.

46. For case studies of the ways in which anthropological methods and concepts can inform

epidemiology, see Janes, Stall, and Gifford, *Anthropology and Epidemiology;* Inhorn and Brown, *The Anthropology of Infectious Disease.*

47. Centers for Disease Control and Prevention, "Diphtheria Outbreak—Russian Federation, 1990–1993."

48. Field, "The Health Crisis in the Former Soviet Union"; Patz et al., "Global Climate Change and Emerging Infectious Diseases."

49. McMichael, "The Health of Persons, Populations, and Planets," p. 634. See also Krieger and Zierler, "Accounting for Health of Women."

50. Garrett, "Public Health and the Mass Media," p. 147. Laurie Garrett's comprehensive and engaging *The Coming Plague* does an excellent job of highlighting many of the social factors central to disease emergence. See also Poinsignon, Marjanovic, and Farge, "Maladies infectieuses nouvelles et résurgentes liées à la pauvreté."

51. In addition to the Institute of Medicine publications, see the statements by the Centers for Disease Control and Prevention (National Center for Infectious Diseases, *Addressing Emerging Infectious Disease Threats*) and by the National Academy of Sciences (Roizman, *Infectious Diseases in an Age of Change*).

52. See Richard Wilkinson's 1996 review (*Unhealthy Societies*) of the mechanisms by which inequality and the resulting lack of social cohesion adversely affect health in "developed" societies. The topic is also explored in Aïach et al., *Les inégalités sociales de santé en France et en Grande-Bretagne;* and Fassin, "Exclusion, Underclass, Marginalidad."

53. Krieger et al., "Racism, Sexism, and Social Class," p. 99. On this topic, see also Navarro, "Race or Class Versus Race and Class"; Marmot, "Social Differentials in Health within and between Populations."

54. Satcher, "Emerging Infections," p. 2.

55. Wilson, "Travel and the Emergence of Infectious Diseases," p. 39.

56. Haggett, "Geographical Aspects of the Emergence of Infectious Diseases."

57. Horton, "Towards the Elimination of Tuberculosis," p. 790.

58. Warner, "Health Issues at the U.S.–Mexican Border," p. 242.

59. Small and Moss, "Molecular Epidemiology and the New Tuberculosis."

60. Levins, "Preparing for Uncertainty," p. 50.

61. Lederberg, Shope, and Oaks, *Emerging Infections*, p. 33.

62. Latour, *The Pasteurization of France*, p. 243.

63. World Health Organization, *Global Health Situation and Projections.*

64. Berkelman and Hughes, "The Conquest of Infectious Diseases," p. 427.

65. Eisenberg and Kleinman, *The Relevance of Social Science for Medicine*, p. 11.

7

Social Scientists and the New Tuberculosis

(1997)

"It seems almost incredible that during this century and the previous one, a single disease, tuberculosis, was responsible for the deaths of approximately a thousand million human beings."[1] So wrote Frank Ryan, looking back in the late twentieth century on the history of efforts to combat that disease. Almost simultaneously, a 1992 review of the world epidemiology of tuberculosis concluded that the disease remained the leading infectious cause of preventable deaths in the world.[2]

Even in some of the fortunate nations where TB mortality had steadily decreased throughout most of the twentieth century, these trends have been reversed. In the United States, the number of active TB cases reported dropped from over 84,000 in 1953 to 22,255 cases in 1984. Since 1984, however, "dramatic changes in TB morbidity trends have occurred, and these changes jeopardize the control of TB," according to the U.S. Centers for Disease Control and Prevention (CDC). Between 1985 and 1991, an 18 percent increase in reported TB cases was registered—approximately 39,000 more cases than would have been expected if the downward trend had continued.[3]

This unsettling reversal has only become more pronounced since 1991. Why has the promise of the 1950s—when experts declared that TB would soon be a disease of the past—failed to come to fruition? Why, when effective chemotherapy exists, does TB remain a leading killer of young adults? Two factors are commonly cited to explain this setback: the advent of HIV, the virus that causes AIDS; and the emergence of TB strains resistant to multiple drugs (multidrug-resistant tuberculosis, or MDRTB). The impact of these two developments has been so great that several leaders in the field have begun to speak of "the new tuberculosis."[4]

Let us take each of these new developments in turn. Through two major mechanisms, HIV and TB exhibit a synergy that is particularly noxious to their human hosts. First, in patients who carry quiescent TB infection—perhaps 1.7 billion persons, roughly a third of the world's population, are thought to fall in this category—subsequent infection with HIV often means that the immune system's ability to keep mycobacteria in check will be lost. In this subgroup of doubly infected persons, dormant TB "reactivates" as cell-mediated immunity wanes; in much of the world, reactivation TB heralds previously unsuspected HIV infection. TB may in fact be the world's most common AIDS-associated opportunistic infection: in late 1992, one leading source observed that, of the 11.8 million persons then estimated to be infected with HIV, 4.6 million of them were co-infected with *Mycobacterium tuberculosis*.[5]

The second mechanism of synergy follows naturally from these epidemiological insights. Unlike many of the opportunistic infections afflicting those with AIDS, and unlike HIV infection itself, the tubercle bacillus may be transmitted without sustained or intimate contact. Viable bacilli are aerosolized by the coughing TB patient; they may remain in the air for hours. Perfectly immunocompetent persons may subsequently inhale these organisms and become infected. If HIV-infected persons are much more likely to develop active pulmonary TB than are controls who are HIV-negative but PPD-positive (suggesting infection with *M. tuberculosis*), then it is obvious that the new disease will have an enormous impact on the old scourge.

Into this already grim scenario comes MDRTB, which develops when naturally occurring mutants become favored during the course of intermittent or poorly conceived therapy. Individuals who have developed MDRTB in this way can then expose others, who suffer a primary infection with a resistant strain.[6] In cities throughout the world, the past decade brought reports of strains resistant to at least the first-line drugs isoniazid and rifampin. Significant U.S. outbreaks of MDRTB have been reported in homeless shelters, prisons, and medical facilities from Washington, D.C., to Boston to San Francisco.

The city of New York has been hit particularly hard by MDRTB, in large part thanks to HIV, but also because the city allowed its TB infrastructure to crumble. In 1968, for example, some $40 million was spent annually to maintain New York City's one thousand designated TB beds, its twenty-one "chest clinics," and the staff of these facilities. Ten years later, the TB beds were gone, and annual funding for TB had been slashed by up to $17 million. Federal monies earmarked for TB control in New York City also decreased. In 1979, TB incidence for the city began to climb for the first time in decades, and it continued to do so until 1992.[7] By 1991, fully a third of the city's reported cases were resistant to at least one first-line drug; almost 20 percent were resistant to both isoniazid and rifampin.[8]

Although some believe the MDR strains to be less virulent than drug-susceptible isolates, the new strains are notoriously difficult to treat. The finest medical care in the world can offer no assurance of cure. In the largest cohort study to date, Marian Goble, Michael Iseman, and coworkers report their experience with 171 patients, all of whom were HIV-negative. TB isolates from this cohort were all resistant to isoniazid and rifampin; most were resistant to three or more first-line agents. These patients were treated with an average of over six drugs per person, had a mean hospital stay of over six months, and received, in certain cases, adjunctive surgery. Treatment lasted, on average, over four years. These heroic measures, which can cost more than $250,000 per patient, yielded an overall response rate of only 56 percent.[9]

The story is even worse for those patients who also have HIV disease. Among the HIV-infected who fall ill with drug-susceptible strains of TB, response to therapy is frequently excellent. When these patients do die, it is usually not from TB—unless they lack access to care. But HIV-positive patients who fall ill with drug-resistant strains of TB have done poorly. "Despite aggressive multidrug treatment," concludes one review, "72 to 89% of more than 200 patients were dead in 4 to 19 weeks, with 38 to 70% of the deaths caused by tuberculosis."[10]

Who is falling ill with these deadly strains of TB? In spite of the theoretical risk to the "general population," the majority of U.S. cases to date have been registered among the inner-city poor, with significant outbreaks confined to prisons, homeless shelters, and public hospitals. This strikingly patterned occurrence of MDRTB speaks to some of the large-scale forces at work in the pandemic. The two factors central to the new TB—the development of drug-resistant strains and the advent of HIV—are ostensibly biological in nature, but are in fact best understood as *sociomedical* phenomena. Arguing that drug-resistant TB is a socially produced biological phenomenon should not be controversial, since it refers to the induction of resistance to chemotherapeutic agents recently created by humans. But the rapid spread of HIV among certain populations has also been shaped by social (political, economic, and cultural) processes—the same processes, in large part, that led to the emergence of MDRTB.

René Dubos, who began his career as a distinguished microbiologist but later turned to the contemplation of the patterns of TB and other epidemic diseases, underlined the social nature of TB almost half a century ago: "Tuberculosis is a social disease, and presents problems that transcend the conventional medical approach . . . its understanding demands that the impact of social and economic factors on the individual be considered as much as the mechanisms by which tubercle bacilli cause damage to the human body."[11]

Anthropologists and other social scientists have long argued that tuberculosis will not be eradicated without attention to these fundamentally social forces. In this sense, then, the arrival of MDRTB is a terrible vindication for the sociomedical sciences. But there is less consensus among the social scientists than meets the eye. *Which* social forces might be involved in the persistence of TB and the emergence of MDRTB? How might these forces be differentially weighted? By what mechanisms, precisely, do large-scale and impersonal forces come to be embodied as individual pathology? As epidemic disease? More to the point, what is the significance of such analyses to interventions to prevent and treat MDRTB?

Indeed, for researchers in a host of disciplines, the emergence of MDRTB poses new challenges and also forcefully brings a number of old questions to the fore. In addition to those just raised are the inevitable and thorny "compliance" questions. "The word compliant," notes Esther Sumartojo in a sophisticated 1993 review of the topic, "has the unfortunate connotation that the patient is docile and subservient to the provider."[12] Even more unfortunately, the term exaggerates patient agency, for it suggests that *all* patients possess the ability to comply—or to refuse to comply—with antituberculous therapies. This makes no sense, if the World Health Organization is correct: as many as half of all cases of active TB are never even diagnosed.[13] Experiences across boundaries of time and place have shown radical differences in the ability of different populations to comply with demanding therapies, whether they consist of admonitions to move to "consumptive climes," as in the past century, or exhortations to take a year's worth of several drugs.

More can be said. The poor have no options but to be at risk for TB and are thus from the outset victims of "structural violence."[14] For many populations, the chances of acquiring infection, developing disease, and lacking access to care are structured by a series of forces that we can now identify. In South Africa, say, these forces include poverty and racism; in other settings, gender inequality conspires with poverty to lead to a higher incidence of TB in poor women.[15] Throughout the United States, increased indices of economic inequity seem to favor epidemics in blighted inner cities, already ravaged by related epidemics of AIDS, injection drug use, homelessness, and racism. Overt political violence and war, themselves usually a reflection of structural violence, have well-known associations with increased rates of TB.

I would like to examine the relationship between structural violence and the emergence of drug-resistant TB by presenting data from Haiti, which currently serves, sadly, as a natural laboratory for the ill effects of such violence on the health of a population. Although TB has usually been termed the leading cause of death in autopsy series of Haitian adults between fifteen and fifty years of age,[16] MDRTB has not yet been reported in Haiti. Indeed, in the only large study in which drug susceptibilities were tested, we read that "no significant resistance to drugs other than isoniazid was seen even though streptomycin and thiacetazone have been widely used."[17]

But the hypotheses generated in this essay would lead us to predict that such strains are present and that they will emerge first among the poor. The case of Robert David, examined in detail here, shows that this prediction has already come true.

CASE STUDY: ROBERT DAVID

In August of 1986, Robert David, then nineteen years old, noticed the onset of a nonproductive cough, night sweats, and intermittent fevers and chills that were more marked in the evenings. Like most impoverished peasant families, the Davids lived in fear of tuberculosis, in part because of its high mortality and in part because of its tendency to leave survivors—or surviving kin—saddled with unpayable debts.[18] And so Robert attempted, at first, to self-treat with readily available herbal remedies. But when his cough gave way to dyspnea (shortness of breath) and marked weight loss, Robert's parents brought him to a referral hospital in the city of Hinche, the district seat of Haiti's Central Plateau. There Robert was diagnosed with pulmonary TB and placed on an unknown two-drug regimen that probably included isoniazid.

In order to receive care in this public facility, Robert had to commute from his home village. By truck, the trip took two hours; by donkey or on foot, it was an overnight trek. In spite of heroic efforts to keep appointments, which included a full day of waiting once inside the clinic, Robert did not respond promptly to treatment. In June 1987, he sought care in a large market town closer to his home village. He was then treated for eighteen months, initially with a three-drug regimen (isoniazid, ethambutol, streptomycin). During this second course of therapy, Robert recalled, he was told that he had organisms in his sputum on "several" occasions, but his regimen was never altered. Throughout this period, he had great difficulty acquiring his medications, even though family members made enormous financial sacrifices—including selling more than half their land—in order to buy the prescribed items.

Robert terminated one and one-half years of irregular treatment in December 1988, but he continued to experience the same symptoms. In January of 1989, he had an episode of massive hemoptysis (coughing up blood) but essentially received no biomedical care for this life-threatening complication. "We didn't have any money," he responded, when asked why he did not seek care, "and the bleeding had stopped by the time we borrowed some."

The other symptoms persisted. In May 1990, Robert traveled to Port-au-Prince, the capital city, where he was admitted to a sanatorium for six months of directly observed therapy with isoniazid, ethambutol, pyrazinamide, and rifampin. He was discharged to complete a total of eight months of this regimen, followed by two more months of isoniazid and ethambutol. Because of political difficulties—including but not limited to the destruction of a key pharmacy by a bomb—

Robert was unable to obtain many of his medications. He did, however, feel "much better" for more than a year.

Robert returned to central Haiti, where he remained until June 1992, when most of his symptoms (cough, weight loss, night sweats) recurred. In September, he was again admitted to a Port-au-Prince sanatorium, where he received only thiazina, the combination of isoniazid and thiacetazone. His symptoms did not lessen substantially, and, again, Robert was often unable to acquire medication because of political disruptions in the capital.

These same political upheavals drove Robert back to the Central Plateau and, eventually, to the Clinique Bon Sauveur. When we first met him, in January 1993, Robert explained that he had been unable to obtain his medications because he had no money. He reported to the clinic seeking relief of his chronic cough, night sweats, and weight loss. A thin young man with minimally labored breathing, Robert then weighed 110 pounds. Physical examination revealed temporal wasting, pale conjunctiva, and severe oropharyngeal candidiasis. His neck was supple with no cervical lymphadenopathy. Examination of his lungs revealed abolition of breath sounds at the left apex. The remainder of his exam was unremarkable. Laboratory studies included examination of his sputum, which was laden with acid-fast bacilli (AFB), signaling the presence of active pulmonary tuberculosis; and a rapid serologic test for HIV, which was negative. We could not perform mycobacterial cultures because we lacked regular electricity.

We found Robert to be a highly motivated young man who wished desperately to recover from his refractory TB. He had made every attempt, he told us, to comply with his physicians' orders. MDRTB was raised as a possibility, although it had not been previously reported in Haiti. The only antituberculous drugs available in Haiti were isoniazid, thiacetazone, pyrazinamide, PAS, streptomycin, and rifampin, all of which were stocked at the Clinique Bon Sauveur. Observing that the patient developed floridly positive sputum on thiazina, we elected to give him a cocktail of *all* the other drugs, although we were aware that PAS was the only drug he had not yet received.

On February 9, 1994, then, Robert began this difficult regimen. The streptomycin was stopped when he complained of a buzzing in his ears; this symptom abated shortly thereafter. In both March and May, Robert had negative sputum exams, but he continued to lose weight, and his pulmonary symptoms diminished only slightly. He attributed his nausea and abdominal pain to the enormous number of pills he was taking each day. A repeat HIV test was again negative.

In August, Robert's sputum was again laden with AFB. A sputum specimen was collected for culture and sensitivity testing, which was performed in the United States. These isolates were found to be resistant to isoniazid, rifampin, ethambutol, streptomycin, and pyrazinamide. The isolate was sensitive to kanamycin, cycloserine, capreomycin, ethionamide, and ciprofloxacin. As none of these latter drugs were readily available in Haiti, arrangements were made to import them, and Robert was eventually started on a four-drug regimen consisting of cycloserine, kanamycin, ethionamide, and ciprofloxacin.

He showed marked clinical improvement—weight gain, decreased shortness of breath and coughing—within two months. His sputum became free of AFB two months after initiation of this therapy and remained so for six months. In August of 1994, however, Robert again began losing weight and coughing. He continued his treatment, in spite of side effects including epigastric pain and, at one point, an abscess at an intramuscular injection site. Repeat tests showed that his MDRTB had recurred and, furthermore, had become resistant to kanamycin. The organism continued to destroy his lungs in spite of his religious compliance with a brutal regimen. In December 1995, Robert David died in his sister's home.[19]

POVERTY AND MDRTB

Robert's story is explored in some depth in the hope that the complex interplay of individual agency and structural violence—central to the emergence of drug resistance—is best illuminated by considering the gritty details of biography. How does his experience speak to the central thesis of this paper, that the emergence of MDRTB (and of the "new" TB in general) is inextricably linked to structural violence? How representative of others' experience of MDRTB was Robert's story?

First, how does the biomedical literature explain the emergence of resistance? In an influential review published in the *New England Journal of Medicine*, Iseman writes: "In the circumstances of monotherapy, erratic drug ingestion, omission of one or more of the prescribed agents, suboptimal dosage, poor drug absorption, or an insufficient number of active agents in a regimen, a susceptible strain of *M. tuberculosis* may become resistant to multiple drugs within a matter of months."[20] In this sentence, Iseman lists a host of risk factors for MDRTB; each of these is inescapably a part of the lives of millions like Robert David— poorly nourished adults who develop reactivation TB, which is treated (when it is treated) with a small number of erratically available drugs. There is, then, a "political economy of MDRTB." That is, there are large-scale forces that make monotherapy and erratic drug ingestion much more likely in settings such as Haiti or Harlem, say, than in the affluent communities where MDRTB has not become a problem.

Like most patients with MDRTB, Robert had been previously treated for TB. He was treated inappropriately—started on a two-drug regimen that he could ill afford. When he relapsed, he was not started on a regimen consisting of drugs that he had never received before. He was deemed "noncompliant"—but how useful is such a term in describing the experience of a young man whose family was willing to sell all its land to treat him? Even while in a sanatorium, he was unable to purchase his medications, a problem worsened by the incessant political violence of the period.

Robert David's lamentable experience brings into relief the complicated relationship between individual agency and structural violence. In most settings where TB is prevalent, the degree to which patients are able to comply is significantly limited by forces quite beyond their control. In reading the biomedical literature, one detects a certain delicacy in discussing this problem. In the largest Haitian series in which drug susceptibilities were examined, we read only that "primary drug resistance in Haiti has many probable causes, including the availability of isoniazid without prescription, past inclusion of isoniazid in cough remedies and a high default rate."[21] Nowhere do we read about the insurmountable barriers to effective biomedical care faced by the overwhelming majority of Haitians.

In theory, MDRTB can often be cured, at least in HIV-negative patients like Robert David. What do the experts recommend as therapy? Empirical five- or six-drug regimens, followed by multidrug regimens after sensitivity data, are available. The recommended duration of these therapies is eighteen to thirty-six months. Careful monitoring of all drug levels is strongly advised, as are directly observed therapy, universal precautions for all those in close contact with patients, and the use of ultraviolet light to protect health care workers. But to whom are these recommendations addressed? Leaving aside the millions now dying from *susceptible* strains of TB, dying for lack of therapy, it must be pointed out that these recommendations for the treatment of MDRTB cannot possibly be addressed to those without access to laboratories, masks, electricity, and up to $250,000 worth of medical care. In other words, the recommendations are not relevant to precisely those persons most likely to acquire MDRTB.

Just as the poor are "at risk" of finding themselves likely to develop or acquire MDRTB, so too are they "at risk" of being unable to find adequate therapy for this disease. In places like Haiti, one sadly concludes, active MDRTB is likely to be fatal.

SOCIAL SCIENCE AND IMMODEST CLAIMS OF CAUSALITY

How have social scientists discussed the various forces that conspire to render certain groups susceptible to TB while shielding others? Let us examine a handful of studies of TB published in the sociomedical or anthropological press. Each was conducted in a poor country, and each makes certain claims of causality in attempting to explain both noncompliance and the persistence of TB as a major cause of mortality in the setting under study. Frequently, the former is held to explain the latter.

In important research conducted in southern Haiti and published in *Social Science and Medicine,* Helen Wiese allots most of the discussion to the "health beliefs" of TB patients and their families, which are certainly a legitimate preoccupation for an anthropologist. She further argues that the failure of a TB control program in the region was largely the result of "the clinic's lack of knowledge about the local culture and consequent failure to operate within it."[22]

One could more easily argue that TB control programs in Haiti have failed not because of cultural insensitivity but rather because of a lack of commitment to the destitute sick. In a study conducted in the Central Plateau, we interviewed one hundred TB patients regarding their own understanding of their illness, which most agreed was TB. Many patients felt that sorcery might have caused their illness. Because both the medical anthropological literature and the Haitian physicians queried predicted that these individuals who cited sorcery as a cause would be more likely than others to abandon antituberculous therapy, we followed all these patients for more than eighteen months. We found that patients' etiologic beliefs did not predict their compliance with chemotherapy.[23] Similar disjunctions are reported elsewhere in the literature. For example, Arthur Rubel and Linda Garro reported high rates of compliance among migrant Mexican farmworkers with TB in California, who attributed their symptoms to disorders ranging from bronchitis to "folk illnesses" such as *susto:* "Interestingly, interviews with these patients show a continued denial of their diagnosis of tuberculosis despite faithful adherence to lengthy treatment regimens and extensive education by clinical staff members."[24]

In Haiti's Central Plateau, what *did* predict adherence to therapy? Among patients who were offered free and convenient care, compliance and outcome were strongly related only to whether or not patients had access to supplemental food and income. We were led to conclude that cultural, political, and economic factors, although inevitably important, cannot be of equal significance in all settings. Whereas cultural considerations, such as the nearly universal stigma attached to TB, may very well be of overriding significance in settings in industrialized countries, we would argue that they are commonly less so in Haiti, where so many factors (initial exposure to mycobacteria, reactivation of exogenous TB infection, complications, access to therapy, length of convalescence, development of resistance, degree of tissue destruction, and, finally, mortality) are determined chiefly by economic forces.[25]

To take an example from South Africa, where blacks of all ethnic backgrounds have much higher rates of TB than whites, an anthropological study identified several reasons for the high default rate seen among Xhosa-speaking patients with TB. Chief among these were the "deep-seated mystical beliefs" of the people under study, including the understanding that TB may be caused by witchcraft and is thus best treated with the help of a diviner who can explain *who* caused the sickness. The author listed several other reasons for noncompliance as well, from the side effects of the medications to the "carelessness" of certain patients, but nowhere was there any mention of the poverty of South African blacks or of apartheid and its effects on the delivery of services. Small wonder, then, that the investigator's conclusions focus so exclusively on patients' cognitive profiles: "As an anthropologist it is therefore possible to plead that health care personnel who treat black patients with tuberculosis be aware that their patients' perceptions of the disease may differ from their own, that the patient may already have consulted a non-western practitioner, or that they are merely seeking time before they embark on a different strategy for seeking a solution for what troubles them."[26]

One could argue instead that, for South African blacks, the proximate cause of increased rates of morbidity and mortality is not their "mystical beliefs" but rather lack of access to resources, as a 1990 study by a team of physicians concluded: "Poverty remains the primary cause of the prevalence of many diseases and widespread hunger and malnutrition among black South Africans. The role of apartheid in creating and maintaining this poverty has been well documented."[27]

Even here, more rigorous social analysis is necessary, for TB is closely linked to a "racial capitalism" far older than apartheid itself. In an important study of TB in South Africa, historian Randall Packard shows that institutionalized apartheid does not in and of itself explain the skewed incidence of the disease. Indeed, these patterns were emerging well before the enactment of apartheid laws, which are merely decades old: "It is not enough to invoke apartheid, racial discrimination, and black poverty, for they themselves are symptoms of more fundamental political and economic transformations that have been associated with the rise of industrial capitalism in South Africa. Ultimately the answer to why TB remains such a serious problem in South Africa lies in understanding the history of these transformations."[28]

Another study, set in Honduras and published in *Medical Anthropology*, begins with a telling vignette:

> One day, in an important health center in Tegucigalpa, the capital city of Honduras, Central America, the general practitioner identified ten patients suffering from symptoms of tuberculosis. He asked them to go up to the laboratory, which was one floor above, then get the authorization for laboratory exams. Only five of them arrived at the laboratory; of those, only three brought the sputum sample the following day. Only one of them returned to pick up his result: it was negative. The results of the other two, who had given false addresses, were positive. They were suffering from tuberculosis. They were never located.[29]

A team of investigators then set off to interview some five hundred Hondurans to uncover the reasons for this noncompliance. The study began with the formulation of six hypotheses that might explain it. None of these hypotheses linked treatment failure to a failure of the public health system or to Honduran society at large; none mentioned poverty or social inequality at all, although those surveyed, in contrast, correctly associated TB with "extreme poverty, filth, and malnutrition."[30]

The researchers found the patients and the public to be full of strange "knowledge, attitudes, and behaviors" as well as a "great lack of education about the disease." When patients were interviewed, many "maintained a careful distance when speaking to the investigators, and seemed fearful and distrustful." (They had, the author speculated, "feelings of isolation . . . accompanied by guilt.") Above all, of course, the patients were noncompliant, "refus[ing] to accept [TB's] existence, and attempt[ing] to remedy the symptoms with self-prescribed medications." Some of the patients were downright refractory "and obstinately refused the visits of health personnel." "Even when the patient can no longer ignore the evidence of his symptoms," the author added, "he is willing to die rather than undergo treatment."[31]

Fortunately, consultants like the author of the study were able to remedy the situation. They designed a flip-chart explaining "the measures that should be taken by the patient and his family" and had sputum cups "printed with attractive and clear illustrations." Sadly enough, "the Ministry [of Health] had not yet improved its tuberculosis program services, and the necessary sample cups were not available in time," nor were the flip-charts. But a series of radio spots, posters, and a pamphlet served to "clear up the patient's immediate confusions about the disease."[32] The author seemed confident that Honduras—which in his account sounds more like Sweden than one of the poorest countries in Latin America—is well on its way to solving its TB problem.

Even in a more thoughtfully conceived investigation, with more robust data, the same circular logic is easily discerned. Working in Wardha District in central India, Florie Barnhoorn and Hans Adriaanse compared fifty-two compliant patients with fifty noncompliant patients in an effort to determine what factors might be responsible for failure to take medications. They found that "three socioeconomic variables, i.e., the monthly income per capita in a family, the type of house in which a family lived, and the monthly family income" were the strongest predictors of compliance with antituberculous chemotherapy. "It is noteworthy," the authors add, "that the highest ratings were followed by three additional socioeconomic variables, i.e., place of residence, fuel used, and education."[33]

In this study, etiologic beliefs about TB did not have striking relevance to compliance. Although a number of "health beliefs" were felt to be strong predictors of compliance, these "beliefs" sound much more like indirect socioeconomic indicators: "Compliers also tended to clean their body, ate good foods, visited a Primary Health Centre, whereas noncompliers tended to isolate themselves and prayed to God for a cure." Similarly, other items classified under "family attitudes" include having someone to prepare meals and "eating breakfast regularly."[34]

In essence, the researchers found that the only strong predictors of compliance were fundamentally economic, not cognitive or cultural. However, their conclusions would seem otherwise: "Concerns with the determinants of [noncompliance] might improve the care of tuberculosis patients by giving directions for *educational interventions*." And although Barnhoorn and Adriaanse insist that socioeconomic obstacles to treatment do exist and are fundamental, these impediments become secondary in much of the discussion: "Before obstacles to a treatment regimen can be cleared away, patients have to develop health beliefs and social norms consistent with it." When the investigators call for the patients to be "liberated," it is not from the structural violence that creates and sustains a significant and growing TB epidemic among the world's poor. Instead, they propose that "future health education programmes aimed at the public at large should be focused on the liberation of the masses from false thoughts and burdens."[35]

In another paper published in *Social Science and Medicine,* a prominent anthropologist reported that, in one city in the Philippines, children's respiratory symptoms are commonly attributed to *piang,* a folk illness best treated by traditional healers: "Such a lay diagnosis *leads to* long delays before tubercular children are brought to a physician."[36] If this claim is true, then little short of changing the culture could lead to a change in compliance. But other researchers, working in a nearby area, were able to double compliance with antituberculous medications merely by making drugs readily available and easy to take.[37]

In East Africa, another region characterized by extreme poverty, a weak medical infrastructure, and high rates of TB, one study claimed that "attribution of tuberculosis symptoms to witchcraft or other folk illnesses is associated with delays in seeking professional treatment as well as remarkably high rates of default once treatment has begun."[38] Similar claims are frequently made in Haiti, where we found no association, except in the minds of most physicians surveyed, between sorcery and TB *outcomes*—although even compliant patients frequently attributed their TB to sorcery.

It is inappropriate, of course, to generalize based on such a small number of papers. But a more thorough review of the sociomedical literature on compliance with antituberculous therapy does little to gainsay the impressions made upon reading the articles cited here. Such research tends to be conducted in settings—called "cultures" in many of these studies—characterized by high rates of tuberculosis and by extreme poverty, which a priori calls into question conclusions regarding the impact of the patients' culture on treatment failures. These patients do not share culture or language. What they share is tuberculosis and poverty. They also share, often enough, spectacularly bad TB services, such as those described by J. Frimodt-Möller, working in rural India: "The treatment began when a sufficient number of patients had been collected to justify sending out a drug-issue team the long distances. To begin with, there was an interval of 2 months from the time the sputum was found positive until treatment began. Forty-seven patients died before the treatment could begin, 14 left the towns, 20 refused treatment from the beginning, 26 stopped after the first or second drug issue, two preferred to take their own drugs."[39]

Strenuous insistence on the causal role of culture or personality in explaining treatment failures runs the risk of conflating cultural (or psychological) difference with structural violence, leading to the immodest claims of causality evident in the studies described here. *Throughout the world, those least likely to comply are those least able to comply.* In theory, it would be necessary to ensure full and facile access to all persons before ascribing blame for the failure to complete treatment to patient-related shortcomings. And in none of the places in which this research was conducted is full and facile access ensured. On the contrary, these settings are crying out for measures to improve the quality of care, not the quality of the patients.[40]

Curiously, many of these studies take it as a matter of faith that educational interventions will have significant effects on rates of TB in a particular population. But no one, as far as I know, has ever shown this to be true. Historical reviews, such as that by Thomas McKeown and R. G. Record, would suggest that, in England and Wales at least, death rates from TB have varied quite independently of patients'—and healers'—understandings about the disease.[41]

In each of the sociomedical studies critiqued here, a well-intentioned effort to incorporate the patients' points of view has served, paradoxically, to shift the blame onto the sick-poor by exaggerating their agency. In so doing, researchers have echoed the received wisdom of many physicians and other providers. Their explanations tend to focus on local actors—most notably, on patients—and local factors. "The most serious problem hampering tuberculosis treatment and control," note three pulmonologists in a 1993 review, "is patient non-compliance with therapy." There is no mention of any structural barriers to therapy. "Potential determinants of compliance," they continue, "include personal characteristics of patients, features of the disease and/or treatment, and patients' beliefs and attitudes."[42]

Sociomedical research shows not merely the expected divorce between patients' and healers' etiologic conceptions of TB but also great dissensus regarding treatment failure.[43] D. A. Collando reported that when Mexican district health officials were asked, "To what do you attribute the problematic nature of tuberculosis control in your jurisdiction?" those surveyed "overwhelmingly laid the blame at the door of their patients' shortcomings: 'poverty,' 'lack of education,' 'poor motivation,' 'superstition,' and 'failure to comprehend the importance of compliance with treatment recommendations.'"[44]

A similar pattern was described in a San Francisco chest clinic, where in the 1960s up to 34 percent of patients failed to keep their appointments. Again, the providers and the patients had very discrepant ideas about this failure. The physicians and nurses tended to focus on the patients' shortcomings—"the social and cultural characteristics of the user population"—while the patients listed structural barriers ranging from the inconvenience of the clinic's hours and location and a "rigidity in taking patients in order of registration regardless of extenuating circumstances" to a failure to treat affected families as a unit, with adults and children seen on different days and by different physicians.[45] Addressing these structural problems by moving the clinics to more convenient times and places, as well as "an improved attitude on the part of the professional staff," led to a decrease in missed appointments from 34 percent to 6 percent after five years.[46]

Anthropologists and other social scientists have long complained that their perspectives have not been incorporated into TB control efforts. While it is true that physicians and their biomedical colleagues have been guilty of underplaying the significance of the social forces at work in the changing epidemiology of TB, a review of the biomedical literature increasingly reveals a willingness to incorporate social factors into their explanations of why TB control has failed. Indeed, specialists from the CDC and from academic departments are all likely, these days, to speak of social and economic determinants. For example, the following assessment is by two TB specialists writing in the journal *Seminars in Respiratory Infections*: "Regaining control of epidemic tuberculosis will be difficult and will require effective approaches to hardcore issues also common to the AIDS epidemic: poverty, homelessness, and substance abuse."[47]

Medical anthropologists have commonly been less willing to incorporate basic biomedical insights, including the following: untreated TB may have a case-fatality rate of over 80 percent; in drug-susceptible TB, at least, over 95 percent can be cured with appropriate therapy. Nonetheless, drug-susceptible TB will kill millions in the coming years, and it will kill them slowly, allowing many of them to serve as culture media for the induction of resistant strains. The obscenity of late-twentieth-century TB lies precisely in this, and not in a failure to incorporate the concept of culture—or the opinions of anthropologists—in efforts to prevent or treat the disease.

These assertions are rooted in the hopeful belief that social science may well hold some of the keys to halting the spread of these new pandemics. But if we are to be other than academic Cassandras, we would do well to acknowledge the largely structural causes of persistent TB and to take stock of why we have not had much influence in past attempts to prevent or treat it. In other words, the research tasks before us are more likely to be accomplished if we can avoid the traps of the past. When I examine my own field—similar exercises would be welcome in each of the sociomedical sciences—five such pitfalls come quickly to mind, discussed in the following sections.

Conflating Structural Violence with Cultural Difference

Each of the sociomedical sciences—medical anthropology, medical sociology, health economics, and so on—tends to stake out its own turf, a focus or emphasis to be regarded as the bailiwick of that particular subspecialty. Representatives of these fields then tend to claim that their disciplinary focus is of paramount importance in explaining the phenomenon under scrutiny—regardless of what that phenomenon happens to be. In medical anthropology, often enough, "culture" is held up as the determinant variable.

Surely these immodest claims of causality amount to inadequate phenomenology and are underpinned by inadequate social theory. Because culture is merely one of several potentially important factors, anthropologists and other researchers who cite cognitivist "cultural" explanations for the poor health of the poor have been the object of legitimate critiques: "Medical anthropologists and sociologists have tended to elevate the cultural component into an omnibus explanation. The emphasis is on cultural determination. Even when social relations receive more than reflexive recognition, medical social scientists restrict the social relations to small 'primary' group settings, such as the family, and factions at the micro unit. . . . Little or no attempt is made to encompass the totality of the larger society's structure."[48]

One side effect of such cognitivist approaches to culture is a conflation of structural violence and cultural difference. Related trends are easily discerned in medical psychology, where personality attributes—the turf of that field—are held to explain risk for such disorders as AIDS, alcoholism, and addiction to drugs.

Minimizing the Role of Poverty

Many anthropologists, regarding their turf as the "cultural piece," have also tended to underplay economic barriers to effective care. Poverty has long been the chief risk factor for both acquiring and dying from TB; this was true long before MDR strains appeared. It was true when the likes of Lord Byron and Keats died from TB, for even then "the white plague" found the great majority of its victims among the poor. Dramatic shifts in local epidemiology aside, a global analysis does not suggest major decreases in the importance of tuberculosis as a cause of death. In fact, tuberculosis may be said to be an "emerging" disease only with significant provisos.[49] Tuberculosis has retreated in certain populations, maintained a steady state in others, and surged forth in still others, remaining, at the time of this writing, the world's leading infectious cause of preventable deaths.[50] Thus tuberculosis has not really emerged so much as *emerged from the ranks of the poor.* One of the implications, clearly, is that one place for diseases to "hide" is among poor people, especially when the poor are socially and medically segregated from those whose deaths might be considered more significant.

Almost unexamined has been the relationship between the social reproduction of inequalities and the persistence of TB. Our failure to discern a political economy of risk both for the development of MDRTB and for suboptimal treatment may be related to a desire to link our (perfectly legitimate) investigations of the shaping of personal experience by culture to (inaccurate) claims of causality.

Exaggerating Patient Agency

The praiseworthy effort to incorporate patients' points of view can serve, at times, to obscure the very real constraints on agency experienced by most, but not all, patients with TB. Clinicians make their own immodest claims. One influential editorial in *Chest* declared "patient compliance" to be "the most serious remaining problem in the control of tuberculosis in the United States."[51] Assumptions regarding human agency are readily discerned in most discussions of treatment failures and noncompliance. In tuberculosis clinics throughout the world, patient-related factors top providers' lists of reasons to explain treatment failures. These lists, as Sumartojo politely and accurately notes, reflect providers' "observations and experience, but [they] exclude environmental, structural, and operational factors that are beyond the patient's control."[52] Calls to change "lifestyle and behavior" are typically directed to precisely those persons whose agency is most constrained. The same exaggerations took place in earlier eras, as historian Barbara Rosenkrantz has observed in examining the elaborate treatment protocols of the turn of the century: "The disease-oriented hygienic regimen dictated by bacteriologic research came to grief when a patient's poverty made it unlikely that such advice would be followed."[53]

Exaggeration of patient agency is particularly marked in the biomedical literature, in part because of medicine's celebrated focus on individual patients, which is inevitably desocializing. But it is social science that has underlined the importance of contextualization, and so our failure to complement clinicians' views with more robustly contextualized ones is all the more significant. A similar critique of modern epidemiology was advanced by Anthony McMichael: "Epidemiology today, in developed countries, thus assigns a primary importance to studying interindividual variations in risk. By concentrating on these specific and presumed free-range individual behaviors, we thereby pay less attention to the underlying social-historical influences on behavioral choices, patterns, and population health."[54]

Romanticizing "Folk Healing"

A strong vein of commentary in medical anthropology depicts folk healing as somehow superior to biomedical therapies. Although these claims have been called into question by some within the field, they have since assumed importance far beyond the boundaries of anthropology.[55] But nonbiomedical treatments for active pulmonary or extrapulmonary TB have thus far proven to be spectacularly ineffective. They do not change case-fatality rates. If folk healing were so effective, the world's wealthy would be monopolizing it. When the privileged do use folk healing and other nonbiomedical modalities, it is as adjunctive therapy, typically for chronic illnesses refractory to biomedical intervention. (As an aside, I cannot count the number of Haitian folk healers that I have personally treated for TB and malaria.) We live in an increasingly interconnected world. Robert David's use of herbal remedies to treat tuberculosis is emblematic not of cultural integrity but of an unfair distribution of the world's resources.

Persisting in Insularity

Medical anthropologists, like other subspecialists, are usually familiar with the arcane debates of our own field. Yet we are too frequently unwilling to learn the basics of infectious disease or epidemiology, even when they are related to our chosen arenas of intervention. This sectarian approach to research can be costly when examining pandemics with demonstrable relation to both biological and social forces. Why, for example, have anthropologists' voices been drowned out in the AIDS pandemic? Perhaps because we too often and too loudly made immodest claims of causality: in the first years of the pandemic, the refrain at many of our professional meetings was that anthropology had "special knowledge" about the "cultural practices" then held to be related to the high incidence of AIDS in certain areas where we worked.[56] Regarding Haiti, for example, there was much talk of the role of voodoo. Long after "exotic" cultural practices proved irrelevant to the spread of HIV, these red herrings continued to figure prominently in our professional meetings. Meanwhile, important multidisciplinary research faltered or was underpinned by slipshod social theory.

FUTURE RESEARCH ON MDRTB

The emergence of MDRTB is a terrible vindication for those who predicted that a social disease could not be eradicated without social responses. But this clairvoyance is no occasion for celebration, nor is it a time for concern about the advancement of our own particular subspecialties. MDRTB is a biologically and socially complex development. To check it, we must understand the forces promoting and retarding its advance. How, more precisely, might anthropology (and the other social sciences) make meaningful contributions to efforts to control the new scourge of MDRTB?

Several research tasks come to mind. First, who better than social scientists to discern the precise mechanisms by which social forces (ranging from racism to political violence) promote or retard the transmission or recrudescence of TB? Since there are likely several mechanisms, it is incumbent on us to offer a hierarchy of factors and to understand how, in different settings, these might be differentially weighted. New research technologies, such as DNA fingerprinting techniques, promise new insight into transmission dynamics[57] but also illuminate new social problems that will demand innovative responses.

Second, ethnographic research will be important in identifying and, again, *ranking* the barriers preventing those afflicted with MDRTB from having access to the best care available. The best available care, regardless of the etiologic beliefs of the patient, seems to consist of multiple-drug regimens, accompanied by adequate nutrition, for at least eighteen months, and probably longer. Adopting a patient-centered approach, though important, is insufficient: "The challenge to researchers is to acknowledge that adherence is influenced by a complex array of factors, many of which are beyond the patient's control, and to begin identifying and describing these factors."[58]

Third, social scientists should become more engaged in multidisciplinary research and trials. We have much to offer those who seek to design programs that increase access to optimal therapies. Comparative trials, not just of directly observed therapy but also of simpler, more dignified, and "user-friendly" regimens, have yet to be widely initiated.

Fourth, research that exposes—and deplores—the precise mechanisms by which entrenched medical inequities are buttressed may help to redress these inequities. In so doing, we would no doubt also be exposing the real co-factors in this emerging epidemic of "social disease."

These suggestions are more crassly utilitarian than those usually heard in calls for social science research, but it is clear that we should act quickly to make common cause with those on the side of the sick-poor, regardless of profession—whether we are community health workers, or folk healers, or physicians, or bench scientists. Certainly, some of these will be stop-gap measures, but such measures matter a great deal to those sick with tuberculosis. "It is useful to remember," remarks Rosenkrantz, "that a 'social disease' typically affects the socially marginal, who can ill afford to wait for the fundamental insights and social transformations that challenge the well-established associations of disadvantage and disease."[59]

NOTES

1. Ryan, *The Forgotten Plague,* p. xxi.

2. Bloom and Murray, "Tuberculosis," p. 1055.

3. Hinman et al., "Meeting the Challenge of Multidrug-Resistant Tuberculosis," p. 52.

4. Snider and Roper, "The New Tuberculosis."

5. Mann, Tarantola, and Netter, *AIDS in the World,* p. 150.

6. A third mechanism, exogenous *reinfection* with a resistant strain, has also been described among those with HIV infection: see Small et al., "Exogenous Reinfection with Multidrug-Resistant *Mycobacterium tuberculosis* in Patients with Advanced HIV Infection." Exogenous reinfection may even occur in immunocompetent patients (Peter Small, personal communication with the author, 1996).

7. Frieden et al., "Tuberculosis in New York City—Turning the Tide"; this report also indicates that "the tide is turning" as a result of improved TB control strategies.

8. For an excellent overview of the effects of these changes in TB policy, see Brudney and Dobkin, "Resurgent Tuberculosis in New York City."

9. Goble et al., "Treatment of 171 Patients with Pulmonary Tuberculosis Resistant to Isoniazid and Rifampin." The CDC reported the case of an individual with MDRTB who exposed nine family members and friends. Care for these ten persons alone exceeded a million dollars (Centers for Disease Control and Prevention, "Outbreak of Multidrug-Resistant Tuberculosis—Texas, California, and Pennsylvania," p. 369).

10. Iseman, "Treatment of Multidrug-Resistant Tuberculosis," p. 785.

11. Dubos and Dubos, *The White Plague,* p. xxxvii.

12. Sumartojo, "When Tuberculosis Treatment Fails," p. 1311. Dr. Sumartojo prefers the term "adherence."

13. World Health Organization, *Treatment of Tuberculosis.*

14. Farmer, "On Suffering and Structural Violence," p. 261.

15. Margono et al., "Tuberculosis among Pregnant Women—New York City, 1985–1992." Although biological universals are important—cell-mediated immunity wanes during pregnancy—TB is strikingly patterned even among pregnant women. Among U.S. women, poor, urban women of color are disproportionately affected. See also Snider, "The Impact of Tuberculosis on Women, Children, and Minorities in the United States."

16. For a review of these data, see Farmer, Robin, et al., "Tuberculosis, Poverty, and 'Compliance.'"

17. Scalcini et al., "Antituberculous Drug Resistance in Central Haiti."

18. For a fuller discussion of Haitian understandings of TB, see Farmer, *AIDS and Accusation.*

19. The case of Robert David led us to search more aggressively for other cases of MDRTB. Two other patients were also discovered to be infected with multiply resistant strains. The resistance patterns of their strains were different from those of the strain infecting Robert.

20. Iseman, "Treatment of Multidrug-Resistant Tuberculosis," p. 784.

21. Scalcini et al., "Antituberculous Drug Resistance in Central Haiti," p. 509.

22. Wiese, "Tuberculosis in Rural Haiti," p. 359.

23. This study is described in Farmer, *Pathologies of Power,* pp. 150–51.

24. Rubel and Garro, "Social and Cultural Factors in the Successful Control of Tuberculosis," p. 627.

25. Farmer, Robin, et al., "Tuberculosis, Poverty, and 'Compliance,'" p. 259. Pierre Chaulet, writing from Algeria, makes a similar point after deriding providers' tendencies to blame patients for treatment failures: "In developing countries, noncompliance with anti-tuberculosis chemotherapy

is less often due to the patient's failure to comply with treatment than to other factors" ("Compliance with Anti-Tuberculosis Chemotherapy in Developing Countries," p. 19).

26. de Villiers, "Tuberculosis in Anthropological Perspective," p. 72.

27. Nightingale et al., "Apartheid Medicine," p. 2098.

28. Packard, *White Plague, Black Labor*, p. xvi.

29. Mata, "Integrating the Client's Perspective in Planning a Tuberculosis Education and Treatment Program in Honduras," p. 57.

30. Ibid., p. 59.

31. Quotations drawn from ibid., pp. 62, 60, 61, 58.

32. Ibid., pp. 62–63.

33. Barnhoorn and Adriaanse, "In Search of Factors Responsible for Noncompliance among Tuberculosis Patients in Wardha District, India," p. 296.

34. Ibid., pp. 299, 302.

35. Ibid., pp. 291, 301, 302.

36. Rubel and Garro, "Social and Cultural Factors in the Successful Control of Tuberculosis," p. 630 (emphasis added) (citing Lieban, "Traditional Medical Beliefs and the Choice of Practitioners in a Philippine City," p. 289).

37. Valeza and McDougall cited in Sumartojo, "When Tuberculosis Treatment Fails," p. 1314.

38. Rubel and Garro, "Social and Cultural Factors in the Successful Control of Tuberculosis," p. 630.

39. Frimodt-Möller, "Domiciliary Drug Therapy of Pulmonary Tuberculosis in a Rural Population in India," p. 22. In most studies, improving the quality of services inevitably results in drastic improvements in outcomes. In a discussion of tuberculous meningitis in urban India, where access to care was significantly better, one large study found that "default was not a very serious problem, despite the fact that about half the patients come from outside Madras City. Patients attended punctually on 90% of occasions. Furthermore, in 95% of the remaining unpunctual occasions, drugs were missed for less than a week which, as there was no proper retrieval action, is very commendable. All those who attended late had valid reasons for their unpunctuality" (Ramachandran and Prabhakar, "Defaults, Defaulter Action, and Retrieval of Patients during Studies on Tuberculous Meningitis in Children," p. 171). See also Grange and Festenstein, "The Human Dimension of Tuberculosis Control."

40. Chaulet puts this sharply in an editorial castigating health care professionals for *their* noncompliance: "It is only after these general measures have been applied that we can turn our attention to improving compliance" ("Compliance with Anti-Tuberculosis Chemotherapy in Developing Countries," p. 20).

41. McKeown and Record, "Reasons for the Decline of Mortality in England and Wales during the Nineteenth Century."

42. Menzies, Rocher, and Vissandjee, "Factors Associated with Compliance in Treatment of Tuberculosis."

43. For sharply divergent interpretations of TB control, see Nachman, "Wasted Lives." Steven Nachman, an anthropologist who briefly worked among Haitians detained by the U.S. Immigration and Naturalization Service, offers compelling ethnography without making immodest claims of causality. For a review stressing the importance of patients' perspectives, see Conrad, "The Meaning of Medications." Too few of the papers reviewed underline the enormous difference between failure to adhere to a 1NH prophylaxis regimen and failure to adhere to treatment for active disease.

44. Collando cited in Rubel and Garro, "Social and Cultural Factors in the Successful Control of Tuberculosis," p. 627.

45. The experience of the San Francisco chest clinic is cited in ibid.

46. Sumartojo, "When Tuberculosis Treatment Fails," p. 1316.

47. Brudney and Dobkin, "A Tale of Two Cities," p. 261.

48. Onoge, "Capitalism and Public Health," p. 221. Medical anthropologists are not the only ones who lend importance to factors that cannot be considered central in the shaping of TB pandemics. While René Dubos was at times hard-bitten in his assessments, calling TB "the first penalty that capitalistic society had to pay for the ruthless exploitation of labor," he saw the disease as a reflection of humans' failure to adapt harmoniously to the environment. The "anonymous gloom of the industrial cities" of the nineteenth century, where TB flourished, contrasted with the pastoral lifestyle that had reigned prior to the industrial revolution: "The most destitute villager in his native land had learned to adorn the dullness and drudgery of existence with bright ribbons and jolly tunes, and with the pageantry of his church". (Dubos and Dubos, *The White Plague*, pp. 207, 202).

49. For an excellent review, see Porter and McAdam, "The Re-Emergence of Tuberculosis."

50. Bloom and Murray, "Tuberculosis."

51. Addington, "Patient Compliance," p. 741.

52. Sumartojo, "When Tuberculosis Treatment Fails," p. 1312.

53. See the excellent commentary by Barbara Rosenkrantz ("Preface," in Dubos and Dubos, *The White Plague*, p. xxi).

54. McMichael, "The Health of Persons, Populations, and Planets," p. 633.

55. See, for example, Patel, "Problems in the Evaluation of Alternative Medicine."

56. Farmer, "New Disorder, Old Dilemmas."

57. See, for example, Small and Moss, "Molecular Epidemiology and the New Tuberculosis."

58. Sumartojo, "When Tuberculosis Treatment Fails," p. 1318.

59. Rosenkrantz, "Preface," p. xxxiv.

8

Optimism and Pessimism
in Tuberculosis Control

Lessons from Rural Haiti

(1999)

What the social world has made,
the social world, armed with knowledge, can undo.

PIERRE BOURDIEU, *LA MISÈRE DU MONDE*

A survey of the current literature reveals discordant views on the question of progress in the control of tuberculosis. On the one hand, optimistic observers point with understandable pride to advances in our understanding of mycobacterial pathogenesis and to the elaboration of shorter but more effective treatment regimens. Recent years have seen a growing consensus that even six-month-long, multidrug regimens will lead to high cure rates if therapy is directly observed by medical personnel or health workers. The World Health Organization's adoption of DOTS—directly observed therapy, short-course—has been hailed as a victory by experts from around the world.[1] Indeed, the WHO claims that DOTS is "the most important public health breakthrough of the decade."[2] The cure for tuberculosis, in this view, has at last been discovered.

Pessimists, on the other hand, call attention to the widening gulf between the advances reported in the scholarly literature and the degree of effective control in those communities hardest hit by the disease. Some point to the increasing microbial resistance to our best drugs; some point to our lack of an effective vaccine. But deaths from tuberculosis, numbering in the millions, are the most compelling rebuke to optimism.

In fact, it is difficult to document any impact of the new treatment regimens on worldwide tuberculosis incidence: in the current decade, an estimated three hundred million people will become infected with tubercle bacilli; ninety million will develop active tuberculosis; and, if access to care does not become a global priority, thirty million will die.[3] In projecting changes in the ranked order of the fifteen leading causes of death, Christopher Murray and Alan Lopez predict that tuberculosis alone will hold its unenviable place for the next thirty years; with the exception of HIV disease, all other infectious diseases are projected to drop in rank over the coming three decades. According to a baseline projection, tuberculosis will be the fourth leading cause of death overall in developing countries by the year 2020. Tuberculosis and HIV, which both afflict young adults disproportionately, are the only infectious diseases expected to cause more life years to be lost in 2020 than they cause now.[4]

Tuberculosis heads the list of diseases dreaded by Haitians, too. "Of all the health problems cited," observes Helen Wiese, "one stands out from the others by virtue of its insidious onset, its tenacity, and its prevalence—pulmonary tuberculosis."[5] The prevalence of tuberculosis in Haiti is estimated to be the highest in the hemisphere. Little is known of the disease's occurrence there during the nineteenth century, but in 1941 James Leyburn wrote that, in a series of seven hundred autopsies performed in the Port-au-Prince General Hospital, 26 percent of the deaths were due to tuberculosis.[6] The United Nations reported that in Haiti in 1944 "tuberculosis was the most important cause of death among hospitalized patients." Linking the high incidence of the disorder to poor sanitation and poverty, the organization predicted that "for many years to come tuberculosis will, it is feared, continue to take a heavy toll of human lives in Haiti."[7]

This prediction has come true. In 1965, the Pan American Health Organization estimated prevalence in Haiti at 3,862 per 100,000 inhabitants.[8] Available data indicate that tuberculosis remains the leading cause of death among individuals between the ages of fifteen and forty-nine. Studies from the Hôpital Albert Schweitzer suggest that, in this age group, tuberculosis causes two to three times as many deaths as the next most common diagnosis.[9]

In recent years, the situation seems to have worsened. The high prevalence of tuberculosis has been further augmented by the advent of HIV. In sanatoriums in urban Haiti during the mid-1980s, some 45 percent of all tuberculosis patients reportedly were co-infected with HIV. In a later survey of over 7,300 ostensibly healthy adults living in a densely populated slum, 70 percent of those screened were tuberculin-positive, and more than 15 percent were HIV-positive. More alarming, community-based screening detected a prevalence of 2,281 *active* pulmonary tuberculosis cases per 100,000 adults. One study conducted in rural regions found that 15 percent of patients diagnosed with tuberculosis disease were also infected with HIV. In another rural setting, at the Hôpital Albert Schweitzer, 24 percent of all patients with tuberculosis were co-infected with HIV.[10]

Added to this noxious synergy is the emergence of resistance to first-line antituberculous drugs. There are very few published studies of drug resistance in

Haiti, in large part because it is difficult to culture *Mycobacterium tuberculosis* in settings with no reliable source of electricity. One of the few large series including culture data revealed that 22 percent of isolates were resistant to at least one first-line drug.[11]

Although drug resistance presents a new and potentially significant problem, most studies of treatment failure agree that the problem is predominantly one of designing and implementing programs that are appropriate to the needs of the population to be served.[12] In one large town in southern Haiti, fully 75 percent of all patients had abandoned treatment by six months after diagnosis, and over 93 percent had abandoned treatment before the end of one year.[13] Since short-course therapy did not exist at the time of this study, we must assume that the majority of patients in this series were left with partially treated disease.

This essay will describe in some detail one community-based organization's efforts to implement a tuberculosis control program that takes into account the crippling poverty that so often plays a central role in determining who does or does not benefit from interventions. In examining this program, I also want to oppose the "either-or" approach that has led some health advocates, tragically, to adopt a Luddite stance.[14] This position holds that it is acceptable to defer tuberculosis treatment while the "root causes" of the disease are addressed through development projects. But health policy is not a zero-sum game. One of the lessons from rural Haiti is that effective tuberculosis-specific interventions are both urgent and inexpensive and should not be regarded as somehow detracting from the broader development efforts that might well serve to reduce tuberculosis incidence.

THE PROJE VEYE SANTE EXPERIENCE

Since it was founded in 1984, Proje Veye Sante has sought to serve the landless peasants and children of the Péligre basin of Haiti's Central Plateau. The program's catchment area includes settlements scattered around a reservoir, which was created by a hydroelectric dam that flooded the basin in 1956. Sector 1 of the catchment area rings the lake; at the time of this study it encompassed approximately twenty-five thousand individuals, almost all of them peasants living in small villages. Sector 2, more loosely demarcated, consists of a large number of outlying villages and towns contiguous to Sector 1.

Although inhabitants of the villages in Sector 2 were offered the same clinical services available in Sector 1 (consultations with a physician, lab work, and all medication for about eighty cents), they were not served by community health workers; nor did they benefit from activities sponsored by Proje Veye Sante such as women's health initiatives, vaccination campaigns, water protection efforts, and adult literacy groups. These interventions, implemented by community health workers, had proven to be a powerful means of addressing malnutrition, diarrheal disease, measles, neonatal tetanus, malaria, and typhoid fever. Through the community activities, the health workers were able to identify the sick and refer them to the clinic, where, it should be noted, all antituberculous medications were free of charge. (Isoniazid, ethambutol, pyrazinamide, and streptomycin were then on formulary at the clinic.)[15]

Although Proje Veye Sante was effective in identifying patients with pulmonary tuberculosis and getting them to the clinic, it became clear during the late 1980s that detection of new cases did not necessarily lead to cure, in spite of our policy of waiving even the eighty-cent fee for any patient diagnosed with tuberculosis. In December of 1988, following the deaths from tuberculosis of three HIV-negative patients, all in their forties, the staff of Proje Veye Sante met to reconsider how the care of these individuals had been managed. How had the staff failed to prevent these deaths?

Responses to this question varied. Some community health workers felt that tuberculosis patients who had poor outcomes were the most economically impoverished and thus the sickest. Others, including the physicians present, attributed poor compliance to widespread beliefs that tuberculosis was a disorder inflicted through sorcery, which led patients to abandon biomedical therapy. Still others hypothesized that patients lost interest in chemotherapy after ridding themselves of the symptoms that had caused them to seek medical advice.

Over the next two months, we devised a plan to improve services to patients with tuberculosis—and to test these discrepant hypotheses. Briefly, the new program embraced the goals of finding cases, offering adequate chemotherapy, and providing close follow-up. Although contact screening and BCG vaccination for infants were included in the program, the staff of Proje Veye Sante was then most concerned with the care of smear-positive and coughing patients—believed by many to be the most important source of community exposure.

The new program was designed to be aggressive and community-based, relying heavily on community health workers for close follow-up. It was also designed to respond to patients' appeals for nutritional assistance. All residents of Sector 1 diagnosed with pulmonary or extrapulmonary tuberculosis would be eligible to participate in a treatment program featuring—during the first month following diagnosis—daily visits from their village health worker. These patients would receive financial aid of thirty dollars per month for the first three months and would also be eligible for nutritional supplements.

Further, these patients were to receive a monthly reminder from their village health worker to attend clinic. Travel expenses (for example, renting a donkey) would be defrayed with a five-dollar honorarium when they came to the clinic. If a Sector 1 patient did not attend, someone from the clinic—often a physician or an auxiliary nurse—would visit the no-show's house. A series of forms, including a detailed initial interview schedule and home-visit reports, regularized these arrangements and replaced the relatively limited forms used for other clinic patients.

During the initial enrollment period, between February of 1989 and September of 1990, fifty Sector 1 patients joined the program.[16] Forty-eight of those identified had pulmonary tuberculosis. Seven individuals also had extrapulmonary tuberculosis (for example, tuberculosis of the spine), and two had cervical lymphadenitis ("scrofula") as their sole manifestation of tuberculosis. During the same period, the clinical staff diagnosed pulmonary tuberculosis in 213 patients from outside Sector 1. Many of these patients were from Sector 2, although a few had traveled even greater distances to seek care at the clinic; at least 168 of these individuals returned to the clinic for further care. The first fifty of these patients to be diagnosed formed the comparison group by which the efficacy of the new interventions would be judged. They were a "control group" only in the sense that they did not benefit from the community-based services and the financial aid; all Sector 2 patients continued to receive free care. To test hypotheses regarding patients' beliefs and clinical outcomes, we interviewed all patients regarding their own explanatory models and their experience of tuberculosis.[17]

The mean age of our patients (forty-two years) and the sex ratio (both groups had significantly more women than men) did not vary significantly between the two groups.[18] But indirect economic indicators (for example, years of school attended, ownership of a radio, access to a latrine, a tin roof rather than a thatched roof) suggested that patients from Sector 2 may have been slightly less poor than those from Sector 1. This is not surprising, as several of the villages in Sector 1 are squatter settlements dating from the year the valley was flooded.

Results

The following discussion explains the findings of the Proje Veye Sante study in some detail. These findings are summarized in table 8.1.

Mortality. One patient from the Sector 1 group died in the year following diagnosis, although she did not die from tuberculosis. Six patients from Sector 2 died, all, it seems, from tuberculosis; one of these was a young woman who was also seropositive for HIV.

Sputum Positivity. The clinical staff attempted to examine sputum for acid-fast bacilli (AFB)[19] whenever patients developed recrudescent symptoms as well as approximately six months after the start of antituberculous therapy. None of the patients from Sector 1 were sputum-positive at six months. One young woman did become sputum-positive during a pregnancy in the subsequent year;

Table 8.1 Characteristics of Tuberculosis in Sector 1 Patients versus Sector 2 Patients

	Sector 1 (N = 50)		Sector 2 (N = 50)	
All-cause mortality (18 months follow-up)	1.0	(2%)	6.0	(12%)
Sputum-positive for AFB after 6 months of treatment	0.0		9.0	(18%)
Persistent pulmonary symptoms after 1 year of treatment	3.0	(6%)	21.0	(42%)
Average weight gained/patient/year (lbs.)	9.8		1.9	
Return to work after 1 year of treatment	46.0	(92%)	24.0	(48%)
Average number of clinic visits/patient/year	11.6		5.4	
Average number of home visits/patient/year	32.0		2.0	
HIV co-infection	2.0	(4%)	3.0	(6%)
Number denying the role of sorcery in their illness	6.0	(12%)	9.0	(18%)
One-year disease-free survival	50.0	(100%)	24.0	(48%)

we found that she was infected with HIV and may have been reinfected with a second strain of tuberculosis. Of the Sector 2 cohort, nine patients had acid-fast bacilli demonstrable in their sputum about six months after the initiation of therapy.

Persistent Pulmonary Symptoms.   After a year of treatment, a thorough history and physical exam were used to screen for persistent pulmonary symptoms such as cough, shortness of breath (dyspnea), and coughing up blood (hemoptysis). Only three patients of the Sector 1 group reported such symptoms, and two of them had developed asthma during the course of their convalescence. Twenty patients in Sector 2, however, continued to complain of cough or other symptoms consistent with persistent or partially treated tuberculosis. One additional patient in this group was an asthmatic without radiographic or other evidence of persistent tuberculosis.

Weight Gained.   Monitoring body weight revealed marked differences between the two sector groups in the amount of weight gained per patient per year. Correcting for fluctuations associated with pregnancy, Sector 1 patients gained an average of nearly ten pounds during the first year of their treatment. Patients from Sector 2 had an average weight gain of about two pounds per person per year.

Return to Work.   The vast majority of patients from both groups were peasant farmers or market women whose families relied on their ability to perform physical labor. It is especially notable, then, that one year after diagnosis, forty-six of the Sector 1 patients stated that they were able to return to their work activities. In Sector 2, fewer than half (twenty-four patients) were able to do so.

Clinic Visits.   As patients were given one month's supply of medication with each visit, the staff of Proje Veye Sante strongly encouraged monthly clinic visits, which served as an indirect measure of a patient's adherence to antituberculous therapy. In the Sector 1 group, the one-visit-per-month ideal was nearly achieved: these patients, who received a small sum for travel expenses, averaged 11.6 visits per year. In the control group, the average number of visits per year was 5.4.

Home Visits.   Our treatment protocol at that time called for at least 30 grams of intramuscular streptomycin during the first two months of therapy, and community health workers were asked to administer these injections to the patients living in their area. Most patients from Sector 2 had their streptomycin administered by local *pikiris,* or injectionists. (Some lived near licensed practical nurses and received this drug in other clinics.) This is perhaps the chief reason that the number of home visits by members of the Proje Veye Sante staff was far higher in the Sector 1 group than in the Sector 2 group: thirty-two visits in the former versus two visits in the latter.

HIV Seroprevalence.   The rate of HIV seroprevalence was not substantially different between the two groups. Only two patients from Sector 1 showed serologic evidence of HIV infection; both had lived in urban Haiti for extended periods. One of these patients became smear-positive for acid-fast bacilli during a pregnancy that occurred over a year after she completed her initial course of therapy. She was treated with a new multidrug regimen and remained asymptomatic some sixty months after her initial tuberculosis diagnosis. In the Sector 2 group, similarly, three patients were seropositive for HIV; all had lived in greater Port-au-Prince.

Etiologic Conceptions about Tuberculosis.   Previous ethnographic research had revealed extremely complex and changing ways of understanding and speaking about tuberculosis among rural Haitians.[20] Open-ended interviews with patients from both sectors permitted us to delineate the dominant explanatory models used by members of both groups. Because several physicians, nurses, and community health workers had hypothesized that a belief in sorcery would lead to higher rates of noncompliance, we took some pains to address this issue with each patient. We learned that few from either group would deny the possibility of sorcery as an etiologic factor in their own illnesses, but we could discern no relationship between avowed adherence to such models and a patient's degree of compliance with a biomedical regimen. The Proje Veye Sante effort demonstrated the relative insignificance of patients' understandings of etiology, when compared to access to financial aid—one marker of the primacy of economic considerations in impoverished settings.

Cure Rate.   In June 1991, forty-eight of the Sector 1 patients remained free of pulmonary symptoms. Two patients with a persistent cough and/or dyspnea did not
meet radiologic or clinical diagnostic criteria for tuberculosis (both had developed bronchospastic disease). Therefore, we judged that none had active pulmonary tuberculosis, giving the participants a cure rate of 100 percent. One of these
patients, as noted earlier, was co-infected with HIV but remained asymptomatic
sixty months after her initial diagnosis of tuberculosis. We could not locate all
the patients from Sector 2, but of the forty patients we examined at more than
one year after diagnosis, only twenty-four could be declared free of active disease
based on clinical, laboratory, and radiographic evaluation. (Six patients from
this group had died during the course of this study.) Even if the four patients lost
to follow-up had in fact been cured, that would have left twenty-six others dead
or with signs and symptoms of persistent tuberculosis—a cure rate of, at best,
48 percent.

Explaining Treatment Outcomes

In an important review of the significance of tuberculosis in developing countries,
Christopher Murray, Karel Styblo, and Annik Rouillon estimate that 26 percent
of avoidable adult deaths in these countries are due to tuberculosis, making it the
greatest cause of avoidable death.[21] The experience of Proje Veye Sante speaks to
the discrepant explanations of this colossal failure, since the majority of these
deaths occur in settings not unlike Haiti. Although our small numbers do not
permit any sweeping conclusions, the project described here suggests that *high
cure rates are possible in settings of extreme poverty in which hospital-based care is
unavailable even for the critically ill.*

Even after so small a study, we can also advance other pragmatic conclusions.
First, projects designed to treat tuberculosis among the very poor must include
financial and nutritional assistance, for many of these patients develop reactivation tuberculosis in the setting of malnutrition or concurrent disease. The Proje
Veye Sante antituberculosis initiative indicates that, in Haiti at least, hunger
and poverty are the prime culprits in treatment failure, just as they are so often
responsible for the reactivation of endogenous infection. The factors that govern
treatment success or failure there—factors such as initial exposure to mycobacteria, reactivation of endogenous tuberculosis infection, complications, access
to therapy, length of convalescence, development of drug resistance, degree of
tissue destruction, and, finally, mortality—are determined chiefly by economic
variables. Countries held in underdevelopment would do well to invest resources
in programs that address patients' nutritional needs while ensuring easy and
reliable access to multidrug regimens.

In fact, these interventions may be more important than the choice of regimen: although we initially used traditional antituberculous therapy, rather than the short-course multidrug regimens shown to be effective in recent studies, our results are as encouraging as those of Styblo and colleagues, who report a 90 percent cure rate when a six-month course of INH and thiacetazone is preceded by two months of an *in-hospital,* strictly supervised three-drug regimen.[22] Given the high costs of hospitalization, a program that includes financial or nutritional aid may be less expensive—and far more feasible—than the tuberculosis control programs now in place in many poor countries. Similarly, although directly observed therapy would seem to be almost always preferable to unobserved therapy, our experience suggests that high cure rates can be achieved even in sparsely settled, difficult terrain where patients are unable to make daily trips to clinics or health posts.

Second, projects designed to prevent tuberculosis among the very poor must keep in mind a central maxim of tuberculosis control: treatment is prevention. Although the priorities of these projects may differ from those of projects designed for low-prevalence, high-income settings, identification and complete treatment of patients with active pulmonary tuberculosis should be the top priority of tuberculosis control in settings like rural Haiti. Similar conclusions have been advanced in a review of data from throughout the developing world.[23] Experience among New York City's poor might also lead to such conclusions, since in one review of patients diagnosed with tuberculosis at Harlem Hospital, only 11 percent could be shown to have completed therapy.[24]

The eradication of tuberculosis would require that we halt transmission and also prevent the reactivation of quiescent TB infection. We have the tools to do both: treatment of all active cases and, in the majority of quiescent cases, "chemoprophylaxis" with isoniazid. Until there are major redistributions in the current partition of the world's wealth, however, chemoprophylaxis of contacts and of asymptomatic but infected patients who show a positive PPD test result has a limited role to play in poverty-stricken areas. Although a community may have a high level of tuberculosis infection—our own survey suggests that 70 percent of rural Haitian adults are PPD-positive—individuals with active pulmonary disease are those most likely to transmit the disease to others. They are also those most likely to die of tuberculosis. Ideally, however, resources available for tuberculosis control would be increased so that even chemoprophylaxis could be administered as directly observed therapy.

In a sense, the high cure rates we achieved also show that debates over whether to treat tuberculosis or to prevent it are essentially false debates, whose costs are borne, as usual, by the poor. Among those who argue (correctly) that in our time poverty is the ultimate cause of tuberculosis, some make a serious error by advocating that development efforts should take precedence over tuberculosis treatment. As noted earlier, this Luddite trap remains a peril of modern tuberculosis control. We know how to treat tuberculosis, but development efforts often go awry. The people of the Péligre area know this well, for the hydroelectric dam that immiserated them, and so increased their tuberculosis risk, was billed as a development project.

NOTES

1. See Third East African/British Medical Research Council Study, "Controlled Clinical Trial of Four Short-Course Regimens of Chemotherapy for Two Durations in the Treatment of Pulmonary Tuberculosis"; Cohn et al., "A 62-Dose, 6-Month Therapy for Pulmonary and Extrapulmonary Tuberculosis"; Hong Kong Chest Service/British Medical Research Council, "Controlled Trial of 4 Three-Times-Weekly Regimens and a Daily Regimen All Given for 6 Months for Pulmonary Tuberculosis"; Snider et al., "Supervised Six-Months Treatment of Newly Diagnosed Pulmonary Tuberculosis Using Isoniazid, Rifampin, and Pyrazinamide with and without Streptomycin"; Singapore Tuberculosis Service/British Medical Research Council, "Five-Year Follow-Up of a Clinical Trial of Three 6-Month Regimens of Chemotherapy Given Intermittently in the Continuation Phase in the Treatment of Pulmonary Tuberculosis."

2. See Kochi, "Tuberculosis Control—Is DOTS the Health Breakthrough of the 1990s?" p. 232.

3. World Health Organization Global Tuberculosis Programme, *TB: WHO Report on the Tuberculosis Epidemic 1997.*

4. Murray and Lopez, *The Global Burden of Disease.*

5. Wiese, "The Interaction of Western and Indigenous Medicine in Haiti in Regard to Tuberculosis," p. 40.

6. Leyburn, *The Haitian People,* p. 275.

7. United Nations, *Mission of Technical Assistance to the Republic of Haiti,* pp. 70–72.

8. Pan American Health Organization, *Reported Cases of Notifiable Diseases in the Americas,* p. 290.

9. For a review of these data, see Feilden et al., "Health, Population, and Nutrition in Haiti."

10. Desormeaux et al., "Widespread HIV Counseling and Testing Linked to a Community-Based Tuberculosis Control Program in a High-Risk Population"; Pape and Johnson, "Epidemiology of AIDS in the Caribbean"; Long et al., "Impact of Human Immunodeficiency Virus Type 1 on Tuberculosis in Rural Haiti."

11. Scalcini et al., "Antituberculous Drug Resistance in Central Haiti." On multidrug-resistant strains in Haiti, see Farmer, Bayona, Becerra, et al., "Poverty, Inequality, and Drug Resistance."

12. Shears, *Tuberculosis Control Programmes in Developing Countries.*

13. Wiese, "Tuberculosis in Rural Haiti."

14. Farmer and Nardell, "Nihilism and Pragmatism in Tuberculosis Control."

15. Rifampin has since replaced streptomycin in the initial treatment of adults with tuberculosis. The clinic also stocks second-line drugs for culture-proven cases of multidrug-resistant tuberculosis.

16. One patient who initially lived in Sector 1 later moved out of the catchment area and was no longer served by a community health worker. This patient, rumored to have died some months after leaving the area, is not considered in any of the data analysis of either group.

17. For a concise review of this methodology, see Kleinman, Eisenberg, and Good, "Culture, Illness, and Care." For an assessment of the methodology's limitations, see Kleinman, *Writing at the Margin,* pp. 5–15.

18. The preponderance of women waned over subsequent years, suggesting a backlog of untreated women facing significant barriers to care.

19. The presence of acid-fast bacilli in a sputum sample usually signals the presence of active pulmonary tuberculosis. Although an imperfect test for tuberculosis—as all patients with extra-pulmonary disease and many with pulmonary disease will have falsely negative smears—sputum microscopy is the standard test in most settings in the developing world, including Haiti.

20. Farmer, "Sending Sickness" (included in this volume as chapter 2).

21. Murray, Styblo, and Rouillon, "Tuberculosis in Developing Countries."

22. Styblo, "Overview and Epidemiological Assessment of the Current Global Tuberculosis Situation."

23. Murray, Styblo, and Rouillon, "Tuberculosis in Developing Countries."

24. Brudney and Dobkin, "Resurgent Tuberculosis in New York City"; Brudney and Dobkin, "A Tale of Two Cities."

Cruel and Unusual

Drug-Resistant Tuberculosis as Punishment

(1999)

CONSUMPTION AS PUNISHMENT

The long and grim history of punishment records many inventive ways of making prisoners suffer. The crudest of these are usually known as penal torture, a practice roundly condemned by all governments—and practiced, nonetheless, by many. This essay addresses the issue of *tuberculosis as punishment*.

Tuberculosis has a long history of association with prisons. In the pre-chemo-therapeutic era, "consumption" was in many settings the major cause of prison mortality. In the mid-nineteenth century, for example, TB was estimated to have caused up to 80 percent of all U.S. prison deaths: in Boston, Philadelphia, and New York, in any case, about 10 percent of all prisoners died from the disease.[1] In our own post-antibiotic era, prisoners continue to endure TB risks well in excess of those faced by individuals outside prison walls. In most countries, rates of five to ten times the national average are not uncommon in prisons, and outbreaks can lead rapidly to TB rates more than a hundred times the national average.[2]

This is not to say that there's nothing new under the sun. On the contrary, it's easy to discern novel developments. We are living in a global economy with its own rapidly changing "geoculture," a transnational social phenomenon that interacts in novel ways with local cultures, themselves rapidly mutating.[3] Alterations in telecommunications and a proliferation of regulations and laws are linked to all manner of human rights discourses, which are in turn linked both to emerging geoculture and to more established cultural traditions. The degree of global travel and trade is unprecedented.

In addition to these changes in society and in human behavior, there are changes in *Mycobacterium tuberculosis,* the organism that causes TB. Multidrug-resistant tuberculosis (MDRTB) is a relatively recent development, emerging only in the past two decades, a frightening concomitant of drug development. Unfortunately, the organism has mutated more quickly than our own ability to respond with new and effective drugs. MDRTB is exceedingly difficult to treat and carries a high case-fatality rate when not treated. It is also stubbornly entrenched in certain prisons.

This essay examines TB—and, particularly, MDRTB—in prisons during an era in which neither prison bars nor national boundaries confine the disease. Ours is an era in which treatment is available for the fortunate few; others, including most prisoners, are summarily informed that their affliction is incurable. Accordingly, I write both as a clinician specializing in the treatment of tuberculosis and as an anthropologist trying to comprehend the myths and mystifications that hamper effective interventions.

KEY CONCEPTS: DOTS, RESISTANCE, AMPLIFICATION

To critically examine the problem at hand, it is necessary to define or explain certain terms and concepts. DOTS (directly observed therapy, short-course) is a mode of treatment delivery designed to prevent the development of drug resistance by ensuring that every required dose is administered on schedule under observation. The term "MDRTB" implies resistance to at least isoniazid (INH) and rifampin (RIF), the most powerful antituberculous drugs. When a patient infected with a TB strain resistant to INH and RIF is treated with a regimen based on these two first-line agents, he or she is unlikely to be cured. Although this may seem obvious, many experts have nonetheless advocated one-size-fits-all empiric regimens based on first-line drugs—even in the middle of MDRTB outbreaks. Such recommendations are made, often enough, because the second-line drugs that might cure patients with MDRTB are deemed too expensive for use in precisely those countries or settings in which they are most needed. They are not "cost-effective," in the confused jargon of our day.

Not only do INH/RIF-based regimens fail to cure patients with MDRTB, but they may also lead to iatrogenic worsening of an individual patient's pattern of resistance. That is, the infecting strain is exposed to brief courses of drugs that cannot kill the microbe but that can induce further resistance, rendering even carefully designed subsequent regimens less effective. In our work, we've called this the "amplifier effect" of short-course chemotherapy.[4] For DOTS to be effective, it must include the drugs that have a chance of killing the microbe.

But there are, of course, other ways to amplify the problem. TB is an airborne pathogen. It is coughed into the air in what are known as "droplet nuclei," and these may be inhaled by anyone who shares air with an infectious person. The number of droplet nuclei coughed into the air and the rate of ventilation (air changes per unit time) are key determinants of the risk of infection. Complex mathematical formulas describe transmission dynamics, but suffice it to say that overcrowded prisons with poor ventilation are particularly effective amplification systems for TB whenever prompt and effective therapy is unavailable. Adding HIV to the equation increases the likelihood that new infections will progress to active and contagious TB, further amplifying outbreaks and driving up mortality.

We also know that prisons are highly permeable institutions, with a great deal of interaction with surrounding communities (the "outside world"). This occurs not only through the guards and other employees but also because detention is frequently brief: in the United States, for example, about ten million people pass through prisons or jails each year. So what goes on inside these institutions is of great relevance to the public's health, as we'll see in examining data from the United States and Russia. It is for all these reasons that certain correctional facilities have been felicitously termed "infectious prisons."[5]

Another bit of terminology bears consideration. "Acquired MDRTB" occurs when TB patients do not or cannot adhere to therapy, and intermittent selective pressures allow naturally occurring, drug-resistant mutants to become the dominant infecting strain. "Primary MDRTB" occurs when others are initially infected with MDR strains and fall ill. When poorly conceived regimens further amplify preexisting resistance, primary MDRTB may be misdiagnosed as acquired MDRTB. This distinction is critical in prisons, as we shall see.

Other generalities about TB in prisons are bandied about, but a review of the literature reveals many discrepant claims about the nature of the prison-tuberculosis association.[6] For example, while one study argues that prisons are "particularly difficult environments" in which to treat TB and that prisoner education is "often hopeless," another more hopefully concludes that, "with on-site services and confined patients, [correctional institutions] are well suited for public health interventions, health professional education and epidemiologic study."[7] And although the literature seems to show that TB treatment outcomes among prisoners are frequently poor, there's little agreement as to why. Few if any studies have examined the contribution of endemic drug resistance to poor clinical outcomes in prisons. Some commentators argue that poor treatment outcomes are the result of the structural constraints of working within underfunded prison systems; others seem to blame the prisoners, focusing on alleged psychological or even "cultural" traits. Still others refer to the fragility of the patient-doctor relationship when the latter works for the system that is punishing the former. Because generalizations are hazardous, allow me to turn to tuberculosis in the prisons of two countries, the United States and Russia.

TAKING A CLOSER LOOK:
THE UNITED STATES AND RUSSIA

The United States and Russia hold world records in many prison statistics, taking the prize, most notably, for the highest per capita rates of imprisonment in the world. For years, the United States was the world leader in detention, but Russia has recently edged ahead. Of every 100,000 U.S. citizens, 619 are in prison; 690 per 100,000 Russians are incarcerated. For the sake of comparison, note that in many European countries fewer than 100 per 100,000 citizens are in prison.[8]

What do we know about epidemics of MDRTB in U.S. prisons? Several of what are termed "nosocomial outbreaks" began in prisons, not hospitals. Take the largest U.S. outbreak, which began in New York City in 1989. Fully 80 percent of all index cases could be traced to jails and prisons.[9] The Centers for Disease Control (CDC) had sounded the alarm even before the New York MDRTB epidemic, reporting the steady and dramatic rise in TB incidence within prisons. In the New York state correctional system, for example, average annual TB incidence went from 15.4 per 100,000 inmates in 1976–78 to 105.5 per 100,000 in 1986.[10] Much of the rise was associated with HIV, but TB transmission within prison walls was clearly affecting HIV-negative inmates, wardens, visitors, and surrounding communities: there were at least eleven prison outbreaks between 1985 and 1989.[11]

These warnings went largely unheeded, as did guidelines to prevent transmission within prisons and jails.[12] By 1991, the Rikers Island jail, which during the 1980s experienced a threefold increase in census, had one of the highest TB case rates in the nation: 400 to 500 cases per 100,000 population.[13] The record shows a dozen more prison epidemics, many with fatalities, between December 1990 and December 1992. By the time the dust settled, it was clear that a strain of M. tuberculosis resistant to all five first-line drugs was implicated in most of the deaths. In the New York prison system, for example, MDRTB was diagnosed in at least thirty-three inmates, of whom 84 percent died of the disease; one correctional officer was fatally afflicted.[14]

The prison epidemics were amplified, certainly, by HIV: at the time of the outbreaks, New York inmates were already saddled with the nation's highest reported rates of HIV infection.[15] But the explosion of TB in prisons was even more intimately tied to government policies, most notably those of the Reagan and Bush administrations. In addition to dismantling the country's TB infrastructure—budgets had been slashed throughout the 1970s as well—the government declared a "War on Drugs" in 1982, which became, in large part, a war on drug users and petty traffickers rather than on those who ran or financed the drug trade. Rates of drug-related arrests and imprisonment skyrocketed during the first decade of the program. In 1980, there were approximately ten thousand new commitments for drug offenses; in 1990, there were over a hundred thousand. The inequalities of U.S. society were mirrored in sentencing: by 1990, some 7.9 percent of all African American adults were interned or on probation or parole.[16] As noted, these trends reflect changes in policy rather than changes in behavior.

By 1990, some 2.35 percent of the U.S. adult population—4.3 million men and women—were in prison or jail or were on probation or parole. This was a 63 percent increase over 1984, and it left most U.S. detention facilities filled well beyond the capacity for which they had been designed. Prisons without proper ventilation were soon crammed with inmates who had high baseline rates of infection with both HIV and *M. tuberculosis*. "Expansion of physical facilities has not kept pace with the doubling of prison and jail populations in the past decade," observe Robert Greifinger, Nancy Heywood, and Jordan Glaser in a 1993 review, "nor did it contemplate the risk of transmission of airborne disease."[17]

Yet the connection between the War on Drugs and drug-resistant tuberculosis was reported early on by those working in the correctional system.[18] Just as detention facilities were not designed to warehouse such large numbers of prisoners, so too was the prison medical system ill prepared to manage the resulting TB crisis. A lack of TB diagnostic capabilities was further compounded by HIV co-infection, which was associated with atypical presentations of active TB.[19] More critically, overburdened providers could not track adherence to anti-TB therapy, and the resulting inconsistent treatment led to increased rates of acquired resistance to first-line drugs. In the sardine-can atmosphere of 1980s prisons, MDRTB transmission soon led to high rates of primary MDRTB infection in a vulnerable and captive population.

HIV and prison are thus two reasons for the predominance of males in U.S. tuberculosis case rates: more than 70 percent of the new "excess" TB cases were diagnosed among men, most of them poor blacks and Latinos living in cities.[20] Among urban African American males, for example, rates of TB jumped *over 1500 percent* between 1985 and 1990.[21] Many of those afflicted shared the social space of prisons, jails, homeless shelters, drug treatment programs, and public hospitals. Molecular epidemiology subsequently showed that TB outbreaks linked such institutions together, the mutant strains working their way rapidly across the nation.[22]

There was little public outcry until prison wardens and health professionals began to fall ill. Then, as Laurie Garrett describes, "panic broke out."[23] Articles began to appear in newspapers and other print media.[24] "This publicity caused such alarm in one upstate New York community," write the authors of one review, "that its hospitals refused to care for inmates, even in life threatening emergencies."[25] With unions of health care workers and prison employees pressing for protection, the Occupational Safety and Health Administration and other regulatory bodies laid down guidelines designed to contain nosocomial and institutional transmission; court-ordered caps on the number of inmates were issued to several of the key prisons and jails.[26] Several detention facilities were upgraded; others were built to permit respiratory isolation.

These tardy interventions were, in the end, effective. But what was the cost of the delay? The MDRTB outbreaks, to an important extent the result of imprudent cost-cutting and ill-advised public policy, led to a massive outlay of public monies, especially in New York City. In addition to treatment costs, the upgrading of hospitals and detention facilities cost big money: a new Rikers Island facility cost $113 million. In a helpful review, Garrett puts it well: "When all the costs of the 1989–94 MDR-TB epidemic were totaled, it was clear that more than $1 billion was spent to rein in the mutant mycobacteria. Saving perhaps $200 million in budget cuts during the 1980s eventually cost America an enormous sum, not only in direct funds but also in lost productivity and, of course, human lives."[27]

The MDRTB misadventures also led many professionals to reevaluate the War on Drugs, widely regarded as totally ineffectual by both medical and jurisprudence communities. "Prisons are terrible institutions," observed Dr. Robert Cohen, whose experience as medical director of the Rikers Island facility forever changed his views on prisons and on drug policy. "The problem of drug abuse is much better approached with a medical model than with a crime-and-punishment model."[28]

Crime-and-punishment models bring us to Russia. There the story is even more grim. In 1990, TB incidence in Moscow was 27 per 100,000 population; by 1993, it had almost doubled, to 50 per 100,000. The situation is worse in Siberia, where incidence went from 43 to 94 per 100,000 during the same period.[29]

And the degradation continues. International health officials announced at a March 24, 1998, news conference in Copenhagen that TB incidence had risen another 50 percent in Russia between 1994 and 1996. "We have never seen such an increase before," commented Arata Kochi, director of the World Health Organization's Global Tuberculosis Programme. About a quarter of a million cases were announced in 1996, and officials further warned that these infections respected no borders: half of all Danish cases from that year were diagnosed in immigrants from the Baltic states or elsewhere in the former Soviet Union.[30]

Russia's increase in TB rates cannot be attributed to HIV or to ill-conceived drug policy. The collapse of the public health system, a part of the broader social disruption registered in Russia, is the heart of the problem; and prisons, it transpires, are central both to the amplification of the TB problem and to the mortality trends. "In the Russian Federation," notes one review, "there is evidence from tuberculosis control programs in the community that a high proportion of patients have served time in prisons, and that having been in jail is a major risk factor for the development of multidrug resistant strains of *M. tuberculosis.*" The same report pegs tuberculosis death rates as high as 24 percent, with the disease causing from 50 to 80 percent of all prison deaths.[31] The problem is not denied by prison officials. As one of them remarked, "The three major problems facing our correctional system are funding, overcrowding, and tuberculosis. Simply being in prison is one of Russia's biggest risk factors for TB."[32]

With so many TB deaths in prison and with such a high rate of imprisonment, it is less surprising to learn that tuberculosis has become the single leading contributor to increased mortality among young Russian men. Why are these patients dying from an eminently treatable disease? Although HIV has only recently been introduced to the formula, it remains, at this writing, a potential contributor to the problem. Some Russian patients die because they have no access to therapy; others die because they have access to the wrong kind of therapy. As in the U.S. outbreaks, many of these prisoners have MDRTB, but in Russia many are being prescribed the very medications to which their infecting strains are already resistant. Still others, it is said, are dispirited enough to give up. Poor conditions in Russian jails and prisons led to prison riots in 1992, but these were harshly repressed. Conditions continue to worsen.

Overcrowding in Russian prisons is now far worse than in U.S. facilities. To combat overcrowding in U.S. prisons, legislation was passed to ensure that each prisoner was allotted 80 square feet of space. In Russia, the space allotment was increased recently from 27 to 43 square feet.[33] But site visits to prisons and jails reveal this actual parameter to be far below 27—especially in pre-trial detention centers, where some three hundred thousand people currently languish. And more and more of those detained have or develop active tuberculosis. In these conditions, even brief pre-trial detainment may amount to intense bombardment with viable TB bacilli. With the average duration of *pre-trial* detention now up to ten months, one journalist has observed that, in these crowded holding centers, "a death sentence stalks people who have not yet been convicted of a crime."[34]

Pre-trial detention, certainly, is more Kafka-esque than Dostoyevskian. For example, Dima Shagina was arrested as a teenager, along with three other boys, for stealing a car. Since that time, he has been in Matrosskaya Tishina, a jail in central Moscow. Built for two thousand prisoners, it currently holds five thousand—no small number of them with active tuberculosis. It took almost three years for Shagina's case to come to trial, by which time he too was sick with active tuberculosis. His mother hopes that his next stop will be a TB penal colony—she "hopes" this because many tuberculosis patients die in Matrosskaya Tishina. Moscow's chief of corrections reports that seventy detainees died in that city in the first nine months of 1996—a majority of them from tuberculosis.[35]

What are the TB penal colonies like? Russia counts some forty-five such colonies; they house almost seventy-one thousand prisoners—half of them under twenty-five years of age. We recently spent a day in a colony located in a town of about thirty thousand inhabitants, about 100 kilometers east of Moscow. After our trip through well-tended fields and thick forests of birch and fir, the colony's dreary barracks seemed depressing and overcrowded: prisoners with TB were allotted 4 square meters per person. But the facility was clean, the guards and correctional officials were cooperative, and the prisoners did not appear malnourished.

The medical director explained that of 909 prisoners, well over 800 suffered from active tuberculosis. Their mean age was forty and falling, even though teenagers were sent to another facility. The prison had been designed, she explained, for patients who had already received the "intensive phase" of treatment and who, smear-negative, were slated to complete therapy in the colony. In recent years, however, patients arrived with nothing more than a diagnosis; they were transferred, smear-positive, from the facility where they'd been diagnosed. To tend to these sick prisoners, she had an ancillary staff of forty-three, most of them from the community and several of them prisoners themselves. HIV was not yet a problem, although hepatitis B and syphilis were endemic among the prisoners. "Our medical capacity," she warned, "is altogether inadequate."

Asked about TB outcomes, the medical director was very forthcoming: cure rates were low. Why? She denied that prisoners showed widespread reluctance to be treated: "On the contrary, the patients are very interested in treatment. They want to recover—especially the younger ones. A very small percentage of them refuse treatment, and usually do so because of some extenuating circumstance or misunderstanding. For example, some patients with liver disease are under the impression that they cannot tolerate the drugs. With a minimal amount of explanation, they too accept TB therapy." Furthermore, all patients, she insisted, received directly observed therapy.

The explanation for low cure rates lay elsewhere: "We know how to manage the cases," she explained wearily, "even the drug-resistant ones. But we don't have the resources." An annual medication budget of 14,000 rubles—not much more than $2,000—meant an irregular supply of first-line drugs and no supply whatsoever of second-line drugs, even though many patients, especially those infected in prison, were known to have drug-resistant disease.[36] Although no survey of drug susceptibility had ever been conducted, the medical director estimated that half of all prisoners had drug-resistant TB.

Just how low are the cure rates? The colony's general plan is to treat patients with active TB and then transfer them back to regular prisons. But fewer than one hundred prisoners were transferred last year, reported the chief warden. Far more common is another scenario: the prisoners remain in the colony until they are released from prison, still with the active disease. The warden informed us that *of thirty prisoners slated for release that month, twenty-seven were known to have active, infectious TB.* "We can't really cure them," added the doctor, "so we do our best to keep them alive."

Post-release care is not under the jurisdiction of the correctional system, and there is little coordination between the Ministry of Interior and the Ministry of Health. "They're released, and many have not finished therapy," continued the prison doctor. "We send them out with prescriptions, rather than the medications. By law, they have a right to the medications for free. But that's on paper. In reality, we know that the medications are no longer available for free. Sometimes they are not available at all." Asked about transmission to family members, she replied, "We have no statistics, but we fear the worst. We certainly have cases in which a father comes here as a convict, and we later meet his son—also a convict, and also with active TB."

Concern about this state of affairs was visible in the prisoners' faces. Take, for example, the case of Viktor, a thirty-two-year-old man arrested in Eastern Siberia in 1988. He is now only four months away from the end of an eleven-year sentence for fraud. He was diagnosed with TB while working in the TB infirmary, a job he earned for good behavior. He was treated but relapsed later in the course of his sentence. He is now slated to return to his wife and children in Siberia, but he's still sick. "Of course I'm worried I won't be better by the time my sentence is up," he said, "and that I will give my illness to my family."

The double jeopardy faced by Russian detainees is not lost on those working on their behalf. One penal reform activist observed that "sometimes, the prison officers and medical staff are doing the best they can, and the inmates understand that poor conditions are not the fault of the prison staff but rather of the whole criminal justice system."[37] A former dissident, also now a prisoners' rights activist, agrees, but his assessment is even more dour: "During my six years in Soviet prisons, I lived through many horrors." But "it is certain," he adds, "that conditions in normal jails were not this bad even under Stalin."[38]

In summary, the collapse of the Soviet Union, with its infamous gulags and "psychiatric prisons," has led to a *worsening* of TB care for prisoners, even as it has increased their risk of contracting the disease. The cost of this degradation is in some ways incalculable, and not merely in terms of human lives. The failure of the safety net and a blatant disregard for human dignity fuel a growing cynicism in Russia, weakening chances for the development of a truly open society.

WHAT SHOULD BE DONE?

There is no doubt, then, that MDRTB in prisons—a subset of the problem of tuberculosis in prisons—is a significant public health problem and also a peculiarly modern human rights challenge. How have the public health and human rights communities responded? It is not hyperbole to argue that much commentary on the problem reveals both a lack of vision and an ignorance of MDRTB management. Many international health experts throw their hands up, as if the ongoing spread of MDRTB and the mounting death toll were reflections of a *force majeure,* beyond the scope of human intervention. Although there is evidence to the contrary, one of the most commonly heard excuses is that MDRTB is simply untreatable.[39] Since drug stockouts are a major problem, it's also argued that drugs are "unavailable" or "too expensive." But is it really a question of drug distribution, when Coca-Cola and McDonald's have introduced their products into the far reaches of Siberia without much difficulty?

Other excuses abound. Here are some heard in Peru, the United States, Geneva, and Russia: the patients refuse treatment; they're noncompliant; they hide drugs in their mouths and spit them out later; they falsify lab results. Some complain that prisoners with TB are simply "too antisocial to be treated." It's also been argued that "prison culture" in Russia undermines efforts to treat. When these excuses are heard from the very persons responsible for addressing tuberculosis in prisons, one fears that hunches and impressions and prejudices are being elevated to the level of public policy. Indeed, segregation of tuberculosis patients and permanent isolation have been proposed as "solutions," with little objection from human rights activists. This is surprising, since cohorting is tantamount to endorsing differential standards of therapy: those already bearing a disproportionate risk of assaults on their rights are in essence being abused even further.

What about those who propose action on behalf of prisoners with tuberculosis? Even in these circles, we're offered long lists of pitfalls. For example, Hernán Reyes and Rudi Coninx report on the Red Cross experience in six Ethiopian prisons, in which a TB program was abandoned because of a high default rate— 62 percent of patients in the Addis Ababa prison defaulted. And these partially treated prisoners were unlikely, adds the report, to receive therapy elsewhere: "the national tuberculosis program for the general population was unable to provide treatment."[40] The situation in Russia is depicted as singularly discouraging: there, even laboratory results must be regarded with suspicion, since "wealthy prisoners" may "put pressure on laboratory technicians to find bacilli in negative sputum samples" in order to have access to antituberculous drugs that can be sold in the prison black market.[41]

Recognizing the gravity of the situation, the International Committee of the Red Cross, working with the World Health Organization, called a meeting last year in Baku, Azerbaijan, where an estimated seven hundred prisoners were sick with TB. Many of them, it is clear, have MDRTB. Disturbingly, 89 percent of the patients whose sputum did not convert after they received first-line drugs were found to have MDRTB. Furthermore, fully 24 percent of all consecutive patients initiating therapy were found to have MDRTB. It is not clear from the report what therapy was offered to these prisoners, but the Baku Declaration, issued at this meeting, called on "governments, ministries of justice and interior and state security and health to work together towards providing prisoners with adequate health care and the means to cure tuberculosis, and Prison health service to implement DOTS."[42] Unfortunately, this strategy will not work well in the Baku prisons: if 24 percent of all comers already have MDRTB, DOTS will not afford a "means to cure tuberculosis." Empiric short-course regimens of first-line drugs are the wrong prescription for what ails a substantial fraction of these prisoners.

A robust human rights discourse must be underpinned by technically correct recommendations. So what, then, is to be done? Alexander Paterson, a British prison commissioner in the 1930s, put it well: "Men are sent to prison *as* punishment, not *for* punishment."[43] Paterson's aphorism reminds us that we're faced with an enormous challenge: to identify prisoners with tuberculosis, to remove them from conditions in which treatment is unrealistic, and to initiate effective therapy. In so doing, we will halt the ongoing transmission of this disease, reducing the risk of making detention tantamount to a sentence of tuberculosis. And we will also respond, at last, to the mandate of protecting the public's health.

Enacting this plan of action requires a great deal of collaboration and goodwill, and it requires important resources. Surveillance of drug resistance is critical, for this alone helps to steer the choice of empiric regimens, when and if empiric regimens are warranted. New field tools for rapid detection of resistance to INH and RIF are becoming available and should be deployed where they are most needed. Once patients with MDRTB are identified, further testing is necessary to design treatment regimens, and technical assistance will be critical to ensure good outcomes. It is difficult to abort prison TB epidemics through effective therapy, but it is possible with no more than the existing tools. This has been proven in the United States, a country hardly known for progressive prison policies: only after the situation got totally out of hand were ample resources made available, but flow they did. Ironically, some prison health experts now deplore a lack of funding for TB *outside* U.S. prisons.[44]

Above all, we must avoid the temptation to throw our hands up, for that is the stance that has led us to the current impasse in Russia and elsewhere. In fact, some years of engagement with this problem leads me to conclude that the biggest pitfall of all may be resignation—not that of the prisoners but rather our own. It's for this reason that we cannot find, either in the published literature or in public health circles, a blueprint for action that would help us respond effectively to the problem of drug-resistant tuberculosis in prisons. Nowhere can we find recommendations arguing that prisoners, precisely because they are wards of the state, must be protected from undue risk of infection. Nowhere can we find recommendations arguing that prisoners have the right to top-of-the-line therapy in part because they are prisoners. Instead, calls for effective therapy for MDRTB are often dismissed as "utopian," "unrealistic," "pie in the sky."

No matter how utopian universal TB care may sound, it is clear that the problem will not improve without it. Most prison officials in Russia and Central Europe insist that they would like to see this problem brought under control. Many prison physicians are competent and, indeed, compassionate advocates for prisoners sick with TB. Furthermore, many of the prisoners are afraid of TB and are more than willing to undergo rigorous treatment. Finally, the propositions now before us—more directly observed therapy with short-course empiric regimens—simply will not work wherever MDRTB is already a problem.

Prison medicine is most legitimate when it is humane. Medical interventions are most powerful when they are effective. Human rights arguments are most powerful if we believe that all humans are equally valuable. When we do believe this, we are less likely to shrug off second-rate interventions, attending instead to remediating the inequalities that are each day brought more clearly into view by a globalizing economy.

CONCLUSION: ON AGENCY AND CONSTRAINT

Allow me to conclude by returning to the concept of tuberculosis as punishment. "Contracting tuberculosis in prison," asserts one report, "is most certainly not part of a prisoner's sentence."[45] But in many places, as we have seen, it most certainly is. As long as prison serves as amplifier, as long as effective treatment is not ensured, tuberculosis is part of the punishment—a package deal of new corporality. In his history of French penology, Michel Foucault charts a "displacement of the very object of the punitive operation" from the body of the offender to his "soul" or "psyche."[46] Does tuberculosis as punishment signal a return to a sort of laissez-faire penal torture, a reembodiment of discipline? Does the state's apparent impotence before the problem mean that no one is to blame for ongoing, fatal outbreaks of drug-resistant tuberculosis in prisons? That such outbreaks are accidents? Freakish natural events, a sort of microbial El Niño?

The state, in all its forms, has always arrogated the power to punish. In all societies, government reserves the right to strip those deemed miscreant of their agency; in some societies, including certain self-declared democracies, it reserves the right to kill criminals. But even prisoners on death row are regarded as having certain rights, including freedom from undue risk of disease. The U.S. Supreme Court has in recent times reminded us that "deliberate indifference to the serious medical needs of prisoners constitutes the unnecessary and wanton infliction of pain proscribed by the Eighth Amendment."[47]

For what it's worth, then, allowing prisoners to die of tuberculosis is illegal in the United States. While many of those who died in U.S. prison outbreaks were the voiceless poor, it did not take long for prisoners' rights groups to see that many detainees had been exposed, through poor planning and carelessness, to unnecessary risks. In 1982, in *Lareau v. Manson*, a group of pre-trial detainees and inmates brought suit against Connecticut's Hartford Community Correctional Center for exposing them to tuberculosis and other transmissible pathogens. A district circuit court ruled that failure to screen detainees for communicable diseases not only violates the Eighth Amendment's due process clause protecting pre-trial detainees but also constitutes "cruel and unusual punishment" for all inmates.[48] The ruling was subsequently upheld by a federal circuit court. In 1992, a group of inmates in Pennsylvania argued that the prison's lack of an adequate TB control strategy violated the rights guaranteed them under the Eighth and Fourteenth Amendments. A federal district court ruled in their favor, mandating the prompt implementation of an effective TB control program.[49]

Greifinger, Heywood, and Glaser have reviewed a large number of similar cases, and many other cases have been filed since their review appeared.[50] The point is simply this: since history reveals our persistent inability to protect prisoners on principle, we must entrap ourselves into decency through public policy. The call for better policy is not an argument against human rights discourse. On the contrary, it is an argument to gird such discourse with the power to enforce.

Ironically, perhaps, it is the globalizing economy that brings into relief the flabby relativism of the public health *realpolitik* that leaves us with a double standard of therapy—prompt, effective MDRTB treatment for those with resources, and no treatment at all for prisoners and the poor with MDRTB. The unacceptability of such double standards was foreseen by the architects of health internationalism. Signed into effect on July 22, 1946, the Constitution of the World Health Organization warned that "unequal development in different countries in the promotion of health and control of disease, especially communicable disease, is a common danger." The only good news, for those ardently opposed to such double standards, is that transnational TB epidemics will at least remind the affluent few that no one is really safe if these epidemics are not brought under control.

NOTES

1. Greifinger, Heywood, and Glaser, "Tuberculosis in Prison."

2. Although careful studies are lacking, TB incidence in prisons in Kazakhstan and other newly independent states of the former Soviet Union may well exceed one hundred times that in surrounding communities (based on data presented at the conference Public Health Implications of Prisons and Jails in Eastern Europe and Central Asia, Budapest, Hungary, June 4–7, 1998). For more data on this association, see Reyes and Coninx, "Pitfalls of Tuberculosis Programmes in Prisons." It's important to add here that nameless millions must somehow live in a pre-antibiotic time warp, since they, whether in or out of detention, continue to die from this disease: worldwide, TB remains

the single leading infectious cause of adult deaths. For a review, see Farmer, *Infections and Inequalities*, chap. 7.

3. I use the term "geoculture" after Immanuel Wallerstein; see, for example, Wolf et al., "Perilous Ideas"; Wallerstein, *After Liberalism*.

4. Farmer, Bayona, Becerra, et al. "Poverty, Inequality, and Drug Resistance."

5. Reyes and Coninx, "Pitfalls of Tuberculosis Programmes in Prisons," p. 1449.

6. The literature on tuberculosis and prisons is of mixed quality. The term "resistance," for example, is misused in several ways. Some social scientists have even poured resources, material and intellectual, into celebrations of prisoners' refusal to take medications as acts of "resistance." For a review, see Farmer, "Social Scientists and the New Tuberculosis" (included in this volume as chapter 7). Physicians and public health specialists, in turn, often attempt to ignore drug resistance in the hope that it will go away.

7. See Reyes and Coninx, "Pitfalls of Tuberculosis Programmes in Prisons," pp. 1447, 1449; compare Greifinger, Heywood, and Glaser, "Tuberculosis in Prison," p. 339. Note, of course, that Reyes and Coninx refer primarily to resource-poor countries, while Greifinger, Heywood, and Glaser refer to U.S. institutions.

8. Stern, *A Sin against the Future.*

9. See, for example, Laurie Garrett's description: "Studies showed that some 80 percent of all MDR-TB index cases in 1989–90 (not including the secondary HIV-positive cases) were injecting drug and crack users, many of whom, as a result of federal and local crackdowns, drifted in and out of the jail and prison system" (*The Coming Plague*, p. 524).

10. Braun et al., "Increasing Incidence of Tuberculosis in a Prison Inmate Population."

11. Centers for Disease Control and Prevention, "Prevention and Control of Tuberculosis in Correctional Institutions."

12. Garrett puts it best: "The emergence of novel strains of multiply drug-resistant TB came amid a host of clangs, whistles, and bells that should have served as ample warning to humanity. But the warning fell on unhearing ears" (*The Coming Plague*, p. 508).

13. Skolnick, "Some Experts Suggest the Nation's 'War on Drugs' Is Helping Tuberculosis Stage a Deadly Comeback."

14. Greifinger, Heywood, and Glaser, "Tuberculosis in Prison," p. 335.

15. As of 1992, "New York has had the highest reported prevalence of HIV infection among inmates: 12 percent of the incoming males and 20 percent of incoming females" (ibid., p. 334).

16. "For the first time, the number of persons admitted for drug offenses was greater than the number admitted for property offenses, violent offenses, or public-order offenses" (ibid., p. 333).

17. Ibid.

18. For example, John Raba, former medical director of the Cook County jail, was quick to link the War on Drugs to outbreaks of MDRTB: "The result is that we are now seeing outbreaks including a number of cases of highly lethal multidrug-resistant TB. We're continuing the nation's program of incarcerating drug users despite the absence of any demonstrated individual or social benefit" (cited in Skolnick, "Some Experts Suggest the Nation's 'War on Drugs' Is Helping Tuberculosis Stage a Deadly Comeback," p. 3177).

19. Many patients later shown to have HIV-associated active TB were AFB smear-negative; many had atypical chest radiographs and disseminated disease.

20. Snider, Salinas, and Kelly, "Tuberculosis," p. 647.

21. Jereb et al., "Tuberculosis Morbidity in the United States," tables SS23–SS27.

22. Bifani et al., "Origin and Interstate Spread of a New York City Multidrug-Resistant Mycobacterium Tuberculosis Clone Family."

23. Garrett, *The Coming Plague*, p. 520.

24. *New York Post* reporter Ann Bolinger was herself infected with *M. tuberculosis* while covering the Rikers Island outbreak; see Skolnick, "Some Experts Suggest the Nation's 'War on Drugs' Is Helping Tuberculosis Stage a Deadly Comeback."

25. Greifinger, Heywood, and Glaser, "Tuberculosis in Prison," p. 335.

26. Robert Cohen, former medical director of the Rikers Island jail, notes: "Court-ordered inmate population caps have been the only thing that has kept correctional institutions in many jurisdictions from collapsing into total chaos" (cited in Skolnick, "Some Experts Suggest the Nation's 'War on Drugs' Is Helping Tuberculosis Stage a Deadly Comeback," p. 3178).

27. Garrett, *The Coming Plague*, p. 523.

28. Cohen cited in Skolnick, "Some Experts Suggest the Nation's 'War on Drugs' Is Helping Tuberculosis Stage a Deadly Comeback," p. 3178.

29. Tayler, Besse, and Healing, "Tuberculosis in Siberia."

30. See Garrett, "TB Surge in Former East Bloc."

31. Reyes and Coninx, "Pitfalls of Tuberculosis Programmes in Prisons," p. 1450, citing Khomenko and Médecins Sans Frontières. Note that in spite of the magnitude of the U.S. problem, deaths from tuberculosis remained relatively rare and did not inflect the country's overall mortality curves. In a sense, the Russian patients have been transported to the "pre-antibiotic time warp" inhabited by the Southern Hemisphere poor.

32. Ivan Nikitovich Simonov, former chief inspector of prisons, and now with the Chief Board of Punishment Execution, Ministry of Internal Affairs, Russian Federation, interview with the author, June 1998.

33. Valery Sergeyev of Penal Reform International, Moscow Bureau, interview with the author, June 1998.

34. See Stanley, "Russians Lament the Crime of Punishment."

35. Ibid.

36. The prison also lacked syringes, masks, and other supplies. As a result, staff morale was low. "We regard this as an especially terrible problem," remarked the facility's medical director. "We have professionals who want to work but don't have the necessary resources."

37. Sergeyev interview.

38. Stanley, "Russians Lament the Crime of Punishment."

39. The experience of Socios En Salud in Peru shows that a majority of patients sick with even highly resistant strains of MDRTB can be cured; see Farmer, Bayona, Shin, et al., "Preliminary Outcomes of Community-Based MDRTB Treatment in Lima, Peru." Also see Turett et al., "Improved Outcomes for Patients with Multidrug-Resistant Tuberculosis."

40. Reyes and Coninx, "Pitfalls of Tuberculosis Programmes in Prisons," p. 1448.

41. Ibid. The irony here is that we're willing to go to war over weapons inspections but throw our hands up in the face of relatively minor challenges such as quality control in prison laboratories.

42. Ibid., p. 1449.

43. Cited in ibid., p. 1447; emphasis added.

44. "Since the outbreak in New York, other outbreaks have been reported in correctional systems in Connecticut, Washington, Ohio, Alabama and California. Following the reports of cases in these states, resources were provided for an appropriate public health response. *In contrast, there has been scant funding for TB control outside the prison walls.* This is unfortunate because TB in prison is solely a symptom of a broader public health problem" (Greifinger, Heywood, and Glaser, "Tuberculosis in Prison," p. 336).

45. Reyes and Coninx, "Pitfalls of Tuberculosis Programmes in Prisons," p. 1447.

46. Foucault, *Surveiller et punir*, p. 38 (translation mine).

47. *Estelle v. Gamble*, 429 U.S. 97 (1976).

48. The court ruled that the "resulting threat to the well-being of the inmates is so serious, and the record so devoid of any justification for the defendant's policy that, under the standard of *Bell v. Wolfish,* this practice constitutes 'punishment' in violation of the Due Process Clause" (cited in Greifinger, Heywood, and Glaser, "Tuberculosis in Prison," p. 338).

49. *Austin v. Pennsylvania Department of Correction,* WL 277511, E.D.Pa. (1992).

50. Greifinger, Heywood, and Glaser, "Tuberculosis in Prison." For example, in late March 1988, a parolee sued a county jail, a prison, and the Colorado Department of Health after developing tuberculosis while in prison for theft (Abbott, "Parolee with Tuberculosis Sues County Jail, State Prison").

The Consumption of the Poor

Tuberculosis in the Twenty-First Century

(2000)

Are you unaware that vast numbers of your fellow men suffer or perish from need of the things that you have to excess, and that you required the explicit and unanimous consent of the whole human race for you to appropriate from the common subsistence anything besides that required for your own?

JEAN-JACQUES ROUSSEAU, *DISCOURSE ON THE ORIGIN OF INEQUALITY*

BACK WITH A VENGEANCE?

The World Health Organization recently announced that in 1999 alone nearly two million persons died of tuberculosis.[1] Not since the turn of the century, when tuberculosis was the leading cause of young adult deaths in most U.S. cities, has the disease claimed so many lives. Tuberculosis, we are told, has returned "with a vengeance."[2] In the language of the day, it is an "emerging infectious disease." In scientific publications and in the popular press, the refrain is the same: tuberculosis, once vanquished, is now resurging to trouble us once again.

Yet tuberculosis has been with us all along; only from a highly particular point of view can it be seen as an emerging, or even "reemerging," disease. "Thinking in terms of a returned tuberculosis," objects Katherine Ott, "obscures the unabated high incidence of tuberculosis worldwide over the decades."[3] Those who experience tuberculosis as an ongoing concern are the world's poor, whose voices have systematically been silenced. Yet they deserve a hearing, if for no other reason than that the poor infected with the tubercle bacillus are legion. Some estimate that as many two billion persons—a third of the world's population—are currently infected with quiescent but viable *Mycobacterium tuberculosis*. This figure corroborates another: tuberculosis remains, at this writing, the world's leading infectious cause of preventable deaths in adults.[4]

Tuberculosis is thus two things at once: a completely curable disease and the leading cause of young adult deaths in much of the world. As we enter a new century, it is instructive to compare our circumstances to the situation that prevailed at the end of the nineteenth century. At that time, Robert Koch had recently identified the tubercle bacillus, but no effective treatment existed. "Consumption" was the leading cause of death and the most feared of diseases. "During the late nineteenth century," notes Frank Ryan, "there was a growing fear that the disease might destroy European civilization."[5]

Although its victims during the eighteenth and nineteenth centuries included members of all classes, TB has always disproportionately affected the poor. For example, English mortuary registers from the 1830s reveal that although tuberculosis deaths were common, they were increasingly so at the lower end of the social ladder: "The proportion of 'consumptive cases' in 'gentlemen, tradesmen and laborers' was 16, 28, and 30 percent respectively."[6] The affluent could "take the cure" in a number of ways—they could travel to different climes or enjoy protein-rich diets—but case-fatality rates were high among all those with "galloping consumption."

With the advent of improved sanitary conditions and the development of food and trade surpluses, tuberculosis incidence declined in the industrializing nations, particularly in those communities and classes that enjoyed the greatest benefits of these transformations. Still, the infection remained widespread yet patterned in its distribution. In 1900, annual death rates from tuberculosis for white Americans approached 200 per 100,000 population. "Among black Americans," adds historian Barbara Rosenkrantz, "the figure was 400 deaths per 100,000, approximately the same level recorded in the middle of the 19th century for the population as a whole."[7] Black Americans were enjoying the fruits of medical progress with a fifty-year lag.

Technology has often been presented as the remedy for social ills, and the development of effective tuberculosis chemotherapy was hailed as the beginning of the end of the disease. But the poor remained much more likely to become infected and ill with *M. tuberculosis*. When they were sick with complications of tuberculosis, they were more likely to receive substandard therapy—or no therapy at all. In the years after the Second World War, those with access to the new antituberculous medications could expect to be cured of their disease. Who had access to streptomycin and PAS (para-aminosalicylic acid, one of the first antituberculous drugs) in the late 1940s? Fortunate citizens of the United States and a handful of European nations, all with well-established and encouraging trends in tuberculosis incidence that predated effective chemotherapy. Thus risk, though never evenly shared, became increasingly polarized.

By mid-century, tuberculosis was still acknowledged as a problem in certain quarters, but it was becoming less and less of a concern. One historian has argued that "TB had all but disappeared from public view by the 1960s."[8] The reasons for this invisibility stem in part from the decreasing absolute incidence in wealthy nations and in part from persistent patterns of differential susceptibility. Writing in 1952, René Dubos and Jean Dubos observed that "while the disease is now only a minor problem in certain parts of the United States, extremely high rates still prevail in the colored population." Nor were poor outcomes distributed merely by race. Within racial categories, differential risk remained the rule. Among whites, these authors noted, the case-fatality rate was "almost seven times higher among unskilled laborers than among professional persons."[9] Ironically, then, *the advent of effective therapy seems to have further entrenched this striking variation in disease distribution and outcomes.* Inequalities operated both locally and globally: the "TB outcome gap" between rich and poor grew, and so too did the outcome gap between rich countries and poor countries.

In short, the "forgotten plague" was forgotten in large part because it ceased to bother the wealthy. In fact, if tuberculosis is reexamined from the point of view of those living in poverty, a radically different picture emerges. In the twentieth century, at least, tuberculosis has not really emerged so much as *reemerged from the ranks of the poor.*[10] One place for diseases like tuberculosis to "hide" is among poor people, especially when the poor are socially and medically segregated from those whose deaths might be considered more significant. Who are these throwaway people? I propose to rethink these issues by drawing on life histories of people afflicted with tuberculosis and by seeking to ground their experience in the political economy of this plague.

For more than a decade, I have worked as both ethnographer of and physician to populations bearing excess burdens of tuberculosis. In central Haiti, where I have worked since 1983, I have conducted hundreds of open-ended interviews with people afflicted with tuberculosis, not only hearing their stories but also coming to understand their own complex views of disease causation. In Peru, I have served as medical director of an effort to treat one of the most dreaded forms of the disease—multidrug-resistant tuberculosis (MDRTB). In the process, I have learned a great deal about how social inequalities come to have pathogenic effects. In the United States, where tuberculosis is a rare disease, I have been privileged to meet those for whom it is far from rare: poor people of color and those newly arrived from areas in which tuberculosis remains endemic. More recently, my work in tuberculosis has taken me to jails and prisons in these countries and to others in Russia, Azerbaijan, and Latvia.[11]

PWATRINÈ IN CENTRAL HAITI: JEAN DUBUISSON

Jean Dubuisson, who has never been sure of his age, lives in a small village in Haiti's Central Plateau, where he farms a tiny plot of land. He shares a two-room hut with his wife, Marie, and their three surviving children. All his life, recounts Jean, he has "known nothing but trouble." His parents lost their land to the Péligre hydroelectric dam, which flooded the valley where they lived—a loss that plunged their large family into misery. Long before Jean became ill, he and Marie were having a hard time feeding their own children: two of them died before their fifth birthdays, and that was before the cost of living became intolerable.

And so it was a bad day when, sometime in 1990, Jean began coughing. For a couple of weeks, he simply ignored his persistent hack, which was followed by an intermittent fever. There was no clinic or dispensary in his home village, and the costs of going to the closest clinic (in a nearby town) are prohibitive enough to keep men like Jean shivering on the dirt floors of their huts. But then he began having night sweats. Night sweats are bad under any conditions, but they are particularly burdensome when you have only one sheet and often sleep in your clothes.

Marie insisted that it was time to seek professional treatment for Jean's illness. But it was already late September, Jean argued, and school would be starting soon. There would be tuition to pay, books and notebooks to buy, school uniforms to sew for the children. Jean did not seek medical care; instead he drank herbal teas as empiric remedies for the *grip,* a term similar to "cold" in North American usage.

Jean's slow decline continued over the course of several months, during which he lost a good deal of weight. The next event, in the story told by Jean and Marie, was when he began to cough up blood, in late December of 1990. This is common in rural Haiti, and most people living there do not believe that the *grip* can cause it. Instead, Jean and his family concluded that he was *pwatrinè*—stricken with tuberculosis—and they knew that he had two options: to travel to a clinic or to seek care from a voodoo priest. These were not mutually exclusive options, but, as Jean had no enemies, he concluded that his tuberculosis was due to "natural causes" rather than to sorcery. Emaciated and anemic, he went to the clinic closest to his home village.

At the clinic, he paid two dollars for multivitamins and the following advice: eat well, drink clean water, sleep in an open room and away from others, and go to a hospital. Jean and Marie recounted this counsel without a hint of sarcasm, but nonetheless evinced a keen appreciation of its total lack of relevance. In order to follow these instructions, the family would have had to sell off its chickens and its pig, and perhaps even what little land they had left. They hesitated, understandably.

Two months later, however, a second, massive episode of hemoptysis sent them to a church-affiliated hospital not far from Port-au-Prince. There Jean, still coughing, was admitted to an open ward. We were unable to review his records, but we know that he stayed for a full two weeks before being referred to a sanatorium. During his stay, Jean was charged four dollars per day for his bed; at the time, the per capita income in rural Haiti was about two hundred dollars per year. When the hospital's staff wrote prescriptions for him, he was required to pay for each medication before it was administered. Thus, although Jean could not tell us what therapies he received while an in-patient, he knew that he actually received less than half of the medicine prescribed. Furthermore, the only meals he ate in the hospital were those prepared by Marie: most Haitian hospitals do not serve food.

Jean continued to lose weight, and he simply discharged himself from the hospital when the family ran out of money and livestock. He did not go to the sanatorium. Needless to say, the cough persisted, as did the night sweats and fever. "We were lucky, though," added Jean. "I stopped coughing up blood."

After reaching home, Jean, bedridden, was visited by a cousin who lived in Bois Joli, a small village served by Proje Veye Sante, a Haitian organization that was then sponsoring a comprehensive tuberculosis treatment project.[12] The program, which included financial aid and regular visits from community health workers, had been designed for people like Jean Dubuisson and for a country like Haiti—that is, it was designed for poor and hungry people with tuberculosis who receive shabby treatment wherever they go. Unfortunately, the project then served the permanent residents of only sixteen villages and was based in a village over two hours from Jean's house. "Several [villagers] had benefited from it," recalled Jean's cousin, "so I suggested that he move to Bois Joli, so then he would be eligible for this assistance."

Marie Dubuisson "took down the house" and moved her husband and children to Bois Joli. "We didn't have a tin roof or good land," she added philosophically, "so it wasn't as bad as it might have been. And Jean needed the treatment." The skeletal man with sunken eyes and severe anemia began therapy in May of 1991. Jean gained eighteen pounds in his first three months of treatment. His oldest daughter was found to have tuberculosis of the lymph nodes, and she too was treated.

Jean was cured of his tuberculosis, but this cure, in many respects, came too late. Although he is now free of active disease, his left lung was almost completely destroyed. He grows short of breath after only minimal exertion. Marie now does most of the household's manual labor, depending on her daughter (who was also cured) for assistance in carrying water and hoeing. "I have a hard time climbing hills," Jean reports, surveying the steep valley before him. "And that's a bad thing when you're trying to get by up in the hills."

MDRTB AND *FUJISHOCK* IN URBAN PERU: CORINA BAYONA

Corina Bayona was born in 1942 in Huánuco, in Peru's Central Sierra. Like most of the region's poorer peasants, her parents found it increasingly difficult to wrest a living from the unforgiving countryside. When Corina married Carlos

Valdivia, both had dreams of escaping the harshness of rural life. A son, Jaime, was born before Corina was twenty.

In 1974, the three of them emigrated to Carabayllo, the new and sprawling slum north of Lima, one of Latin America's most rapidly growing cities. The edges of the settlement consisted of "*invasiones*"—dry and dusty slopes dotted with ramshackle shelters built first of straw and cardboard and plastic, and then rebuilt in dun-colored brick years later, when the squatters no longer feared that they would be removed by force. To settlers and to visitors alike, the steep and treeless fringes of Carabayllo looked like the surface of the moon.

Soon Corina, Carlos, and Jaime moved into a one-room house. During the 1970s and 1980s, Corina worked as a maid in a schoolteacher's house; Carlos worked as a night watchman in the industrial area south of Lima. Their house eventually had electricity, if no running water, and Corina and Carlos were able to send Jaime to high school. Carlos recalls this time as relatively secure, despite the political violence that often struck the city. Unemployment was high in Carabayllo, although not as high as it would later become, and they were lucky to have two jobs, especially since their son's new wife and baby precipitously added two more mouths to feed in the mid-1980s.

At some point in 1989, Corina began coughing. Initially, she attempted to treat herself with herbal remedies, primarily because she was unable to visit the clinic. Although a public health post was based nearby, it was closed during the hours that Corina was in Carabayllo. What Corina lacked most was time: it took her more than two hours on public buses to commute to work each day. When her cough worsened, she finally went to the post, where a doctor raised the possibility of tuberculosis. A smear of her sputum revealed the tubercle bacillus, and she began standard antituberculous therapy.

In August of 1990, shortly after Alberto Fujimori was elected president of Peru, the urban poor underwent what they later termed *fujishock*—the rapid implementation of one of the most draconian structural adjustment policies in the hemisphere. Inflation spiraled, and public services, including health care, were trimmed back sharply.[13] Soon Carlos was out of work.

Implemented in 1990 under pressure from the World Bank, the International Monetary Fund, the United Nations, and other multilateral agencies, the "shock therapy" administered for Peru's inflationary crisis created an economic recession by imposing a number of new economic policies: the government ended price supports for fuel and food, devalued the currency, and imposed a 14 percent sales tax on all domestic purchases. Another key component of the reform plan involved privatization of state industries; by 1997, these reforms had expanded to encompass the health sector. Whatever the long-term budgetary advantages reaped by this drastic and sudden overhaul of the Peruvian economy, the poor have continued to bear the brunt of these reforms. Just one year after *fujishock* was implemented, the number of people officially classified as "poor" increased from seven to twelve million, while a signal decrease in social funding hobbled the state's ability to support this burgeoning number of impoverished citizens. Although their numbers later decreased as Peru's economy rebounded, these policies had already taken their toll on the Peruvian poor.

In the midst of all these problems, Corina began coughing again. More sputum was collected for a smear, which was positive, and for culture. When Carlos later returned for the culture results, however, he was informed that the specimen had been misplaced. In April of 1991, after more delays and worsening symptoms, Corina was formally diagnosed with relapsed pulmonary tuberculosis. Given the health post's inconvenient hours and long waits—and also, as one of her doctors noted, the significant stigma associated with tuberculosis—she began receiving treatment at a private clinic.

What Corina gained in privacy and convenience she lost in increased costs. As was not uncommon in those months after *fujishock,* the family's meager savings were soon expended; Corina was unable to complete her treatment. As her husband recalls it, they could afford to buy only two of the four drugs prescribed.[14] Corina became sicker and soon could no longer work. When she next sought care, this time in a public health center in Carabayllo, physicians there discovered that she did not respond to standard therapy. When her condition worsened still further, in April of 1991, she was advised to seek care in a hospital.

Corina first presented to a private university teaching hospital, but she could not afford to purchase the medications and supplies prescribed. She was referred to the public facility not far away. At the private hospital, Corina had been told that she would have to pay for supplies; at the public facility, where supplies were extremely scarce, she was told that she must bring her own—including syringes, gloves, and gauze. Further, Corina had the ill fortune to arrive at this hospital just before the national health workers' strike, which was called in response to the new government's massive cuts in public spending. During the strike, most ambulatory treatment was simply suspended; Corina received, in essence, no care for her tuberculosis during this time.

In August of 1991, shortly after the strike ended, Corina returned for her medications. A physician roundly upbraided her: "Señora, it's your own fault that you did not complete your treatment. Why didn't you come before?" Brusquely, he sent her to yet another facility, complaining that she was not from his hospital's catchment area. This third hospital, though close to the Valdivia household, was not highly regarded, and Corina complained that there too she received a cool welcome. She was summarily referred back to the local health post for her care.

Dr. Raúl García, director of the Peruvian community-based organization Socios En Salud, had just initiated a health survey of Carabayllo. He met Corina in the course of inquiring about drug-resistant tuberculosis in the area. She was, he recalls, scarred by her interactions with the health care system. "Every time she went to the hospital, the physicians were mean or impolite to her. They had labeled her as noncompliant." Thus branded, Corina "felt attacked." "She was filled with fear," continued Dr. García. "She resolved not to return to seek care at the health center."

Carlos Valdivia was troubled by this resolution, for Corina continued to deteriorate. She coughed incessantly and became short of breath, even at rest. Her son, still living at home, worried for his mother. "You should go back to the health center," he pleaded, "so that they will cure you." But soon Jaime began to cough as well. "He didn't want to go either," recalled Dr. García, "because he didn't want to be treated the way they had treated his mother." Eventually Jaime sought treatment at the local post, but he too failed to respond to standard therapy.

For the next three years, Corina and Jaime lived with active pulmonary tuberculosis. Their household, wracked by coughing, was increasingly tense. Jaime's wife left, leaving behind their two infants, and Carlos began to drink. Late in the summer of 1994, Corina began to cough up blood. When at last she sought care for this condition, it was documented that her infecting strain had become resistant to all first-line antituberculous drugs except ethambutol. For reasons that remain unclear, the doctors then prescribed those very same medications for her again. Corina of course failed to respond to these agents—and, worse, she had a life-threatening reaction to one of them in November. Shortly thereafter, she was advised to give up completely on her "futile" efforts to treat her disease.

But Corina and her family were not so easily dissuaded. Upon inquiring, they learned that other drugs were available but that the public health system could not provide them free of charge. Among the drugs prescribed by a pulmonologist were two new agents, ciprofloxacin and ethionamide, with an estimated cost of 500 *soles* a month—eight times her husband's income when he'd been fortunate enough to have a job.

Carlos Valdivia, seeing his family dying before him, each month searched high and low for 500 *soles* for his wife and for his son, because by then it had become clear that Jaime also had drug-resistant tuberculosis. Sometimes Carlos succeeded; often he did not. "What unemployed person in Carabayllo could find 1000 *soles* a month?" reflected Carlos sadly. His son died in December of 1995, leaving behind the two small children.

Corina, finding herself the primary caretaker for her grandchildren, found new reasons to fight for survival. Dr. García recalls her saying, "I thought that I'd lived long enough until I had these two children to take care of. All I ask is for God to let me live in order to care for them." Through the efforts of a local community-based organization, Corina eventually received therapy with a multidrug regimen designed for resistant tuberculosis disease. The medications were provided for free, but she soon had another adverse reaction: bruises erupted on her legs. A pulmonologist advised her to stop taking all of her medications and recommended another culture of her sputum.

In February 1996, one week before Corina died, Carlos went to the health post with yet another sputum sample. The plan, he knew, was to find other medications that his wife might be able to take. Suddenly, however, Corina became severely short of breath. Carlos took her to the clinic, and an auxiliary nurse subsequently tried to place her in two different hospitals. In the emergency room of the teaching hospital, the staff informed Corina: "We have nothing we can do for you; your case is too chronic." After that, Corina stated that she would not return to the local public hospital, to which she had been again referred. "I would rather wait for the end at home than go back there," she said. She did not have long to wait.

FROM HARLEM TO VIETNAM AND BACK: CALVIN LOACH

Calvin Loach was born in New York City in 1951. His parents were both from the Carolinas. Shortly before Calvin's birth, they had emigrated to the city hoping to find steady work and respite from the racism that had so limited their economic opportunities in the South. New York, they found, was not much better. As Calvin and his two sisters were growing up, their father toiled in a series of unrewarding and short-lived jobs; later, and for many years, their mother worked in the medical records department of a Brooklyn hospital.

Calvin attended public high school, where his academic performance was fairly unremarkable, and graduated in 1969. There was talk, at the time, of his attending a local community college, but Calvin never completed an application. In the second month of his second job, at age nineteen, he was drafted into the U.S. Army.

Calvin spoke rarely about his tour of duty in Vietnam. He saw active combat in April 1971 and was part of a platoon that sustained heavy fire and loss of life. Calvin was not wounded by gunfire, but during a march in rough terrain he sustained a penetrating wound to the sole of his right foot. This injury soon became infected, eventually requiring surgery and intravenous antibiotics. It subsequently became the source of many problems for him.

Another problem stemming from Calvin's tour of duty concerned heroin. In one telling, the former soldier linked the use of opiates to the chronic pain that resulted from his injury; in another account, his regular use of heroin preceded this injury by several months. In any case, it was in Vietnam, and not in New York, that Calvin first used the drug, which was inexpensive, readily available, and (according to many) widely used by the increasingly demoralized U.S. soldiers.

In 1972, Calvin returned to New York City, where he lived with his mother and one of his sisters; his father had returned to North Carolina. Although he did drink and smoke, sometimes heavily, Calvin initially did not use heroin in the United States; upon returning, he knew no one else who was involved with the drug. It was during a visit to Boston, where his mother's cousins owned part of a convenience store, that Calvin was reintroduced to heroin and also to cocaine. From the late 1970s until 1992, Calvin used heroin, sometimes steadily and sometimes intermittently.

Most social histories obtained from his medical records suggested that Calvin never had a steady job after Vietnam, but a more thorough interview, by a social worker at a Boston-area Veterans Administration hospital, documented over three years of full-time employment in a furniture warehouse. At the time, Calvin was living with a woman who had previously worked for his cousins. His girlfriend told another social worker that Calvin had turned again to heroin after he lost this job in 1982. This girlfriend strongly discouraged his drug use, and it led her to leave him.

In 1991, Calvin was hospitalized for an episode of staphylococcal endocarditis, which permanently damaged one of his heart valves. During this hospitalization, Calvin's old foot injury became increasingly painful and began to drain pus. He was diagnosed with osteomyelitis (infection of the bone) and received two months of therapy for the infection.

It was during this hospital stay, which lasted almost a month, that Calvin developed a dislike for the hospital milieu. The feeling, it seems, was mutual: medical records describe Calvin as "difficult" and, in one instance, "verbally abusive." The word "noncompliant" is found throughout his records, although it is not entirely clear why, since Calvin was well on his way to completing difficult therapy for endocarditis and osteomyelitis, and in the previous year he had used an antihypertensive medication with regularity.

By the time Calvin was referred for expert management of his addiction, he had already spent a month withdrawing from narcotics, without the help of opiates or benzodiazepines. By his account, he did not use heroin again, although he later received methadone.

Some months later, in the spring of 1992, Calvin began to cough. As a heavy smoker, he initially attributed the cough to bronchitis, which he'd had intermittently for years. He was reluctant to return to the VA clinic. When he began to experience fevers and drenching sweats, Calvin was sure that he had AIDS; this made him even less enthusiastic about seeking medical care. These symptoms eventually drove him to the emergency room, however, and there he was promptly diagnosed not with AIDS but with pulmonary tuberculosis.

Calvin initially responded to a three-drug regimen, which he took for several weeks. He felt that one drug—it's not clear which one, though it was not isoniazid—made him itch, and so he stopped taking it. Cultures later revealed that his infecting strain was resistant to isoniazid. Thus, although public health officials believed that Calvin was taking two effective agents, he was actually taking only one. It is difficult to know, in retrospect, how much of the incorrect treatment Calvin received was physician-directed. It is clear that he reported his distressing itch to his private physician and was instructed to "take pyridoxine with isoniazid"—even though it had been demonstrated by then that his strain of TB was resistant to isoniazid. Calvin also received conflicting information regarding the interaction of methadone with his antituberculous drugs: the public health nurse, who seemed more concerned and better informed than his doctor, worried about such an interaction; his internist dismissed this possibility.

About six months into therapy, Calvin noted that his cough was worsening. A chest radiograph suggested relapse, although sputum studies, urged by a tuberculosis outreach worker, did not reveal the tubercle bacillus in his lungs. His internist then added another drug to Calvin's regimen. Although his laboratory results were reviewed, his documented resistance to isoniazid must have been missed again, because the drug was continued.

Calvin felt better, but his improvement was short-lived. By December 1992, reported the tuberculosis outreach worker, Calvin "felt as sick as he had ever been." He continued to take his medications but did not return to either the public health clinic or the VA clinic. In January, quite possibly with active pulmonary disease, Calvin "took off," by bus or by train, for New York City.

Calvin's internist, an affable but busy man, subsequently attributed his patient's poor response to "his HIV infection." When reminded that, in fact, multiple serologies had revealed Calvin to be HIV-negative, the physician recalled that his patient's infecting strain of M. tuberculosis was "mildly resistant." He further ventured that Calvin, "notoriously noncompliant," was just "not with the program." In any case, Calvin's doctor never heard from him again. When New York public health authorities created a central information bank about tuberculosis patients, Calvin Loach's name was not among those listed.

MAKING SENSE OF MISERY:
FROM ETHNOGRAPHY TO POLITICAL ECONOMY

Jean, Corina, and Calvin all had unfavorable outcomes. At what point in the trajectories of their lives were their fates sealed? Were their experiences typical of what it's like to have tuberculosis at the end of the twentieth century?

Dr. García, who met Corina near the end of her life, remarked that her experience revealed to him "the significance of external factors and their effects on the lives of poor people. These factors determined whether Corina lived or died." Critical perspectives on tuberculosis must link ethnography to political economy and ask how large-scale social forces become manifest in the morbidity of unequally positioned individuals in increasingly interconnected populations. Poverty, social inequality, economic policy, war, discrimination along lines of race and gender and class, medical incompetence—which forces were significant in structuring the risks faced by Jean, Corina, and Calvin, as well as their poor outcomes?

Take the cases one by one. Much could be said about Jean's experience in rural Haiti. Looking at ethnographic literature reveals that much has been said, but most anthropologists have focused on "voodoo" and sorcery accusations. After a decade of living in the same region, I was accustomed to ferreting out accusations of sorcery and had previously spent some years trying to make sense of them. And that, paradoxically, is the primary function of such accusations: to make sense of suffering. But the causes of that suffering are less often commented upon.

As Haiti produces few nonagricultural products, it is safe to say that Jean is a member of its only truly productive class: the rural peasantry. But membership in that class brought certain "birthrights." For example, Jean is, de facto, a member of the poorest class in the hemisphere. From the day he was born, he was guaranteed the "right" not to attend school, to have no access to electricity or safe drinking water, and to have little access to medical care. Jean was also guaranteed no role whatsoever in the running of the country he and those like him were supporting. He was born, as the Haitians say, with a *baboukèt,* a muzzle, on his mouth. In fact, Jean fared better than many Haitian peasants, since tuberculosis is the leading cause of death in his age group. But delays in therapy meant permanent damage to Jean's lungs, forever compromising his ability to feed his family—a precarious enough enterprise in contemporary Haiti, even for the hardy.

Corina similarly typifies the experience of Latin Americans living with multi-drug-resistant tuberculosis. Although she may have been originally infected with a drug-resistant strain of *M. tuberculosis,* it is equally probable that her disease became resistant during the course of intermittent and poorly conceived therapy. Her son, Jaime, however, was likely to have been infected with a drug-resistant strain from the beginning. How common are such experiences in Peru? The country has been praised for its greatly improved tuberculosis control program, which has systematized the diagnosis and treatment of the disease, made first-line medications more widely available, and instituted directly observed therapy.[15] But Corina did not fit into the prevailing algorithm, which does not take account of increasing drug resistance on the part of the bacillus; subsidized retreatment schemes, while available, are inadequate for patients like her.

Indeed, while attention is focused on the detection and control of susceptible tuberculosis disease, cases such as Corina's will inevitably take on greater epidemiological significance. Corina was sick and infectious for at least six years, as Jaime's tragic death reveals. She worked during most of those years, taking crowded buses across Lima twice a day. At this writing, hundreds of cases of highly resistant tuberculosis have been documented in northern Lima; only a few of these patients are receiving appropriate therapy. All of them may be presumed to be infectious.

What of Calvin's experience in the United States, a country vastly more wealthy than Peru (although Peru itself boasts a per capita income ten times higher than that of rural Haiti)? Calvin was probably registered as one of the thousands of "excess cases"[16] reported to the U.S. Centers for Disease Control in 1991. As an African American and an injection drug user, he fits the bill: the brunt of the recent epidemic has been borne by U.S. citizens living in poverty, many of them people of color, as a review by David McBride makes clear.[17]

Nor was Calvin's clinical course atypical of the lot of the U.S. poor with tuberculosis. Although his fate is unknown, he clearly received inappropriate care and was "lost to follow-up." This is much less common in Massachusetts than in New York, where dismantling of the tuberculosis control program had made it difficult to ensure successful completion of therapy. In 1989, for example, fewer than 50 percent of New York tuberculosis patients who began treatment could be declared cured.[18] In one study conducted in Harlem Hospital, almost 90 percent of patients did not complete therapy for their disease.[19] An overview from the New York City Department of Health painted a grim picture: "By 1992, the situation in New York City looked bleak. The number of cases of tuberculosis had nearly tripled in 15 years. In central Harlem, the case rate of 222 per 100,000 people exceeded that of many Third World countries. Outbreaks of multidrug-resistant tuberculosis had been documented in more than half a dozen hospitals, with case fatality rates greater than 80 percent, and health care workers were becoming ill and dying of this disease."[20]

Did Calvin also have multidrug-resistant tuberculosis? Although resistance to more than one drug was never documented, Calvin was put at high risk of developing resistance and of infecting others when his physician continued to give him a medication to which the strain was resistant and later added a single drug to an already failing regimen—a well-known recipe for generating drug resistance. In reviewing the histories of patients with drug-resistant tuberculosis who had been referred to a leading hospital in Colorado, Artin Mahmoudi and Michael Iseman discovered an average of 3.9 physician-directed errors per patient.[21]

Medical errors are readily discerned in the other cases as well, and this mismanagement is linked to the patients' poverty. Jean saw a nurse and two physicians and spent two weeks (along with all his family's savings) in a hospital before receiving effective antituberculous therapy elsewhere. Furthermore, the long duration of his active disease, including his time on an open ward, helps to explain why transmission continues apace in settings like Haiti. Corina's initial sputum sample was lost, and her providers mistook drug resistance for non-compliance. When she was at last correctly diagnosed, she was prescribed an inadequate regimen, which she took when she could afford it—a good way to engender resistance to even second-line drugs.

In all these cases, the patients were blamed for their failure to respond to therapy. In every case, the patients' agency—their ability to comply with costly and difficult regimens—was exaggerated. Certainly patients may be noncompliant. But how relevant is such a notion in the case of Jean Dubuisson? Biomedical practitioners told him to eat well. He "refused." They told him to drink clean water, and yet he persisted in drinking from the only stream near his village. He was instructed to sleep in an open room and away from others, and here again he was "noncompliant," as he built no such addition on to his two-room hut. Most important, he was instructed to go to a hospital. Jean was "grossly negligent" and dragged his feet for months.

Can we, in good conscience, blame our patients for a failure to make new technologies available? Is the locus of blame to be found in the hearts and minds of the sick? Can we claim that personal motivation or cultural beliefs will determine the efficacy of medical interventions, when we can readily document that economic and logistical barriers to access continue to play a major role in the delivery of health care?

A broad view of tuberculosis brings into relief the political, cultural, and economic barriers to effective tuberculosis treatment (and chemoprophylaxis). Such a view reveals "compliance" to be an analytically flimsy, even vacuous, concept in countries such as Haiti, where the poor are systematically put at risk of tuberculosis and then denied access to adequate care. Richard Horton writes of the "institutional inertia" impeding effective tuberculosis control, identifying not patients but rather national governments, science policymakers, the market, and national health infrastructures as the chief impediments.[22] Yet all too often, the notion of patient noncompliance is used as a means of explaining away program failure. Patient-dependent failure should be a "diagnosis of exclusion"—invoked only *after* poor program design and lack of access are excluded.

One can also exaggerate the effects of medical mismanagement, which does not by itself explain skewed rates of tuberculosis distribution. Physician-directed errors do not create poverty or social inequalities, and it is along these lines that rates of tuberculosis vary. Other questions raised by these cases are harder to answer but nonetheless worth considering. For example, did Peru's structural adjustment plan increase Corina's risk of a tuberculosis death? Corina was driven from the Peruvian Central Sierra by the collapse of the agrarian order and other complex economic transformations. But once in Carabayllo, she and her family were subjected to a new set of vagaries: they were beset no longer by drought and storm but rather by equally uncontrollable, and even less predictable, shifts in economic policy. Decisions made in far-off World Bank headquarters, for example, led to significant changes in the employment structure of Lima and to massive fluctuations in the price of key commodities. Corina soon found herself the maid to a woman who would eventually become only slightly less poor than she was—*fujishock* took its toll on schoolteachers, too. When Corina became ill with drug-resistant tuberculosis, she and her family were in essence helpless to combat it.

In Calvin's experience, what role did racism play? He wondered more than once about its contribution to his care. In the VA hospital, he felt punished because of his history of drug use, and he was irritated by the predominantly white staff's relative tolerance of alcoholism—the ranking substance-abuse problem of most of the other patients, who were largely white. But the more important effects of racial discrimination may have been those that led to his becoming infected with tuberculosis in the first place. As a black Vietnam veteran living in the inner city and injecting drugs, Calvin was certainly in a high-risk group. Furthermore, conscription for this war was to some extent distributed by the very same forces that had driven his parents out of the Jim Crow South, as the army ranks were disproportionately filled with young African Americans. And among the troops, those with the grimmest prospects back home seemed to be those most likely to use heroin or opium.

FROM ETHNOGRAPHY TO SOCIAL HISTORY

Reflecting on tuberculosis mortality in the world today brings a troubling question to the fore: does TB's association with poverty damn it to irrelevance in the eyes of the powerful, who, after all, control funding for everything from treatment to research? In August 1994, an official of the International Union against Tuberculosis and Lung Disease seemed to say as much. "You never hear about TB in North America," he commented to a journalist, "because of who gets it these days: immigrants, natives, poor people and AIDS patients for the most part."[23] It would appear that diseases predominantly afflicting the poor are unlikely to garner funding—unless they begin to "emerge" into the consciousness and space of the nonpoor.

A look back over past professional commentary on the differential distribution of tuberculosis reveals that this neglect was not always the case. A huge literature documents the pernicious synergy between poverty and tuberculosis. During its first 150 or so years, the United States, like Europe, counted tuberculosis as its number one killer. Lemuel Shattuck's *Report of the Sanitary Commission of Massachusetts, 1850,* named "consumption" as the leading cause of U.S. deaths, and this remained true even in the latter part of the century, when rates began to fall sharply.[24] But tuberculosis rates differed variably between the sexes, and reliably along lines of race and class.

Perhaps not surprisingly, given TB's importance, differences in mortality and susceptibility among various social groups occasioned much comment. In fact, according to historian Georgina Feldberg, "concern about differential susceptibility *dominated* American discussions of tuberculosis from the mid-nineteenth century onward." But interpretations of these differences, continues Feldberg, depended on the social perspectives of the commentators: "As each generation attempted to make sense of this preferential, or differential, susceptibility, the explanations they offered reflected and reinforced their uncertainties about a changing scientific and social order."[25]

For example, "Southerners commonly believed that blacks suffered from a distinctive form of consumption, known as 'negro consumption.'"[26] Susceptibility, in this view, was genetically determined. This construct not only demonstrated a vested interest in an agrarian, slave-holding social order but also reflected, to some extent, prevailing medical views. An 1844 editorial in the *Boston Medical and Surgical Journal* asserted that the "reality of hereditary influence on the production of phthisis [as tuberculosis was then known] is so universally admitted, that it would seem a sort of scientific heresy to doubt it."[27] Feldberg summarizes these views: "The hereditarian/environmental debate persisted as Northern commentators regularly attributed excessive mortality to the 'general insalubrity of the sections of the city inhabited by [blacks], the crowded conditions of their dwellings, insufficient nourishment, and the other influences of poverty,' while Southerners more typically cited the 'habitual improvidence' of the black races."[28]

Similar theories abounded in discussions of why such great numbers of Native Americans died of tuberculosis. Although solid evidence from Peru documents TB's pre-Columbian existence in the hemisphere, there is less evidence of tuberculosis among the native population in North America before the arrival of the Europeans, and there is little doubt that rates increased dramatically after contact. But TB's rise among the native peoples was so clearly linked to a rapid decline in their standard of living that hereditary arguments were widely seen as less compelling.[29]

The belief that tuberculosis was hereditary was dealt a near-lethal blow by Robert Koch's discovery of the tubercle bacillus in 1882. "One has been accustomed until now to regard tuberculosis as the outcome of social misery," Koch wrote, "and to hope by relief of distress to diminish the disease. But in the future struggle against this dreadful plague of the human race one will no longer have to contend with an indefinite something, but with an actual parasite."[30]

Paradoxically, perhaps, but fortuitously, the idea of tuberculosis as "the outcome of social misery" was not undermined by the discovery of its etiology. In the latter part of the century, persistent poverty and rising inequality were increasingly believed to contribute to differential mortality. One prominent physician "venture[d] to assert that the necessary privations of poverty on the one hand, and the absurd excesses of wealth on the other, tend more to the formation of tubercles in children than all other causes combined."[31] By 1900, observe Dubos and Dubos, "it had become obvious that tuberculosis was most prevalent and most destructive in the poorest elements of the population, and that healthy living could mitigate its harmful effects. Reformers could attack the disease from two directions, by improving the individual life of man and by correcting social evils."[32] Both of these approaches, never neatly demarcated, were advocated by public health officials, most of whom were physicians.

Many in the nascent antituberculosis movement, which in the earlier part of the twentieth century was linked to the establishment of sanatoriums, believed that education was the key to curing the disease. One side effect of this belief was a habit of infantilizing the sufferers. Reformers wrote of "careless consumptives" who needed above all to be trained. As one classic statement of this view would have it: "People are now infected by consumption through ignorance on the part of those who give and receive infection. Each man whose habits have been corrected, even by a short residence in the sanatorium will neither do nor willingly permit to be done by others acts which before would have seemed perfectly natural."[33]

But other medical reformers continued to argue that "tuberculosis is closely associated with all the social problems of housing, food, wages, rest, clothing, and insurance and can in no way be separated from them."[34] Feldberg, whose excellent work has restored to the historical score the voices of physicians whose understanding of tuberculosis was firmly biosocial, points out that "well into the twentieth century, American physicians held fast to an etiology that included microbes but also found room for malnutrition, unemployment, crowding, the living conditions in slums, and other social ills." As one example, she cites a 1921 publication by pathologist Allen Krause, director of the Johns Hopkins University tuberculosis laboratories: "The solution of the tuberculosis problem is partly dependent on the removal of other evils and inequalities which constitute, no doubt, a more fundamental problem than does tuberculosis itself."[35]

Hybrids of these positions also emerged. Barbara Rosenkrantz writes of Ellen N. LaMotte's *The Tuberculosis Nurse (A Handbook for Practical Workers in the Tuberculosis Campaign)*, published in 1915:

> LaMotte assembled facts showing that tuberculosis was principally a disease of the poor, afflicting both those who were "financially handicapped and so unable to control their environment," and "those who are mentally and morally poor, and lack intelligence, will power, and self control." Her conclusion that "People of this sort . . . constitute almost the entire problem—otherwise the situation would be so simple that the word problem would not apply" conflicted uncomfortably with her intention of encouraging nurses to go forth and help the poor to defend themselves against tuberculosis.[36]

The increased susceptibility of the African American population continued to engender racial speculations. John Bessner Huber's popular 1906 text derided discriminatory "phthisophobia" but argued that "the negro's small lung capacity, as compared with that of the white, and his deficient brain capacity render him less resistant to the disease when once acquired." Huber concluded by warning that "unless the hygienic and moral surroundings of the race are improved there is danger of its extinction."[37] In a 1926 paper called "Vital Capacity of the Negro Race," two Alabama physicians published their findings (based on research conducted on prisoners and children) that "low vital capacity is a racial characteristic, and that vital capacity standards applied to white people cannot be directly applied to the negro race."[38]

When anatomic considerations could not be invoked, commentators speculated about the "bizarre beliefs" of the afflicted. In seeking to explain the persistence of tuberculosis among the urban poor, Edward Livingston Trudeau wrote of "the blind love of 'the average proletarian . . . for the chorus of city life.'"[39] High rates of tuberculosis among immigrants were commonly blamed on their "lifestyles" and lack of cleanliness.[40] It was widely argued that "superstition" and "conjuring" were to some extent responsible for poor health outcomes among African Americans, views that were echoed even among black professionals. For example, a survey entitled "Superstition and Health," conducted in 1926 by the National Urban League, cites a young black physician practicing in New York: "Ignorance, cherished superstitions and false knowledge often govern Negroes in illnesses and hamper recoveries. Young Negroes show patriarchal obeisance to the aged—the aged are, in a large measure, fatalists. They are willing to leave all to whatever their fate may be, the fatalism that has cursed the Orient for centuries. This fatalism exasperates the physician, for it ties his hands and tends to nullify his efforts."[41]

Strong associations between tuberculosis and race and class did not weaken as the century progressed, but calling attention to such associations did not typically lead to compassionate responses. Changing conceptions of tuberculosis transmission—due in part to the frenetic campaign against spitting in public places—led many to regard with hostility and fear those who were popularly held to have high rates of tuberculosis, such as black people and foreigners.[42] In a 1923 address to a state medical society, one physician observed that "tuberculosis continues to be a serious problem with [Negroes], and because of their association with whites . . . as cooks, nurses, maids, [and] laundresses," black people represented a "menace to whites."[43] Such interpretations were common well into the 1960s. "In the South," McBride points out, "segregationists attempted to turn blacks' excessive tuberculosis mortality rates into justification for keeping white and black youths from attending integrated schools."[44]

Racial differentials, tightly tied to class divisions, became further entrenched

Table 10.1 Leading Causes of Death by Age and Race, United States, 1940
(per 100,000 population)

Nonwhites, Ages 25–34		Whites, Ages 25–34	
Cause of Death	Rate	Cause of Death	Rate
1. Tuberculosis	196.3	Tuberculosis	40.0
2. Major cardiovascular-renal diseases	120.6	Major cardiovascular-renal diseases	39.3
3. Homicide	75.2	Other accidents (nonvehicular)	25.3
4. Influenza and pneumonia	57.6	Motor vehicle accidents	24.4
5. Other accidents (nonvehicular)	44.1	Malignant neoplasms	16.3

SOURCE: Grove and Hetzel, *Vital Statistics Rates in the United States, 1940–1960.*

as effective therapies were developed (see table 10.1). Although tuberculosis continued to decline among all U.S. citizens, rates among blacks remained relatively high, particularly among young black adults, for whom tuberculosis remained the leading cause of death even during the Second World War. A 1946 study by Jacob Yerushalmy found that, although tuberculosis mortality in relation to overall mortality in whites declined substantially in the period 1900–1940, no such encouraging progress was reported for nonwhites.[45] In fact, not only was mortality from tuberculosis among nonwhites not declining as rapidly as overall mortality, but in 1938 a three-decade downward trend was reversed, and by 1943 the tuberculosis death ratios surpassed those from 1930. Deaths were highly concentrated in the large industrial cities to which blacks had been drawn throughout the first decades of the century: "From 1938 to 1939 black TB mortality rose in New York City from 949 deaths to 1,036. In numerous other major cities, blacks were more than one-half of those dead from TB in 1939. That year blacks suffered 50 percent of the TB deaths in Baltimore; 58 percent in New Orleans; 72 in Washington, D.C.; 78 in Birmingham; 78 in Atlanta; and 79 in Memphis. Nationally, blacks suffered 5,925 deaths or 32 percent of the TB deaths reported in the nation's 46 largest cities."[46]

In 1946, one prominent Harlem physician took city, state, and federal authorities to task for ignoring the tuberculosis problem among African Americans, which during the war years had claimed thousands of lives: "Here is a contagious disease killing people in the low income brackets at an outrageous rate, yet health authorities don't get excited. Several days ago, a plane flew experts from Boston to Texas because of 5 children ill with infantile paralysis—not a death but just becoming ill. They wanted to protect the other children. We in Harlem want protection too, not from just a paralyzed limb but from death itself."[47]

But afflicted communities had never been less likely to be construed as such. With the development of effective therapy, which began in 1943, energies turned increasingly toward treatment of the *individual* case. "At the national meetings of public health officials and TB experts," recounts McBride, "this optimistic and narrow concept of public health, which focused on the patient and not groups at risk or conditions and social behaviors that created this risk, prevailed."[48] By the late 1950s, tuberculosis was regarded as a disease well on its way to being eradicated, and little interest remained in attacking the disease at its roots.

If individuals, and not the conditions endured by entire communities or classes, are increasingly seen as the sole repositories of risk, has there at least been a corresponding decrease in the differential risk so well described for the pre-antibiotic era? On the contrary, inequalities of risk seem to be increasing. For example, tuberculosis rates have dropped substantially among Native Americans, but less rapidly than among other groups. J. M. Michael and M. A. Michael, in reviewing the health status of contemporary Native Americans, report, as do others, increased morbidity and decreased life expectancy.[49] And although tuberculosis plays a small role in these grim figures, it takes on a new significance if disparities of risk become the focus. In looking at age-adjusted mortality rates, 1987 tuberculosis deaths among Native Americans exceeded those among "all races" by 400 percent. Thus tuberculosis still tops the list of disorders *disproportionately* killing Native Americans.

The story is similar for other minorities in the United States, where "the decrease [in tuberculosis] has been considerably greater among whites than nonwhites. As a result, the ratio of the annual risk of tuberculosis among nonwhites to the risk among whites has risen from 2.9 in 1953 to 5.3 in 1987."[50] Increasing inequalities of risk belie the claim of a "national problem" of excess cases; they reveal, rather, a scenario in which longstanding inequalities of risk are now being further accentuated.

Similarly desocialized readings of tuberculosis continue to hold sway today. The reasons for treatment failures and for TB's persistence are often sought in the psychological traits of individual "defaulters" or in the cultural attributes of groups held to be "at risk." And yet in no instance has it been clearly demonstrated that rates of tuberculosis vary by beliefs or by psychological makeup. In no instance have educational interventions for those deemed "at risk" been shown to inflect trends in tuberculosis incidence. The occurrence of tuberculosis has varied primarily with economic development; tuberculosis case-fatality rates have varied with ready access to effective therapy. Pierre Chaulet puts it well: as an "index of poverty, [tuberculosis] underlines inequalities of income and in the distribution of wealth. . . . In a world both off-track and 'deregulated,' TB persists and spreads, striking always the poor."[51]

MODEST INTERVENTIONS AND PRAGMATIC SOLIDARITY

As a new century opens, we are challenged not only to explain the uneven distribution of tuberculosis but also to explain poor therapeutic outcomes in a time when effective treatments have existed for decades. Between 1943, when Selman Waksman and coworkers discovered streptomycin, and the late 1970s, over a dozen drugs with demonstrable effectiveness against tuberculosis were developed. New diagnostic methods, including immune-fluorescence staining and new culture methods, are equally impressive. In fact, in 1997 the U.S. Food and Drug Administration approved a test that can identify and amplify myco-bacterial gene sequences in a matter of minutes. Now in the pipeline are tools that might identify resistant strains in less than twenty-four hours. We have the scientific knowledge—but the hard truth is that the "we" in question does not include the vast majority of the two million people who died from tuberculosis in 1999. We must acknowledge that our guilt surpasses that of earlier generations, who lacked our resources: Michael Iseman, one of the world's leading authorities on tuberculosis, is right to use the word "shameful" in describing our failure to touch tuberculosis prevalence in much of the world.[52]

Looking to the future, it is difficult to muster optimism. The arrival of strains of *M. tuberculosis* resistant to all first-line and many second-line drugs is surely a harbinger of pan-resistant strains to come. And HIV looms: ever-increasing numbers of co-infected individuals, most of them poor, promise millions of cases of reactivation tuberculosis. These "excess cases" will in turn infect tens of millions. The failure to curb tuberculosis prior to these truly novel problems slammed shut a window of opportunity.

Although tuberculosis is inextricably tied to poverty and inequality, experi-ence shows that modest interventions have effected dramatic changes in out-come. In Haiti, we showed that listening to people with tuberculosis meant listening to stories not only of sorcery but of hunger and bad harvests and leaky roofs and dirt floors. We discovered that attending to these problems during the course of treatment could double cure rates.[53] We knew that merely listening to such stories could be termed solidarity, but we came to believe that *pragmatic solidarity* is what the afflicted were demanding.

Pragmatic solidarity means increased funding for tuberculosis control and treatment. It means making therapy available in a systematic and committed way. For example, we now know that short-course, multidrug regimens can lead to excellent outcomes in even the most miserable settings. Even in settings of relative affluence, the impact of modest interventions can be substantial. In San Francisco, one project addressed poor attendance at tuberculosis clinics by moving the clinics to the times and places desired by the patients and by replac-ing staff who placed the blame for poor outcomes on the patients.[54] In New York, where the chances of compliance among injection drug users with tuberculosis were wearily dismissed as hopeless, one clinic more than trebled rates of completion. Much of the success was due to directly observed therapy, but a comprehensive, convenient, and user-friendly approach clearly had an impact, too.[55] Especially critical—and important to underline when confronted with claims that treating susceptible disease will somehow make MDRTB go away—were efforts in New York to speed the rate at which resistant strains were identified and treated with antibiotics to which they had demonstrated susceptibility.[56]

Pragmatic solidarity means preventing the emergence of drug resistance whenever possible, but it also means treating people like Corina Valdivia. Currently, a massive pandemic of MDRTB in Russia and other countries of the former Soviet Union is becoming even more massive—with minimal public comment and even less public action.[57] Problems of this dimension call for public subsidies of costly second-line drugs as well as for the development of new drugs.[58]

In identifying the microbiological cause of consumption, Koch had hoped to end the era in which tuberculosis could be addressed only "by relief of distress." But tuberculosis remains, at this writing, "the outcome of social misery." If it is true, as Feldberg argues, that "scientific professionalism ... fundamentally eroded the therapeutic impulse to social reform,"[59] surely it would be an error to divorce efforts to confront tuberculosis from broader efforts to confront social misery. We still have something to learn from the analysis of those who did not have our tools at their disposal. In 1923, pathologist Allen Krause made the following observation: "More or less poverty in a community will mean more or less tuberculosis, so will more or less crowding and improper housing, more or less unhygienic occupations and industry."[60] This statement remains as true today as it was seventy-five years ago.

At the same time, it is necessary to avoid "public health nihilism."[61] Even if we lack the formulas necessary to "cure" poverty and social inequalities, we do have at our disposal the cure for almost all cases of tuberculosis. Those who remain committed to addressing tuberculosis by championing increased access to effective drugs must resist restricting their field of analysis of the tuberculosis problem. We are told to choose, in Haiti and in much of Africa, between treating tuberculosis and treating malnutrition. We are told to choose, in Peru, between treating those with susceptible and resistant strains. We are told to choose, in Harlem, between more funding for tuberculosis and more funding for affordable housing. Calls for more ambitious interventions are trumped by a peculiarly bounded utilitarianism: such interventions, we are told, are not "cost-effective." The inadequacies, the multiple ironies, of such analyses are not lost on the poor. In Peru, for example, it is impossible to ignore that a much-praised tuberculosis program is funded in part by the World Bank, one of the institutions that mandated the structural adjustment program that led to increased suffering—and perhaps increased tuberculosis risk—for the Peruvian poor.

It is possible, of course, to exaggerate the significance of any one policy change. To cite Dr. García again: "If there had not been *fujishock,* it would have been something else. In Peru, there's always something beating down the poor." Although Dubos and Dubos mistakenly identify tuberculosis with a time—the nineteenth century—rather than with the inhuman conditions faced by billions on this planet, on another score they are right: "It is only through gross errors in social organization, and mismanagement of individual life, that tuberculosis could reach the catastrophic levels that prevailed in Europe and North America during the nineteenth century, and that still prevail in Asia and much of Latin America today."[62]

As decision-making power—about social organization *and* about individual life—comes to be increasingly concentrated in the hands of a very few, we must ask: Who gets to determine the boundaries of analysis? Who is to determine what is "cost-effective" and what is not? As a global economy is "restructured," is there no room for alternative strategies of development—alternative visions of providing health care to the poor? Increasingly, it is the pharmaceutical and insurance and health care industries, and also international agencies (including, most prominently, financial institutions), that determine who will have access to effective medical care. But the power of technological advancement stems not merely from the wonders of science. It stems, too, from the power of moral persuasion. We can call for certain measures not because they are "cost-effective"—the current and unchallenged mantra—but because they are the best we can do for the sick.

A focus on complex epidemics—including not only tuberculosis but also HIV—offers a stinging rebuke to the "cost-effectiveness" argument advanced in public policy debates. At least four sets of reasons—one clinical, one epidemiological, one analytic, and one moral—lead us to conclude that ignoring these plagues is an unacceptable strategy. The clinical reasons are straightforward—we have effective therapies to cure even drug-resistant strains of tuberculosis, and the anti-HIV armamentarium is expanding rapidly. People like Jean, Corina, and Calvin exist, and they matter. Cost-effectiveness arguments against treating such maladies are also epidemiologically flawed: in this era of increasing global travel, "local" epidemics rarely remain local for very long.

The oft-heard insistence that it is too expensive to treat MDRTB in poor countries is additionally a failure of social analysis in at least two ways. First, the hypothesis that we lack sufficient means to cure all tuberculosis cases, everywhere, is unsupported by data. In fact, the degree of accumulated world wealth is altogether unprecedented. Second, such a head-in-the-sand approach represents a failure of ethnographic analysis. As we have seen, and as social scientists who study the therapeutic itineraries of tuberculosis patients know, a slow death from the disease is not quietly accepted by the young adults who are its chief victims. Thanks to increased access to information, patients and their loved ones know that MDRTB can be treated with second-line drugs, just as AIDS patients in many poor countries now know about the existence of effective antiviral therapies. In middle-income countries such as Peru, which are in reality inegalitarian settings where wealth and poverty are in close juxtaposition, second-line antituberculous drugs are in fact already available—for sale at exorbitant prices.

Finally, arguments against treating disease in settings of poverty are morally unsound. Through analytic chicanery—the claim that the world is composed of discretely bounded nation-states, some rich, some poor—we are asked to swallow what is, ultimately, a story of growing inequality and our willingness to countenance it. But careful systemic analysis of pandemic disease leads us to see *links, not disjunctures.* When these failures of analysis are pointed out, the real reason that MDRTB and HIV are treatable in the United States and "untreatable" in Peru or Haiti comes into view. Opposition to the aggressive treatment of such afflictions in developing countries may be justified as "sensible" or "pragmatic," but, as a policy, it is tantamount to the differential valuation of human life, since those advocating it, regardless of their nationality, would never accept such a death sentence for themselves. It is because the afflicted tend to be poor, and also from marginalized and stigmatized groups more generally—and thus less valuable—that such policies appear reasonable.

Addressing these issues may get at the heart of the meaning of tuberculosis as we begin the twenty-first century. If tuberculosis could once be termed "the first penalty that capitalistic society had to pay for the ruthless exploitation of labor,"[63] what does it mean now? Is it perpetually the lot of the poor to pay this penance?

NOTES

1. Stop TB Initiative, *Tuberculosis and Sustainable Development.*
2. "TB Returns with a Vengeance," *Washington Post.*
3. Ott, *Fevered Lives*, p. 157.
4. Bloom and Murray, "Tuberculosis."
5. Ryan, *The Forgotten Plague*, p. 8.
6. Rosenkrantz, "Preface," in Dubos and Dubos, *The White Plague*, pp. xiv–xv, n. 1.
7. Ibid., p. xxi.
8. Feldberg, *Disease and Class*, p. 1.
9. Dubos and Dubos, *The White Plague*, p. 22.
10. See Farmer, Robin, et al., "Tuberculosis, Poverty, and 'Compliance'"; also Spence et al., "Tuberculosis and Poverty."
11. This work has been explored in a number of books and articles: Farmer, *AIDS and Accusation;* Farmer, *Infections and Inequalities;* Farmer, Bayona, Becerra, Furin, et al., "The Dilemma of MDR-TB in the Global Era"; Farmer, Furin, and Shin, "Managing Multidrug-Resistant Tubercu-

losis." See also Becerra et al., "Using Treatment Failure under Effective Directly Observed Short-Course Chemotherapy Programs to Identify Patients with Multidrug-Resistant Tuberculosis."

12. On the antituberculosis efforts of Proje Veye Sante, see Farmer, *Infections and Inequalities*, pp. 211–27 (also included in this volume as chapter 8).

13. For an in-depth exploration of the effects of *fujishock* on the health of Peru's urban poor, see Kim, Shakow, Bayona, et al., "Sickness amidst Recovery."

14. Current standards would favor initiation of empiric treatment with four drugs to avoid the development of resistant strains of *M. tuberculosis*.

15. World Health Organization Global Tuberculosis Programme, *Groups at Risk*.

16. "Excess cases" was the term used by the U.S. public health officials who calculated the difference between the number of cases predicted (if downward trends had persisted) and those actually reported; see, for example, Grove and Hetzel, *Vital Statistics Rates in the United States, 1940–1960*.

17. McBride, *From TB to AIDS*.

18. Frieden et al., "Tuberculosis in New York City—Turning the Tide."

19. Brudney and Dobkin, "Resurgent Tuberculosis in New York City."

20. Frieden et al., "Tuberculosis in New York City—Turning the Tide," p. 229.

21. Mahmoudi and Iseman, "Pitfalls in the Care of Patients with Tuberculosis."

22. Horton, "Towards the Elimination of Tuberculosis."

23. Cited in Feldberg, *Disease and Class*, p. 214.

24. "Whether as a result of changing definitions of disease, new methods of record-keeping, or actual changes in mortality, the number of recorded deaths dropped by almost one-third between 1850 and 1890" (ibid., p. 13).

25. Ibid., pp. 11–12; emphasis added.

26. Ibid., p. 23. Georgina Feldberg further notes that many southern antebellum physicians "believed that the physician could make no greater error than to treat 'negroes' as though they were 'white men in black skins'" (pp. 24–25). For a more thorough review of this subject, see McBride, *From TB to AIDS*.

27. Editorial cited in Feldberg, *Disease and Class*, p. 14.

28. Ibid., p. 26. Not all southern physicians shared the locally dominant explanatory models, however. Feldberg notes that in 1873 one doctor from Richmond, Virginia, trenchantly observed that "the most marked difference between the diseases of the two races is in the far greater prevalence and mortality of tubercular diseases amongst the blacks" (p. 26).

29. For a review, see Rieder, "Tuberculosis among American Indians of the Contiguous United States."

30. Koch cited in Feldberg, *Disease and Class*, p. 439.

31. Henry Wiley cited in ibid., p. 30.

32. Dubos and Dubos, *The White Plague*, p. 210.

33. Cited in Feldberg, *Disease and Class*, p. 101.

34. Cited in ibid., p. 105.

35. Ibid., p. 4.

36. Rosenkrantz, "Preface," p. xxii.

37. Huber cited in ibid., pp. xxv–xxvi.

38. Smillie and Augustine, "Vital Capacity of the Negro Race," p. 2058.

39. Trudeau cited in Feldberg, *Disease and Class*, p. 48.

40. Kraut, *Silent Travelers*.

41. Cited in McBride, *From TB to AIDS*, p. 46.

42. On the relationship between xenophobia and tuberculosis, see Kraut, *Silent Travelers*.

43. Cited in McBride, *From TB to AIDS*, p. 61.

44. Ibid., p. 51.

45. Yerushalmy, "The Increase in Tuberculosis Proportionate Mortality among Non-White Young Adults."

46. McBride, *From TB to AIDS*, p. 126.

47. Cited in ibid., p. 129. Preferential attention to polio continued, as Feldberg notes: "In 1949, as polio cases rose to the 'epidemic' rate of 30/100,000, the tuberculous case rate exceeded 90/100,000; in 1951 alone, there were 119,000 new cases of tuberculosis. Tuberculous mortality also exceeded that for polio almost threefold" (*Disease and Class*, p. 2).

48. McBride, *From TB to AIDS*, p. 151.

49. Michael and Michael, "Health Status of the Australian Aboriginal People and the Native Americans—A Summary Comparison."

50. Snider, Salinas, and Kelly, "Tuberculosis," p. 647.

51. Chaulet, "Les nouveaux tuberculeux," p. 7. The impact of neoliberal economic policies on the health of the poor has been described in Kim, Millen, et al., *Dying for Growth*, which includes case studies from Haiti, Peru, Mexico, Senegal, Cuba, Russia, and El Salvador. In each setting, a decline in social spending has been associated with dramatic erosion in the health status of people living in poverty.

52. Iseman, "Tailoring a Time-Bomb."

53. Farmer, Robin, et al., "Tuberculosis, Poverty, and 'Compliance.'"

54. Curry, "Neighborhood Clinics for More Effective Outpatient Treatment of Tuberculosis."

55. Frieden et al., "Tuberculosis in New York City—Turning the Tide."

56. Telzak et al., "Multidrug-Resistant Tuberculosis in Patients without HIV Infection."

57. For a comprehensive review of the problem of tuberculosis and MDRTB in Russia, see Farmer, Kononets, et al., "Recrudescent Tuberculosis in the Russian Federation"; Farmer, "Cruel and Unusual" (included in this volume as chapter 9); Farmer, "Managerial Successes, Clinical Failures"; and Farmer, "TB Superbugs."

58. "No new antituberculous compounds have been developed by the pharmaceutical industry since the 1970s" (Cole and Telenti, "Drug Resistance in Mycobacterium Tuberculosis," p. 701S). However, researchers have serendipitously found certain antibiotics that act against *M. tuberculosis*. Lee Reichman sounds a pessimistic note: "Most of the drug companies that publicly announced a quest for TB drugs at the time of the recent resurgence have been noticeably quiet. Few have even shown interest in developing such drugs" ("Tuberculosis Elimination—What's to Stop Us?" p. 7).

59. Feldberg, *Disease and Class*, p. 38.

60. Krause cited in ibid., p. 107.

61. The term "public health nihilism" was coined by Ron Bayer of Columbia University; this concept in regard to tuberculosis is discussed in Farmer and Nardell, "Nihilism and Pragmatism in Tuberculosis Control."

62. Dubos and Dubos, *The White Plague*, p. 225.

63. Ibid., p. 207.

Social Medicine and the Challenge of Biosocial Research

(2000)

The sociology of knowledge must concern itself with whatever passes
for "knowledge" in a society, regardless of the ultimate validity or
invalidity (by whatever criteria) of such "knowledge." And in so far
as all human "knowledge" is developed, transmitted and maintained
in social situations, the sociology of knowledge must seek to understand
the processes by which this is done in such a way that a taken-for-granted
"reality" congeals for the man in the street. In other words, we contend
that the sociology of knowledge is concerned with the analysis of the social
construction of reality.

PETER BERGER AND THOMAS LUCKMANN,
THE SOCIAL CONSTRUCTION OF REALITY

This essay examines social medicine as a necessarily interdisciplinary enterprise. It draws on examples from clinical practice in the area of infectious diseases and also from my work as an anthropologist seeking to understand the ways in which culture determines how health problems are construed as solvable or intractable. But this is neither a clinical review nor an ethnographic study; instead, I want to address a couple of vexing medical problems from a sociology-of-science point of view.[1] That is, I will look at the rise of antibiotic-resistant microbes—indisputably a biological process with social roots—and then examine critically a number of claims that have been staked in the medical and public health literature.

Any social scientist examining the production and dissemination of knowledge about tuberculosis—a classic "social disease," with deep roots in Europe—would agree that we need the tools wielded by sociologists of science if we are to understand complex biosocial phenomena such as the emergence of drug resistance. These tools encourage us to take a step back and ask: What are the epistemological frameworks driving clinical and public health practice as well as basic science research? What frameworks drive health policy? What are the historical underpinnings of these frameworks and how are they institutional-ized? We need the contextualizing tools of sociology and anthropology if we are to understand what is happening right now with tuberculosis. Although the disease has plagued humanity for centuries, it is now changing rapidly on an epidemiological and a molecular level.

Social medicine, informed by a properly biosocial perspective, is well placed to understand complex and rapidly changing epidemics. The Department of Social Medicine at Harvard Medical School has long been interdisciplinary and trans-disciplinary. In this department are surgeons, historians, philosophers, inter-nists, and anthropologists; qualitative and quantitative methods are welcome. Many of the faculty are trained in medicine as well as in social science. In this setting, anthropologists and other social scientists are encouraged to study the development of scientific knowledge and policy as socially constructed entities.[2] In fact, anthropology in itself is considered a "basic science" at Harvard Medical School, a fact that amuses some on the other side of the Charles River, where the Faculty of Arts and Sciences is found.

Anthropologists are famous for adopting their tribes. Many have noted, and not in a flattering manner, the "my-tribe syndrome" in anthropology: every social event or process is compared to its analogue within the culture of the "tribe" with whom the anthropologist has done long-term fieldwork. I have spent over fifteen years working in rural Haiti as an anthropologist and as a physician, so my "tribe" was for years the Haitian peasantry. But in more recent years I began to study another tribe, one based in the world's capitals—Geneva, London, New York, Washington. It is hard to discern the social outlines of this tribe, at least initially. But those who set international "health policy" have a great deal in common. Although this tribe speaks many different languages, it has shared, elaborate representations of what it is trying to do; and so its members come to learn a common language and complex culture, which may best be described as transnational. In other words, I try, never taking off my doctor hat, to look at international health policy as an anthropologist might. Needless to say, this is not always welcome. This is not unlike what a historian of science does or tries to do, with the difference being that I am something of an ethnographer of science, or the lack of science, in the international health arena. Obviously I am engaged in a specific way, since, when considering the health problems of the poor, I am also a clinician who treats the disease in question.

I should therefore like to examine a specific problem, tuberculosis, in three ways. First, I will follow others in examining "problem choice." Why did this problem present itself to me personally and to our group, which is very much an interdisciplinary group? Why do so many who are ill with tuberculosis die of this perfectly treatable disease? I will then address the emergence of drug-resistant tuberculosis as a problem that is itself resistant to disciplinary perspectives: no single discipline can hope to unravel the dynamics of what is fundamentally a socially induced molecular change. Finally, I want to look at some solutions in a very pragmatic and perhaps almost prosaic sense. In so doing, I hope to show that the production, content, and dispersal of "scientific knowledge" about this disease is shaped by ideology and by a series of hegemonic (and thus often unexamined) ideologies tied tightly to neoliberal economics.

PROBLEM CHOICE IN RESEARCH

Tuberculosis is as compelling a research topic now as it was over one hundred years ago, when it was one of the classic diseases studied by social medicine. Indeed, tuberculosis and "venereal" diseases were long called "social diseases." Well over a century after the work of Rudolf Virchow—considered by many to be the father of social medicine—tuberculosis and a sexually transmitted pathogen, HIV, are the leading infectious causes of adult deaths in the world today.[3] Then, as now, poverty and social inequalities sculpted the contours of a global pandemic. But there is something new under the sun: the development of antibiotics that, if used promptly and correctly, cure almost every case of tuberculosis. There are also treatments that can transform AIDS from an inevitably lethal condition to a chronic but treatable disease. The late-twentieth-century development of antibiotics also underscores the need, in contemporary twenty-first-century epidemics, for a properly biosocial analysis.

In rural Haiti, where I have worked since 1983, tuberculosis is still probably the single leading infectious cause of adult deaths, one hundred and ten years after Robert Koch's famous discovery of the tubercle bacillus. It is therefore very interesting, from the perspective of a sociologist of science, to hear tuberculosis termed an "emerging" infectious disease or a "reemerging" disease. Tuberculosis never went away. Some people escaped it, that is all. The mortality rates globally have not shifted that significantly, although of course there have been massive local shifts. Only from a highly particularistic point of view—that of the wealthy nations—could one speak of tuberculosis as a disease that disappeared and then came back.

Haiti is known to some of you as the poorest country in the Americas. With a gross national product of about four hundred dollars per person per year, all of Haiti is poor. The area where I work is poor even by Haitian standards, a rocky hilltop farmed by people who were displaced by a hydroelectric dam built in 1956. One of the diseases that has most plagued this displaced community is tuberculosis in all its forms. Most patients have pulmonary tuberculosis, a disease that can be diagnosed and treated expeditiously and cheaply. Pulmonary TB is the contagious form of the disease. Extrapulmonary tuberculosis, however, is harder to diagnose and sometimes harder to treat. But it is often just as lethal.

Let us look at an instructive case, that of a young woman who came to the Clinique Bon Sauveur in central Haiti. She had been sick for many months with weight loss, shortness of breath, and, later, fever. Her hair fell out, and she eventually became so fatigued she could hardly stand. She had almost given up her quest for medical care. International health policy offers a set of very clear guidelines as to how to diagnose a case of tuberculosis. Most important, according to international guidelines, the patient must have what is called in the jargon a "positive smear." (Some programs require *three* positive smears.) Specifically, microscopic examination of the patient's sputum, dyed with special stains, must show evidence of the microbe. One reason I bring up this specific test is that it is only marginally different from the one developed by Koch over a century ago.[4] Perhaps, one may imagine, this is because the technology did not need to be improved. But this is not at all the case. In fact, the Ziehl-Neelsen smear is an insensitive and nonspecific test; it is not easy to perform and could use a great deal of improvement. Nor have new antituberculous agents been developed in over thirty years.[5]

The absence of new tests, new diagnostics, and new therapies for tuberculosis is not related to the overall need for better tests, nor could it be related to the global burden of disease. Here we see how "problem choice" in research may be related to the perceived purchasing power of the afflicted.[6] Although research and development institutions are quite willing to provide funding for projects such as the hydroelectric dam mentioned earlier, funding for research into the diagnosis and treatment of tuberculosis is pitifully limited.[7] These again are the sorts of ironies that make the modern tuberculosis epidemic interesting from a sociological perspective as well as from local, medical, or even ethnographic perspectives.

Other questions arise: How good are the guidelines, how good are the diagnostics, and how good are the therapeutics for patients like this young woman in Haiti? How well is she served by existing policy? The answer is, not very well at all. This patient, it turned out, had extrapulmonary tuberculosis, undetectable by smear microscopy of the sputum. According to certain international guidelines, she therefore did not have tuberculosis. I am overstating this, of course, but tuberculosis programs in poor countries are instructed to restrict diagnostic testing to smear microscopy of the sputum on the grounds that it will detect the majority of infectious cases. Yet the young woman responded immediately and spectacularly to empiric tuberculosis therapy. Existing guidelines and algorithms designed to diagnose and treat tuberculosis did not serve her well. The justification for restricting "problem choice" to the identification of smear-positive pulmonary tuberculosis is that this approach is inexpensive and that the pulmonary patients are the ones who infect others. But, as we shall see in examining a form of pulmonary (infectious) tuberculosis that is difficult and expensive to treat, the public health mandate is not the mandate most honored in international public health. Rather, the most important mandate is to decrease expenditures in settings in which "cost recovery" cannot occur.

POLICY, EVIDENCE, AND
MULTIDRUG-RESISTANT TUBERCULOSIS

The case I present next is also a transnational case. A dam and certain health policies are transnational phenomena in that they are developed in one place (Washington, say, or Geneva) and implemented in another, very different setting (for example, rural Haiti). But what happens when the double standards are challenged because a single person, afflicted with hard-to-treat tuberculosis, moves from a place in which low-cost cure is the rule to one in which the sky is the limit, in terms of medical costs? In 1994, a relief worker returned to the United States from Peru with what appeared to be active tuberculosis. This American did, in fact, have disseminated tuberculosis. He was admitted to a Harvard teaching hospital, where he was treated with four powerful antituberculous agents: rifampin, isoniazid, ethambutol, and pyrazinamide. These are termed "first-line" antituberculous drugs. They are powerful, they are off-patent, and they are very inexpensive. Like the diagnostic stains just mentioned, this treatment regimen has not changed in a long time; all these drugs are thirty to fifty years old. But this patient died shortly thereafter, and cultures of his sputum and his blood revealed a strain of *Mycobacterium tuberculosis* resistant to those four drugs. In other words, this U.S. citizen died in Boston of multidrug-resistant tuberculosis (MDRTB) acquired in Peru.

What is to be done next in such a situation? A tuberculosis specialist might suggest "active case-finding"—that is, tracing the close contacts of the patient who died in order to see if other deaths might be averted through rapid case detection and treatment. But the patient had come directly from Peru, and the public health authorities in Massachusetts were not about to do international case-finding. Nonetheless, just a few years after some in Massachusetts judged such measures heroic and beyond the scope of their obligations, it was reported that more than 60 percent of Massachusetts tuberculosis patients were foreign-born.[8] Transnational epidemics are common; transnational solutions, less so.

What do we know about tuberculosis in Peru? I mentioned earlier that I had turned my attention from the tribe based in rural Haiti to the tribe based in cities like Geneva, Paris, and Boston. The World Health Organization's *TB Treatment Observer*, a representative artifact of that tribe's culture, offers the following epidemiological forecast: it is raining MDRTB over Colombia, but in Peru "tuberculosis is being defeated by a model DOTS program."[9] DOTS means "directly observed therapy, short-course." DOTS is the treatment and management strategy favored by international tuberculosis experts, and it is effective at diagnosing and treating cases of smear-positive pulmonary tuberculosis caused by strains of *M. tuberculosis* that are susceptible to all first-line drugs. But what about extrapulmonary tuberculosis, as in the first case I presented, that of the young woman in Haiti? What about tuberculosis caused by drug-resistant strains? The forecast for such patients is much less favorable, to say the least.

When my colleagues and I arrived in Peru, we found little to confirm the sunny picture reported in the WHO's publication. The man who died in Boston had been working in an urban slum in northern Lima. Rates of tuberculosis among young adults were as high in the slums of Lima as in Haiti or even in sub-Saharan Africa.[10] Furthermore, some of the patients who had been treated with DOTS were still sick with active, infectious pulmonary tuberculosis. When we took sputum samples from these patients and grew them in the lab (again, more or less the same way it was done one hundred years ago) and then tested these isolates for susceptibility to first-line drugs, 93.8 percent of the 160 cases tested were shown to have multidrug-resistant tuberculosis.[11] Multidrug-resistant tuberculosis is defined by convention as any strain of *M. tuberculosis* resistant to at least the two most powerful first-line drugs, isoniazid and rifampin.

What will happen next, if hundreds of patients living in a crowded slum are sick with untreated MDRTB? In an editorial in the *European Journal of Public Health*, we argued, tongue in cheek, that we expect MDRTB will spread because we believe it to be an infectious, airborne disease.[12] As one might expect from looking at the Peruvian households we investigated, what happens inside them is that everyone becomes infected; many people become sick and die (see figure 11.1).[13] We also argued that current recommendations—which call for treating *all* patients with first-line drugs only—need to be updated, as the organism has been "updated" genetically.[14] The idea of a transnational epidemic and the need for transdisciplinary and innovative interventions based on epidemiology should not have been shocking, but they were in fact received as heresy by some in international health circles. As mentioned earlier, what drives forward many policies and algorithms is less the imperative of protecting the majority and more a desire to reduce expenditures. MDRTB makes this point more clearly than any other disease—unlike extrapulmonary TB, it *is* contagious and is not treatable with standardized, first-line regimens.

Let me return to a sociology-of-science perspective and examine some rather emphatic statements regarding drug-resistant tuberculosis from the architects of international tuberculosis policy. I would like to "unpack" some of these statements: for example, the assertion that "DOTS is our only available hope for preventing a plague of incurable drug-resistant tuberculosis from worsening to terrifying and unimaginable proportions."[15] This is strong language. It singles out one particular intervention not only as the *best* but as the *only rational* treatment. In Haiti, DOTS is exactly the strategy that we use, because it is very effective wherever rates of drug resistance are low. The cure rates among patients with smear-positive pulmonary tuberculosis are well over 95 percent in the catchment area around the clinic where we work.[16] Mine is therefore not a critique of a partic-

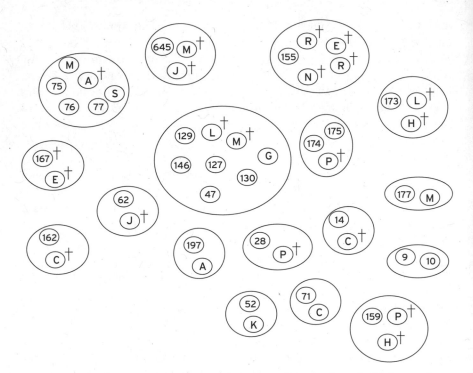

FIGURE 11.1. A schematic representation of seventeen Peruvian household clusters that include patients with MDRTB. Bubbles with numbers denote TB sufferers examined in the course of the study who had failed to respond to at least one first-line drug. Letters denote individuals not directly examined but whose stories were relayed to the investigators by their relatives; in most cases, drug resistance in these individuals could not be confirmed. Crosses mark patients who died, most of them before the study began: only one patient (167) began treatment too late for recovery. Based on data from Becerra-Valdivia, "Epidemiology of Tuberculosis in the Northern Shantytowns of Lima, Peru."

ular intervention; rather, it is a step back to look for second-order objectification, and the ideology and hegemony that underpin it, in international health policy.[17]

DOTS is effective, as I just said, where rates of drug resistance are low. But in many environments, drug resistance is a persistent concern. The short-course chemotherapy (SCC) that is integral to DOTS is based on isoniazid and rifampin. But, by definition, someone who has MDRTB is sick with strains resistant to those drugs. It logically follows that if drug resistance is high and only DOTS is used, cure rates are going to be low.

In the former Soviet Union, we see ample evidence of this. A remarkable study, not yet commented upon by sociologists of knowledge (to say nothing of ethicists), shows that there is, in a certain Russian oblast, a 5 percent cure rate of documented MDRTB when SCC is used.[18] This is interesting because it means that the culture results and susceptibility data were available prior to (or during) therapy, and yet SCC was given anyway. Even more interesting, the laboratory results were reported in a U.S. publication, since this was a transnational project to show that DOTS was the cure for Russia's TB problem.[19] Although data and good sense both indicate that one would not want to use SCC for patients who are resistant to the two main drugs in the treatment regimen, this is precisely what happens when DOTS is pushed as the sole TB treatment strategy. A 5 percent cure rate means that most of the remaining patients either died or remained sick—and infectious. Using this particular strategy, blessed by the international health community for *all* patients, may have been termed a managerial success, but it also meant clinical failure.[20] For most people—patients, family members, doctors, nurses, and others—managerial success is not the ultimate goal of clinical practice. Clinical success is.

Other emphatic statements made by international experts suggest that this ostensibly arcane debate is indeed a subject worthy of the attention of sociologists and historians of science: for example, "DOTS makes it virtually impossible to cause patients to develop incurable forms of tuberculosis that are becoming more common."[21] Another interesting claim: "Other treatment strategies are actually causing multidrug-resistant tuberculosis and may be doing more harm than good."[22] With regard to the first claim, it is simply false, as we know from empirical research and experience. DOTS can sometimes "amplify" preexisting resistance. In that regard, it is no different from "other treatment strategies." A second round of SCC for those who fail the first course—again, strongly recommended by international health experts—can further amplify drug resistance. This is not a mere theoretical model. We know patients who present with drug-resistant disease, receive DOTS, acquire more resistance to more drugs, and then get the officially recommended retreatment regimen, only to pick up resistance to a fourth or fifth drug.

Many infectious-disease clinicians would predict this outcome. But it is not that clinicians deserve praise in this realm; they have their own sorry history of dealing with tuberculosis, a failure that is already the subject of a good deal of commentary. It is simply that clinical concerns are not driving these policies forward; managers and health economists are. Nor is protection of public health the paramount concern. It is, rather, the reduction of public health expenditures that figures prominently in the era of "cost-effectiveness."

Neoliberal ideology is shaping not only the dissemination of knowledge—through the promotion of officially condoned treatment strategies for tuberculosis—but also the very construction of our categories of evidence. Take the example of smear microscopy, discussed earlier, as a gauge of cure. MDRTB is only transiently suppressed in many patients said to be cured by DOTS, and they

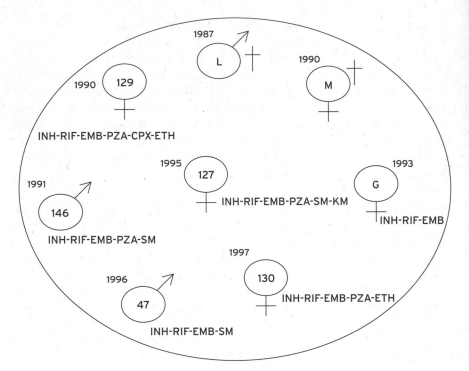

FIGURE 11.2. A schematic depiction of one household from figure 11.1, containing eight individuals who either have MDRTB or have died from it. Patients 127, 129, 130, L, M, and G are siblings; patients 47 and 146 are married to two of the sisters. The year when each individual was first treated for TB is indicated. Also indicated are the last available results from drug-susceptibility testing: patient 127, for example, has demonstrated resistance to six of the first- and second-line medications. Based on data from Becerra-Valdivia, "Epidemiology of Tuberculosis in the Northern Shantytowns of Lima, Peru."

relapse as soon as therapy stops, or shortly thereafter. On official records in the DOTS system, even patients who are smear-negative but culture-positive—that is, with viable mycobacteria in their sputum—were labeled as cured. In Peru, some of those who became our own patients, sick with MDRTB after completing DOTS, figure among the published percentages "cured" by DOTS.[23] Thus are categories of knowledge, and results also, sculpted by what can only be described as zealous application of a particular management strategy.

Let us consider this problem of evidence categories at the level of the family. Valeria, who suffers from MDRTB, comes from what is called a "TB family." Eight of her close relatives (six siblings and two brothers-in-law) either have MDRTB or have died from it (see figure 11.2). Following an initial and ineffective round of therapy, Valeria even changed her name in order to obtain treatment again, after being told that she was a "problem patient." Her husband, Chalo, who had been caring for her, became ill with cough and weight loss. When acid-fast bacilli were found in his sputum, many assumed that he would also have MDRTB. In order to avoid amplification of resistance, and, more important, in order to cure him, it would have been wise to initiate therapy as if he did have MDRTB, awaiting confirmation by laboratory testing. He was, however, given the same empiric DOTS regimen, because that was what the public health community insisted should be done for all newly diagnosed patients. In Peru, all new smear-positive cases received the same treatment, regardless of their history of exposure to drug-resistant strains of M. tuberculosis.

Managerially, this is certainly an easier strategy than considering the subtleties of each case. But in this simple strategy, clinical outcomes and other data are dismissed as irrelevant when an algorithm is elevated to the level of hegemonic discourse. Every month Chalo would go in and have his smear checked, and he would still be positive—not surprising considering that he had MDRTB and was receiving a treatment that could not cure it.

Also to no one's surprise, Chalo wanted to stop the treatment that could not cure him. When he said that he was no longer going to take first-line antituberculous drugs, he was forced to sign a document that read: "I am not going to take my therapy any more because it makes me feel sick, nauseated, and I am withdrawing from treatment." This twist in the story is relevant on several levels. Obviously the experience is relevant on the level of human suffering. (Both his own medical care and the possibility of transmitting the disease to his children may profitably be discussed at this level.) It is important on the level of policy. It is also important on the level of recording data. A patient with a piece of paper like this in his file is considered to be, like Valeria, a "problem patient."

But there are two ways to fall ill with MDRTB. One is to acquire it through inappropriate treatment—usually attributed to the "noncompliance" of the problem patients—and this was the framework at play in this case. This is termed "secondary" or "acquired MDRTB." But another possibility is to be infected with a drug-resistant strain: this is called "primary MDRTB." Now, this young man will, of course, never be counted as having primary MDRTB. By definition—as the piece of paper in his file shows—Chalo is a treatment "defaulter," a problem patient who has *acquired* MDRTB through noncompliance. But we have evidence that this was not the case. When we tested the strain causing his sickness, we found DNA "fingerprints" similar to those of the strains that were causing sickness among other members of the family (figure 11.3). This evidence strongly supports our contention that this patient became ill with primary MDRTB by being in close contact with his wife and eight in-laws, all sick with the same strains of the disease.

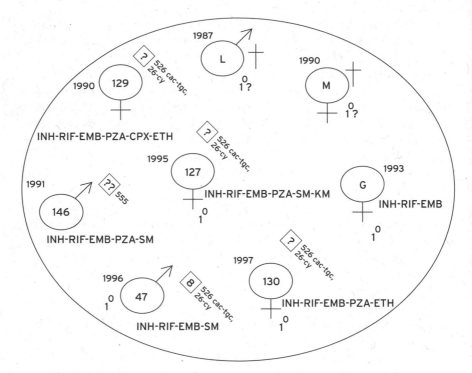

FIGURE 11.3. This schematic depicts the same family shown in figure 11.2. Tests for mutations associated with rifampin resistance indicate the likelihood that patients 47, 127, 129, and 130 were infected with similar strains of *Mycobacterium tuberculosis*. Results for patient 146 were not conclusive; patients L, M, and G were not available for this study. The symbol 1° indicates a patient whose TB has never responded to a first-line medication; it is probable that these patients were originally infected with an already drug-resistant strain of TB rather than developing resistance in the course of treatment. Based on data from Becerra-Valdivia, "Epidemiology of Tuberculosis in the Northern Shantytowns of Lima, Peru."

I would call this a *biosocial* analysis, as it moves from sociology and political economy to the molecular level. Such analysis is possible when a transdisciplinary, multidisciplinary team (composed of clinicians, anthropologists, epidemiologists, and bench scientists doing the molecular epidemiology) collects and analyzes the data in all its richness and complexity. The shortcomings of both the policies and the therapies might otherwise not have been apparent. It now appears that conventional epidemiology quite significantly underestimates the levels of epidemic transmission of MDRTB, as gauged by using molecular diagnostics. The last thing that we would want to be, in the sociology of science, is Luddites who reject new technologies (in this case, molecular diagnostics).

They come in handy when we are attempting to understand such a complex set of biosocial processes. And the broader the net is cast, the more likely that our analyses will lead us back to the political economics of international health.

THE IDEOLOGY OF COST-EFFECTIVENESS

Let me return to my tribe. The specific public health strategies described here, such as insisting on DOTS as the sole intervention, are commonly guided by larger epistemological frameworks with ideologies behind them. We would like to know what these frameworks and ideologies might be. What are the competing agendas here? The most common response to this question is that there is a struggle between clinical and public health approaches to the problem of tuberculosis. The public health approach would necessarily be focused on preventing transmission above all, which is the reason that extrapulmonary tuberculosis tends to be ignored in the public health literature. But, as the example from Peru suggests, prevention of transmission is not always the primary concern of those arguing that DOTS will suffice for MDRTB. *Reducing costs* is the primary concern in certain circles. This is stated quite explicitly by the WHO: "In many high TB prevalence countries, second-line drugs are prohibitively expensive and unavailable. . . . Multidrug-resistant TB is therefore often untreatable."[24] Some very interesting hypotheses underpin these assertions. Let us look at one of the central assertions, that MDRTB is an untreatable disease in a "resource-poor setting." ("Resource-poor," by the way, is the latest euphemism for settings of poverty.)

Is MDRTB really untreatable in poor countries? A group of concerned people, some of them slum-dwellers and patients themselves, have tried to answer the question by building a coalition to respond to the problem of MDRTB. In Peru, youths from the barrio were trained as outreach workers in a new program of directly observed therapy (DOT). It was not the DOTS approach, since the standard short-course chemotherapy was not prescribed for those ill from strains of *M. tuberculosis* resistant to SCC. When the correct drugs were used for these MDRTB patients, what cure rates were obtained? Far from being zero, as had been suggested by officialdom, the cure rates of the "incurable" chronic MDRTB patients exceeded 80 percent.[25] Furthermore, despite the predictions of skeptics, the majority of patients did not abandon therapy because of side effects: only 7 percent of the first cohort of seventy-four patients abandoned the difficult and prolonged therapy. In later cohorts, the percentage of patients who dropped out decreased further, as patients became aware that effective therapy for drug-resistant disease was, in fact, accessible. Through this small-scale project alone, multiple hypotheses presented as facts by powerful organizations in the international health policy arena were cast in doubt.

Considering the high cure rates among our patients, we believed that ours was a good intervention, and we thought that perhaps we would get a pat on the back for it. It was appreciated by the patients whose lives were saved and by their loved ones. It certainly had a large impact on the community, training people who were otherwise unemployed and making use of local resources. It restored faith in the broader public health agenda, a faith that had been undermined for many who had watched their neighbors die of tuberculosis while listening to the media claim that the tuberculosis program in Peru was the best in the world. But for years we did not receive unstinting praise for this effort and for years did not get the public health approbation needed to "scale up" this approach and serve other populations.

So our group spent a lot of time thinking about why so many were saying that MDRTB (and HIV as well—another story) cannot be treated in settings of poverty. We even took to calling what we were doing "DOTS-Plus" in an effort to win approval from the international TB community, which seemed to be obdurately focused on advancing a single agenda for tuberculosis treatment. We started studying all the objections. First, it was supposed to be too expensive. But the second-line drugs had also been off-patent for decades. Pooled procurement and other innovations could and did drop drug prices dramatically.[26] We looked at other claims regarding epidemics elsewhere in the world. For example, it was argued that DOTS alone had sufficed to turn around the MDRTB epidemic in New York City. This was not true. Careful reanalysis of the epidemic there showed that more than a single strategy was used; there had been multiple interventions, and people with MDRTB were treated with the right drugs.[27] Fewer than half of the New York patients received DOTS before the epidemic began to decline. And it would of course have been considered unethical to give Americans drugs to which their infecting strains were resistant.

DOTS was supposedly sufficient in resource-poor settings. But in the former Soviet Union, newly declared as a resource-poor area, DOTS does not give high cure rates, even in projects supervised by the international experts of the tuberculosis world. In the past decade, rates of tuberculosis rose sharply in Russia as cure rates fell. During the first five years after the collapse of the Soviet Union, it was easy to blame the Russians, and many international tuberculosis experts were happy to do so. But in more recent years it has been harder to attribute failure to Russian TB experts because DOTS programs, in partnership with the international organizations, have also had low cure rates. This is in large part the result of drug resistance.

Another objection to DOTS-Plus was that it was too difficult technically. But we did it in Peru and Haiti, and if you can do something in Haiti, I think you can make the argument that it can be done just about anywhere. Finally, what about the argument that DOTS-Plus is not cost-effective? The idea that treating MDRTB in resource-poor settings is not cost-effective obviously depends wholly on two things: cost and efficacy or effectiveness. We had documented that repeated empiric regimens—that is, getting the same medicines again and again—were both ineffective and costly. These treatments were also a source of acquired drug resistance, both by changing the genetics of the microbe and by changing the host, the human, whose lungs were damaged badly by ineffectively treated tuberculosis. These patients were not cured but did continue to transmit increasingly resistant strains to others.

Allow me to reexamine the problem from the point of view of what is boldly called "management science." Take the example of one second-line drug manufactured by a giant pharmaceutical company. On a given day, this drug in a Boston teaching hospital costs thirty dollars a gram. In Peru, it is twenty-one dollars. In France shortly thereafter, it is sold for less than seven dollars per gram. Same company, same drug: how can this be considered rational drug pricing? Since TB is a disease that has not affected many people in affluent settings, there is no vocal lobby agitating around it. There are no organized patient groups. This in itself is sobering, since TB is the world's leading infectious killer. But the patients are poor and marginalized and therefore do not constitute an effective lobby. What would happen if one tried to organize a task-force solution and make common cause with the World Health Organization, Médecins Sans Frontières, and other international groups? Would the prices drop? We began organizing such a coalition to negotiate for lower prices with pharmaceutical companies selling both generic and "branded" medications. It took a few years to get the right people on board, but we were together able to drop the prices quite significantly in the space of one year.[28]

Drug-resistant tuberculosis is not a problem that can be ignored much longer in Europe, because the largest epidemics reach into Europe. After the collapse of the Soviet Union, life expectancy began to drop, especially for men. In recent years, deaths from cardiovascular disease have started to decline again, and the mortality crisis in general has started to improve. But tuberculosis remains a problem in Russia. Tuberculosis continued to increase in incidence and prevalence every year for the last ten years of the twentieth century, until it reached levels five times those seen elsewhere in Western Europe and three times the levels registered in the former Soviet Union.[29] This is a fairly recent epidemic. It is prison-seated, just as the New York MDRTB epidemic once was. It affects a patient population similar to those we treated in New York: young adults, mostly men. In the prisons of the former Soviet Union, the mean age of tuberculosis patients is twenty-nine and dropping. Their crimes are typically crimes against property—petty larceny, for example—and related to the social upheaval occurring throughout the region. The big difference is that the Russian epidemic is so much larger than the one in the urban United States. Most prisoners with tuberculosis who have drug-susceptibility tests performed on their sputum are revealed to be sick with drug-resistant disease. Therefore this is not only an epidemic of tuberculosis in Europe—it is also an epidemic of drug-resistant tuberculosis. MDRTB cannot be wished away.

PUBLIC HEALTH AND
THE SOCIOLOGY OF MANAGING INEQUALITY

To understand the state of the socially constructed universe at any given time, or its change over time, one must understand the social organization that permits the definers to do their defining. Put a little crudely, it is essential to keep pushing questions about the historically available conceptualizations of reality from the abstract "What?" to the socially concrete "Says who?"

PETER BERGER AND THOMAS LUCKMANN,
THE SOCIAL CONSTRUCTION OF REALITY

The sociology of science often shows us how knowledge held to be scientific arises instead from unacknowledged ideological frameworks. Like other forms of knowledge, science is socially constructed: everything from research problem choice to the interpretation of data is influenced by the factors that influence other human affairs. What is true of the natural sciences is even more so for those arenas of inquiry termed "social sciences." Clinical medicine sits between the basic sciences and the social sciences. Lewis Thomas once called medicine "the youngest science."[30] Only recently has the scientific method made its way into what had long been deemed an art. Public health, for all its obsession with quantification, is similarly vulnerable to distortion.

I have attempted to apply a sociology-of-knowledge approach to recent claims about how best to understand, and to manage, a new variation on an old disease. Tuberculosis has long been a scourge of the poor, but a number of fundamentally biosocial events have changed the stakes in recent years. First, the advent of effective therapy changed mortality rates for those who had access to diagnosis and care, removing tuberculosis from the list of potentially fatal infections for the affluent even as it remained the leading infectious cause of adult deaths in the poor world. The advent of antibiotics led, as it did with other infectious pathogens, to the emergence of drug-resistant strains. Then came HIV, which changed the stakes further: co-infection with HIV often awakens quiescent infection with *M. tuberculosis*. Clearly, biosocial events such as these—which reflect the ever-changing interplay between the large-scale social forces that shape the distribution and outcome of disease and also genetic changes in the microbes—are not readily understood without interdisciplinary research. Nor are the health and research policies that reflect and aggravate growing social inequalities. Even as tuberculosis and AIDS top the list of infectious pathogens causing millions of deaths annually, there are no new antituberculous drugs and too few plans to move anti-HIV drugs to places in which they are needed most.

The examples I use here are meant not to impugn the architects of global tuberculosis control policies but rather to show how ideological templates come to sculpt these policies and how they play out in the poor communities where tuberculosis takes its toll. Why would policies ignore drug-resistant and extra-pulmonary tuberculosis? I argued here that the recent debates about difficult-to-treat chronic infectious diseases are less about competing agendas between medicine and public health and more about the struggle to reduce expenditures on the health of the poor. Indeed, it is an unchallenged truism that "we are living in a time of limited resources" and thus must "make hard choices." It is rarely remarked, in response to such confident claims, that resources are less limited now than ever before in human history. As science and technology become domi-nant forces in medicine and public health, they are improving outcomes for the fortunate few. For the others, we are reduced to managing inequality.

The leading calculus of these times, at least in international public health, is "cost-effectiveness." Presented as scientific and "evidence-based," the cost-effectiveness approach attempts to gauge the health impact of particular expen-ditures and, increasingly, to reserve public investments in health in poor com-munities for interventions that are deemed affordable. The World Bank and other international institutions have promoted certain approaches and interventions as "excellent investments," frequently using economic arguments to justify health outlays.

The idea that such discourses and tools for analysis might themselves be more ideological than evidence-based is one that is met with a good deal of resistance in international health circles. Too often, complex therapies, whether for infec-tious diseases, for malignancies, or for mental illness, are not considered cost-effective in an era in which money is worshipped so ardently that it is difficult to attack market logic without being called misguided or irresponsible.

The revolution that occurred in physics over a century ago is at last happen-ing in medicine and, to some extent, in public health. But there was no social revolution to accompany the scientific one. As a result, we now live in a world in which several different standards of care may be advocated for the same disease. For those with chronic infectious diseases, including tuberculosis and AIDS, these standards include excellent treatment for some, ineffective treatment for others, and no treatment for most. Ironically, perhaps, the reality that hundreds of millions live without any access to effective therapy at all serves to justify the setting of double standards, with the excuse that any care is an improvement over current conditions. But the use of scientific language and "evidence-based approaches" to public health cannot mask the fact that managing inequality has been our approach to the great plagues of our times.

NOTES

1. Taking a sociology-of-science approach to this problem offers a unique opportunity to examine the ideologies driving knowledge production and dispersal. As many philosophers have argued, knowledge, including scientific knowledge, cannot be created in an ideological void. The perspectives of people involved in all facets of knowledge production—from research to funding to policy—influence what becomes a part of accepted scholarly knowledge. For useful edited volumes that discuss studies of the link between scientific knowledge production and ideology, see Meja and Stehr, *The Sociology of Knowledge*; and Meja and Stehr, *Knowledge and Politics*.

2. I use the term "socially constructed" following Berger and Luckmann, *The Social Construction of Reality*.

3. Farmer, *Infections and Inequalities*. For a short review of Rudolf Virchow's extensive contributions to the field of social medicine, see Eisenberg, "Rudolf Ludwig Karl Virchow, Where Are You Now That We Need You?"

4. Robert Koch discovered the tubercle bacillus in 1882. "One has been accustomed until now to regard tuberculosis as the outcome of social misery," Koch wrote, "and to hope by relief of distress to diminish the disease. But in the future struggle against this dreadful plague of the human race one will no longer have to contend with an indefinite something, but with an actual parasite" (cited in Feldberg, *Disease and Class,* p. 439).

5. Associated Press, "Experimental Drug Gives Researchers Optimism for New Treatment for TB."

6. Between 1975 and 1996, 1,233 new chemical entities were registered. Of that number, only eleven were medications to treat tropical diseases such as tuberculosis and malaria. For more on this, see Pfeifer, "Public-Private Partnership Attacks Tuberculosis—Aim Is to Spur Development of New Drugs."

7. Tuberculosis funding by the National Institutes of Health—an institution at the forefront of research efforts in the United States and, with a total budget in excess of $23 billion, the major funder of domestic medical research—reached only $87 million this year, despite the disease's standing as the second leading infectious cause of adult deaths worldwide. This $87 million is nonetheless a marked increase from the $3 million allocated to TB-related research in 1989. Since 1999, funding for TB research has risen, although it is still far from adequate, considering the disease burden. Much of this increased funding has been led by the Bill and Melinda Gates Foundation, which has invested over $200 million in TB and malaria research since its inception. For more details, see Shadid, "Fighting Scourges with Funds."

8. Centers for Disease Control and Prevention, *Reported Tuberculosis in the United States, 1999.* The national rate stood at 41.6 percent in 1998, an increase of more than 10 percent since 1993, with six states reporting greater than 70 percent of cases occurring among the foreign-born (Talbot et al., "Tuberculosis among Foreign-Born Persons in the United States, 1993–1998").

9. See the illustration caption in issue 2 of the World Health Organization Global Tuberculosis Programme's *TB Treatment Observer* (1997).

10. Prevalence of TB is estimated at about 300 per 100,000 population for the district (Farmer, Bayona, Becerra, Furin, et al., "The Dilemma of MDR-TB in the Global Era"). In the hardest-hit regions of Africa, estimates fall between approximately 300 and 550 cases per 100,000 population (World Health Organization, *Global Tuberculosis Control*).

11. Becerra et al., "Using Treatment Failure under Effective Directly Observed Short-Course Chemotherapy Programs to Identify Patients with Multidrug-Resistant Tuberculosis."

12. Farmer and Kim, "Resurgent TB in Russia."

13. Becerra-Valdivia, "Epidemiology of Tuberculosis in the Northern Shantytowns of Lima, Peru."

14. Farmer, Bayona, Becerra, Furin, et al., "The Dilemma of MDR-TB in the Global Era."

15. World Health Organization Global Tuberculosis Programme, *WHO Report on the Tuberculosis Epidemic, 1995.*

16. Farmer, Robin, et al., "Tuberculosis, Poverty, and 'Compliance.'"

17. "Legitimation as a process is best described as a 'second-order' objectification of meaning. Legitimation produces new meanings that serve to integrate the meanings already attached to disparate institutional processes. The function of legitimation is to make objectively available and subjectively plausible the 'first-order' objectifications that have been institutionalized" (Berger and Luckmann, *The Social Construction of Reality*, p. 110).

18. Centers for Disease Control and Prevention, "Primary Multidrug-Resistant Tuberculosis— Ivanovo Oblast, Russia, 1999."

19. Using First World diagnostics and Third World therapeutics is, unfortunately, not uncommon in medical research and is also not limited to MDRTB studies. Research universities and development agencies now have global reach, and, just as epidemics are transnational, so too, increasingly, is research. But although the pathogens readily cross borders, the fruits of research are often delayed in customs. For example, it will not go unnoticed that it proved easy enough to use First World diagnostics in the contentious HIV study conducted in Uganda by Thomas Quinn and colleagues in 2000—for example, sophisticated assays of viral load were available—even though antiretroviral therapy was deemed unfeasible, too difficult, or "cost-ineffective" (Quinn et al., "Viral Load and Heterosexual Transmission of Human Immunodeficiency Virus Type 1"). In defending their decision not to treat HIV-infected study participants, Quinn and colleagues write: "Most important, neither we nor the Ugandan government had, or currently have, the clinical capacity to manage antiretroviral treatment, including side effects and compliance" (Gray et al., "The Ethics of Research in Developing Countries," p. 361). It is in fact this attitude (which is not Quinn's, but rather is the regnant philosophy in international health) that I, and many of those who wrote letters voicing their objections to the study, argue is wrong. Critiquing the oft-used argument that weak infrastructure makes treating the sick an impossibility in poor countries, Vinh-Kim Nguyen retorts, "Using the 'weak-infrastructure' excuse to not do anything is equivalent to refusing to offer someone CPR because cutbacks have closed the local intensive-care unit" ("The Shape of Things to Come?").

20. Farmer, "Managerial Successes, Clinical Failures."

21. World Health Organization Global Tuberculosis Programme, *WHO Report on the Tuberculosis Epidemic, 1995*, p. 2.

22. Ibid.

23. Espinal et al., "Standard Short-Course Chemotherapy for Drug-Resistant Tuberculosis."

24. Harries and Maher, *TB/HIV*, p. 89.

25. For more on our treatment results, see Farmer, Kim, et al., "Responding to Outbreaks of Multidrug-Resistant Tuberculosis." The WHO aims for an 85 percent cure rate with DOTS (World Health Organization, *Global Tuberculosis Control*).

26. Gupta et al., "Responding to Market Failures in Tuberculosis Control."

27. For a summary of New York's TB outbreak, see Garrett, *The Coming Plague;* and Frieden et al., "Tuberculosis in New York City—Turning the Tide." For a critical commentary on the relative contribution of DOTS, see Farmer and Nardell, "Nihilism and Pragmatism in Tuberculosis Control." And see Bayer et al., "Directly Observed Therapy and Treatment Completion for Tuberculosis in the United States."

28. Gupta et al., "Responding to Market Failures in Tuberculosis Control."

29. Farmer, Kononets, et al., "Recrudescent Tuberculosis in the Russian Federation."

30. Thomas, *The Youngest Science.*

12

The Major Infectious Diseases in the World—To Treat or Not to Treat?

(2001)

In the July 2001 issue of the *New England Journal of Medicine,* Kemal Tahaoğlu and coworkers report on their experience in treating a cohort of patients infected with strains of *Mycobacterium tuberculosis* that are resistant to powerful anti-tuberculosis drugs. Tuberculosis caused by strains that are resistant to at least isoniazid and rifampin is, by convention, termed "multidrug-resistant tuberculosis."[1] The authors of this report work in a referral center in Turkey that has available a full complement of clinical, laboratory, and surgical services, including multidrug treatment regimens given for eighteen to twenty-four months, resources for the management of side effects, adjuvant surgery when necessary, and full financial and nutritional support. Tahaoğlu and coworkers show that with a high standard of care, the treatment of multidrug-resistant tuberculosis can have excellent results, especially among younger patients without serious coexisting conditions.

This study is important for several reasons. It has already been documented that multidrug-resistant tuberculosis is a pandemic. Drug-resistant cases of tuberculosis have been reported in every country surveyed.[2] *M. tuberculosis* is an airborne pathogen, and persons with active pulmonary tuberculosis caused by a multidrug-resistant strain can transmit the disease to others as long as they are alive and coughing. For the hundreds of thousands who are sick with multidrug-resistant tuberculosis, the Tahaoğlu report should come as welcome news. Throughout the world, most patients with multidrug-resistant tuberculosis are like the majority of those in the Turkish study: young and middle-aged adults who are not infected with the human immunodeficiency virus (HIV) and who do not have serious coexisting conditions. Almost none of these patients, however, are receiving effective therapy, and most remain infectious.

Some *Journal* readers may be surprised to learn that the great majority of patients with multidrug-resistant tuberculosis throughout the world are not receiving effective therapy. The need for such therapy in "resource-poor settings"— the latest euphemism for poverty—is disputed in international tuberculosis control circles, where it is argued that multidrug-resistant tuberculosis is too expensive and too difficult to treat. The authors of the current study take note of the debate about "whether to consider multidrug-resistant tuberculosis treatable or untreatable, given the often limited resources available." Some have claimed that multidrug-resistant tuberculosis can be treated with a short course of chemotherapy (that is, treatment based on isoniazid and rifampin, the very drugs to which multidrug-resistant strains of *M. tuberculosis* are, by definition, resistant). It was not until last year that this misconception was put to rest. In a six-country study, the cure rates among patients with laboratory-documented, multidrug-resistant tuberculosis were well under 50 percent in most settings.[3] In a study in Ivanovo Oblast, in Russia, only 5 percent of patients with multidrug-resistant tuberculosis were cured by short-course chemotherapy.[4]

It is not surprising that patients infected with multidrug-resistant strains of *M. tuberculosis* are not cured by treatment with the drugs to which the strains are resistant. Moreover, delays in establishing the diagnosis and initiating effective therapy are associated with poor outcomes, even when patients do finally receive effective therapy. In accordance with the current public health convention, all patients in Turkey who have smear-positive pulmonary tuberculosis receive empirical short-course chemotherapy based on isoniazid and rifampin. In the Tahaoğlu study, drug-susceptibility testing was performed on specimens obtained from patients at the outset of therapy, and the results were then ignored. The delay in initiating effective therapy might have been reduced if the results of these tests had been taken into account.

It is not standard practice in North America or in Europe to perform such laboratory tests and then disregard the results. Why would such a procedure be followed? In most resource-poor settings, all patients receive empirical, standardized short-course chemotherapy, and it is assumed that drug-susceptibility testing is not available. Turkey is not a resource-poor country but geopolitically a part of Europe. At the facility described in this report, although it is perhaps not as handsomely equipped as a referral center in the United States, doctors have far more resources at hand than do the beleaguered doctors trying to battle tuberculosis in Latin America, the former Soviet Union, and other regions where multidrug-resistant tuberculosis is a major problem. The Tahaoğlu report shows that multidrug-resistant tuberculosis is treatable, at least where there are centers of excellence to deal with the problem.

What about countries where there are no centers of excellence? In a squatter settlement in Haiti and in a slum in Peru, my colleagues and I have obtained similar cure rates in treating patients with chronic multidrug-resistant tuberculosis.[5] Many communicable diseases can now be cured. Others, although still incurable, can be suppressed effectively with therapy. That patients with multidrug-resistant tuberculosis are going untreated raises the general question of the standards of care for patients with chronic infectious diseases who have the misfortune to live in impoverished countries. The assumption that these diseases are treatable in some places and not in others is widely accepted. A lack of infrastructure is commonly cited as the justification for lower standards of care in some countries, but the real issue is cost. It has been argued that the high cost of "second-line" antituberculosis medications makes the treatment of multidrug-resistant tuberculosis problematic in poor countries. However, the prices of these medications, which have long been off-patent, are exorbitant because there has not been a concerted effort to treat patients who have tuberculosis and who live in poverty.[6] The destitute sick generate no perceptible demand in the medical marketplace.

The most important question facing modern medicine involves human rights. We are witnessing a growing "outcome gap." Some populations have access to increasingly effective interventions; others are left out in the cold. The more effective the treatment, the greater the injustice meted out to those who do not have access to care.

The question of global injustice applies directly to AIDS, which has recently overtaken tuberculosis as the world's leading infectious cause of death among adults. Over the past five years, deaths from AIDS in the United States have dropped sharply, as have admissions related to HIV infection in U.S. hospitals, because of widespread use of highly active therapy against the virus. But these advances, like those in the treatment of multidrug-resistant tuberculosis, have served only a tiny minority of persons throughout the world who could benefit from them. For most HIV-infected persons, these lifesaving drugs are unavailable. We hear all kinds of excuses. Efforts to treat AIDS and multidrug-resistant tuberculosis in areas such as Africa and Haiti, which lack a health care infrastructure, are dismissed as "unsustainable" or "not appropriate technology." Antiviral therapy and complex antituberculosis treatments are considered impermissible where market conditions do not support the sale of such medical services, clear evidence of economic imperatives trumping medical concerns.

In too many policy discussions, the argument that treatment is not cost-effective is largely a means of ending unwelcome discussions about the destitute sick. A high-ranking official in the U.S. Department of the Treasury once objected to a strategy that would make anti-HIV drugs available on the continent where they are most needed. He is quoted as saying that Africans lack the necessary "concept of time," implying that the drugs would be ineffective because of the required schedule of administration.[7] Despite the absence of data that support these claims—and much experience to the contrary—they are persuasive within the elite circles where decisions are made that affect the health and fate of millions of the world's sick.

Prevention is, of course, always preferable to treatment. But epidemics of treatable infectious diseases should remind us that although science has revolutionized medicine, we still need a plan for ensuring equal access to care. As study after study shows the power of effective therapies to alter the course of infectious disease, we should be increasingly reluctant to reserve these therapies for the affluent, low-incidence regions of the world where most medical resources are concentrated. Excellence without equity looms as the chief human rights dilemma of health care in the twenty-first century.

NOTES

1. Tahaoğlu et al., "The Treatment of Multidrug-Resistant Tuberculosis in Turkey."

2. See Pablos-Méndez et al., "Global Surveillance for Anti-Tuberculosis Drug Resistance, 1994–1997." See also Harvard Medical School and Open Society Institute, *The Global Impact of Drug-Resistant Tuberculosis;* Espinal et al., "Global Trends in Resistance to Antituberculosis Drugs."

3. Espinal et al., "Standard Short-Course Chemotherapy for Drug-Resistant Tuberculosis."

4. Centers for Disease Control and Prevention, "Primary Multidrug-Resistant Tuberculosis—Ivanovo Oblast, Russia, 1999."

5. Farmer, Bayona, Shin, et al., "Preliminary Outcomes of Community-Based MDRTB Treatment in Lima, Peru"; see also Farmer, Furin, and Shin, "Managing Multidrug-Resistant Tuberculosis."

6. Kim, Furin, et al., "Treatment of Multidrug-Resistant Tuberculosis (MDR-TB)."

7. Kahn, "Rich Nations Consider Fund of Billions to Fight AIDS."

13

Integrated HIV Prevention and Care Strengthens Primary Health Care

Lessons from Rural Haiti

(2004)

David A. Walton, Paul Farmer, Wesler Lambert,
Fernet Léandre, Serena P. Koenig, and Joia S. Mukherjee

The Declaration of Alma-Ata, signed by World Health Organization member states in 1978, constitutes a major milestone in the contemporary primary health care movement. The goal was lofty—"health care for all by the year 2000"—and close attention was paid to the specific means by which that goal might be reached.[1] The plans that emerged from the meeting—from improved vaccination coverage to decreased malnutrition—were deemed feasible by the signatories. Yet these objectives have not been met in many of the very countries where such victories were most needed. Worse, the promotion of health care as a right provoked violent reactions in some settings. Writing from Guatemala, where community health workers had been targeted for government repression and worse, Kris Heggenhougen surveyed the fates of local community health activists and asked, simply enough, "Will primary health care efforts be allowed to succeed?"[2] Thus, although many countries were able to meet certain goals set in Alma-Ata, many more were not; some of the poorest countries, in fact, experienced worsening health indices. As the year 2000 approached, the Alma-Ata slogan became the butt of ridicule in international health circles. The slogan contained a typographical error, went the joke: the rallying cry was in fact "health care for all by the year 3000."

If we afford ourselves another millennium in which to remediate growing inequalities of access to something as basic as primary health care, we are certain to see a growing gap in health outcomes. New and improved diagnostics and therapeutics mean longer lives for those who have access to modern medicine; not so for the world's poor. The United Nations Food and Agriculture Organization recently reported that more than 840 million people in more than thirty countries are going hungry, while in many industrialized nations obesity ranks among the leading causes of morbidity and mortality.[3] Such ironies are not lost on those living and working in what are now termed "resource-poor settings." They are asked to do more and more with less and less. This "mission impossible" has led to deep discouragement within the primary health care movement. Self-described pragmatists have argued that we must lower our expectations and that only interventions deemed "cost-effective" should be encouraged.[4] Health care systems falter where they are most needed, and it is clear that the world's poorest billion inhabitants are far from obtaining even the most basic primary health care.

Into this grim situation comes a series of transformed or newly described pathogens. Most malaria infections are now resistant to chloroquine, and drug-resistant tuberculosis is on the rise throughout the world; the most frightening newly described pathogen is HIV.[5] Each of these three diseases can be managed with multidrug regimens, but an effective vaccine exists for none of them. AIDS, especially, has spawned a number of questionable public health clichés—for example, "education is the only vaccine." Despite two decades of experience using information and education as the primary tools in HIV prevention, there have been, until very recently, no careful studies of the efficacy of these interventions. One review of information and education campaigns concluded that, "somewhat surprisingly, towards the end of the second decade of the AIDS pandemic, we still have no good evidence that primary prevention works."[6] There is increasing agreement that these tools, though of great importance, are of limited efficacy in precisely those settings where they are most needed—settings where social vulnerability, and not cognitive deficits or ignorance, is the primary determinant of risk for HIV infection.[7]

A dispirited international health movement, the advent of new and complex epidemics, and struggles over the scant resources dedicated to improving the health of the poor have led to great debate about AIDS. One major UN-affiliated organization last year canceled a program to provide breast milk supplements to HIV-positive mothers, arguing that it was neither cost-effective nor feasible, given the lack of potable water with which to prepare the supplements. A high-ranking UNICEF official asserted that, in impoverished settings, "provision of infant formula was creating dependence."[8] Unbelievably, continued reliance on HIV-positive breast milk was deemed the "realistic" approach for women and infants living with poverty and HIV.[9]

The debate about universal provision of highly active antiretroviral therapy, sometimes termed "HAART," has been even more contentious. Many public health experts contend that these drugs—the only agents shown to prolong survival among patients with advanced HIV disease[10]—are too expensive and complex for patients in resource-poor settings. A 2002 paper argued that prevention was "28 times more cost-effective than HAART,"[11] as if these were mutually exclusive and competing activities. Still others have insisted that AIDS care will draw resources away from primary health care. Such views tend to remove AIDS treatment from the priority list.

Drawing on our experience in one of the poorest parts of rural Haiti, we have found, in contrast, that improving HIV care can in fact strengthen primary health care goals. In what has been described as the world's third hungriest nation, we launched a small pilot project that integrated AIDS care with robust prevention efforts.[12] In seeking to scale up this effort, we discovered that such projects are replicable and may enhance rather than take away resources from primary health care. This essay describes the "minimum basic package" of integrated HIV prevention and care in the hope that others may find this approach useful, now that novel funding mechanisms, including the Global Fund to Fight AIDS, Tuberculosis, and Malaria (GFATM) and the U.S. President's Emergency Plan for AIDS Relief (PEPFAR), make it possible to tackle the world's leading infectious killers.

SETTING

Haiti is Latin America's oldest independent nation, born of a slave revolt that began in 1791. More than 95 percent of its population is descended from African slaves, and its history has been characterized by ongoing political strife. Haiti, far and away the most impoverished nation in the Western Hemisphere, is, not coincidentally, the country with the region's largest burden of HIV. The World Health Organization estimates that more than 6 percent of the adult population is already infected with HIV.[13] AIDS is believed to be the reason that life expectancy is dropping in Haiti, with the WHO estimating average life expectancy at 43.8 years.[14] With a population of 8.3 million, Haiti accounts for only 25 percent of the Caribbean population but has more than 60 percent of the HIV/AIDS cases.[15] The introduction of HIV to Haiti occurred more than twenty-five years ago, and Haiti's is considered a mature epidemic. Some have termed it "generalized," because it has long been difficult to identify anything resembling discrete risk groups; as a further indication of the disease's spread into the general population, young women now account for half of all HIV cases.[16] Poverty and gender inequality are the leading co-factors for the dissemination of HIV in Haiti, and precisely these forces render existing prevention methods less effective.[17]

The history of the Haitian HIV epidemic, which began in the early 1980s in urban Haiti and was linked to the larger epidemic in North America, has been reviewed elsewhere.[18] During subsequent years, HIV worked its way along major trading routes into the rural regions, where most Haitians live. It is important to note that many prevention efforts were launched in the difficult years between the introduction of the virus and the advent of effective therapy. Although these efforts met with a measure of success, much of the transmission was occurring in urban Haiti, wracked during the past two decades by political violence and growing poverty.

The Central Plateau is one of the poorest parts of Haiti. With over 550,000 inhabitants, most of them living in villages and small towns, the Central Plateau lacks potable water, paved roads, and electricity; the region also lacks basic health infrastructure.[19] In 1988, working in a clinic in Cange, a squatter settlement in the lower Central Plateau, the Partners In Health/Zanmi Lasante team introduced what is now termed "voluntary counseling and testing." Although serologic tests were and remain free to patients, few, at the outset, came to us asking to be tested. Pregnant women, among others, were unlikely to accept voluntary counseling and testing. The great majority of tests performed had been recommended by clinicians seeking to confirm a presumptive diagnosis of advanced HIV disease. As a result, the majority of all tests performed between 1988 and 1995 were positive.

When in-patient capacity was added to the ambulatory clinic in Cange, the proportion of HIV-associated admissions, whether for bacterial pneumonia, tuberculosis, or acute or chronic enteropathy, continued to rise. One survey of all in-patients conducted in the early 1990s, a time of great social upheaval in Haiti, revealed that more than 40 percent were seropositive.[20] The majority of these patients were returning from the urban slums of Haiti's capital, Port-au-Prince. The clinic's overwhelmed medical staff did its best to manage opportunistic infections, but morale was then at an all-time low.[21] There were simply too few tools to stave off death. AIDS had become the leading infectious cause of young adult mortality in rural Haiti.

A handful of errors and discoveries made during these difficult years led, however, to the establishment of one of the world's first community-based AIDS care programs. The first discovery was that voluntary counseling and testing remained unappealing in the absence of effective therapy.

The second discovery concerned the nature of presenting opportunistic infections. During 1993–95, a careful study of two hundred consecutive HIV diagnoses revealed that nearly half of these patients were judged by clinicians to have active tuberculosis (figure 13.1).[22] Most patients treated for HIV-associated tuberculosis with directly observed, short-course chemotherapy for tuberculosis (DOTS) showed marked clinical improvement when clinical care was associated with social support.[23] Although diagnoses were made in clinics, village health workers called *accompagnateurs* provided the great majority of all tuberculosis care. Most of the *accompagnateurs* were local residents caring for their own neighbors and receiving a modest stipend to do so. Patients were given medications and follow-up care free of charge. In addition, families affected by tuberculosis were eligible for social services.[24]

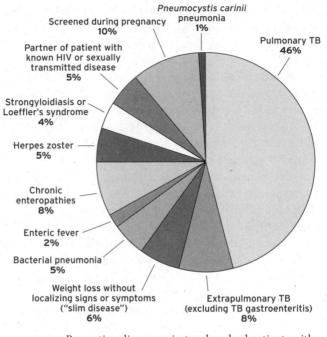

FIGURE 13.1. Presenting diagnoses in two hundred patients with HIV disease, Clinique Bon Sauveur, 1993–95.

A third discovery was made near the end of 1995, when the Cange facility became Haiti's first clinic to introduce AZT for the prevention of mother-to-child transmission of HIV. Rates of voluntary counseling and testing in the prenatal clinic skyrocketed from around 30 percent to over 90 percent in the course of the ensuing year. For the first time, the great majority of HIV serologies performed were negative.

A decade of experience with a successful community-based tuberculosis program, later termed DOTS (directly observed treatment with short-course chemotherapy), and the substantial overlap between the AIDS and tuberculosis epidemics led our Haiti team to decide in 1998 to deliver AIDS care via the same model used to treat tuberculosis: "DOTS" became "DOT-HAART" as village health workers used antiretroviral therapy rather than, or in addition to, antituberculous drugs. From 1999 to 2002, the team relied on clinical algorithms—CD$_4$ counts and viral loads were unavailable—to identify AIDS patients who would not survive long without antiretroviral therapy.[25] During the early years of the program, there was a significant rise in demand for voluntary counseling and testing, itself temporally associated with a large number of equally dramatic clinical responses to antiretroviral therapy. We noted that the "Lazarus effect," as it became known locally, led to a sharp decline in AIDS-related stigma.

A corollary lesson was that AIDS prevention and AIDS care go hand in hand. The rate-limiting factors from 1999 to 2002 were always the same: an inability to find funding for staff and for antiretrovirals.

Other lessons emerged in the course of implementing this program in scores of villages. To improve AIDS care, the team was not only serving HIV-affected families but also increasing its ability to identify and treat patients with other diseases, most notably tuberculosis and sexually transmitted infections.[26] Expanding capacity for prevention of mother-to-child transmission enhanced the quality not only of prenatal care but of all women's health services. Introducing comprehensive AIDS care improved staff morale and increased the flow of essential medications and vaccines to treat and prevent other infections. In other words, improving AIDS prevention and care led in at least one part of central Haiti to a dramatic improvement in the quality of primary health care in general.

Could this exercise be replicated elsewhere? Working with the *accompagnateurs,* the program directors attempted to identify the essential elements of the project, those without which we could not deliver integrated HIV prevention and care that would, at the same time, strengthen public health capacity. This list outlines the six program elements we identified as the "basic minimum package" for a complex health intervention:

- Training and capacity-building for voluntary counseling and testing
- Training and capacity-building for staging (whether with clinical or laboratory criteria) and clinical management
- Community-based care delivered by village health workers
- Training of village health workers in side-effect management and referral
- Program capacity for diagnosis and care of tuberculosis and sexually transmitted diseases
- Program capacity for prenatal care and women's health

In addition, we designated four functions as central to program success, referring to them as "pillars" propping up primary health care:

- HIV prevention and care
- Tuberculosis diagnosis and case-holding
- Case-finding and treatment of sexually transmitted diseases
- Women's health services

The sum of these interventions was deemed a public good and thus was supported by donor funds and by Haiti's Ministry of Health. Because each of these components of care was delivered in large part by village health workers, local training became critical to the effort. Approximately thirty essential medications were judged necessary for the program to succeed, as were a small number of laboratory tests—important components of primary health care even in resource-poor settings.

FROM PILOT PROJECT TO SCALE-UP: BUILDING ON THE FOUR PILLARS

Having identified the key lessons we had learned during the first three years of operations, from 1999 to 2002, and noting the synergy between AIDS services and primary health care, we addressed the next question: could these lessons be applied elsewhere in the region? In 2002, when Haiti's application to the Global Fund to Fight AIDS, Tuberculosis, and Malaria received a high rating in the first round of proposals,[27] the Partners In Health/Zanmi Lasante team decided to replicate the Cange program of prevention and care elsewhere in Haiti. In addition to the "four pillars," our approach included a careful assessment of the social conditions of patients and their families, as basic social services could be offered as part of the minimum package of services for AIDS and TB patients. Since cases were to be found and care delivered largely by village health workers, scale-up of training efforts would also be necessary.

In August 2002, we performed a needs assessment for the town of Lascahobas, a commune of over 55,000 inhabitants abutting Haiti's border with the Dominican Republic. Unlike Cange, which is a small and recently settled squatter encampment of landless peasants, Lascahobas is a large and long-established town with a central square, a market, a public high school, a police station, a courthouse, and a large number of churches. The town is predominantly an agricultural market center, without industry or tourism. Trade occurs across the Dominican border, and there is daily traffic between Lascahobas and Port-au-Prince, three to four hours to the south and west. In some ways, Cange and Lascahobas are strikingly different settings, but both places are saddled with a large burden of tuberculosis, AIDS, and primary health care problems.

Our preliminary assessment found the Lascahobas public clinic to be nearly empty in the morning and closed by noon. We found a demoralized staff (there were no doctors) with very little in the way of tools. As for HIV prevention and care, no services were being offered at all: the absence of serologic tests meant that even voluntary counseling and testing and prevention of mother-to-child transmission were unavailable. On paper, at least, diagnosis and care of tuberculosis were provided free of charge to patients. But in the year preceding scale-up, only nine cases of tuberculosis had been diagnosed in Lascahobas, and roughly half of these were lost to follow-up. Incidence data from the Cange region would have predicted closer to 180 patients each year presenting with active tuberculosis.[28]

METHODS

Ours is a retrospective observational study and relies on a number of quantitative and qualitative methodologies, ranging from participant-observation to active case-finding; this report also relies on the monitoring of key health indices during the first fourteen months of operations in Lascahobas. The health indices that we followed include the number of diagnoses of tuberculosis, HIV infection, and sexually transmitted infections; the number of prenatal visits; and detailed encounter reporting by services (pediatrics, women's health, and so on) within the ambulatory clinic. Reports of services were compiled daily by local staff trained to use computers and basic spreadsheet software; some learned how to use Epi-Info. We submitted monthly distillations of information to Haiti's Ministry of Health, which provided oversight of the project and also basic clinical operations. Partners In Health/Zanmi Lasante staff worked closely with Ministry of Health staff to deliver the basic minimum package described earlier. These services were provided free to patients, with most fees defrayed by the GFATM; other expenditures were covered by Partners In Health and the Ministry of Health.

RESULTS

Our experience in central Haiti suggests that scale-up of community-based care for advanced HIV disease is feasible. Less than a year after the four pillars were implemented, Lascahobas's health center had been radically transformed by what was ostensibly an "AIDS project." Introducing all four pillars meant introducing thirty new essential drugs to the formulary, establishing a small laboratory, training and paying stipends for community heath workers, and complementing Ministry of Health personnel with staff trained by Partners In Health/Zanmi Lasante.

The impact of these efforts was profound. Hundreds of people living with HIV came forward for evaluation and care; within a year, over 120 patients were receiving supervised therapy with ARVs (DOT-HAART). In Lascahobas, as in Cange, almost all prenatal care came to include voluntary counseling and HIV testing. Algorithmic management of sexually transmitted infections was introduced. Aggressive HIV prevention efforts took place within the clinic, in area churches and schools, and in the villages served by the *accompagnateurs*. Within fourteen months after we initiated scale-up, more than 200 tuberculosis patients had been identified and began receiving DOTS. A small in-patient unit was built.

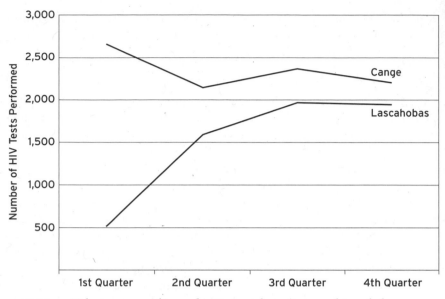

FIGURE 13.2. Voluntary counseling and testing uptake in Cange and Lascahobas, July 2002 through September 2003.

In April 2003, rural Haiti's second AIDS clinic, with equipment comparable to that available in Cange, was dedicated in a ceremony that drew hundreds of local well-wishers. The naysayers who had argued that stigma would prevent the success of such a clinic were proven wrong, as the AIDS clinic is the most active part of what is now one of rural Haiti's busiest health centers.

We can quantify many of the trends documented during the first fourteen months of the scale-up, including those services central to primary health care. The pace of voluntary counseling and testing uptake, shown in figure 13.2, has been striking. Voluntary counseling and testing have long been available in Cange, but prior to August 2002 HIV testing was not available in the commune of Lascahobas. Only a year after scale-up began, almost two thousand serologic tests were being performed there each month. Concordantly, the number of HIV-positive serologies has also increased, as shown in figure 13.3.

Figure 13.4 illustrates the dramatic rise in ambulatory visits to the Lascahobas primary health clinic since the four pillars were implemented; staff there now routinely see more than 300 patients per day. Tuberculosis diagnoses also display a rapid rise (see figure 13.5), peaking in December 2002, demonstrating the "first pass effect" of tuberculosis case-finding in endemic regions that previously had limited or no access to care. Routine screening for all symptomatic patients, with

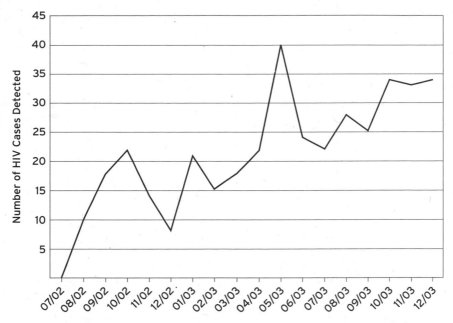

FIGURE 13.3. HIV case detection (number of HIV-positive serologies) in Lascahobas, July 2002 through December 2003.

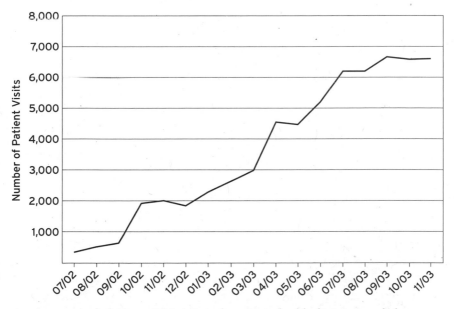

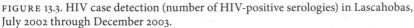

FIGURE 13.4. Ambulatory patient visits to the primary health clinic in Lascahobas, July 2002 through November 2003.

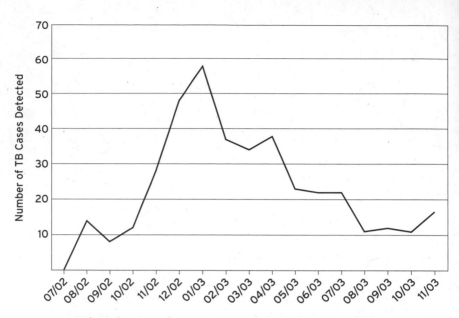

FIGURE 13.5. Tuberculosis case detection in Lascahobas, July 2002 through November 2003. The peak in December 2002 represents the "first pass effect" of case-finding in regions that previously had little or no access to care.

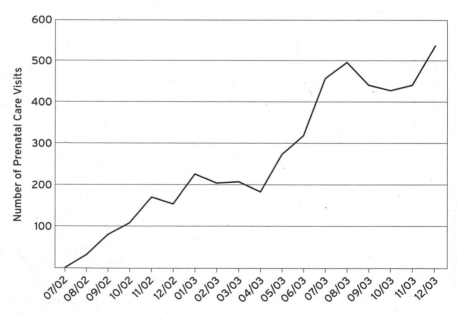

FIGURE 13.6. Prenatal care visits to the clinic in Lascahobas, July 2002 through December 2003.

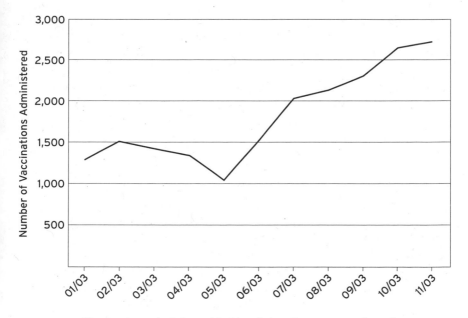

FIGURE 13.7. Vaccinations administered in Lascahobas, January 2003 through November 2003.

smear microscopy and chest radiography, is now central to the services offered in Lascahobas.

Prenatal care, not offered in the clinic prior to scale-up, has seen a similarly dramatic rise (see figure 13.6) since our program of HIV prevention and care has been integrated into the primary health services offered in the town. Even vaccinations, ostensibly unrelated to HIV prevention and care, have become more readily available through the Lascahobas clinic: figure 13.7 shows the secular trend in vaccinations performed in the course of clinic operations.

Less easily quantified results include, as in Cange, improved staff morale and greater community participation. Both are indispensable to the success of primary health care. The lessons of scale-up have shown us that improving AIDS care, far from diverting resources, has in fact strengthened primary health care throughout Haiti's lower Central Plateau.

EPIDEMIC DISEASE AND PRIMARY HEALTH CARE

In April 2003, with monies from the Global Fund to Fight AIDS, Tuberculosis, and Malaria, the Partners In Health/Zanmi Lasante team set out to replicate this experience in three other large towns across rural Haiti. In each setting, the Partners In Health/Zanmi Lasante team chose to work with understaffed and underfunded public clinics, believing that such public-private partnerships are central to rebuilding dilapidated and neglected public health infrastructure. In each setting, we integrated the "four pillars" of such a program: linking quality HIV care, including antiretroviral therapy for those with advanced disease, to HIV prevention efforts; aggressive case-finding and supervised treatment of tuberculosis, the leading opportunistic infection in Haiti; aggressive case-finding and algorithmic treatment of all sexually transmitted infections; and improving women's health services. In each setting, although we have relied on village health workers, rather than physicians or nurses, to provide the bulk of care, we have recruited and retained a large number of young physicians and nurses happy to work in the rural reaches of their country as long as they have access to the tools of their trade.

With a modicum of technical and financial assistance, implementing the four pillars is within the reach of many institutions, including ministries of health and nongovernmental organizations now operating in the heavily HIV-burdened regions of Africa and Latin America. Our own experience leads us to believe that each of these pillars is a necessary component of a robust AIDS prevention and care program. Just as AIDS prevention is hampered by a lack of AIDS care, so too will such a program fail if tuberculosis is the leading opportunistic infection but does not figure in the planning of those designing AIDS interventions. Similarly, a prenatal care program that offers only voluntary counseling and testing and prevention of mother-to-child transmission of HIV but is unable to treat mothers with advanced HIV disease will soon find itself attending to many young HIV-negative orphans, and many pregnant women will decline testing in the absence of treatment. Because untreated sexually transmitted infections can enhance transmission of HIV,[29] it is also important that AIDS programs be prepared to diagnose, treat, and prevent all sexually transmitted infections.

Lessons learned in attempting to respond to another chronic infectious disease afflicting the poor disproportionately, tuberculosis, offer insights regarding the synergy between AIDS programs and primary health care. These lessons include, first, the integration of prevention and care activities. The prevention of tuberculosis is no longer based on sequestering people for years in sanatoriums; rather, prevention is based on prompt diagnosis and ambulatory treatment, because an effectively treated patient is no longer infectious.[30] This insight has relevance even for a sexually transmitted pathogen: in rural Haiti, we soon discovered that improving HIV care helped to destigmatize what had been considered a fatal and "untreatable" disease—untreatable because of the poverty of the patients. Since the introduction of antiretroviral therapy and community-based care to central Haiti, we have seen an enormous increase in demand for voluntary counseling and testing. Now, of course, the majority of these tests are negative, affording health care workers a chance to do a better job of preventing new infections. Research from Uganda suggests that the risk of transmission between serodiscordant couples varies with viral load.[31] It is not unreasonable to argue that those with undetectable viral loads—again, effectively treated patients—are less infectious.[32] In our programs, people receiving antiretroviral therapy have daily contact with an *accompagnateur* and monthly contact with clinic staff. Such exchanges afford all involved, including those living with HIV, a chance to work harder on secondary prevention.

A second lesson from tuberculosis control concerns the delivery of care. Evidence from around the globe suggests that the most successful tuberculosis treatment outcomes are seen when supervised community-based care is offered to patients.[33] In parts of rural Haiti, *accompagnateurs* began supervising therapy for tuberculosis in 1988 and soon saw the end of deaths from that disease. A decade later, the *accompagnateurs* added antiretrovirals (along with other therapies for chronic disease) to their armamentarium, providing essentially the same services for a different disease. Village health workers also serve as a vital link between village and clinic and help attend to the pressing social problems that the majority of our patients face. Although this approach was pioneered in rural Haiti, it was exported successfully to a slum in Peru[34] and more recently to poor neighborhoods in Siberia and in Boston. Our experience in very different settings permits us to argue that this model may be adapted widely. *Accompagnateurs* can serve as the chief purveyors of primary health care services in resource-poor settings.[35]

Third, AIDS prevention and care must be seen as a "public good."[36] Tuberculosis is again paradigmatic: an airborne disease, it has long been considered a public health responsibility. Throughout the world, the most successful tuberculosis control programs, regardless of funding, are public ones, which provide services to all those who might benefit from them, regardless of social standing or ability to pay. AIDS prevention and care should be considered a public good for many reasons, the most important being that HIV kills more young adults than any other single pathogen. Many of the countries most beleaguered by AIDS no longer have the capacity, financial or infrastructural, to confront this pandemic with public funds. But the answer in these instances is not to further privatize these efforts; the answer is to reinforce or rebuild public infrastructures and to do what it takes to make sure that populations in need have access to both prevention and treatment.[37] In a place like rural Haiti, this means that the cost of care cannot be borne by the patients. Slowing the pandemic, and stopping senseless deaths, requires that public-private partnerships make resources available in the poorest and most heavily burdened regions. Such transfers of wealth are not only possible but necessary if we are to break the cycle of poverty and disease. This was the spirit in which primary health care was advanced in 1978 as a central goal of public health.

Fourth, and perhaps most significant, good AIDS prevention and care programs do not drain resources away from primary health care. On the contrary, our experience in central Haiti suggests just the opposite. Writing of this experience, Joia Mukherjee notes that "providing a comprehensive HIV treatment program has necessitated revitalizing the public health infrastructure, and improving the delivery of essentials, such as vaccinations, sanitation, and clean water."[38] To the degree that public health goals prove to support, rather than exclude, each other, the rhetoric of "limited resources" and "cost-efficiency" begs for reexamination.

NOTES

1. "Declaration of Alma-Ata," International Conference on Primary Health Care.

2. Heggenhougen, "Will Primary Health Care Efforts Be Allowed to Succeed?"

3. United Nations Food and Agriculture Organization, "The State of Food Insecurity in the World"; U.S. Department of Health and Human Services, "The Surgeon General's Call to Action to Prevent and Decrease Overweight and Obesity."

4. In a 2003 speech, Craig Calhoun, president of the Social Science Research Council, argued that cost-effectiveness models do not begin to capture the complex web of benefits resulting from AIDS treatment:

> Take the statement that antiretroviral drugs are expensive. This is surely true, whether or not the ARVs in question are generics, and whether or not drug companies need additional income to support new research. But it obscures another question: compared to what? If ARVs ward off opportunistic infections that would result in expensive hospital visits, how much does that save? If they help employers maintain skilled labor forces, how much does that save? If they keep schoolteachers alive so that more don't have to be trained, how much does that save? If they provide potential orphans with real, living parents, how much does that save? . . . These are not just rhetorical questions. I mean them seriously. How much is saved? How do we integrate these factors into macroeconomic models in a meaningful way so that ministers of health and ministers of finance and ministers of education can be on the same page? ("U.S. and Multilateral Efforts to Fight HIV/AIDS")

5. On malaria, see Talisuna, Bloland, and D'Alessandro, "History, Dynamics, and Public Health Importance of Malaria Parasite Resistance." On the rise of drug-resistant tuberculosis, see Harvard Medical School and Open Society Institute, *The Global Impact of Drug-Resistant Tuberculosis;* and World Health Organization Global Tuberculosis Programme, *Anti-Tuberculosis Drug Resistance in the World, Third Global Report.*

6. Mayaud, Hawkes, and Mabey, "Advances in Control of Sexually Transmitted Diseases in Developing Countries," p. 32.

7. Farmer, *Infections and Inequalities.*

8. "Uganda: HIV Project Runs Out of Infant Milk," *The New Vision.*

9. UNICEF, *HIV and Infant Feeding.*

10. Fauci, "The AIDS Epidemic—Considerations for the 21st Century."

11. Marseille, Hofmann, and Kahn, "HIV Prevention before HAART in Sub-Saharan Africa," p. 1851.

12. On hunger in Haiti, see United Nations Food and Agriculture Organization, "The State of Food Insecurity in the World." For description and details of this pilot project, see Farmer and Walton, "Condoms, Coups, and Ideology of Prevention"; and Mukherjee et al., *Access to Antiretroviral Treatment and Care.*

13. UNAIDS, "2002 Report on the Global HIV Epidemic."

14. World Health Organization, *The World Health Report, 2003.*

15. Based on case estimates at the end of 2001. See UNAIDS, "2002 Report on the Global HIV Epidemic."

16. See Pape et al., "Characteristics of the Acquired Immunodeficiency Syndrome (AIDS) in Haiti"; Desvarieux and Pape, "HIV and AIDS in Haiti"; UNAIDS, "2002 Report on the Global HIV Epidemic."

17. Farmer, *AIDS and Accusation.*

18. Ibid.; Guérin et al., "Acquired Immune Deficiency Syndrome"; Pape and Johnson, "AIDS in Haiti."

19. The Département du Centre (along with Grand-Anse, in the south) has the lowest ratio of physicians to population and the smallest number of hospital beds per population (Haitian Ministry of Health and Population, "AIDS"). A 1998 study estimated that 66.1 percent of the population lived in poverty, with 33 percent in "extreme poverty" ("Enquête: Projet de marketing social").

20. Zanmi Lasante, "Rapport trimestriel des données de base."

21. Farmer, "Haiti's Lost Years."

22. Farmer, "Letter from Haiti."

23. Farmer, Léandre, Mukherjee, Gupta, et al., "Community-Based Treatment of Advanced HIV Disease."

24. Farmer, Robin, et al., "Tuberculosis, Poverty, and 'Compliance.'"

25. Farmer, Léandre, Mukherjee, Claude, et al., "Community-Based Approaches to HIV Treatment in Resource-Poor Settings."

26. Smith Fawzi et al., "Prevalence and Risk Factors of STDs in Rural Haiti." On treatment methods and broader social outcomes, see Mukherjee, *The PIH Guide to the Community-Based Treatment of HIV in Resource-Poor Settings.*

27. For complete details about Haiti's proposal to the Global Fund, see Global Fund to Fight AIDS, Tuberculosis, and Malaria, "Haiti's Response to HIV/AIDS."

28. Farmer, Léandre, Bayona, et al., "DOTS-Plus for the Poorest of the Poor."

29. Laga et al., "Non-Ulcerative Sexually Transmitted Diseases as Risk Factors for HIV-1 Transmission in Women"; Gilson et al., "Cost-Effectiveness of Improved Treatment Services for Sexually Transmitted Diseases in Preventing HIV-1 Infection in Mwanza Region, Tanzania."

30. Crofton, "The Contribution of Treatment to the Prevention of Tuberculosis."

31. Quinn et al., "Viral Load and Heterosexual Transmission of Human Immunodeficiency Virus Type 1."

32. Blower et al., "Predicting the Impact of Antiretrovirals in Resource-Poor Settings."

33. World Health Organization, *WHO Tuberculosis Programme.*

34. Mitnick et al., "Community-Based Therapy for Multidrug-Resistant Tuberculosis in Lima, Peru."

35. Cufino Svitone et al., "Primary Health Care Lessons from the Northeast of Brazil."

36. Kim, Shakow, Castro, et al., "Tuberculosis Control."

37. World Health Organization, *The World Health Report, 2003.*

38. Mukherjee, "HIV-1 Care in Resource-Poor Settings," p. 994.

14

AIDS in 2006—
Moving toward One World, One Hope?

(2006)

Jim Yong Kim and Paul Farmer

For the past two decades, AIDS experts—clinicians, epidemiologists, policymakers, activists, and scientists—have gathered every two years to confer about what is now the world's leading infectious cause of death among young adults. This year, the International AIDS Society is hosting the meeting in Toronto from August 13 through 18. The last time the conference was held in Canada, in 1996, its theme was "One World, One Hope." But it was evident to conferees from the poorer reaches of the world that the price tag of the era's great hope—combination antiretroviral therapy—rendered it out of their reach. Indeed, some African participants that year made a banner reading "One World, No Hope."

Today, the global picture is quite different. The claims that have been made for the efficacy of antiretroviral therapy have proved to be well founded: in the United States, such therapy has prolonged life by an estimated thirteen years[1]—a success rate that would compare favorably with that of almost any treatment for cancer or complications of coronary artery disease. In addition, a number of lessons, with implications for policy and action, have emerged from efforts that are well under way in the developing world. During the past decade, we have gleaned these lessons from our work in setting global AIDS policies at the World Health Organization in Geneva and in implementing integrated programs for AIDS prevention and care in places such as rural Haiti and Rwanda. As vastly different as these places may be, they are part of one world, and we believe that ambitious policy goals, adequate funding, and knowledge about implementation can move us toward the elusive goal of shared hope.

The first lesson is that charging for AIDS prevention and care will pose insurmountable problems for people living in poverty, since there will always be those unable to pay even modest amounts for services or medications, whether generic or branded. Like efforts to battle airborne tuberculosis, such services should be seen as a public good for public health. Policymakers and public health officials, especially in heavily burdened regions, should adopt universal-access plans and waive fees for HIV care. Initially, this approach will require sustained donor contributions, but many African countries have recently set targets for increased national investments in health, a pledge that could render ambitious programs sustainable in the long run.

As local investments increase, the price of AIDS care is decreasing. The development of generic medications means that antiretroviral therapy can now cost less than fifty cents per day, and costs continue to decrease to affordable levels for public health officials in developing countries. All antiretroviral medications—first-line, second-line, and third-line—must be made available at such prices. Manufacturers of generic drugs in China, India, and other developing countries stand ready to provide the full range of drugs. Whether through negotiated agreements or use of the full flexibilities of the Agreement on Trade-Related Aspects of Intellectual Property Rights, full access to all available antiretroviral drugs must quickly become the standard in all countries.

Second, the effective scale-up of pilot projects will require the strengthening and even rebuilding of health care systems, including those charged with delivering primary care. In the past, the lack of a health care infrastructure has been a barrier to antiretroviral therapy; we must now marshal AIDS resources, which are at last considerable, to rebuild public health systems in sub-Saharan Africa and other HIV-burdened regions. These efforts will not weaken efforts to address other problems—malaria and other diseases of poverty, maternal mortality, and insufficient vaccination coverage—if they are planned deliberately with the public sector in mind.[2] Only the public sector, not nongovernmental organizations, can offer health care as a right.

Third, a lack of trained health care personnel, most notably doctors, is invoked as a reason for the failure to treat AIDS in poor countries. The lack is real, and the brain drain continues. But one reason doctors flee Africa is that they lack the tools of their trade. AIDS funding offers us a chance not only to recruit physicians and nurses to underserved regions but also to train community health care workers to supervise care, for AIDS and many other diseases, within their home villages and neighborhoods. Such training should be undertaken even in places where physicians are abundant, since community-based, closely supervised care represents the highest standard of care for chronic disease,[3] whether in the First World or the Third. And community health care workers must be compensated for their labor if these programs are to be sustainable.

Fourth, extreme poverty makes it difficult for many patients to comply with antiretroviral therapy. Indeed, poverty is far and away the greatest barrier to the scale-up of treatment and prevention programs. Our experience in Haiti and Rwanda has shown us that it is possible to remove many of the social and economic barriers to adherence, but only with what are sometimes termed "wrap-around services": food supplements for the hungry, help with transportation to clinics, child care, and housing. In many rural regions of Africa, hunger is the major coexisting condition in patients with AIDS or tuberculosis, and these consumptive diseases cannot be treated effectively without food supplementation.[4] Coordination among initiatives such as the President's Emergency Plan for AIDS Relief, the Global Fund to Fight AIDS, Tuberculosis, and Malaria, and the World Food Program of the United Nations can help in the short term; fair trade agreements and support of African farmers will help in the long run.

Fifth, investments in efforts to combat the global epidemics of AIDS and tuberculosis are much more generous than they were five years ago, but funding must be increased and sustained if we are to slow these increasingly complex epidemics. One of the most ominous recent developments is the advent of highly drug-resistant strains of both causative pathogens. "Extensively drug-resistant tuberculosis" has been reported in the United States, Eastern Europe, Asia, South Africa, and elsewhere; in each of these settings, the copresence of HIV has amplified local epidemics of these almost untreatable strains. Drug-resistant malaria is now common worldwide, extensively drug-resistant HIV disease will surely follow, and massive efforts to diagnose and treat these diseases ethically and effectively will be needed. We have already learned a great deal about how best to expand access to second-line antituberculous drugs while increasing control over their use;[5] these lessons must be applied in the struggles against AIDS, malaria, and other infectious pathogens. The most effective way to slow the inevitable rise of drug resistance is to insist on supervised, community-based care.

Finally, there is a need for a renewed basic science commitment to vaccine development, more reliable diagnostics (the hundred-year-old tests widely used to diagnose tuberculosis are neither specific nor sensitive), and new classes of therapeutics. The research-based pharmaceutical industry has a critical role to play in drug development, even if the overall goal is a segmented market, with higher prices in developed countries and generic production with affordable prices in developing countries.

There has been a heartening increase in basic science investments for tuberculosis and malaria; funding for HIV research at the National Institutes of Health remains robust. Yet the fruits of such research will not arrive in time for those now living with, and dying from, AIDS and tuberculosis. New tools to prevent, diagnose, and treat the diseases of poverty will be added to the stockpile of other potentially lifesaving products that do not reach the poorest people, unless we develop an equity plan to provide them. Right now, our focus must be on improving access to the therapies that are available in high-income countries. The past few years have shown us that we can make these services available to millions, even in the poorest reaches of the world.

The unglamorous and difficult process of increasing access to prevention and care needs to be our primary focus if we are to move toward the lofty goal of equitably distributed medical services in a world riven by inequality. Without such goals, the slogan "One World, One Hope" will remain nothing more than a dream.

NOTES

1. Walensky et al., "The Survival Benefits of AIDS Treatment in the United States."

2. Walton et al., "Integrated HIV Prevention and Care Strengthens Primary Health Care."

3. Behforouz, Farmer, and Mukherjee, "From Directly Observed Therapy to *Accompagnateurs.*"

4. Paton et al., "The Impact of Malnutrition on Survival and the CD4 Count Response in HIV-Infected Patients Starting Antiretroviral Therapy."

5. Gupta et al., "Responding to Market Failures in Tuberculosis Control."

Structural Violence

Introduction to Part 3

Paul Farmer

To talk of the twentieth-century atrocities is in one way misleading. It is a myth that barbarism is unique to the twentieth century: the whole of human history includes wars, massacres, and every kind of torture and cruelty: there are grounds for thinking that over much of the world the changes of the last hundred years or so may have been towards a psychological climate more humane than at any previous time.

But it is still right that much of twentieth-century history has been a very unpleasant surprise. Technology has made a difference. The decisions of a few people can mean horror and death for hundreds of thousands, even millions, of other people.

JONATHAN GLOVER, *HUMANITY*

Part 3, "Structural Violence," stems from an abiding interest in (possibly an obsession with) the ways in which epic poverty and inequality, with their deep histories, become *embodied* and experienced as violence. With Haiti in mind, it's easy to see that socioeconomic processes, such as the entrenchment of chattel slavery in the eighteenth and nineteenth centuries and the violent responses to it, are still experienced as violence by those most affected, well after the lash is gone. Thus would the Haitians cited in these pages assure me that Haiti's everyday travails during the late twentieth century were the direct result of previous ones. Similar explanatory frameworks are common elsewhere, as I later discovered during visits to other places in Latin America. Returning to social theory, it was clear enough that, romantic notions about "resistance" aside, severe poverty constrained personal and collective agency and was experienced as violent and grossly unfair: the lash wasn't gone so much as transformed.

This understanding remains conceptual bedrock for me two decades after my first foray into writing for academic publications and university presses. But it wasn't easy to write and teach about such insights: how could the violence of poverty be compared, say, to that of war or slavery? In the early nineties, taking a cue from liberation theology, I began to write about "structural violence." Some years later, I was lucky enough to deliver the Sidney Mintz Lecture, "An Anthropology of Structural Violence," which is included in this reader (chapter 17). My remarks appeared in *Current Anthropology,* where the format required brief commentary from luminaries in the field.[1] These comments were generally encouraging, although one of my favorite sociologists argued that structural violence, which almost a decade previously had found its way into the title of a book I edited, was not a very useful construct. In graduate school, those would have been fighting words; but I thought, upon reading these critiques, "Hey, it's only a theoretical construct! We'll come up with some others."

That said, I haven't yet found a better phrase to convey the impact, through processes of embodiment and other mechanisms, of social disparities and poverty. Although the discussion of the Mintz Lecture took place in a specialized academic journal, all the participants took it seriously as more than an academic issue. I knew that many wars of ideas—not the shallow "culture wars" we read about in the United States, as described by Todd Gitlin and many others, but rather (and again) claims of causality about violence and suffering—were matters of life and death. It's a shame that we attribute to Henry Kissinger the clever aphorism about academic feuds being so bitter because the stakes are so low. It's not always true.

For example, claims of causality regarding the roots of Haiti's intransigent poverty and violence determine the movement of hundreds of millions of dollars' worth of capital, termed "aid"—which very often goes to the wrong recipients or the wrong projects. Claims of causality about why AIDS was, in the 1980s and 1990s, a major scourge in Haiti led to funding for some prevention efforts and not others. To claim that poverty, gender inequality, and the collapse of the agrarian economy were the chief co-factors in the epidemic, as I have here, was to watch funding opportunities disappear: who wants to fund efforts to lessen structural violence as an AIDS prevention method? (Answer: no foundation yet known.) Who wants to take on labor migration in southern Africa when it's easier, and cheaper, to pretend that the problem is cognitive rather than social and economic? If the problem of risk is in the heads and cultures of far-off peoples, let's invest in changing their "knowledge, attitudes, beliefs, and practices"—already called "KABP" in aid circles—rather than investing in labor practices that do not dissolve families and promote anomie. (Weber would be turning in his grave if he knew that anomie was rarely, if ever, considered in modern risk assessment, to say nothing of epidemiology.)

We once did a study of rates of sexually transmitted infections among pregnant women in rural Haiti and found that having such an infection was most strongly associated with three factors: being unemployed, having spent time in the city as a domestic servant, or being the sexual partner of a landless peasant seeking work across the border—in other words, increasingly typical conditions of young women in poverty.[2] But in the rapidly expanding world of global health, it's more fashionable to argue that risk resides largely in poor people's ignorance about such matters as the modes of transmission of various plagues.

How could shaky claims of causality be made with such confidence? One mechanism that allows this is desocialization: that is, erasing history and political economy and any notions of deep culture and cosmology (these latter also rooted, at the very least, in history and political economy). It's perfectly fine to strip affect from journal articles when the topic is the outcome of laboratory research (even though we know from studies such as those by Bruno Latour and Steve Woolgar that laboratory work itself is also shaped, often fundamentally, by social forces).[3] But the desocialization is extreme in much sociomedical literature, and with untoward effect. I found a paper in a pediatric journal that explored child survival in Rwanda just prior to the 1994 genocide, though published some time after it, and neither genocide nor political violence was mentioned at all, except obliquely, in the acknowledgements, when it was lamented that many of the authors' Rwandan coworkers had been killed.

Similarly desocialized are most studies of drug-resistant infections, a matter with which I've been occupied for two decades. You'd think that it would be difficult to credit studies of widespread drug resistance, which has emerged only since humans introduced antibiotics less than a century ago, that are *not* biosocial. What could be less "natural" or more biosocial than an epidemic of, say, drug-resistant tuberculosis spreading from prisons to the civilian population? Yet it is very difficult to receive substantial funding for properly biosocial research on this topic and much easier to find subsidies for desocialized research that does not broach such messy topics as social inequalities and access to medical care, prison conditions, or prescribers' views on wise antibiotic use. (Studies of the views of those who need their services are more common.) To invoke "the political economy of drug-resistant disease" makes it likely that your NIH grant won't even be reviewed, much less funded.

Desocialized understandings of social phenomena—I take it that epidemics are by definition social phenomena—are a major source of error and a significant reason for poorly prioritized investments in clinical medicine, public health, and attempts to intervene in the cycle of poverty and disease. I've written about "immodest claims of causality" in most of my books and in some of the essays included here. Most of these claims are immodest because they are not supported by knowledge of the history and political economy of the places in which epidemics progress or recede.

Structural violence under a purported rule of law requires justification, and so its maintenance leaves both normative code and a paper trail. Concerning slavery, for example, we need only review the Code Noir (France's rulebook for the traffic in human beings; all slaving nations, including mine, had one) and the meticulous records kept by the slave traders and their customers. Concerning more recent genocidal sprees in Guatemala, we can find handbooks and public statements by military officials; a huge cache of documentation of police and military activities is just now proving useful in prosecuting some of those involved in killing civilians. The same is true in Rwanda, where the mass media, especially the radio, played a prescriptive role.

It's a long way from slavery and genocide to formal acceptance of "the way the world is" (this expression often precedes a call for impunity or for the erasure of history). But it's difficult to imagine how widespread apathy regarding the short lives lived by some could reign without some sort of rationalization that is regarded as compelling. In our day, these rationalizations tend to be economic or pseudoeconomic, rather than religious or racial: actions deemed "reasonable" in polite circles must these days bear a stamp of approval such as "cost-effective," "sustainable," "transparent," or "measurable." All of these terms are used in international circles and enjoy enormous prestige in what some are now calling "audit cultures." "Procedures for assessment have social consequences, locking up time, personnel and resources, as well as locking into the morality of public management," Marilyn Strathern writes, discerning in this practice "the contours of a distinct cultural artifact."[4] It's not wise to say you're against accountability and measurement, but we didn't need the collapse of Wall Street finance to show us that "procedures for assessment" are not the exact science that the paladins of audits would suggest. The great majority of resources needed for such procedures are of course controlled by those who control other resources, so the ground rules of contemporary audit culture are *related,* at the very least, to the audit cultures of previous epochs, including colonialism.

In addition to crude similarities, it is clear that some interventions in public health are legitimated simply because of alleged quantification. I believe it's for this reason that modern audit culture rarely questions the veracity of cost-effectiveness analysis—as if either cost or effectiveness were easy to assess and quantify. As Peter Berger and Thomas Luckmann observe in *The Social Construction of Reality,* "legitimation justifies the institutional order by giving a normative dignity to its practical imperatives." Cost-effectiveness analyses are too seldom challenged, in part because they benefit from a normative dignity they too rarely merit. Berger and Luckmann also remind us that "to understand the state of the socially constructed universe at any given time, or its change over time, one must understand the social organization that permits the definers to do their defining. Put a little crudely, it is essential to keep pushing questions about the historically available conceptualizations of reality from the abstract 'What?' to the socially concrete 'Says who?'"[5]

Says who, indeed. It might not be a huge leap to argue that, in part because of desocialization and legitimation, audit cultures may become intimately related to what Michel Foucault termed "biopower." He wrote: "One might say that the ancient right to *take* life or *let* live was replaced by a power to *foster* life or *disallow* it to the point of death."[6] Biopower as such is difficult to discern when you're in the middle of events, as opposed to looking back as a historian, but imagine what a properly biosocial critique of cost-effectiveness analysis might reveal about power over approval or rejection of life-saving interventions.

The ways in which human life may be differentially valued, with some lives worth more than others, serve to introduce other topics in this section, including the relationship between different kinds of violence. Although the everyday indignities of structural violence do not usually involve weapons in the conventional sense, it's important to note the connection between structural violence and war or other forms of mass violence, such as genocide. This connection strikes me as undeniable and in need of investigation. It's important here to think about myths and mystifications, since we all live in a world in which it's acceptable, or accepted, to think up devious ways in which massive military expenditures might be considered normal or even necessary. It's in this context that land mines are made to look innocuous or even to mimic toys (the topic of chapter 20). Look at the U.S. military budget and at the justifications for wars we've seen just in the past few years, decades after we were warned about the "military-industrial complex" by no less a radical than Dwight Eisenhower. Eisenhower observed that the growth of this complex (which has its own, often arcane, audit culture) was sure to lead to a warping of collective priorities. He pointed out that "every gun that is made, every warship launched, every rocket fired signifies, in the final sense, a theft from those who hunger and are not fed, those who are cold and not clothed. This world in arms is not spending money alone. It is spending the sweat of its laborers, the genius of its scientists, the hope of its children."[7]

NOTES

1. Farmer, "An Anthropology of Structural Violence (Sidney W. Mintz Lecture for 2001)"; Bourgois et al., "Commentary on Farmer, Paul, 'An Anthropology of Structural Violence.'"

2. Farmer, "Ethnography, Social Analysis, and the Prevention of Sexually Transmitted HIV Infection among Poor Women in Haiti" (included in this volume as chapter 4).

3. Latour and Woolgar, *Laboratory Life*.

4. Strathern, *Audit Cultures*, p. 3.

5. Berger and Luckmann, *The Social Construction of Reality*, p. 93.

6. Foucault, *The History of Sexuality*, pp. 138, 139.

7. Eisenhower, "The Chance for Peace."

15

Women, Poverty, and AIDS

(1996)

*These days, whenever someone says the word "women" to me, my mind
goes blank. What "women"? What is this "women" thing you're talking
about? Does that mean me? Does that mean my mother, my roommates,
the white woman next door, the checkout clerk at the supermarket, my
aunts in Korea, half the world's population?*

JEEYEUN LEE, "BEYOND BEAN COUNTING"

*Macroeconomic conditions operating in a context of pervasive gender
inequality have different effects upon the lives of women in different
regional, class, and family circumstances. Different circumstances also
produce different negotiating strengths among women as well as different
HIV risks.*

BROOKE SCHOEPF, "GENDER, DEVELOPMENT, AND AIDS"

AIDS was first recognized as a distinct physical syndrome in the summer of 1981, when physicians in California and New York noted clusterings of unusual infections and cancers in their patients. All of these patients were young, gay men, a group not previously known to have such opportunistic infections. In August, a mere two months after the first cases were reported in men, the same syndrome was identified in a woman.[1] Within a year, AIDS cases were registered among men and women who injected drugs, among hemophiliacs and some of their sexual partners, and among women and men from poor countries, including Haiti, who seemed to share none of the risk factors seen in the other patients.

Since that time, both AIDS and commentary on it have swept the globe. Never before has a single sickness been the subject of such intense and sustained scrutiny. Given the intensity of public awareness and fear of AIDS, it is not surprising that so many myths and misunderstandings about this illness have thrived and even proliferated. Though surely there is a compelling interest in getting the facts right and developing appropriate responses on the basis of accurate research, fantasies and junk science have often dominated public discussions of AIDS.

The initial misunderstanding—that AIDS was a disease of men—can be attributed, perhaps, to historical accident: the new disease was first characterized in the technologically advanced United States, where it did, initially at least, primarily afflict men.[2] But from the outset of the world pandemic it was apparent that women were also vulnerable to AIDS, and, within a year or two, data began to suggest that women were at least as likely as men to become infected.

Evidently, however, AIDS cases involving women did not count for much. In 1985, a cover story in *Discover,* a popular science magazine, dismissed the idea of a major epidemic in women. The story claimed that because the "rugged vagina," in contrast to the "vulnerable anus," was designed for the wear and tear of intercourse and birthing, it was unlikely that large numbers of women would ever be infected through heterosexual intercourse. AIDS, we were informed, "is now—and is likely to remain—largely the fatal price one can pay for anal intercourse."[3]

Such mistaken verdicts were slowly called into question. By late 1986, it was becoming clear that AIDS incidence was declining among gay men even as it was climbing among those classified as the "heterosexual exposure group."[4] "Suddenly," proclaimed the cover of *U.S. News and World Report* in January 1987, "the disease of them is the disease of us." The accompanying illustration depicted the "us" in question as a white, yuppie couple.[5] (The image was epidemiologically inaccurate as far as HIV was concerned—white, yuppie couples were not those falling ill with heterosexually acquired HIV infection—but was probably accurate in its depiction of which "us" concerned the editors of the magazine.)

In her study of the gradual evolution of U.S. AIDS discourse, Paula Treichler discerns a "diversification" of commentary about women and AIDS in the spring of 1987.[6] Nonetheless, one still heard voices maintaining that women would never constitute a significant proportion of AIDS victims. *The Myth of Heterosexual AIDS,* released in 1990 by a commercial publisher with strong ties to the conservative movement, typifies that sort of thinking: "Among the great wide percentage of the nation the media calls 'the general population,' that section the media and the public health authorities has [sic] tried desperately to terrify, there is no epidemic. AIDS will pick off a person here and there in this group, but the original infected partner will be one of the two groups in which the disease is epidemic. Most heterosexuals will continue to have more to fear from bathtub drowning than from AIDS."[7]

The irony here is not one of false predictions. Even as such projections were being written, millions of women—whose partners were neither bisexual men nor intravenous drug users—had already been "picked off" by HIV. Even in the United States, where the epidemic among women had initially been closely linked to injection drug use, the proportion of women reported to have been exposed by a partner whose risk was not specified—in other words, not an inject-ing drug user—quintupled between 1983–84 and 1989–90. In the five years pre-ceding the publication of *The Myth of Heterosexual AIDS*, the percentage increase in annual AIDS incidence was greater among the "heterosexually acquired" exposure group than in any other.[8] By 1991, AIDS was the leading killer of young women in most large U.S. cities.[9]

The mismatch between reality and representation led Paula Treichler to pose the following question in 1988: "Given the intense concern with the human body that any conceptualization of AIDS entails, how can we account for the striking silence, until very recently, on the topic of women in AIDS discourse (includ-ing biomedical journals, mainstream news publications, public health literature, women's magazines, and the gay and feminist press)?"[10] In other words, why did many continue to think of AIDS as a disease of men? More poignantly, perhaps, why were the voices of women with AIDS absent from scientific and popular commentary a full decade into the pandemic?[11]

One explanation is that the majority of women with AIDS had been robbed of their voices long before HIV appeared to further complicate their lives. In settings of entrenched elitism, they have been poor. In settings of entrenched racism, they have been women of color. In settings of entrenched sexism, they have been, of course, women.

If it is finally recognized that AIDS poses enormous threats to poor women, this wisdom comes too late. Throughout the world, millions of women are already sick with complications of HIV infection. In the United States and in Latin America, the epidemics among women are increasing at a rate much higher than those registered among other groups: AIDS is already the leading cause of death among young African American women living in the United States.[12] In Mexico, the male:female ratio of HIV infection went from 25:1 in 1984 to 4:1 in 1990. In São Paulo, Brazil, seroprevalence among pregnant women increased sixfold in only three years.[13]

Similarly disturbing trends are reported elsewhere in the world, particularly in developing countries, where 90 percent of all adults and 98 percent of all children infected with HIV live.[14] In many sub-Saharan African nations, there are already more new infections among women than among men. In 1992, the United Nations Development Programme estimated that "each day a further three thousand women become infected, and five hundred infected women die. Most are between 15 and 35 years old."[15] The World Health Organization has predicted that, during the course of the 365 days of the year 2000, between six and eight million women will become infected with HIV.[16]

Once we begin to see the extent of these problems, further questions emerge. By what mechanisms did most seropositive women come to be infected with HIV? If not all women are at high risk, which groups of women are most likely to be exposed to the virus? How is women's risk similar in vastly different settings? How is it different? Has scholarly research—whether clinical investigation, epidemiology, or social science—kept pace with the advancing AIDS pandemic? Finally, what effects have persistent misunderstandings about women and AIDS had on the allocation of resources designed to prevent, detect, or treat the complications of HIV infection?

To answer these questions, we begin by examining the experience of three women living with HIV. These women are from very different backgrounds: "Darlene" is an African American woman from Harlem; "Guylène" is the daughter of poor peasants from rural Haiti; "Lata" was living in a rural Indian village when, at the age of fifteen, she was sold into prostitution in Bombay. Their stories, similar in some ways and different in others, speak to many of the questions raised here.

DARLENE

Darlene Johnson was born in Central Harlem in 1955, one of three children of a woman who was chronically homeless, leaving her husband and children for long periods of time. Darlene remembers her parents having terrible fights in which her father hit her mother and her mother "cried for days." When Darlene was five, her mother sent her to Alabama to live with her maternal grandmother.

Darlene was shuttled back to New York City when she was eleven and was left in the care of her brother, who was ten years older. Darlene's brother, angry that this new burden narrowed his own life chances, beat her frequently. With no other means of support, Darlene lived with her abusive brother until after eleventh grade, when she married a "hardworking man." The couple soon had two children. "No welfare," she says. "We never did it, not even when things were hard."

Things were often hard. The couple had many problems. Chief among them was their mutual passion, not for each other, but for heroin: "I didn't love him," she recalls. "He beat me, sometimes in front of the kids. It was drugs." After six years of abuse, Darlene found a way to leave. She and her children went to live with her estranged father.

A short while after moving in with her father, Darlene met her second husband. This marriage was for love. Her husband, also a heroin user, worked. They had two sons. Her two older children also loved this man, and things were looking up. Although she used heroin, Darlene insists that it didn't interfere with taking care of her children: "It just made things smooth," she says.

In 1987, her stepbrother, also a heroin user, was diagnosed with AIDS. "He just died," Darlene states; no mess, no fuss. Everyone in the family was stunned. Shortly thereafter, Darlene's stepfather had a fatal heart attack. An autopsy disclosed that he too had been HIV-infected.

Darlene grieved but was determined to keep her family together. Then her husband began to have high fevers and night sweats. He refused to go to the doctor, but Darlene knew it must be AIDS. By this time, she was tortured by the memory of all the times that she, her husband, and her stepbrother had shared needles. Darlene was tested and learned that she was indeed HIV-positive.

Her husband died two months later. Alone with four children, Darlene was heartbroken: she had lost her husband, her stepbrother, and her stepfather in a single year. Two women who were her baby's godparents and who had also shared needles became ill, and they too died.

Darlene was not only heartbroken. She was also broke, forced to add the constant struggle to make ends meet to the struggle to overcome her grief. Her children kept her going. She suspected that her youngest son, sick from birth with one thing or another, was also infected. His first serious bout with pneumonia made everything clear: "I didn't know he had it till they took my baby to the hospital." At this time, Darlene was, by her own account, in a state of shock. "Too many close people" had died.

Darlene decided to set up her home to care for her son. She didn't want to abandon him in the hospital, and so she learned to do everything she could for him. When her older children began to act up, cutting school and hanging out in the streets, Darlene tried to get them help, to no avail. There was nothing for them. The counselors in their schools couldn't be trusted not to divulge information about her illness and that of her son.

Soon the children were completely out of hand. By this time, the baby stared at Darlene as if he didn't know who she was. Crack, she explains, came to be the only way she could find to ease her pain. But, as always, there was a price to pay. She began to lose patience with her children. She yelled often; she didn't cook regular meals for them. She was relieved when they were away. Darlene felt she had nothing but pain:

> This social worker was telling everybody I had the virus. . . . The police came looking for me when my little son ran away, he ran away with my big son; my big son brought him home. When I came downstairs, the cops jumped all the way down the stairs. "Oh, you supposed to be in the hospital 'cause you got AIDS." Everybody on the street was looking at me. . . . [The social worker] told my kids' friends, their parents. A little boy was up in the fire escape, he said, "Oh, look—there's David's mother; she got AIDS."

Darlene concluded that her children were suffering and neglected. She felt there was no family; everyone had died. So she turned to the Department of Social Services and asked that her three oldest children be placed in foster care while she tried to care for the youngest, now dying of AIDS. "I just didn't want to live anymore, and I didn't want the kids to be running in the street, to be hungry."

The children were placed in separate homes. The oldest was sent to a home in the Bronx, but he ran away to live with a friend of Darlene's who wanted him and who was willing to support him. Darlene also wanted the child to be with her friend, but she knew city authorities would never grant custody to this woman, so she said nothing. Darlene's daughter was placed with a woman Darlene knew to be a drug user: "They put my daughter in a house where they sell drugs, crack. My daughter watches this lady's kids." Darlene is powerless to change the placement.

Her third child was placed in New Jersey with a family that Darlene likes. He is well cared for, and she expects the family to adopt him when she dies. She is grateful for them and wants the adoption to happen. She attends family therapy sessions with this family. This son, she feels, will be all right.

Having given her children to foster care, and now left alone with her youngest, Darlene found it painful to care for him. The little boy suffered terribly, she recalls. His stomach became more and more distended, and he stopped responding to her. Finally, one night as he lay in bed with her, he stopped breathing. This death "took me out completely," Darlene says. "He was three years old. It took him six months to die." Now six people in her life had died in a single year.

Darlene gave in to crack completely and hit rock bottom. She lived on the streets for three months but was desperate "not to die that way." The children counted on seeing her. She went into the hospital to detoxify from crack and enrolled in a methadone program. Once in the program, she saw a doctor. All during the year of deaths, she had never gone to a doctor for herself. She thinks she must have been very depressed.

Darlene, too, has been diagnosed with AIDS, but mostly she worries about her two oldest children. She could have used some help with them when all the deaths began. Darlene sees the two children who live near her every day. She visits the son who lives in New Jersey every week. She says she'll see them this way until she dies. She only hopes she doesn't linger.[17]

GUYLÈNE

Guylène Adrien was born in Savanette, a dusty village in the middle of Haiti's infertile Central Plateau. Like other families in the region, the Adriens fed their children by working a small plot of land and selling produce in regional markets. Like other families, the Adriens were poor, but Guylène recalls that they "had enough to get by."

She was the third of four children, a small family by Haitian standards. It was to become smaller still: Guylène's younger sister died in adolescence of cerebral malaria. Guylène's oldest sister is said to be somewhere in the Dominican Republic, where she has been living, if she is living, for over a dozen years.

Guylène's other surviving sister lives with her mother and two children, working the family plot of land for ever-diminishing returns.

Guylène recounts her own conjugal history in the sad voice reserved for retrospection. When she was a teenager—"perhaps fourteen or fifteen"—a family acquaintance, Occident Dorzin, took to dropping by to visit. A fairly successful peasant farmer, Dorzin had two or three small plots of land in the area. In the course of these visits, he made it clear to Guylène that he was attracted to her. "But he was already married, and I was a child. When he placed his hand on my arm, I slapped him and swore at him and hid in the garden."

Dorzin was not so easily dissuaded, however, and eventually approached Guylène's father to ask for her hand—not in marriage, but in *plasaj*, a potentially stable form of union widespread in rural Haiti. Before she was sixteen, Guylène moved with Dorzin, a man twenty years her senior, to a village about an hour away from her parents. She was soon pregnant. Dorzin's wife, who was significantly older than Guylène, was not at all pleased, and friction between the two women eventually led to dissolution of the newer union. In the interim, however, Guylène gave birth to two children, a girl and then a boy.

After the break with Dorzin, Guylène and her nursing son returned to her father's house. She remained in Savanette for five months, passing through the village of Do Kay on her way to the market in Domond or to visit her daughter, who remained in Dorzin's care. It was during these travels that she met a young man named Osner, who worked intermittently in Port-au-Prince, the capital city, as a laborer or a mechanic. One day he simply struck up a conversation with Guylène as she visited a friend in Do Kay. "Less than a month later," she recalls, "Osner sent his father to speak to my father. My father agreed." Leaving her toddler son in her parents' household, Guylène set off to try conjugal life a second time, this time in Do Kay.

The subsequent months were difficult. Guylène's father died later that year, and her son, cared for largely by her sister, was frequently ill. Guylène was already pregnant with her third child, and she and Osner lacked almost everything that might have made their new life together easier. Osner did not have steady work in Port-au-Prince, though he was occasionally able to find part-time jobs as a mechanic.

After the baby was born, in 1985, they decided to move to the city: Osner would find work in a garage, and Guylène would become involved in the marketplace. Failing that, she could always work as a maid. In the interim, Osner's mother would care for the baby, as Do Kay was safer for an infant than was Port-au-Prince.

Osner and Guylène spent almost three years in the city. These were hard times. Political violence was resurgent, especially in their neighborhood of Cité Soleil, a vast and notorious slum on the northern fringes of the city. The couple was often short of work: he worked only irregularly as a mechanic; she split her time between jobs as a maid and selling fried food on the wharf in Cité Soleil. Guylène much preferred the latter:

> Whenever I had a little money, I worked for myself selling, trying to make [my business] last as long as I could. When we were broke, I worked in ladies' houses. . . . If the work is good, and they pay you well, or the person is not too bad, treats you well, you might stay there as long as six or seven months. But if the person treats you poorly, you won't even stay a month. Perhaps you only go for a single day and then you quit. . . . Rich women often hate poor women, so I always had trouble working for them.

When asked what she meant by decent pay, Guylène stated that the equivalent of twenty dollars a month was passable, as long as you were able to eat something at work.

In 1987 (Darlene Johnson's year of losses), three "unhappy occurrences" came to pass in quick succession in Guylène's life. A neighbor was shot and killed during one of the military's regular nighttime incursions into the slum; bullets pierced the thin walls of Guylène and Osner's house. A few weeks later, Guylène received word that her son had died abruptly. The cause of death was never clear. And, finally, Osner became gravely ill. It started, Guylène recalls, with weight loss and a persistent cough.

Osner returned to the clinic in Do Kay a number of times in the course of his illness, which began with pulmonary tuberculosis. In the case of a young man returning from Port-au-Prince with tuberculosis, it was routine practice to consider HIV infection in the differential diagnosis, and it was suggested as a possibility at that time. In the clinic, Osner reported a lifetime total of seven sexual partners, including Guylène. With one exception, each of these unions had been monogamous, if short-lived.

When Osner did not respond, except transiently, to biomedical interventions, many in the village began to raise the possibility of AIDS. At his death in September 1988, it was widely believed that he had died from the new disease. His doctors concurred.

Guylène subsequently returned to Savanette, to a cousin's house. She tried selling produce in local markets, but she could not even support herself, much less the child she had left in the care of Osner's mother. She was humiliated, she says, by having to ask her mother-in-law for financial assistance, even though she informed the older woman that she was pregnant with Osner's child. Finally, a full year after Osner's death, the fetus "frozen in her womb" (as she put it) began to develop. It was, she insisted, Osner's baby. (Others identified a man from her hometown of Savanette as the child's father.) She had the baby, a girl, in November of 1989. Osner's mother always referred to the child as her granddaughter.

A month after her confinement, Guylène returned to Savanette with the baby. She was unemployed; her mother and sister were barely making ends meet. Guylène and others in the household frequently went hungry. Believing herself to be a burden, Guylène finally went to the coastal town of Saint-Marc, where she had cousins. She worked as a servant in their house until the baby became ill; Guylène, too, felt exhausted. Since medical care was readily available only in Do Kay, she returned again to the home of Osner's mother. Guylène and Osner's first child had already started school there, and Osner's mother allowed that she could always find food for two more.

By early June 1992, Guylène was ill: she had lost weight and become amenorrheic. Later that month, a doctor at the clinic heard her story with some alarm. Yes, Guylène acknowledged, she had heard of AIDS; some had even claimed that Osner had died from it, but she knew that was not true. After reviewing Osner's chart, the physician encouraged her to be tested for HIV. She was leaving for Port-au-Prince, Guylène informed him, but would return for the results. The child's physical exam was unremarkable except for pallor and a slightly enlarged liver. The baby was treated, empirically, for worms and also for anemia and sent home.

The next day, Guylène returned to Port-au-Prince. She worked a few days as a maid but found the conditions intolerable. She tried selling cigarettes and candy, but she remained hungry and fatigued. The city was in the throes of its worst economic depression in recent decades. "I was ready to try anything," she remembers.

Shortly thereafter, Guylène's fourth baby died quite suddenly of cardiac failure, presumed secondary to HIV cardiomyopathy. Although the child had never been tested for antibodies to the virus, Guylène's test had come back positive a few days prior to the tragedy.

Guylène was informed of her positive serology on the day following her return; she listened impassively as a physician went through the possible significance of the test and made plans to repeat it. Careful physical examination and history suggested that Guylène had not yet had a serious opportunistic infection. Her only manifestations of HIV infection at that time were severe anemia, amenorrhea, weight loss, occasional fevers, and some swelling of her lymph nodes.

Guylène began visiting the clinic regularly following confirmation of her positive HIV serology. Her doctors spoke with her regularly—"too often," she once remarked—about HIV infection and its implications. She was placed on prophylactic isoniazid, an iron supplement and multivitamins, and also a protein supplement. Guylène did not return to Port-au-Prince; instead, she rented a house with the financial aid she received through an AIDS treatment program based in the village.

Although Guylène experienced significant improvement in less than a month, she remained depressed and withdrawn. A young man named René had been visiting her, but Guylène discouraged him, and he disappeared—"he went to Santo Domingo, I think, because I never heard from him again." In mid-November, however, Guylène responded to the advances of a soldier stationed in Péligre. A native of a large town near the Dominican border, with a wife and two children there, the soldier had been in the region for only about a month. Although residents of Péligre reported that he had a regular partner in that village as well, Guylène insists that she was his only partner in the region:

> He saw me here, at home. He saw me only a couple of times, spoke to me only a couple of times, before announcing that he cared for me. After that, he came to visit me often. I didn't think much of it until he started staying over. I got pregnant at about the time they announced that he was being transferred back to [his hometown]. He said he'd be back, but I never saw or heard from him again.

Because Guylène's physicians had gone to some trouble to advise her against unprotected sexual intercourse, they were anxious to know how conversations about this subject may have figured in her decision to conceive another child, if indeed the pregnancy was the result of a decision. That Guylène understood what it meant to be an asymptomatic carrier of HIV seemed clear from a metaphor she used to describe herself: "You can be walking around big and pretty, and you've got a problem inside. When you see a house that's well built, inside it's still got ugly rocks, mud, sand—all the ugly, hidden things. What's nice on the outside might not be nice on the inside."

Guylène understands, too, that her child might well be infected with HIV. But she is impatient with questions, tired of talking about sadness and death: "Will the baby be sick? Sure, he could be sick. People are never *not* sick. I'm sick . . . he might be sick too. It's in God's hands."

Now Guylène draws near to the close of her fifth pregnancy, which may well culminate in another death. Two of her children are dead; two others have long looked to a father or grandmother for most of their parenting. Guylène's own sisters are dead, missing, or beaten into submission by the hardness of Haiti. Few of her nephews and nieces have survived into adulthood. Guylène assures her physicians that she is without symptoms, but she seems inhabited by a persistent lassitude.[18]

LATA

When Lata first entered the world somewhere in rural Maharastra, in a small thatched hut lit only by lanterns, her mother began weeping—tears not of joy but of shame that she had brought yet another daughter into the world. "God must not have been very happy with me that day," she said. Lata does not know what month she was born into her untouchable Harijan family with two sisters and three brothers, but the year was 1967. Her father farmed a very small plot in Solapur, a small agricultural village. As Lata remembers it, her mother did nearly all of the remaining work:

> So much of my childhood is a blur to me. I remember when my father would return home he would beat my mother for her cooking or because one of us was crying. And if he had drunk too much, he would beat my sister and me, the whole time my mother running around to prepare better food or make us quiet so father could eat. It seems every day passed like this, the only difference being that father got meaner as he grew older.

Never permitted to attend school, Lata by the age of six was tilling and weeding with her father. "Years passed like this," she remarks, examining her hands as if for traces of blisters. Her two elder sisters were married at the ages of fifteen and sixteen, and both weddings came at a heavy price to Lata's family. One sister's dowry totaled 10,000 rupees—almost twice her father's earnings for that year. Predictably, both marriages forced the family to turn to the local moneylender, a man who maintained interest rates as high as 25 percent—compounded quarterly. Lata's father, already faced with selling off more of his tiny plot in order to service his debt, lived in fear of another wedding.

Lack of rainfall during the 1982 monsoon season brought a poor harvest, leaving the family in the worst financial state it had ever experienced. "My father was drinking more every day," Lata says. "Sometimes I recall him not even going out to the fields, yet forcing us to go, and beating us more than he ever had. I know he was worried about my getting married, and when he was drunk he would curse my mother, blaming her for bringing him yet another daughter."

In this context, the arrival of a man who would take Lata from the despair of her village life was regarded as a godsend. Like so many other *dalals* ("middlemen," many of whom are women) who come from Bombay, Prasant had for some years been making a "decent" living in the flesh trade. As he worked a route from the villages of southern Maharastra to the bordellos of Bombay, his scheme was identical in almost every settlement. Upon arrival in a village, Prasant would seek out a local moneylender and, often with the help of a small bribe, extract information about area families with young daughters and heavy debt. Prasant, like other *dalals,* then approached the male heads of families, claiming to have work for their daughters as servants or seamstresses in Bombay. In Lata's case, her father was told that she would be given work as a dishwasher:

> After [Prasant] arrived, my father took my mother aside and told her that jobs were available in Bombay, and this man would give him 11,000 rupees as a payment for me washing dishes and housecleaning. He said I would be able to mail money home every month and allowed to visit Solapur after six months of work. Not for one moment did anyone suspect or question what he told us.

Desperate, hungry, facing the most acute poverty his family had ever experienced, Lata's father saw opportunity and relief in his daughter's departure. A few hours after he and Prasant spoke, Lata was told to pack her two cotton saris, her bangles, and sandals. She would leave for Bombay in the morning.

A frail and frightened fifteen-year-old, Lata had difficulty holding back tears as she waved goodbye. Her father's gaze was stoic, while tears streamed down her mother's face. It was the last time she would ever see her parents.

She remembers nothing of her trip to Bombay, although it was her first train ride. Her inability to recollect, she suspects, was the result of a drug she had been given. The next memory she has is of a taxi in Bombay. Lata was entering the city's red-light district. Barely awake, she was brought to Number 27, Falkland Road, where Prasant sold her to a pimp for 15,000 rupees—about five hundred dollars. His tidy profit of 4,000 rupees was more than enough to carry him through the month.

Lata had arrived in the Kamathipura district of Bombay, and she was about to become one of its thirty thousand sex workers. She remembers regaining complete consciousness in a "cage"—a cramped room full of girls putting on makeup, oiling their hair, and tightening their petticoats and blouses. Lata had no comprehension of where she was:

> I saw all of these girls wearing nothing but colored blouses, makeup, and skirts, and asked the madam, "What is this?" She told me it was a place for working girls. I still didn't understand, frightened by the very clothes these women wore. Sapna, the madam, told me I would be staying with her and ordered me to put on clothes that lay on the floor for me and then stand outside. I began crying and told her I couldn't stay. She slapped me hard, and I remember I couldn't stop crying. I told her to let me go, and she looked me straight in the eye and said, "You want to leave, fine. Give me 15,000 rupees and you're free. Until then, get dressed and start paying back your *kurja*."

Lata's *kurja* was her debt, the mechanism by which she was indeed trapped as if in a cage. She did not join the other girls on the street that day, nor the day after. She slept and lay in the corner of the room, pretending to be ill, eating the food she was given, and listening to the other girls call out to customers on Falkland Road. She watched the parade of men and girls in and out of the adjacent room, furnished only with a bed. On Lata's third day in Bombay, Sapna's patience had been exhausted: she ordered one of her managers to "break Lata in."

No matter how many years pass, Lata says she always has trouble recounting this part of her story. Arun, a manager whose main responsibility was to bring in new customers, also had the duty of making sure the girls were bringing in enough money and "working" hard. As one madam put it, "There are times when they won't listen to us, so the managers and pimps keep the girls in line." Lata recalls:

> I had been sitting in the same corner for days, pretending I was not feeling well, frightened, and wishing Sapna would let me go. Finally Arun came to me and pulled me by my ear, telling me to put on the clothes and stand outside. I was a fifteen-year-old village girl and didn't even know what sex was, let alone prostitution. How could I understand what was going on? He took me to the room with the bed and closed the door and forced me to have sex with him. Afterwards, he said, "Now do you understand?" and laughed and told me to get to work. I remember being silent while the other girls stared at me when I came out. I'm sure they knew what he did. And for the first time I began to accept that there was no way out—I was here to stay.

That day, Lata, clad in a purple blouse and pink petticoat, nervously joined the thousands of prostitutes of Bombay's red-light districts. It was her first night on the streets and the beginning of a long and painful career.

Unlike most other girls, who stand in front of the cages, beckoning to passing men, Lata stood quietly, receiving no business during her first three days out. The days were long: bathing at around 10 in the morning, out on Falkland Road by 11, lunch at 4 P.M., and back on the street until 2 or 3 A.M., with dinner if she was lucky. On an average day, a Bombay prostitute may see four to five customers a day. Times may vary, but generally late evening is when they are busiest. Early in the afternoon of her fourth day, Lata was finally approached:

> An Arab man came, and after seeing me spoke with the madam for some time and wanted to take me to the Taj Hotel for three days. I saw him give her many hundred rupee notes, and then he took me into his taxi and to the hotel. I was terrified of being alone with him; you have to remember that he was my first customer and I had no idea what to do. The first night we slept in separate beds, and the next day he took me to sari and jewelry shops, buying me clothes and gold. When he would go out in the day, he would lock me in the room. But the more he bought, the more scared I became of what he would expect. On the second night, he told me to dress in all of the clothes he bought for me. Frightened as I was, I knew that I had no choice. At that moment, I remember saying to myself, "This is now my life," truly accepting it for the first time. . . . No longer willing to fight him or my own self, I had sex with him.

Upon her return to Falkland Road, Lata settled into the routine of a Bombay prostitute. Slowly, she came to know the stories of the girls in her brothel and others nearby. Although they hailed from many villages and even from Nepal, most had similar experiences. Like the others, she gave half of her daily earnings to the madam as repayment for her *kurja*. Yet Lata knew that she, and all girls sold into prostitution, had little hope of ever buying her freedom; her initial debt of 15,000 rupees was accruing interest at a rate of 20 to 25 percent a month. If a pimp brought a customer to her, she owed him 25 percent. And in most areas, police regularly extorted money from sex workers with the threat of jail. With an average of four or five customers per day, each paying about 20 to 30 rupees, she could be left with as little as 20 rupees to cover food, clothing, and other basic needs.

At this writing, Lata has been in Bombay for thirteen years. She is a well-known figure at Number 27, Falkland Road, a small brothel sandwiched between a tea stall and a large pink building brimming with Nepali girls. Proudly wearing her gold bangles, her hair always neatly oiled and braided, Lata is now a respected "veteran" of the red-light community. At twenty-eight years of age, she continues to see an average of four or five customers a day.

Rumor of AIDS did not reach the red-light district of Bombay until 1989 or so—surely well after the virus itself had arrived. "Back then, I and other people on Falkland Road started to know about AIDS, but we did not take it seriously. Then the Indian Health Organization people came and gave us free condoms."

In 1991, Lata became one of the first sex workers to volunteer as an AIDS peer educator, and she pushes her fellow prostitutes to demand that their clients use condoms: "I tell the girls, it's your life. If he refuses to wear one, send him away. And even if he offers you one million for sex without a condom, you don't do it. But I know this is hard. There are too many hungry girls. Too many scared girls. And the madams are always watching, putting on pressure."

Preventive messages came too late for Lata, who now knows that she is infected with HIV. She continues to work as both an AIDS outreach worker and a prostitute.[19]

SEX, DRUGS, AND STRUCTURAL VIOLENCE

The stories of Darlene, Guylène, and Lata—recounted in detail in order to bring into relief the forces constraining their options—reveal both differences and commonalities. But how locally representative is each woman's history?

Darlene Johnson's tragic experiences are all too commonplace among African American women. Because she was a heroin user, a habit clearly tied to a poverty structured by racism, her chances of avoiding HIV were slim, even if she had wanted to quit using prior to her diagnosis. In 1987, the year that Darlene's world was burst asunder by AIDS, only 338,365 treatment slots were available to the nation's estimated four million addicts, and most of these programs predominantly served men; as a pregnant woman, Darlene would have found it next to impossible to find treatment for her addiction.[20] Writing about women of color who are addicted and live in poverty, Janet Mitchell and coworkers point out that "access to care and services has traditionally been marginal for women with any one of these three criteria. Any two of these . . . essentially put women in the extremely limited access category. Women with all three of these characteristics fall into the no access category."[21]

In the United States, HIV has moved, almost unimpeded, through poor communities of color. By 1991, African Americans, who constitute approximately 12 percent of the U.S. population, accounted for 30 percent of all reported AIDS cases. During the 1980s, the cumulative incidence of AIDS was more than eleven times higher for black women than for white women. Although many early cases were among those who injected drugs, the epidemic is fast expanding among women with no such history. As noted earlier, AIDS is the leading cause of death among African American women between the ages of twenty-five and forty-four; for Latinas in this age group, it is now the third leading cause of death.[22] When the first multicenter study of AIDS among U.S. women was funded, almost 78 percent of over thirteen hundred patients recruited were women of color.[23]

Understanding the strikingly patterned U.S. epidemic is less a matter of knowing one's geography and more a matter of understanding a limited number of events and processes—the "synergism of plagues" discussed by Rodrick Wallace—that range from unemployment to the destruction of housing by fires.[24] "Urban poverty in the United States has created the perfect machinery for the continued propagation of HIV," writes Robert Fullilove. "Inner city poor neighborhoods often shelter a vigorous drug trade, numerous opportunities for strangers to engage in drug-mediated, unprotected sex, and numerous locations where these and other risk behaviors go virtually unchallenged."[25] Darlene's lamentable experience is all too typical.

In Haiti, similarly, young women are driven into domestic service and unfavorable unions by poverty; like Guylène, they have little choice about their acceptance of risk.[26] Indeed, their testimony calls into question facile notions of "consensual sex."

Lata's painful experience also exemplifies that of hundreds of thousands of poor girls in India, Nepal, and elsewhere. It has been estimated that up to 50 percent of Bombay's prostitutes were recruited through trickery or abduction.[27] Although no real population-based surveys have yet been conducted, it is highly likely that most of India's prostitutes have high rates of HIV infection. In the late 1980s, some seven hundred sex workers were arrested and forcibly taken to the city of Madras, where 70 percent of them were found to have antibodies to HIV. Many of these women were jailed or subjected to other forms of harassment, including having their names publicly listed.[28]

In short, the experiences of Darlene, Guylène, and Lata are all too typical. One clear lesson is that both the immediate and systemic causes of increased risk need to be elucidated. For example, heroin use—and needle sharing—put Darlene at increased risk of HIV infection. Sex work—or, rather, unprotected sex work—put Lata at risk of HIV infection. But in Harlem and Bombay, it seems fair to assert that the decisions these women made were linked to their impoverishment and their subordinate status as women. Furthermore, it is important to remember that

Darlene and Guylène and Lata were born into poverty. Their attempts to escape poverty were long bets that failed—and AIDS was the form their failure took.

The stories recounted here force a difficult question: how many girls are, from birth, at inordinate risk of AIDS or some other dreadful destiny? "For some women," explains the founder of an AIDS support group for women, "HIV is the first major disaster in their lives. For many more, AIDS is just one more problem on top of many others."[29] In fact, those in the former category—women for whom HIV is an altogether unprecedented misfortune—are in the minority. Attentiveness to the life stories of women with AIDS usually reveals that their illness is the latest in a string of tragedies. "For poor women," observes anthropologist Martha Ward, "AIDS is just another problem they are blamed for and have to take responsibility for. They ask, 'How am I going to take care of my family?' 'I have to put food on the table now.' 'You think AIDS is a problem! Let me tell you—I got real problems!'"[30]

Millions of women living in similar circumstances—but with very different psychological profiles and cultural backgrounds—can expect to meet similar fates. Their sickness may be thought of as a result of structural violence: neither nature nor pure individual will is at fault; rather, historically given (and often economically driven) processes and forces conspire to constrain individual agency.[31] Structural violence is visited on all those whose social status denies them access to the fruits of scientific and social advances.

If meaningful responses to AIDS are to be presented, the differential political economy of risk must be revealed. Structural violence means that some women are, from the outset, at high risk of HIV infection, while other women are shielded from risk. Reflecting on the experiences detailed here and adopting this point of view—that we can describe a political economy of risk and that this exercise helps to explain where the AIDS pandemic is moving and how quickly—we begin to see why similar stories are legion in sub-Saharan Africa and India and fast becoming commonplace in Thailand and other parts of Asia. The experiences recounted here may be considered textbook cases of vulnerability, but their moral is deciphered only if we clearly understand that these women have been rendered vulnerable to AIDS through social processes—that is, through the economic, political, and cultural forces that shape the dynamics of HIV transmission. Anthropologist Brooke Schoepf, writing from Zaïre, explains how AIDS has "transformed many women's survival strategies into death strategies":

> Women, who often lack access to cash, credit, land or jobs, engage in "off-the-books" activities in the informal sector. Some exchange sex for the means of subsistence. Others enter sex work at the behest of their families, to obtain cash to purchase land or building materials, to pay a brother's school fees, or to settle a debt. Still others supplement meager incomes with occasional resort to sex with

multiple partners. Married or not, the deepening economic crisis propels many to seek "spare tires" or "shock absorbers" to make ends meet.[32]

Taken together, the dynamics of HIV infection among women and the responses to its advance reveal much about the complex relationship between power/powerlessness and sexuality. All sexually active women share biological risk to some extent, but the AIDS pandemic among women is clearly patterned along social, not biological, lines. And many questions remain unanswered. For example, by what mechanisms, precisely, do social forces (such as poverty, sexism, and other forms of discrimination) become embodied as personal risk? What role does inequality per se play in promoting HIV transmission?

Like all societies characterized by extreme inequality or structural violence, the linked societies of Darlene, Guylène, and Lata require other kinds of violence in order to maintain the status quo, which is so unbearable for the majority. In the United States, the enormous number of African Americans in prisons reflects this violence, as do death squads in Haiti and police brutality in Bombay. Other forms of structural violence are more strikingly gendered: for instance, a political economy favoring the import of poor Nepali girls to the economic powerhouse that is India.

HIV and direct violence against women are intimately linked. Among sex workers, risk of assault and risk of HIV are both highest among the poorest prostitutes.[33] Many of the estimated four million U.S. women who are assaulted by their male partners are precisely those at heightened risk for HIV. As Sally Zierler points out, "This figure, awful as it is, obscures the fact that some women are more at risk than others. For like HIV's distribution, partner violence against women follows social divisions marked by class position, and race/ethnicity, creating strata of extreme vulnerability to violence victimization."[34]

In an era of widespread and instantaneous communication, symbolic violence is also used to accomplish these ends: structural violence requires its apologists, witting or unwitting. We now turn to the role played by researchers and other opinion shapers in buttressing the myths and mystifications related to the topic of women and AIDS.

WOMEN AND AIDS: MYTHS AND MYSTIFICATIONS

Throughout the world, the majority of women with HIV infection are poor. They are denied access not merely to resources and services but also to symbolic capital. In her thoughtful examination of the gendering of American AIDS discourse, Paula Treichler asks, "Why were women so unprepared? And why do they continue to take it so quietly?" She responds to her own question with a candor that is all too rare:

As evidence of AIDS in women mounted, speculations linked the disease to prostitutes, intravenous drug users, and women in the Third World (primarily Haiti and countries in central Africa). It was not that these three groups were synonymous but, rather, that their differentness of race, class, or national origin made speculation about transmission possible—unlike middle-class American feminists, for example. American feminists also by this point had considerable access to public forums from which to protest ways in which they were represented, while these other groups of women were, for all practical purposes, silenced categorically so far as public or biomedical discourse was concerned.[35]

This silencing refers to the absence of the voices of poor women in public forums ranging from conferences to published material. But they have not, in fact, been silent—they have simply been unheard. In rural Haiti, for example, a group of poor women committed to preventing AIDS worked together in 1991 to generate a list of common myths about women and AIDS. The document prepared by the group made reference to the following myths:

AIDS is a disease of men. The data are overwhelming: AIDS was never a disease of men. Given transmission dynamics, AIDS may in fact become a disease afflicting predominantly women.

"Heterosexual AIDS" won't happen. Heterosexual AIDS has already happened. Indeed, in many parts of the world, AIDS is the leading cause of death among young women.

Women's promiscuity causes AIDS. Most women with AIDS do not have multiple sexual partners; they have never used i.v. drugs; they have not received tainted blood transfusions. Their major risk factor is being poor. For others, the risk is being married and unable to control not only their husbands but also what jobs their husbands have to perform to make a living.

Women are AIDS vectors. Women are too often perceived as agents of transmission who infect men and innocent babies. Prostitutes have been particularly hard hit by such propaganda, but prostitutes are far more vulnerable to infection than to infecting: AIDS is an occupational risk of commercial sex work, especially in settings in which sex workers cannot safely demand that clients use condoms.[36]

Condoms are the panacea. Gender inequality calls into question the utility of condoms in settings in which women's ability to insist on "safe sex" is undermined by a host of less easily confronted forces. Furthermore, many HIV-positive women choose to conceive children, which means that barrier methods that prevent conception are not the answer for many. Woman-controlled viricidal preventive strategies are necessary, if women's wishes are to be respected.

While these were the myths deemed salient in rural Haiti, other, related mystifications are to be found in every setting in which poor women must now add HIV to a long list of quotidian threats. In the United States, Martha Ward complains of "urban folklore" about mothers with AIDS: "'Those women' have food stamps. They buy alcohol or luxury items. They have infected their innocent babies. They should use birth control, get abortions, get a job, finish school, use condoms, and say 'no' to drugs."[37]

What many of the dominant myths and mystifications have in common is an exaggeration of personal agency, typically through highlighting certain psychological or cultural attributes, even though it is not at all clear that these attributes are in any way related to women's risk for HIV infection. Condoms are a classic case in point. Several studies have revealed that most U.S. women at high risk of HIV infection are already aware that condoms can prevent transmission, but many of these women are unable to insist that condoms be used. Although most acknowledge the link between poverty and low rates of condom use, few studies have carefully explored the association. A study conducted among African American women in Los Angeles showed that couples in which the woman depended on her male partner for rent money were less likely to use condoms than couples in which the woman had more financial independence.[38]

There is nothing wrong with underlining personal agency, but there is something unfair about using personal agency as a basis for assigning blame while simultaneously denying those who are being blamed the opportunity to exert agency in their lives. "A patronage that simultaneously grants 'victims' powerlessness and then assigns them blame for that powerlessness is nothing new," argues Jan Grover. "It is therefore important to make connections between the construction of AIDS victimhood and similar constructions of the poor, who also suffer the triple curse of objectification, institutionalized powerlessness, and blame for their condition."[39]

The objectification of "the poor" is, of course, a risk run by any who use the term, but striving to understand a person's material constraints is hardly tantamount to a refusal to recognize the salience of personal experience. Recognizing a commonality of constraint—in addition to, say, a commonality of psychology or of culture—is an important part of unraveling the nature of risk. Indeed, failure to see individual risk in its larger context of social and economic determinants is often synonymous with intense focus on personal psychology or "deviant subcultures."

Among the myriad mystifications important in obscuring the nature of women's risk, three are recurrent. One is the focus on local factors and local actors to the exclusion of broader analyses that would implicate powerful forces and powerful actors outside the field of view. A second is the conflation of structural violence and cultural difference. A third, centrally related to the others, is the absence of serious considerations of social class.[40] These are not infrequently the mechanisms by which personal agency is exaggerated in both scholarly and popular commentary. To cite Brooke Schoepf again: "the structure of the wider political economy establishes the situations and restricts the options that people can choose as a means of survival. A focus on 'subcultures,' as on individual behaviors, tends to obscure the underlying causes of social interaction."[41]

These expedient erasures and exaggerations are buttressed, rather than challenged or exposed, by research published in a host of key journals. For example, a review of the ever-enlarging epidemiological literature reveals that although racism, sexism, and powerlessness go unmentioned, we usually do find mention of culture. Take a study conducted by Adeline Nyamathi and coworkers in the Los Angeles area among 1,173 women between the ages of eighteen and seventy-five. Half were African Americans; half were designated as Latinas and described as either "high-acculturated" or "low-acculturated." Recruited through homeless shelters or drug treatment programs, all of these women had histories of using drugs, being the sexual partner of an injecting drug user, being homeless, or having a sexually transmitted disease (STD). Some had histories of sex work; some had multiple sexual partners. A survey of these women revealed that "African-American and Latina women were equally knowledgeable about AIDS symptomatology; the etiologic agent of AIDS; and behaviors known to reduce risk of HIV infection, such as using condoms and cleaning works used by intravenous drug users."[42] Greater differences existed concerning how much the women knew about modes of transmission, but the women tended to overestimate transmissibility, not to underestimate it.

In a sense, then, what the researchers found was that ignorance about HIV was not really the issue for these women. What put them at risk for HIV was something other than cognitive deficits. But the researchers' interpretation of their findings, published in the influential *American Journal of Public Health*, was not in keeping with the data: "These findings suggest the need for culturally sensitive education programs that cover common problems relating to drug use and unprotected sex and, in addition, offer sessions for women of different ethnic groups to address problematic areas of concern."[43] Was this truly a key implication of the research? By the researchers' own standards, these women were by and large fully aware that HIV could be transmitted through injection drug use and unprotected sex. Moreover, the more often women had used drugs or had multiple sexual partners, the more likely they were to perceive themselves, correctly, as being at increased risk of HIV infection.

By insisting that "culturally sensitive education programs" have a large role to play in protecting poor women from AIDS, the authors are asserting, all evidence to the contrary, that ignorance of the facts is centrally related to high HIV risk and that, consequently, the way to diminish risk is through increasing knowledge. Through this cognitivist legerdemain, we have expediently moved the locus of the problem—and thus the interventions—away from certain features of an inegalitarian society and toward the women deemed "at risk." The problem is inherent in the women; therefore the interventions should be designed to change the women.

The cost of all this desocialization might well be significant, for cognitivist, behaviorist, or culturist assumptions often privilege effects over cause. Immodest claims of causality, and even undue focus on the psychological or cultural peculiarities of those with AIDS, are not only incorrect emphases; they also serve to expediently deflect attention away from the real engines of the AIDS pandemic. Thus when the *éminences grises* of STD control examine the possibilities for effective AIDS control in developing countries, their list of interventions ranges from public lectures to "long-term psychotherapy for HIV-positive individuals" and "group therapy for commercial sex workers."[44]

Similar themes are widely echoed in a society known for its obsession with individualism. It is not surprising, then, to hear the same exaggerations of agency even from those most committed to preventing AIDS. Often, we hear about a certain community's "denial" of risk or about the epidemic of "low self-esteem" among those living with HIV infection. These cultural and psychological factors are then granted etiologic power: rather than being understood as effects, they are construed as the source of increased risk.

Sadly, if predictably, the same calculus of causality can be found in the comments of those afflicted by AIDS. The founder of one group for women living with HIV put it this way: "Low self-esteem is a significant 'co-factor' that led many women to be at risk of acquiring HIV."[45] Surely there are co-factors for "low self-esteem"—and poverty, otherwise known in post-welfare America as hunger and homelessness, is the obvious leader among them. Other variations on this theme of inequality, including racism and sexism, are also high on the list.

Such immodest claims of causality serve to deflect attention away from structural violence. No wonder U.S. Republicans and their friends among the Democrats have had so little difficulty promoting the same hypotheses. In the recently promulgated "Personal Responsibility Act," recipients of Aid to Families with Dependent Children (AFDC) are called to work a minimum of thirty-five hours per week in a designated "work slot." Since these women, unlike the authors of the act, have more than a passing knowledge of math, they know that with a median disbursement of $366 per month and an hourly wage in such "slots" of well under $3, they will be unable to assemble the funds necessary to provide day care, let alone health care and safe housing, for their children. Even in cities with modest costs of living, a single mother of two children would need an hourly wage of $10 in order to cross the poverty line.[46] We are left to surmise that these women's infants and toddlers will prepare their own formula and meals. As Valerie Polakow, who interviewed scores of single American mothers, bitterly states, this experience should give these babies an early lesson in the importance of personal responsibility. "As . . . rhetoric against won't-work mothers and promiscuous teens escalates," concludes Polakow, "it advances the pernicious idea that poverty is a private affair, that destitution and homelessness are simply products of bad personal choices."[47]

From typhoid to tuberculosis and AIDS, blaming the victim is a recurrent theme in the history of epidemic disease.[48] In case after case, analysis can lead researchers to focus on the patients' shortcomings (failure to drink pure water, failure to use condoms, ignorance about public health and hygiene) or on the conditions that structure people's risk (lack of access to potable water, lack of economic opportunities for women, unfair distribution of the world's resources). The results are not indifferent. One of the chief benefits of choosing to see illness in global-systemic terms is that it encourages physicians (and others concerned to protect or promote health) to make common cause with people who are both poor and sick. In addition, analyses that resolutely embed personal experience in the larger social fields in which such experience takes on its meaning have far more explanatory power in examining epidemics of infectious disease—particularly those such as AIDS, which move along the fault lines of our interlinked societies.

In conclusion, the most frequently encountered and easily circulated theories about women and AIDS are far more likely to include punitive images of women as purveyors of infection—prostitutes, for example, or mothers who "contaminate" their innocent offspring—than to include images of homelessness, barriers to medical care, a social service network that doesn't work, and an absence of jobs and housing. Dominant readings are likely to suggest that women with AIDS have had large numbers of sexual partners, but are less likely to show how girls like Lata are abducted into the flesh trade and are even less likely to reveal how political and structural violence—for example, the increasing landlessness among the rural poor and the gearing of economies to favor export—come to be important in the AIDS pandemic today.

For women most at risk of HIV infection, life choices are limited by racism, sexism, political violence, and grinding poverty. It is a wonder, then, that discussions of AIDS so rarely focus on these issues. Complex indeed are the mechanisms by which such structural violence can be effaced and the apparent significance of personal choice (or cultural difference) inflated. But when dominant myths about women and AIDS are contrasted with the experiences of Darlene and Guylène and Lata, we are forced to call into question many of these understandings.

WHAT NOW?

In rural Haiti in 1991, a group of poor women, some of them living with HIV, met to consider AIDS and its effects on their communities. They agreed that although many were infected with HIV through means well beyond their own control, not enough had been done to educate the people in the region. How could they join forces to make up for this deficiency? It was out of the question to use written materials in a setting of nearly universal illiteracy, and the military government had just taken control of many of the area's radio stations. In the end, these women—who had never had electricity in their homes and had never owned televisions—decided to produce a videotape that told a story very similar to Guylène's. They then worked with Partners In Health to acquire a portable generator, a video projector, and a screen. Condom demonstrations and community discussion accompanied each showing of the video.[49]

Proud of their success, the women subsequently spoke of their experience at a number of meetings and conferences held in rural Haiti. In one of these conferences, a Haitian physician (herself not unsympathetic to the trials of the women who had made the video) listened to a presentation by one of the women and saw the video. During the discussion, the doctor faced the project participant, who had proudly introduced herself as a *malerez*, a "poor woman," and asked, "So what? In other words, if we are manifestly failing to prevent HIV transmission in this region, what is the significance of your project?"

The *malerez* lost no time in answering: "Doctor, when all around you liars are the only cocks crowing, telling the truth is a victory."

Telling the truth about the nature of women's risk would be no mean feat in the current climate.

A second, and related, set of tasks concerns prevention. Making condoms readily available is an altogether insufficient response. Getting the right message across remains a priority, now and in the future, as HIV is unlikely to be eradicated soon. Adolescents everywhere in the world simply must learn about STDs before becoming sexually active. Universal HIV education needs to become part of growing up, which might also help to attenuate AIDS-related stigma. Clearly, such efforts will need to be different in different settings, but the universal finality and obstinacy of AIDS have changed the way we think about sexuality and sexism. Teens throughout the world need to learn about the relationship between HIV transmission and social forces such as poverty and gender inequality.

A third set of activities might be targeted toward specific groups of those at risk for HIV infection. In northern Tanzania, for example, improving the quality and accessibility of treatment for STDs reduced the incidence of HIV by 42 percent.[50] Injecting drug users need ready access to drug treatment programs, but we know that needle-exchange efforts can decrease the incidence of new infections even in the absence of adequate clinical treatment.[51]

Stopping prostitution will require addressing poverty, gender inequality, and racism, but in the absence of serious societal programs aimed at doing that, public health authorities can make a priority of protecting, rather than punishing, sex workers.[52] Commercial sex workers have benefited from high-quality medical care, especially when it is provided with their well-being—rather than that of their clients—in mind. "It is important," one advocate emphasizes, "that a full range of health care services, including health care for their children and not just STD services, be made more accessible—and more acceptable—to prostitutes."[53] Attacking AIDS-related stigma will require attacking the stigmatization of sex workers, gays, and other scapegoated groups.

For women already living with HIV disease, improved clinical services are critical. This means, among other things, educating health care professionals about women and AIDS.[54] HIV infection is underrecognized in women, with many cases diagnosed during pregnancy—or at autopsy. When AIDS case definitions were changed to include, among other conditions, invasive cervical cancer, the number of AIDS diagnoses in U.S. women doubled in a single year.[55]

Improving services further implies the removal of barriers that currently prevent poor women, regardless of their HIV status, from obtaining much-needed resources. These resources range from access to certain medications to safe housing. Although data are incomplete, the 1996 HIV Epidemiologic Research Study conducted in the urban United States indicates that in one large cohort of women, the majority of patients with advanced HIV disease were not receiving *Pneumocystis* prophylaxis, to say nothing of antiretroviral therapy. In the same cohort, most women did not have housing security; almost 20 percent stated that they had "no safe place to live."[56] Given that HIV-positive Americans face AIDS-related discrimination ranging from insults to loss of jobs and housing, the tasks before us in this country are indeed challenging, if less so than the tasks facing those who would change the frightful conditions endured by poor women living in poor countries. Scrupulous attention to these matters could, in principle, prolong the lives of millions of women already infected.[57]

Finally, it is important to recall that women are also affected by AIDS in indirect ways, for it is women who bear the brunt of caring for the sick, regardless of age or gender.[58] For this reason, improving the quality of care for all people living with AIDS will improve the lives of the women who care for them.

Through these three sets of tasks alone—that is, setting the record straight, rethinking prevention activities, and improving the array of services available to women and to all persons with AIDS—much can be done to strengthen the hand of women living in poverty. With perseverance and commitment, such measures might eventually result in the slowing of the rate of HIV transmission to poor women.

As important as these AIDS-focused activities are, they largely attack the symptoms of a deeper malaise. Endeavors focused on AIDS, though crucial, must be linked to efforts to empower poor women. The much-abused term "empower" is not meant vaguely here; it is not a matter of self-esteem or even parliamentary representation. Those choosing to make common cause with poor women must seek to give them control over their own lives. Control of lives is related to the control of land, systems of production, and the formal political and legal structures in which lives are enmeshed. In each of these arenas, poor people are already laboring at a vast disadvantage; poor women's voices are almost unheard.

The occurrence of HIV in wealthy countries, where even those living in poverty control more resources than women like Guylène and Lata do, reminds us that HIV tracks along steep gradients of power. In many settings, HIV risks are enhanced not so much by poverty in and of itself but by inequality. Increasingly, what people with AIDS share are not personal or psychological attributes. They do not share culture or language or a certain racial identity. They do not share sexual preference or an absolute income bracket. What they share, rather, is a social position—the bottom rung of the ladder in inegalitarian societies. Writing from Bombay, Sarthak Das underlines similarities in the experience of the untouchable castes of India and poor people of color in U.S. cities: "We need only replace the categories of 'Black' and 'Hispanic' with the low caste, untouchable titles of *Harijan* and *Sudra* in order to observe a parallel epidemiological pattern on the subcontinent."[59]

This is why efforts to promote pragmatic solidarity must engage not only local inequalities but also global ones. The trials of women like Guylène and Lata pose challenges to women—and, of course, to all people of goodwill—in the rich countries. Can we somehow lessen the huge and growing disparities that characterize our world? Within rich countries, the struggles of women like Darlene Johnson are even more of a rebuke, challenging facile notions of sisterhood and solidarity. Unlike Guylène and Lata, Darlene lives within a mile of a world-class medical center. At key points in her experience, however, that center might as well have been half a world away. Without insurance, Darlene did not have ready access to it.

The rapidly growing literature on women and AIDS is well stocked with pieties about solidarity, but the progress of this disease among women seems to take particular advantage of the lack of solidarity among the members of an AIDS-affected society. Very often, when solidarity fails, the reasons are less about color and more about class. A working-class lesbian writes that "HIV makes a mockery of pretend unity and sisterhood." Those most affected, she points out, are women of color and poor white women, many of whom are "struggling with long histories of shooting drugs or fucking men for the money to get those drugs. These are not the women usually identified as the women the feminist movement or the lesbian movement most value and try to organize to create a progressive political agenda."[60] Guylène reserved some of her harshest commentary for the women for whom she worked as a servant: "Rich women often hate poor women, so I always had trouble working for them." In Bombay, not only are the madams, of course, women, but so are many of the *dalals* who abduct teenage girls from their home villages.

One of the contributors to *Listen Up,* a collection of feminist essays, observes: "Many feminists seem to find the issues of class the most difficult to address; we are always faced with the fundamental inequalities inherent in late-twentieth-century multinational capitalism and our unavoidable implication in its structures."[61] Whose interests are served by writing of one group of women with AIDS while ignoring millions of others because of nationality? Clearly, HIV cares little for national boundaries. If inequality is an important co-factor in this pandemic, then stopping AIDS will require a more ambitious agenda, one that calls for the fundamental transformation of our world. What is at stake in these tasks is well expressed by Brooke Schoepf: "Unless the underlying struggles of millions to survive in the midst of poverty, powerlessness, and hopelessness are addressed, and the meanings of AIDS understood in the context of gender relations, HIV will continue to spread."[62]

NOTES

1. Centers for Disease Control and Prevention, "*Pneumocystis* Pneumonia—Los Angeles."

2. For a review of how data gathering was structured in the early years of the epidemic, see Oppenheimer, "In the Eye of the Storm."

3. Langone, "AIDS," p. 52. As Paula Treichler notes of this essay, "Though more vivid and apodictic (i.e., presented as unarguable), Langone's conclusion parallels the conclusion of many scientists" ("AIDS, Gender, and Biomedical Discourse," p. 250, n. 72).

4. For a review of data documenting these trends, see Slutzker et al., "Trends in the United States and Europe," pp. 610–14. It should be noted, however, that changing AIDS incidence was patterned among gay men: although decreases were registered among white, middle-class gay men, this was not the case among poorer gay men and gays of color. See Lemp et al., "Survival for Women and Men with AIDS"; Osmond et al., "HIV Infection in Homosexual and Bisexual Men 18 to 29 Years of Age."

5. *U.S. News and World Report* cited in Treichler, "AIDS, Gender, and Biomedical Discourse," p. 193.

6. Treichler, "AIDS, Gender, and Biomedical Discourse: An Epidemic of Signification," pp. 193, 196.

7. Fumento, *The Myth of Heterosexual AIDS,* p. 32. The first edition was published in 1990. The 1993 paperback edition is prefaced with unrepentant claims that heterosexual AIDS remains a myth.

8. Slutzker et al., "Trends in the United States and Europe," pp. 612–13.

9. See Selik, Chu, and Buehler, "HIV Infection as Leading Cause of Death among Young Adults in U.S. Cities and States." In 1991, the Centers for Disease Control reported that in fifteen U.S. cities,

AIDS had become the leading cause of death among women between the ages of twenty-five and forty-four.

10. Treichler, "AIDS, Gender, and Biomedical Discourse," p. 193.

11. A 1994 editorial in the *American Journal of Public Health* would seem to support these claims, as it notes that only at the 1994 HIV/AIDS conference in Yokohama were women's voices at last heard (Stein, "What Was New at Yokohama—Women's Voices at the 1994 International HIV/AIDS Conference").

12. Centers for Disease Control and Prevention, "Update: AIDS among Women—United States, 1994"; see also Gwinn et al., "Prevalence of HIV Infection in Childbearing Women in the United States"; Wasser, Gwinn, and Fleming, "Urban-Nonurban Distribution of HIV Infection in Childbearing Women in the United States."

13. These figures are taken from reports by the U.S. Centers for Disease Control and Prevention and from Mann, Tarantola, and Netter, *AIDS in the World,* which provides an excellent overview.

14. Global AIDS Policy Coalition, *Status and Trends of the HIV/AIDS Pandemic as of January 1, 1995;* Global AIDS Policy Coalition, *Status and Trends of the HIV/AIDS Pandemic as of January 1, 1996.*

15. United Nations Development Programme, *Young Women,* p. 2.

16. World Health Organization, *The World Health Report, 1995.*

17. For studies of social settings akin to Darlene's, see Pivnick, "HIV Infection and the Meaning of Condoms"; Pivnick et al., "Reproductive Decisions among HIV-Infected, Drug-Using Women." The sociography of AIDS in New York is compellingly detailed in the following works, among others: Fullilove et al., "Black Women and AIDS Prevention"; Fullilove, Lown, and Fullilove, "Crack 'Hos and Skeezers"; Fullilove, "Community Disintegration and Public Health"; Fullilove et al., "Trauma, Crack, and HIV Risk"; Clatts, "All the King's Horses and All the King's Men" and "Disembodied Acts"; Waterston, *Street Addicts in the Political Economy;* Friedman, Des Jarlais, and Sotheran, "AIDS Health Education for Intravenous Drug Users"; Friedman and Des Jarlais, "HIV among Drug Injectors"; Worth, "Sexual Decision-Making and AIDS" and "Minority Women and AIDS"; as well as four studies by Rodrick Wallace: "A Synergism of Plagues"; "Urban Desertification, Public Health, and Public Order"; "Social Disintegration and the Spread of AIDS"; and "Social Disintegration and the Spread of AIDS—II."

18. For more details on the nature of HIV transmission in Haiti, see Farmer, "Sending Sickness" (included in this volume as chapter 2); Farmer, *AIDS and Accusation;* Farmer, "Culture, Society, and the Dynamics of HIV Transmission in Rural Haiti."

19. See the fine ethnographic study "AIDS in India," by Sarthak Das, who collected the material presented here. For overviews of the AIDS situation in India, see Naik et al., "Intravenous Drug Users—A New High-Risk Group for HIV Infection in India"; Mathai et al., "HIV Seropositivity among Patients with Sexually Transmitted Diseases in Vellore."

20. See Hunter, "Complications of Gender," p. 37.

21. Mitchell et al., "HIV and Women"; cited in Schneider and Stoller, *Women Resisting AIDS,* p. 4.

22. Centers for Disease Control and Prevention, "Update: AIDS among Women—United States, 1994." For a review of these data, see Lewis, "African-American Women at Risk," p. 57.

23. Data from the HIV Epidemiologic Research Study (HERS) suggest that 60 percent were African American, 17.5 percent Latina, and 21.5 percent white. See the section on HERS in the summary available at http://aspe.hhs.gov/health/reports/hivdatabases/cdc01.html (accessed July 2, 2009).

24. Wallace, "A Synergism of Plagues." See also Singer, "AIDS and the Health Crisis of the U.S. Urban Poor."

25. See Fullilove, "Community Disintegration and Public Health," p. 96; Fullilove et al., "Black

Women and AIDS Prevention." The Fulliloves draw heavily on the work of Rodrick Wallace. See also McCord and Freeman, "Excess Mortality in Harlem," which reports that, for some groups, age-specific mortality rates are higher in Harlem than in Bangladesh. For an excellent and responsible ethnographic account of injection drug users in New York, see the work of Anitra Pivnick (Pivnick, "HIV Infection and the Meaning of Condoms"; Pivnick et al., "Reproductive Decisions among HIV-Infected, Drug-Using Women"). For an overview of AIDS in African American communities and public health responses, see Wilson and Pounds, "AIDS in African-American Communities and the Public Health Response."

26. For an overview of the study, see Farmer, "Culture, Society, and the Dynamics of HIV Transmission in Rural Haiti."

27. See Das, "AIDS in India."

28. Nataraj, "Indian Prostitutes Highlight AIDS Dilemmas." See also the helpful review in Alexander, "Sex Workers Fight against AIDS."

29. Denison, "Call Us Survivors!" p. 205.

30. Ward, "Poor and Positive," p. 61.

31. For more on structural violence, see Farmer, "On Suffering and Structural Violence" (included in this volume as chapter 16).

32. Schoepf, "Gender, Development, and AIDS," p. 57.

33. See, for example, Miller, "'Your Life Is on the Line Every Night You're on the Streets.'"

34. Zierler, "Hitting Hard," p. 209. Sally Zierler later humanely adds: "These strangling forces of disenfranchisement are likely to include partners of women as well, given class and racial/ethnic distribution of women most at risk for HIV and violence. People who are violent against women may have experienced assaults against their own humanity, through racial discrimination, economic impoverishment and the social alienation that accompanies it" (p. 217).

35. Treichler, "AIDS, Gender, and Biomedical Discourse," pp. 194, 207.

36. Many other assessments concur: "It is worth noting that despite the portrayal of prostitute-as-vector, as of January 1989, in the United States, ' . . . there [had] been no documented cases of men becoming infected through contact with a specific prostitute'" (Carovano, "More Than Mothers and Whores," p. 136).

37. Ward, "Poor and Positive," p. 60.

38. Wyatt, "Transaction Sex and HIV Risks."

39. Grover, "AIDS," p. 30.

40. The effects of these (witting and unwitting) obfuscations on explorations of suffering are examined in Farmer, "On Suffering and Structural Violence" (chapter 16 of this volume). For an overview on the inattention to class in U.S. health data, see Krieger and Fee, "Social Class"; Navarro, "Race or Class versus Race and Class."

41. Schoepf, "Gender, Development, and AIDS," p. 59. For a similarly critical examination of the literature on drug addicts in the United States, see Waterston, *Street Addicts in the Political Economy.*

42. Nyamathi et al., "AIDS-Related Knowledge, Perceptions, and Behaviors among Impoverished Minority Women," p. 68.

43. Ibid., p. 70.

44. Holmes and Aral, "Behavioral Interventions in Developing Countries," p. 337. It should be noted, however, that these interventions do not really square with these authors' excellent analysis of the nature of the problem.

45. Denison, "Call Us Survivors!" p. 205. This phenomenon is by no means unique to AIDS. Alisse Waterston has powerfully argued that street addicts, too, "have, de facto, joined hands with the larger public in believing the ideology of deviance and the myth of the defiant dope fiend. As

such, their roles in social reproduction are obscured, actual resistance is subverted, and other alternatives are suppressed" (*Street Addicts in the Political Economy*, p. 245). See also Connors, "The Politics of Marginalization."

46. A 1994 study conducted in the state of Nebraska revealed that a single woman with two children needed an annual income greater than $21,887 to make ends meet—about $9,000 dollars more than the 1994 federal poverty level. "These numbers are a conservative estimate of a decent but no-frills standard of living," the report's author summarizes. "There's no room here for savings to buy a home, pay for college or build up a nest egg for retirement—all items which have typically defined a middle-class standard of living" ("Federal Poverty Level Not Realistic," *Omaha World-Herald*).

47. Polakow, "Lives of Welfare Mothers," p. 592. See also Polakow, *Lives on the Edge*.

48. See Ryan, *Blaming the Victim;* Farmer, *AIDS and Accusation,* especially part 4.

49. For a fuller account of this project, see Farmer, "Ethnography, Social Analysis, and the Prevention of Sexually Transmitted HIV Infection among Poor Women in Haiti" (included in this volume as chapter 4).

50. See "Improved STD Treatment," *AIDS Analysis Africa.*

51. Don Des Jarlais and coworkers provide an overview of these studies, which come from both Europe and North America; see, for example, Des Jarlais and Friedman, "Needle Sharing among IVDUs at Risk for AIDS"; Des Jarlais, Friedman, and Casriel, "Target Groups for Preventing AIDS among Intravenous Drug Users"; Des Jarlais, Friedman, and Sotheran, "The First City"; Des Jarlais et al., "International Epidemiology of HIV and AIDS among Injecting Drug Users"; Des Jarlais, Friedman, and Ward, "Harm Reduction"; Des Jarlais et al., "AIDS Risk Reduction and Reduced HIV Seroconversion among Injection Drug Users in Bangkok."

52. For examples of AIDS-related repression against sex workers and for insights concerning the importance of organization among prostitutes, see Alexander, *Prostitutes Prevent AIDS;* Alexander, "Sex Workers Fight against AIDS"; Lockett, "CAL-PEP." The differences in the constraints faced by sex workers in different settings warrant emphasis. As Priscilla Alexander shows ("Sex Workers Fight against AIDS," pp. 107–13), prostitutes have had an easier time organizing in Europe, North America, and Australia; in poor countries, the lot of women in the sex industry has been far bleaker. Within these countries, there is also immense variation in the nature of sex work.

53. Alexander, "Sex Workers Fight against AIDS," p. 105. Alexander offers an overview of the effects of providing poor care to sex workers.

54. There are several investigations of the underrecognition of HIV infection among poor women living in the United States; see, for example, Schoenbaum and Webber, "The Underrecognition of HIV Infection in Women in an Inner-City Emergency Room," which showed that in one Bronx emergency room serving the poor, only 11 percent of women were assessed for HIV risks. Other studies continue to reveal significant variation in the knowledge of AIDS management in the United States, with the expected attendant results.

55. Centers for Disease Control and Prevention, "Update: AIDS among Women—United States, 1994."

56. See the section on HERS in the summary available at http://aspe.hhs.gov/health/reports/hivdatabases/cdc01.html (accessed July 2, 2009).

57. A study by Richard Chaisson, Jeanne Keruly, and Richard Moore suggests that if first-rate HIV care is provided to a cohort of poor persons, then "access to medical care is a more important predictor of survival than are sex, race, and income level" ("Race, Sex, Drug Use, and Progression of Human Immunodeficiency Virus Disease," p. 755). This is a remarkable claim and, if true, heartening news for physicians and other providers. It is particularly important coming from one of the groups that in 1991 reported significant race-based differences in outcomes; see Easterbrook et al.,

"Racial and Ethnic Differences in Outcome in Zidovudine-Treated Patients with Advanced HIV Disease."

58. See Schiller, "The Invisible Women."

59. Das, "AIDS in India," p. 8.

60. Hollibaugh, "Lesbian Denial and Lesbian Leadership in the AIDS Epidemic," p. 225. This essay does not cite data showing that lesbians of color account for a large number of the U.S. women living with HIV, but the author's comments are helpful in their clarity and candor. Other writers do underscore divisions between white and black feminists. "When it came down to it," notes Veronica Chambers, an African American feminist, "I could not trust most white women to have my back" ("Betrayal Feminism," p. 25).

61. Lee, "Beyond Bean Counting," p. 211. Nancy Krieger and Sally Zierler note that "although women, as a group, may share experiences of being biologically female, these experiences occur in diverse gendered societies, located within a global economy, and simultaneously split, internally, by social class, race/ethnicity, and other social divisions" ("Accounting for Health of Women," p. 251).

62. Schoepf, "Gender, Development, and AIDS," p. 70.

16

On Suffering and
Structural Violence

Social and Economic Rights in the Global Era

(1996, 2003)

*Growth of GNP or of industrial incomes can, of course, be very important
as means to expanding the freedoms enjoyed by the members of the society.
But freedoms depend also on other determinants, such as social and
economic arrangements (for example, facilities for education and health
care) as well as political and civil rights (for example, the liberty to
participate in public discussion and scrutiny).*

AMARTYA SEN, *DEVELOPMENT AS FREEDOM*

*Where do people earn the Per Capita Income? More than one poor
starving soul would like to know.*

*In our countries, numbers live better than people. How many
people prosper in times of prosperity? How many people find their
lives developed by development?*

EDUARDO GALEANO, "THOSE LITTLE NUMBERS AND PEOPLE"

Everyone knows that suffering, violence, and misery exist. How to define them?
Given that each person's pain has for him or her a degree of reality that the
pain of others can surely never approach, is widespread agreement on the subject
possible? And yet people do agree, as often as not, on what constitutes extreme
suffering: premature and painful illnesses, say, as well as torture and rape. More
insidious assaults on dignity, such as institutionalized racism and gender inequality, are also acknowledged by most to cause great and unjust injury.

So suffering is a fact. Now a number of corollary questions come to the fore.
Whenever we talk about medicine or policy, a "hierarchy of suffering" begins to
take shape, for it is impossible to relieve every case at once. Can we identify the
worst assaults? Those individuals most at risk of great suffering? Among persons

whose suffering is not fatal, who is most at risk of sustaining permanent and disabling damage? Are victims of certain "event" assaults, such as torture or rape, more likely to experience later sequelae than persons who endure sustained and insidious suffering, such as the pain born of deep poverty or racism? Are certain forms of insidious discrimination demonstrably more noxious than others?

Anthropologists and others who adopt these as research questions study both individual experience and the larger social matrix in which it is embedded in order to see how various social processes and events come to be translated into personal distress and disease. By what mechanisms, precisely, do social forces ranging from poverty to racism become *embodied* as individual experience?[1] This has been the focus of most of my own research in Haiti, where political and economic forces have structured risk for AIDS, tuberculosis, and, indeed, most other infectious and parasitic diseases. Social forces at work there have also structured risk for most forms of extreme suffering, from hunger to torture and rape.

Working in contemporary Haiti, where in recent decades political violence has been added to the worst poverty in the hemisphere, one learns a great deal about suffering. In fact, the country has long constituted a sort of living laboratory for the study of affliction, no matter how it is defined. The biggest problem, of course, is unimaginable poverty, as a long succession of dictatorial governments have been more engaged in pillaging than in protecting the rights of workers, even on paper. As Eduardo Galeano noted in 1973, at the height of the Duvalier dictatorship, "The wages Haiti requires by law belong in the department of science fiction: actual wages on coffee plantations vary from $.07 to $.15 a day."[2] When international health and population experts devised a "human suffering index" in 1991, by examining several measures of human welfare ranging from life expectancy to political freedom, 27 of 141 countries were characterized by "extreme human suffering."[3] Only one of them, Haiti, was located in the Western Hemisphere. In only three countries on earth was suffering judged to be more extreme than that endured in Haiti; each of these three countries was in the midst of an internationally recognized civil war.

Suffering is certainly a recurrent and expected condition in Haiti's Central Plateau, where everyday life has felt, often enough, like war. "You get up in the morning," observed one young widow with four children, "and it's the fight for food and wood and water." If initially struck by the austere beauty of the region's steep mountains and clement weather, long-term visitors come to see the Central Plateau in much the same manner as its inhabitants do: a chalky and arid land hostile to the best efforts of the peasant farmers who live here. Landlessness is widespread and so, consequently, is hunger. All the standard measures reveal how tenuous is the peasantry's hold on survival. Life expectancy at birth is less than fifty years, in large part because as many as two of every ten infants die before their first birthday.

Against that background of generalized suffering, the specific experiences of patients recorded in my case histories are inscribed. The stories of two Haitian sufferers in particular, Acéphie Joseph and Chouchou Louis, seem to me to convey more effectively than statistics or graphs the affliction and powerlessness that fill the days of the world's poor.[4] Since any example begs the question of its relevance, I will argue at the outset that the stories of Acéphie and Chouchou are anything but "anecdotal." In the eyes of the epidemiologist as well as the political analyst, they suffered and died in exemplary fashion. Millions of people living in similar circumstances can expect to meet similar fates. What these victims, past and present, share are not personal or psychological attributes. They do not share culture or language or a certain race. What they share, rather, is the experience of occupying the bottom rung of the social ladder in inegalitarian societies.

ACÉPHIE'S STORY

Acéphie Joseph died of AIDS in 1991. She was from an impoverished family of "water refugees" who had lost their home and land years earlier when their valley was flooded by a hydroelectric dam. Acéphie attended primary school in a banana-thatched and open shelter in which children and young adults received the rudiments of literacy in Kay. "She was the nicest of the Joseph sisters," recalled one of her classmates. "And she was as pretty as she was nice."

Acéphie's beauty—she was tall and fine-featured, with enormous dark eyes—and her vulnerability may have sealed her fate as early as 1984. Though still in primary school then, she was already nineteen years old; it was time for her to help generate income for her family, which was sinking deeper and deeper into poverty. Acéphie began to help her mother by carrying produce to a local market on Friday mornings. On foot or with a donkey, it took over an hour and a half to reach the market, and the road led right through Péligre, site of the dam and a military barracks. The soldiers liked to watch the parade of women on Friday mornings. Sometimes they taxed them, literally, with haphazardly imposed fines; sometimes they levied a toll of flirtatious banter.

Such flirtation is seldom rejected, at least openly. In rural Haiti, entrenched poverty made the soldiers—the region's only salaried men—ever so much more attractive. Hunger was a near-daily occurrence for the Joseph family; the times were as bad as those right after the flooding of the valley. And so when Acéphie's good looks caught the eye of Captain Jacques Honorat, a native of Belladère, formerly stationed in Port-au-Prince, she returned his gaze.

Acéphie knew, as did everyone in the area, that Honorat had a wife and children. He was known, in fact, to have more than one regular partner. But Acéphie was taken in by his persistence, and when he went to speak to her parents, a long-term liaison was, from the outset, a serious possibility:

What would you have me do? I could tell that the old people were uncomfortable, worried; but they didn't say no. They didn't tell me to stay away from him. I wish they had, but how could they have known? . . . I knew it was a bad idea then, but I just didn't know why. I never dreamed he would give me a bad illness, never! I looked around and saw how poor we all were, how the old people were finished . . . What would you have me do? It was a way out, that's how I saw it.

Acéphie and Honorat were sexual partners only briefly—for less than a month, according to Acéphie. Shortly thereafter, Honorat fell ill with unexplained fevers and kept to the company of his wife in Péligre. As Acéphie was looking for a *moun prensipal*—a "main man"—she tried to forget about the soldier. Still, it was shocking to hear, a few months after they parted, that he was dead.

Acéphie was at a crucial juncture in her life. Returning to school was out of the question. After some casting about, she went to Mirebalais, the nearest town, and began a course in what she euphemistically termed a "cooking school." The school—really just an ambitious woman's courtyard—prepared poor girls like Acéphie for their inevitable turn as servants in the city. Indeed, becoming a maid was fast developing into one of the rare growth industries in Haiti, and, as much as Acéphie's proud mother hated to think of her daughter reduced to servitude, she could offer no viable alternative.

And so Acéphie, twenty-two years old, went off to Port-au-Prince, where she found a job as a housekeeper for a middle-class Haitian woman who worked for the U.S. embassy. Acéphie's looks and manners kept her out of the backyard, the traditional milieu of Haitian servants. She was designated as the maid who, in addition to cleaning, answered the door and the phone. Although Acéphie was not paid well—she received thirty dollars each month—she recalled the gnawing hunger in her home village and managed to save a bit of money for her parents and siblings.

Still looking for a *moun prensipal,* Acéphie began seeing Blanco Nerette, a young man with origins similar to her own: Blanco's parents were also "water refugees," and Acéphie had known him when they were both attending the parochial school in Kay. Blanco had done well for himself, by Kay standards: he chauffeured a small bus between the Central Plateau and the capital. In a setting in which the unemployment rate was greater than 60 percent, he could command considerable respect, and he turned his attentions to Acéphie. They planned to marry, she later recalled, and started pooling their resources.

Acéphie remained at the "embassy woman's" house for more than three years, staying until she discovered that she was pregnant. As soon as she told Blanco, she could see him becoming skittish. Nor was her employer pleased: it is considered unsightly to have a pregnant servant. And so Acéphie returned to Kay, where she had a difficult pregnancy. Blanco came to see her once or twice. They had a disagreement, and then she heard nothing more from him. Following the birth of her daughter, Acéphie was sapped by repeated infections. A regular visitor to our clinic, she was soon diagnosed with AIDS.

Within months of her daughter's birth, Acéphie's life was consumed with managing her own drenching night sweats and debilitating diarrhea while attempting to care for the child. "We both need diapers now," she remarked bitterly, toward the end of her life. As political violence hampered her doctors' ability to open the clinic, Acéphie was faced each day not only with diarrhea but also with a persistent lassitude. As she became more and more gaunt, some villagers suggested that Acéphie was the victim of sorcery. Others recalled her liaison with the soldier and her work as a servant in the city, by then widely considered to be risk factors for AIDS. Acéphie herself knew that she had AIDS, although she was more apt to refer to herself as suffering from a disorder brought on by her work as a servant: "All that ironing, and then opening a refrigerator." She died far from refrigerators or other amenities as her family and caregivers stood by helplessly.

But this is not simply the story of Acéphie and her daughter, also infected with the virus. There is also Jacques Honorat's first wife, who each year grows thinner. After Honorat's death, she found herself desperate, with no means of feeding her five hungry children, two of whom were also ill. Her subsequent union was again with a soldier. Honorat had at least two other partners, both of them poor peasant women, in the Central Plateau. One is HIV-positive and has two sickly children. And there is Blanco, still a handsome young man, apparently in good health, plying the roads from Mirebalais to Port-au-Prince. Who knows if he carries the virus? As a chauffeur, he has plenty of girlfriends.

Nor is this simply the story of those infected with HIV. The pain felt by Acéphie's mother and twin brother was manifestly intense. But few understood her father's anguish. Shortly after Acéphie's death, he hanged himself with a length of rope.

CHOUCHOU'S STORY

Chouchou Louis, a young man from the same rural area, died in 1992. He grew up not far from Kay, in another small village in the steep and infertile highlands of Haiti's Central Plateau. He attended primary school for a couple of years but was forced to drop out when his mother died. Then, in his early teens, Chouchou joined his father and an older sister in tending their hillside garden. In short, there was nothing remarkable about Chouchou's childhood. It was brief and harsh, like most in rural Haiti.

Throughout the 1980s, church activities formed Chouchou's sole distraction. These were hard years for the Haitian poor, beaten down by a family dictatorship well into its third decade. The Duvaliers, father and son, ruled through violence, largely directed at people whose conditions of existence were similar to those of Chouchou Louis. Although many tried to flee, often by boat, U.S. policy maintained that Haitian asylum-seekers were "economic refugees." As part of a 1981 agreement between the administrations of Ronald Reagan and Jean-Claude Duvalier (known as "Baby Doc"), refugees seized by the U.S. Coast Guard on the high seas were summarily returned to Haiti. During the first ten years of the accord, approximately twenty-three thousand Haitians applied for political asylum in the United States. Eight applications were approved.

A growing Haitian pro-democracy movement led to the flight of Duvalier in February 1986. Chouchou Louis, who must have been about twenty years old when "Baby Doc" fell, shortly thereafter acquired a small radio. "All he did," recalled his wife, years later, "was work the land, listen to the radio, and go to church." On the radio, Chouchou heard about the people who took over after Duvalier fled. Like many in rural Haiti, Chouchou was distressed to hear that power had been handed to the military, led by hardened *duvaliéristes*. It was this army that the U.S. government termed "Haiti's best bet for democracy." (Hardly a disinterested judgment: the United States had created the modern Haitian army in 1916.) In the eighteen months following Duvalier's departure, more than $200 million in U.S. aid passed through the hands of the junta.

In early 1989, Chouchou moved in with Chantal Brisé, who was pregnant. They were living together when Father Jean-Bertrand Aristide—by then considered the leader of the pro-democracy movement—declared his candidacy for the presidency in the internationally monitored elections of 1990. In December of that year, almost 70 percent of the voters chose Father Aristide from a field of nearly a dozen presidential candidates. No run-off election was required—Aristide won this plurality in the first round.

Like most rural Haitians, Chouchou and Chantal welcomed Aristide's election with great joy. For the first time, the poor—Haiti's overwhelming majority, formerly silent—felt they had someone representing their interests in the presidential palace. This is why the subsequent military coup d'état of September 1991 stirred great anger in the countryside, where most Haitians live. Anger was soon followed by sadness, then fear, as the country's repressive machinery, which had been held at bay during the seven months of Aristide's tenure, was speedily reactivated under the patronage of the army.

One day during the month after the coup, Chouchou was sitting in a truck en route to the town of Hinche. Chouchou offered for the consideration of his fellow passengers what Haitians call a *pwen,* a pointed remark intended to say something other than what it literally means. As they bounced along, he began complaining about the conditions of the roads, observing that, "if things were as they should be, these roads would have been repaired already." One eyewitness later told me that at no point in the commentary was Aristide's name invoked.

But his fellow passengers recognized Chouchou's observations as veiled language deploring the coup. Unfortunately for Chouchou, one of the passengers was an out-of-uniform soldier. At the next checkpoint, the soldier had him seized and dragged from the truck. There, a group of soldiers and their lackeys—their *attachés,* to use the epithet then in favor—immediately began beating Chouchou, in front of the other passengers; they continued to beat him as they brought him to the military barracks in Hinche. A scar on his right temple was a souvenir of his several days' stay there.

In rural Haiti, any scrape with the law (that is, the military) led to a certain blacklisting. For men like Chouchou, staying out of jail involved keeping the local *attachés* happy, and he did this by avoiding his home village. But Chouchou lived in fear of a second arrest, his wife later told me, and his fears proved to be well founded.

On January 22, 1992, Chouchou was visiting his sister when he was arrested by two *attachés.* No reason was given for the arrest, and Chouchou's sister regarded as ominous the seizure of the young man's watch and radio. He was roughly marched to the nearest military checkpoint, where he was tortured by soldiers and the *attachés.* One area resident later told us that the prisoner's screams made her children weep with terror.

On January 25, Chouchou was dumped in a ditch to die. The army scarcely took the trouble to circulate the *canard* that he had stolen some bananas. (The Haitian press, by then thoroughly muzzled, did not even broadcast this false version of events; fatal beatings in the countryside did not count as news.) Relatives carried Chouchou back to Chantal and their daughter under the cover of night. By early on the morning of January 26, when I arrived, Chouchou was scarcely recognizable. His face, especially his left temple, was deformed, swollen, and lacerated; his right temple was also scarred. His mouth was a coagulated pool of dark blood. Lower down, his neck was peculiarly swollen, his throat collared with bruises left by a gun butt. His chest and sides were badly bruised, and he had several fractured ribs. His genitals had been mutilated.

That was his front side; presumably, the brunt of the beatings had come from behind. Chouchou's back and thighs were striped with deep lash marks. His buttocks were macerated, the skin flayed down to the exposed gluteal muscles. Already some of these wounds appeared to be infected.

Chouchou coughed up more than a liter of blood in his agonal moments. Although I am not a forensic pathologist, my guess is that the proximate cause of his death was pulmonary hemorrhage. Given his respiratory difficulties and the amount of blood he coughed up, it is likely that the beatings caused him to bleed, slowly at first, then catastrophically, into his lungs. His head injuries had not robbed him of his faculties, although it might have been better for him had they done so. It took Chouchou three days to die.

EXPLAINING VERSUS MAKING SENSE OF SUFFERING

Are these stories of suffering emblematic of something other than two tragic and premature deaths? If so, how representative is either of these experiences? Little about Acéphie's story is unique; it brings to the foreground many of the forces restricting not only her options but those of most Haitian women. What about the murder of Chouchou Louis? International human rights groups estimate that more than three thousand Haitians were killed in the year after the September 1991 coup that overthrew Haiti's first democratically elected government and forced its president, Father Jean Bertrand Aristide, into exile. Almost all were civilians who, like Chouchou, fell into the hands of the military or paramilitary forces. The vast majority of victims were poor peasants, like Chouchou, or urban slum dwellers. But note that the figures just cited are conservative estimates; I can testify that no journalist or human rights observer ever came to count the body of Chouchou Louis.[5]

Thus the agony of Acéphie and Chouchou was, in a sense, "modal" suffering. In Haiti, AIDS and political violence are two leading causes of death among young adults. These afflictions are not the result of accident or a *force majeure;* they are the consequence, direct or indirect, of human agency. When the Artibonite Valley was flooded, depriving families like the Josephs of their land, a human decision was behind it; when the Haitian army was endowed with money and unfettered power, human decisions were behind that, too. In fact, some of the same decision makers may have been involved in both cases.

If bureaucrats and soldiers seemed to have unconstrained sway over the lives of the rural poor, the agency of Acéphie and Chouchou was, correspondingly, curbed at every turn. Their grim biographies suggest that the social and economic forces that have helped to shape the AIDS epidemic are, in every sense, the same forces that led to Chouchou's death and to the larger repression by which it was eclipsed. What's more, both of these individuals were "at risk" of such a fate long before they met the soldiers who altered their destinies. They were both, from the outset, victims of structural violence. The term is apt because such suffering is "structured" by processes and forces that conspire—whether through routine, ritual, or, more commonly, the hard surfaces of economics and politics—to constrain agency.[6] For many, including most of my patients and informants, choices both large and small are limited by racism, sexism, political violence, *and* grinding poverty.

While certain kinds of suffering are readily observable—and the subject of countless films, novels, and poems—structural violence all too frequently defeats those who would describe it. There are at least three reasons. First, the "exoticization" of suffering as lurid as that endured by Acéphie and Chouchou distances it. The suffering of individuals whose lives and struggles recall our own tends to move us; the suffering of those who are "remote," whether because of geography or culture, is usually less affecting.

Second, the sheer weight of the suffering makes it all the more difficult to render: "Knowledge of suffering cannot be conveyed in pure facts and figures, reportings that objectify the suffering of countless persons. The horror of suffering is not only its immensity but the faces of the anonymous victims who have little voice, let alone rights, in history."[7]

Third, the dynamics and distribution of suffering are still poorly understood. Physicians, when fortunate, can alleviate the suffering of the sick. But explaining its distribution requires many minds and resources. Case studies of individuals reveal suffering, telling us what happens to one or many people; but to explain suffering, one must embed individual biography in the larger matrix of culture, history, and political economy.

In short, it is one thing to make sense of extreme suffering—a universal activity, surely—and quite another to explain it. Life experiences such as those of Acéphie and Chouchou, and of other Haitians living in poverty who share similar social conditions, must be embedded in ethnography if we are to understand their representativeness. These local understandings must be embedded, in turn, in the historical system of which Haiti is a part.[8] The weakness of such analyses is, of course, their great distance from personal experience. But the social and economic forces that dictate life choices in Haiti's Central Plateau affect many millions of individuals, and it is in the context of these global forces that the suffering of individuals acquires its own appropriate context.

Similar insights are central to liberation theology, which preoccupies itself with the suffering of the poor. In *The Praxis of Suffering,* Rebecca Chopp states, "In a variety of forms, liberation theology speaks with those who, through their suffering, call into question the meaning and truth of human history."[9] Unlike most previous theologies, unlike much modern philosophy, liberation theology attempts to use social analysis both to explain and to deplore human suffering. Its key texts draw our attention not merely to the suffering of the wretched of the earth but also to the forces that promote that suffering. Theologian Leonardo Boff, commenting on one of these texts, observes that it "moves immediately to the structural analysis of these forces and denounces the systems, structures, and mechanisms that 'create a situation where the rich get richer at the expense of the poor, who get even poorer.'"[10]

Put simply, few liberation theologians reflect on suffering without attempting to understand the mechanisms that produce it. Theirs is a theology that underlines connections. Robert McAfee Brown has these connections, and also the poor, in mind when, paraphrasing the Uruguayan Jesuit Juan Luis Segundo, he observes that "the world that is satisfying to us is the same world that is utterly devastating to them."[11]

MAKING SENSE OF STRUCTURAL VIOLENCE

Events of massive, public suffering defy quantitative analysis. How can one really understand statistics citing the death of six million Jews or graphs of third-world starvation? Do numbers really reveal the agony, the interruption, the questions that these victims put to the meaning and nature of our individual lives and life as a whole?

REBECCA CHOPP, *THE PRAXIS OF SUFFERING*

My apologies to chance for calling it necessity
My apologies to necessity if I'm mistaken, after all.
Please, don't be angry, happiness, that I take you as my due.
May my dead be patient with the way my memories fade.
My apologies to time for all the world I overlook each second.

WISŁAWA SZYMBORSKA, "UNDER ONE SMALL STAR"

How might we discern the nature of structural violence and explore its contribution to human suffering? Can we devise an analytic model, one with explanatory and predictive power, for understanding suffering in a global context? This task, though daunting, is both urgent and feasible if we are to protect and promote human rights.

Our cursory examination of AIDS and political violence in Haiti suggests that such an analysis must, first, be *geographically broad*. The world as we know it is becoming increasingly interconnected. A corollary of this fact is that extreme suffering—especially when on a grand scale, as in genocide—is seldom divorced from the actions of the powerful.[12] The analysis must also be *historically deep:* not merely deep enough to remind us of events and decisions such as those that deprived Acéphie's parents of their land and founded the Haitian military, but deep enough to recall that modern-day Haitians are the descendants of a people kidnapped from Africa in order to provide our forebears with sugar, sago, coffee, and cotton.[13]

Social factors including gender, ethnicity ("race"), and socioeconomic status may each play a role in rendering individuals and groups vulnerable to extreme human suffering. But in most settings these factors by themselves have limited explanatory power. To discern a political economy of brutality, *simultaneous* consideration of various social "axes" is imperative. Furthermore, such social factors are differentially weighted in different settings and in different times, as even a brief consideration of their contributions to extreme suffering suggests.

In an essay entitled "Mortality as an Indicator of Economic Success and Failure," Amartya Sen reminds us of the need to move beyond "the cold and often inarticulate statistics of low incomes" to look at the various ways in which agency—what he terms the "capabilities of each person"—is constrained. He writes: "There is, of course, plenty of [poverty] in the world in which we live. But more awful is the fact that so many people—including children from disadvantaged backgrounds—are forced to lead miserable and precarious lives and to die prematurely. That predicament relates in general to low incomes, but not just to that. It also reflects inadequate public health provisions and nutritional support, deficiency of social security arrangements, and the absence of social responsibility and of caring governance."[14]

To understand the relationship between structural violence and human rights, we must avoid reductionistic analyses. Sen is understandably concerned to avoid economic reductionism, an occupational hazard in his field. But numerous other analytic traps can also hinder the quest for a sound analytic purchase on the dynamics of human suffering.

The Axis of Gender

Acéphie Joseph and Chouchou Louis shared a similar social status, and each died after contact with the Haitian military. Gender helps to explain why Acéphie died of AIDS and Chouchou from torture. Gender inequality helps to explain why the suffering of Acéphie is much more commonplace than that of Chouchou. Throughout the world, women are confronted with sexism, an ideology that situates them as inferior to men. In 1974, when a group of feminist anthropologists surveyed the status of women living in disparate settings, they could agree that, in every society studied, men dominated political, legal, and economic institutions to varying degrees; in no culture was the status of women genuinely equal, much less superior, to that of men.[15]

This power differential has meant that women's rights are violated in innumerable ways. Although male victims are clearly preponderant in studies of torture, females almost exclusively endure the much more common crimes of domestic violence and rape. In the United States alone, the number of such aggressions is staggering. Taking into account sexual assaults by both intimates and strangers, "one in four women has been the victim of a completed rape and one in four women has been physically battered, according to the results of recent community-based studies."[16] In many societies, crimes of domestic violence and rape are not even discussed and are thus invisible.

In most settings, however, gender alone does not define risk for such assaults on dignity. It is *poor* women who are least well defended against these assaults.[17] This is true not only of domestic violence and rape but also of AIDS and its distribution, as anthropologist Martha Ward points out: "The collection of statistics by ethnicity rather than by socio-economic status obscures the fact that the majority of women with AIDS in the United States are poor. Women are at risk for HIV not because they are African-American or speak Spanish; women are at risk because poverty is the primary and determining condition of their lives."[18]

Similarly, only women can experience maternal mortality, a cause of anguish around the world. More than half a million women die each year in childbirth, but not all women face a high risk of this fate. In fact, according to analyses of 1995 statistics, 99.8 percent of these deaths occurred in developing countries.[19] Recent reported maternal mortality rates for Haiti vary, depending on the source, with numbers ranging from 523 deaths per 100,000 live births to the much higher rates of 1,100 and even as high as 1,400 deaths per 100,000 live births. Needless to say, these deaths are registered almost entirely among the poor.[20] Gender bias, as Sen points out, "is a general problem that applies even in Europe and North America in a variety of fields (such as division of family chores, the provision of support for higher training, and so on), but in poorer countries, the disadvantage of women may even apply to the basic fields of health care, nutritional support, and elementary education."[21]

The Axis of "Race" or Ethnicity

The idea of "race," which most anthropologists and demographers consider to be a biologically insignificant term, has enormous social currency. Racial classifications have been used to deprive many groups of basic rights and therefore have an important place in considerations of human inequality and suffering. The history of Rwanda and Burundi shows that once-minor ethnic categories—Hutu and Tutsi share language and culture and kinship systems—were lent weight and social meaning by colonial administrators who divided and conquered, deepening social inequalities and then fueling nascent ethnic rivalry. In South Africa, one of the clearest examples of the long-term effects of racism, epidemiologists report that the infant mortality rate among blacks may be as much as ten times higher than that of whites. For black people in South Africa, the proximate cause of increased rates of morbidity and mortality is lack of access to resources: "*Poverty* remains the primary cause of the prevalence of many diseases and widespread hunger and malnutrition among black South Africans."[22] The dismantling of the apartheid regime has not yet brought the dismantling of the structures of oppression and inequality in South Africa, and persistent social inequality is no doubt the primary reason that HIV has spread so rapidly in sub-Saharan Africa's wealthiest nation.[23]

Significant mortality differentials between blacks and whites are also registered in the United States, which shares with South Africa the distinction of being one of the two industrialized countries failing to record mortality data by socioeconomic status. In 1988 in the United States, life expectancy at birth was 75.5 years for whites, 69.5 years for blacks. In the following decade, although U.S. life expectancies increased across the board, the gap between whites and blacks widened by another 0.6 years.[24] While these racial differentials in mortality have provoked a certain amount of discussion, public health expert Vicente Navarro recently pointed to the "deafening silence" on the topic of class differentials in mortality in the United States, where "race is used as a *substitute* for class." But in 1986, on "one of the few occasions that the U.S. government collected information on mortality rates (for heart and cerebrovascular disease) by class, the results showed that, by whatever indicators of class one might choose (level of education, income, or occupation), mortality rates are related to social class."[25]

Indeed, where the major causes of death (heart disease and cerebrovascular disease) are concerned, class standing is a clearer indicator than racial classification. "The growing mortality differentials between whites and blacks," Navarro concludes, "cannot be understood by looking only at race; they are part and parcel of larger mortality differentials—class differentials."[26] Sociologist William Julius Wilson makes a similar point in his landmark study *The Declining Significance of Race,* where he argues that "trained and educated blacks, like trained and educated whites, will continue to enjoy the advantages and privileges of their class status."[27] Although new studies show that race differentials persist even among the privileged, it is important to emphasize that it is the African American poor—and an analysis of the mechanisms of their impoverishment— who are being left out. At the same time, U.S. national aggregate income data that do not consider differential mortality by race and place completely miss the fact that African American men in Harlem have shorter life expectancies than Bangladeshi men.[28] Again, as Sen remarks, race-based differences in life expectancy have policy implications, and these in turn are related to social and economic rights:

> If the relative deprivation of blacks transcends income differentials so robustly, the remedying of this inequality has to involve policy matters that go well beyond just creating income opportunities for the black population. It is necessary to address such matters as public health services, educational facilities, hazards of urban life, and other social and economic parameters that influence survival chances. The picture of mortality differentials presents an entry into the problem of racial inequality in the United States that would be wholly missed if our economic analysis were to be confined only to traditional economic variables.[29]

Other Axes of Oppression

Any distinguishing characteristic, whether social or biological, can serve as a pretext for discrimination and thus as a cause of suffering. Refugee or immigrant status is one that readily comes to mind, when thinking of the poor and the powerless. Sexual preference is another obvious example; homosexuality is stigmatized to varying degrees in many settings. "Gay bashing," like other forms of violent criminal victimization, is sure to have long-term effects. But crimes against gay men and women are again felt largely among the poor.

Questions about the relationship between homophobia and mortality patterns have come to the fore during the AIDS pandemic. In regard to HIV disease, homophobia may lead to adverse outcomes if it "drives underground" people who would otherwise stand to benefit from preventive campaigns. But gay communities, at least middle-class ones in affluent nations, have been singularly effective in organizing a response to AIDS, and those most closely integrated into these communities are among the most informed consumers of AIDS-related messages in the world.[30]

Homophobia may be said to hasten the development of AIDS if it denies services to those already infected with HIV. But this phenomenon has not been widely observed in the United States, where an "AIDS deficit"—fewer cases than predicted—has been noted among gay men, though not in other groups disproportionately afflicted with HIV disease in the early years of the epidemic: injection drug users, inner-city people of color, and persons originally from poor countries in sub-Saharan Africa or the Caribbean.[31] Nor have those engaged in sex work benefited from the AIDS deficit. However, males involved in prostitution are almost universally poor, and it may be their poverty, rather than their sexual preference, that puts them at risk of HIV infection. Many men involved in homosexual prostitution, particularly minority adolescents, do not necessarily identify themselves as gay.

None of this is to deny the ill effects of homophobia, even in a country as wealthy as the United States. The point is rather to call for more fine-grained, more systemic analyses of power and privilege in discussions about who is likely to have their rights violated and in what ways. We did not need the AIDS pandemic to teach us this. In his novel *Maurice,* E.M. Forster explores both English class politics and the affective experience of Maurice, an upper-middle-class man who falls in love with Clive, an aristocrat with the expected political ambitions. Maurice's liberation, it would seem, comes from his relationship with Alec, a servant on Clive's family estate. In a postscript to the book, Forster deplores the persecution of gays in England, predicting that "police prosecutions will continue and Clive on the bench will continue to sentence Alec on the dock. Maurice may get off."[32]

The Conflation of Structural Violence and Cultural Difference

Awareness of cultural differences has long complicated discussion of human suffering. Some anthropologists have argued that what outside observers construe as obvious assaults on dignity may in fact be longstanding cultural institutions highly valued by a society. Often-cited examples range from female circumcision in the Sudan to headhunting in the Philippines. Such discussions invariably appeal to the concept of cultural relativism, which has a long and checkered history in anthropology. Is every culture a law unto itself and answerable to nothing other than itself? In recent decades, confidence in reflexive cultural relativism faltered as anthropologists turned their attention to "complex societies" characterized by extremely inegalitarian social structures. Many found themselves unwilling to condone social inequity merely because it was buttressed by cultural beliefs, no matter how ancient or picturesque. Citizens of the former colonies also questioned cultural relativism as part of a broader critique of anthropology: for them, it appeared to be a mechanism for rationalizing and perpetuating inequalities between First and Third Worlds.[33]

But this question has not yet eroded a tendency, evident in many of the social sciences but perhaps particularly in anthropology, to confuse structural violence with cultural difference. In far too many ethnographies, poverty and inequality, the end results of a long historical process, are conflated with "otherness." Typically, such myopia comes down not to motives but rather, as Talal Asad has suggested, to our "mode of perceiving and objectifying alien societies."[34] Part of the problem may be the ways in which the term "culture" is used. "The idea of culture," explains Roy Wagner approvingly in a book on the subject, "places the researcher in a position of equality with his subjects: each 'belongs to a culture.'"[35] The tragedy, of course, is that this equality, however comforting to the researcher, is entirely illusory. Anthropology has usually "studied down" steep gradients of power.

Such illusions provide an important means of sustaining other misreadings—most notably, the conflation of poverty and cultural difference—for they suggest that the anthropologist and "his" subject, being *from* different cultures, are *of* different worlds and *of* different times.[36] These sorts of misreadings, innocent enough when kept among scholars, are finding a more insidious utility within elite culture as it becomes increasingly *transnational*. Concepts of cultural relativism, and even arguments to reinstate the dignity of different cultures and "races," have been easily adopted and turned to profit by some of the very agencies that perpetuate extreme suffering.[37] The abuse of the concept of cultural specificity is particularly insidious in discussions of suffering in general and of human rights abuses specifically: cultural difference, verging on cultural determinism, is one of several forms of essentialism used to explain away assaults on dignity and suffering. Practices including torture are said to be "part of their culture" or "in their nature"—"their" designating either the victims, or the perpetrators, or both, as may be expedient.[38]

Such analytic vices are rarely questioned, even though systemic studies of extreme suffering indicate that the concept of culture should enjoy only an exceedingly limited role in explaining the *distribution* of misery. The role of cultural boundary lines in enabling, perpetuating, justifying, and interpreting suffering is subordinate to (though well integrated with) the national and international mechanisms that create and deepen inequalities. "Culture" does not explain suffering; it may at worst furnish an alibi.[39]

STRUCTURAL VIOLENCE AND EXTREME SUFFERING

At night I listen to their phantoms
shouting in my ear
shaking me out of lethargy
issuing me commands
I think of their tattered lives
of their feverish hands
reaching out to seize ours.
It's not that they're begging
they're demanding
they've earned the right to order us
to break up our sleep
to come awake
to shake off once and for all
this lassitude.

CLARIBEL ALEGRÍA, "NOCTURNAL VISITS"

Clearly, no single axis can fully define increased risk for extreme human suffering. Efforts to attribute explanatory efficacy to one variable lead to immodest claims of causality, for wealth and power have often protected individual women, gays, and ethnic minorities from the suffering and adverse outcomes associated with assaults on dignity. Similarly, poverty can efface the "protective" effects of status based on gender, race, or sexual orientation. Leonardo Boff and Clodovis Boff, liberation theologians writing from Brazil, insist on the primacy of the economic:

> We have to observe that the socioeconomically oppressed (the poor) do not simply exist alongside other oppressed groups, such as blacks, indigenous peoples, women— to take the three major categories in the Third World. No, the "class-oppressed"— the socioeconomically poor—are the infrastructural expression of the process of oppression. The other groups represent "superstructural" expressions of oppression and because of this are deeply conditioned by the infrastructural. It is one thing to be a black taxi-driver, quite another to be a black football idol; it is one thing to be a woman working as a domestic servant, quite another to be the first lady of the land; it is one thing to be an Amerindian thrown off your land, quite another to be an Amerindian owning your own farm.[40]

This is not to deny that sexism or racism has serious negative consequences, even in the wealthy countries of North America and Europe. The point is simply to call for more honest discussions of who is likely to suffer and in what ways.

The capacity to suffer is, clearly, a part of being human. But not all suffering is equivalent, in spite of pernicious and often self-serving identity politics that suggest otherwise. Physicians practice triage and referral daily. What suffering needs to be taken care of first and with what resources? It *is* possible to speak of extreme human suffering, and an inordinate share of this sort of pain is currently endured by those living in poverty. Take, for example, illness and premature death, the leading cause of extreme suffering in many places in the world. In a striking departure from previous, staid reports, the World Health Organization now acknowledges that poverty is the world's greatest killer: "Poverty wields its destructive influence at every stage of human life, from the moment of conception to the grave. It conspires with the most deadly and painful diseases to bring a wretched existence to all those who suffer from it."[41]

Today, the world's poor are the chief victims of structural violence—a violence that has thus far defied the analysis of many who seek to understand the nature and distribution of extreme suffering. Why might this be so? One answer is that the poor are not only more likely to suffer; they are also less likely to have their suffering noticed, as Chilean theologian Pablo Richard, noting the fall of the Berlin Wall, has warned: "We are aware that another gigantic wall is being constructed in the Third World, to hide the reality of the poor majorities. A wall between the rich and poor is being built, so that poverty does not annoy the powerful and the poor are obliged to die in the silence of history."[42]

The task at hand, if this silence is to be broken, is to identify the forces conspiring to promote suffering, with the understanding that these are differentially weighted in different settings. If we do this, we stand a chance of discerning the causes of extreme suffering and also the forces that put some at risk for human rights abuses, while others are shielded from risk. No honest assessment of the current state of human rights can omit an analysis of structural violence.

NOTES

1. The embodiment paradigm, for which we are to some extent indebted to Maurice Merleau-Ponty (see, for example, *Phénoménologie de la perception*), has been used widely in medical anthropology. For a helpful review, see Csordas, "Embodiment as a Paradigm for Anthropology"; and Csordas, *Embodiment and Experience*.

2. Galeano, *Open Veins of Latin America*, p. 112. It's worth noting that people with miserable jobs are nonetheless considered fortunate in a country where unemployment is estimated, by the omniscient CIA, at 70 percent (U.S. Central Intelligence Agency, "Haiti" [*World Factbook 2001*]). It's no wonder that the CIA is interested in the matter: Haiti was, until quite recently, one of the world's leading assemblers of U.S. goods. On the conditions of Haitian workers in U.S.-owned offshore assembly plants, see Kernaghan, *Haiti after the Coup*. Of course, U.S. industries are not alone in exploiting cheap Haitian labor.

3. In addition to standard indices of well-being and development, the human suffering index takes into account such factors as access to clean drinking water, daily caloric intake, religious and political freedom, respect for civil rights, and degree of gender inequality.

4. I tell the stories of Acéphie Joseph and Chouchou Louis in more detail in Farmer, *The Uses of Haiti,* pp. 244–82.

5. For an overview of the human rights situation after the 1991 coup led by General Raoul Cédras, see Americas Watch and National Coalition for Haitian Refugees, *Silencing a People;* and O'Neill, "The Roots of Human Rights Violations in Haiti." For a review of these and other reports, see Farmer, *The Uses of Haiti.* See also Inter-American Commission on Human Rights, *Report on the Situation of Human Rights in Haiti, 1995;* United Nations Commission on Human Rights, *Situation of Human Rights in Haiti;* Human Rights Watch/Americas, Jesuit Refugee Service, and National Coalition for Haitian Refugees, *Fugitives from Injustice.*

Toward the end of the coup, which led to thousands of outright murders, the army and paramilitary began a campaign of politically motivated rape. One survey terms this campaign "arguably the greatest crime against womankind in the Caribbean since slavery" (Rey, "Junta, Rape, and Religion in Haiti," p. 74). See also Human Rights Watch/Americas and National Coalition for Haitian Refugees, *Terror Prevails in Haiti.* It was during these years that our clinic received its first rape victims; see Farmer, "Haiti's Lost Years." One of my patients went on to testify about politically motivated rapes in a hearing on this topic held by the Organization of American States.

6. Some would argue that the relationship between individual agency and supraindividual structures forms the central problematic of contemporary social theory. I have tried, in this discussion, to avoid what Pierre Bourdieu has termed "the absurd opposition between individual and society," and here acknowledge the influence of Bourdieu, who has contributed enormously to the debate on structure and agency. For a concise statement of his (often revised) views on this subject, see Bourdieu, *In Other Words.* That a supple and fundamentally nondeterministic model of agency would have such a deterministic—and pessimistic—"feel" is largely a reflection of my topic, suffering, and my "fieldwork site," which is Haiti.

The relationship between agency and human rights is traced by Michael Ignatieff, among others: "We know from historical experience that when human beings have defensible rights—when their agency as individuals is protected and enhanced—they are less likely to be abused and oppressed. On these grounds, we count the diffusion of human rights instruments as progress even if there remains an unconscionable gap between the instruments and the actual practices of states charged to comply with them" (*Human Rights as Politics and Idolatry,* p. 4).

7. Chopp, *The Praxis of Suffering,* p. 2.

8. I have made this argument at greater length elsewhere; see Farmer, *AIDS and Accusation,* chap. 22.

9. Chopp, *The Praxis of Suffering,* p. 2. See also the works of Gustavo Gutiérrez (for example, *A Theology of Liberation;* and *The Power of the Poor in History*), who has written a great deal about the meaning of suffering in the twentieth century. For an anthropological study of liberation theology in social context, see Burdick, *Looking for God in Brazil.* Also see Lancaster, *Thanks to God and the Revolution.*

10. Boff, *Faith on the Edge,* p. 20.

11. Brown, *Liberation Theology,* p. 44.

12. The political economy of genocide is explored in Simpson, *The Splendid Blond Beast.* See also Aly, Chroust, and Pross, *Cleansing the Fatherland.* On the transnational political economy of human rights abuses, see Chomsky and Herman, *After the Cataclysm;* Chomsky and Herman, *The Washington Connection and Third World Fascism.* When Mike Davis explores "late Victorian holocausts," which led to some fifty million deaths, he concludes that "we are not dealing, in other words, with 'lands of famine' becalmed in stagnant backwaters of world history, but with the fate of tropical humanity at the precise moment (1870–1914) when its labor and products were being dynamically conscripted into a London-centered world economy. Millions died, not outside the 'modern world system,' but in the very process of being forcibly incorporated into its economic and political structures" (*Late Victorian Holocausts,* p. 9).

13. For historical background on Haiti, see James, *The Black Jacobins;* Mintz, "The Caribbean Region"; Trouillot, *Haiti, State against Nation.*

14. Sen, "Mortality as an Indicator of Economic Success and Failure," p. 2.

15. Rosaldo and Lamphere, *Woman, Culture, and Society.* For differing views, see Leacock, *Myths of Male Dominance.*

16. Koss, Koss, and Woodruff, "Deleterious Effects of Criminal Victimization on Women's Health and Medical Utilization," p. 342. From November 1995 to May 1996, the National Institute of Justice and the Centers for Disease Control and Prevention jointly conducted a national telephone survey that confirmed the high rates of assault against U.S. women (Tjaden and Thoennes, *Prevalence, Incidence, and Consequences of Violence against Women*). See also Bachman and Saltzman, *Violence against Women.*

17. It is important to note, however, that in many societies upper-class or upper-caste women are also subject to laws that virtually efface marital rape. The study by Mary Koss, Paul Koss, and Joy Woodruff includes this crime with other forms of criminal victimization, but such information is collected only through community-based surveys ("Deleterious Effects of Criminal Victimization on Women's Health and Medical Utilization").

18. Ward, "A Different Disease," p. 414.

19. A recent joint report by the WHO, UNICEF, and UNFPA on estimated maternal mortality for 1995 notes that of the 515,000 estimated maternal deaths worldwide, only 0.2 percent, or 1,200, occurred in industrialized countries. The lifetime risk of maternal death for women in such countries is calculated at 1:4,085, whereas for women in developing nations, the risk is much higher, at 1:61. In fact, for the subgroup of countries characterized as "least developed"—of which Haiti is one—the estimated risk of maternal death is, tragically, even higher, at 1:16 (World Health Organization, United Nations Children's Fund, and United Nations Population Fund, *Maternal Mortality in 1995,* p. 48).

20. The maternal mortality rate (MMR) of 523 deaths is for the year 2000 and is based on reports from the national health authority to PAHO; see Pan American Health Organization, "Country Health Profile: Haiti, 2001." The much higher rate of 1,100 maternal deaths per 100,000 live births is reported in World Health Organization, United Nations Children's Fund, and United Nations Population Fund, *Maternal Mortality in 1995,* p. 44. These numbers are likely to be even higher if one measures maternal mortality at the community level. The only community-based survey done in Haiti, conducted in 1985 around the town of Jacmel in southern Haiti, found that maternal mortality was 1,400 per 100,000 live births (Jean-Louis, "Diagnostic de l'état de santé en Haïti"). During that same period, "official" statistics reported much lower rates for Haiti, ranging from an MMR of 230 for the years 1980–87 (United Nations Development Programme, *Human Development Report 1990*) and an MMR of 340 for 1980–85 to a higher estimate in the years that followed, 1987–92, of 600 maternal deaths per 100,000 live births (World Bank, *Social Indicators of Development, 1994,* p. 148). For additional maternal mortality data from that period, see World Health Organization, "Maternal Mortality."

21. Sen, "Mortality as an Indicator of Economic Success and Failure," p. 13. For an in-depth discussion of the population-based impact of gender bias in poor countries, see Sen's classic essay, "Missing Women."

Sen summarizes the potential impact of public action in poor regions by examining Kerala state:

> Kerala's experience suggests that "gender bias" against females can be radically changed by public action—involving both the government and the public itself—especially through female education, opportunities for women to have responsible jobs, women's legal rights on property, and by enlightened egalitarian politics. Correspondingly, the problem of "missing women" can also be largely solved through social policy and political radicalism. Women's

movements can play a very important part in bringing about this type of change, and in making the political process in poor countries pay serious attention to the deep inequalities from which women suffer. It is also interesting to note, in this context, that the narrowly economic variables, such as GNP or GDP per head, on which so much of standard development economics concentrates, give a very misleading picture of economic and social progress ("Mortality as an Indicator of Economic Success and Failure," p. 15).

22. Nightingale et al., "Apartheid Medicine," p. 2098; emphasis added. For a more in-depth account and a more complicated view of the mechanisms by which apartheid and the South African economy are related to disease causation, see Packard, *White Plague, Black Labor*.

23. Although HIV is said to have recently "taken off" among South Africa's black population, it has been, from the beginning, an epidemic disproportionately affecting black people in that country. South African data indicate that in 1994, when seventeen white women were diagnosed with AIDS, almost fifteen hundred black women—nearly one hundred times as many—had the disease (Republic of South Africa, Department of National Health, *Health Trends in South Africa, 1994*, p. 67).

Even after the dismantling of the apartheid system, HIV continues to disproportionately affect black South Africans; see Lurie et al., "Circular Migration and Sexual Networking in Rural Kwazulu/Natal." As Audrey Chapman and Leonard Rubenstein note in a report for the American Association for the Advancement of Science and Physicians for Human Rights, "the epidemiology of the HIV/AIDS epidemic . . . demonstrates the link between poverty, low status and vulnerability to infection" (*Human Rights and Health*, p. 20). They report the "rigid segregation of health facilities; grossly disproportionate spending on the health of whites as compared to blacks, resulting in world-class medical care for whites while blacks were usually relegated to overcrowded and filthy facilities; public health policies that ignored diseases primarily affecting black people; and the denial of basic sanitation, clean water supply, and other components of public health to homelands and townships" (ibid., p. xix).

As Lurie and colleagues point out, "migrant labour was a central tenet of apartheid, which sought to create a steady flow of cheap black labour to South Africa's mines, industries and farms. A myriad of laws prohibited black South Africans from settling permanently in 'whites only' areas, and as a result, migration patterns in South Africa tend to be circular, with men maintaining close links with their rural homesteads" ("Circular Migration and Sexual Networking in Rural Kwazulu/Natal," p. 18).

This forced system of migration has had a distinct impact on the shaping of the AIDS epidemic. As Carol Kaufman explains, "the system of labor migration remains deeply entrenched, and women who have partners involved in labor circulation are especially vulnerable to unprotected sexual intercourse as well as STDs and HIV/AIDS transmission" ("Contraceptive Use in South Africa under Apartheid," p. 432). Quarraisha Abdool Karim and Salim Abdool Karim cite a 1998 study conducted in rural South Africa which found that "women whose partners spent 10 or fewer nights per month at home had an HIV prevalence of 13.7% compared with 0% in women who spent more than 10 nights in a month with their partners" ("South Africa," p. 139). For further documentation of this link, see Lurie et al., "Circular Migration and Sexual Networking in Rural Kwazulu/Natal." Furthermore, data from 1994 reveal that poverty is rampant in South Africa, with close to two-thirds of black households surviving below the minimum subsistence level (Chapman and Rubenstein, *Human Rights and Health*, p. 20).

24. The National Center for Health Statistics reported life expectancies at birth in 1996 as 76.8 years for whites and 70.2 years for blacks (*Health, United States, 1998, with Socioeconomic Status and Health Chartbook*, p. 206, table 29). Two years later, the same sources suggest a heartening trend: reported life expectancies increased to 77.3 for whites and 71.3 for blacks (National Center for Health Statistics, *Health, United States, 2000, with Adolescent Health Chartbook*, p. 169, table 28). But the

discrepancy is still on the order of 9 to 10 percent of lifespan. For a detailed discussion of recent health status disparities and leading causes of death for African Americans, see Byrd and Clayton, *An American Health Dilemma*, vol. 2, pp. 519–45.

25. Navarro, "Race or Class versus Race and Class," p. 1238.

26. Ibid., p. 1240.

27. Wilson, *The Declining Significance of Race*, p. 178.

28. McCord and Freeman, "Excess Mortality in Harlem."

29. Sen, "Mortality as an Indicator of Economic Success and Failure," p. 17.

30. Although class differences between physicians and university students are not as significant as others examined here, it is notable that a study reported in the *American Journal of Psychiatry* observed that gay psychiatrists were much more likely than students to adopt effective risk reduction (Klein et al., "Changes in AIDS Risk Behaviors among Homosexual Male Physicians and University Students"). For gay men in France, one study suggests that economic status is important in determining access to information and services (Pollak, *Les homosexuels et le SIDA*).

31. These data are reviewed in Farmer, Walton, and Furin, "The Changing Face of AIDS." See also Aalen et al., "New Therapy Explains the Fall in AIDS Incidence with a Substantial Rise in Number of Persons on Treatment Expected."

32. Forster, *Maurice*, p. 255.

33. See Hatch, *Culture and Morality*; Gellner, *Relativism and the Social Sciences*. Of course, the discussion of violence and cultural difference is vastly more complicated than that presented here. One consideration is that anthropological confidence in cultural relativism failed not only as part of the shift to studying "complex societies" but also as a result of shifting demographics within anthropology itself. By the 1990s, it was no longer unusual to hear comments such as that made by Nancy Scheper-Hughes: "Anthropological relativism is no longer appropriate to the violent, vexed and contested political world in which we now live" ("An Essay," p. 991). At the same time, however, argues William Roseberry, the "profoundly conservative reaction in politics and culture, marked politically by the Reagan victory in 1980," has had its echoes within anthropology: "What has fallen out of favor? In practice, it seems to be any work that is too ethnographic, too sociological, too structural, too political, too economic, or too processual" ("The Unbearable Lightness of Anthropology," pp. 17, 21).

34. Asad, *Anthropology and the Colonial Encounter*, p. 17.

35. Wagner, *The Invention of Culture*, p. 2.

36. Johannes Fabian has argued that this "denial of coevalness" is much ingrained in our discipline. Not to be dismissed as an issue of style, such a denial contributes to the blindness of the anthropologist: "Either he submits to the condition of coevalness and produces ethnographic knowledge, or he deludes himself into temporal distance and *misses the object of his search*" (*Time and the Other*, p. 32; emphasis added). See also Starn, "Missing the Revolution."

37. For a penetrating examination of the appropriation of identity politics by big business, see Kauffman, "The Diversity Game." For a broad and sophisticated study of the same topic, see Klein, *No Logo*.

38. Again, this chapter's discussion necessarily gives short shrift to the complexities of these debates. For a revealing example, see Amede Obiora's "Bridges and Barricades," which explores "polemics and intransigence in the campaign against female circumcision."

39. An example of the conflation of structural violence and cultural difference is found in the long lists of reasons given by those who do not believe that AIDS treatment is possible in Africa. Officially sanctioned justifications and explanations for structural violence come most often, however, from the reading and writing classes—that is, us. The Guatemalan poet Otto René Castillo,

who was killed by the Guatemalan army on March 19, 1967, avers that the "apolitical intellectuals" of his country will one day be judged harshly by the poor:

> "What did you do when the poor
> suffered, when tenderness and life
> were dangerously burning out in them?"
> Apolitical intellectuals
> of my sweet country,
> you will have nothing to say.
> A vulture of silence
> will eat your guts.
> Your own misery
> will gnaw at your souls.
> And you will be mute
> in your shame.
>   (Castillo, "Apolitical Intellectuals")

40. Boff and Boff, *Introducing Liberation Theology,* p. 29.
41. World Health Organization, *The World Health Report, 1995,* p. 5.
42. Richard is cited in Nelson-Pallmeyer, *Brave New World Order,* p. 14.

17

An Anthropology of
Structural Violence

(2001, 2004)

The ethnographically visible, central Haiti, September 2000: Most hospitals in the region are empty. This is not because of a local lack of treatable pathology; rather, patients have no money to pay for care. But one hospital—situated in a squatter settlement just 8 kilometers from a hydroelectric dam that decades ago flooded a fertile valley—is crowded. Medicines and laboratory studies are free. Every bed is filled, and the courtyard in front of the clinic is mobbed with patients waiting to be seen. Over a hundred slept on the grounds last night and are now struggling to smooth out wrinkles in hand-me-down dresses or pants or shirts; hats are being adjusted, and some people are massaging painful cricks in the neck. The queue of those waiting to have a new medical record created is long, snaking toward the infectious-disease clinic I am hoping to reach. First, however, it is better to scan the crowd for those who should be seen immediately.

Less ethnographically visible is the fact that Haiti is now under democratic rule. For the first time in almost two centuries, democratic elections are planned and could result in a historic precedent: President René Préval, elected some years earlier, could actually survive his presidency to transfer power to another democratically elected president. (In 2001, Préval succeeded in being the first and so far only president in Haitian history to serve out his mandate, not a day more, not a day less.)

To local eyes, this victory for democratic process is overwhelmed by the deprivation inscribed into the very seams of Haitian society. For the rural poor, most of them peasants, poverty means erosion and lower crop yields; it means hunger and sickness. And every morning the crowd in front of the clinic seems to grow.

To foreign eyes, the Haitian story has become a confused skein of tragedies, most of them seen as local. Poverty, crime, accidents, disease, death—and more often than not their causes—are also seen as problems locally derived. The transnational tale of slavery, debt, and turmoil is lost in Haiti's vivid poverty, the understanding of which seems to defeat the analyses of journalists and even many anthropologists, focused as we are on the ethnographically visible, what is there in front of us.

Making my way through this crowd has become a daily chore, and triage—seeking out the sickest—a ritual in the years since I became medical director of the clinic. Now the morning sun angles into the courtyard, but the patients are shaded by tall ficus trees, planted there years before. The clinic and hospital were built into the hillside over the previous fifteen years, but the dense foliage gives the impression that the buildings have been there for decades.

I see two patients on makeshift stretchers; both are being examined by auxiliary nurses armed with stethoscopes and blood-pressure cuffs. Perhaps this morning it will take less than an hour to cross the 600 or so yards that separate me from another crowd of patients, those already diagnosed with tuberculosis or AIDS. These are the patients I am hoping to see, but it is also my duty to see to the larger crowd, which promises, on this warm Wednesday morning, to overwhelm the small Haitian medical staff.

A young woman takes my arm in a common enough gesture in rural Haiti. "Look at this, doctor." She lifts a left breast mass. The tumor is not at all like the ones I was taught to search for during my medical training in Boston. This lesion started as an occult lump, perhaps, but by this September day it has almost completely replaced the normal breast. It is a "fungating mass," in medical jargon, and clear yellow fluid weeps down the front of a light blue dress. Flies are drawn to the diseased tissue, and the woman waves them away mechanically. On either side of her, a man and a woman help her with this task—not kin, simply other patients waiting in line.

"Good morning," I say, although I know that she is expecting me to say next to nothing and wants to be the speaker. She lifts the tumor toward me and begins talking rapidly.

"It's hard and painful," she says. "Touch it and see how hard it is." Instead, I lift my hand to her axilla and find large, hard lymph nodes there—likely advanced and metastatic cancer—and I interrupt her as politely as I can. If only this were a neglected infection, I think. Not impossible, only very unlikely. I need to know how long this woman has been ill.

But the woman, whose name is Anite, will have none of it. She is going to tell the story properly, and I will have to listen. We are surrounded by hundreds, and at least forty can hear every word of the exchange. I move to pull her from the line, but she wants to talk in front of her fellow sufferers. For years I have studied and written about these peculiarly Haitian modes of declaiming about one's travails, learning how such jeremiads are crafted for a host of situations and audiences. There is so much to complain about. Now I have time only to see patients as a physician and precious little time for interviewing them. Although I miss this part of my work, and I want to hear Anite's story, I want even more to attend to her illness. And to do that properly will require a surgeon, unless she has come with a diagnosis made elsewhere.

I look away from the tumor. She carries, in addition to a hat and a small bundle of oddments, a white vinyl purse. Please, I think, let there be useful information in there. Surely she has seen other doctors for a disease process that is, at a minimum, months along?

I interrupt again to ask her where she has come from and if she has sought care elsewhere. We do not have a surgeon on staff just now. We have been promised, according to a weary functionary at the Ministry of Health, that the Cuban government will soon be sending us a surgeon and a pediatrician. But for this woman, Anite, time has run out.

"I was about to tell you that, doctor." She had let go of my arm to lift the mass, but now she grips it again. "I am from near Jérémie," she says, referring to a small city on the tip of Haiti's southern peninsula—about as far from our clinic as one could be and still be in Haiti. To reach us, Anite must have passed through Port-au-Prince, with its private clinics, surgeons, and oncologists.

"I first noticed a lump in my breast after falling down. I was carrying a basket of millet on my head. It was not heavy, but it was large, and I had packed it poorly, perhaps. The path was steep, but it had not rained on that day, so I don't know why I fell. It makes you wonder, though." At least a dozen heads in line nod in assent, and some of Anite's fellow patients make noises encouraging her to continue.

"How long ago was that?" I ask again.

"I went to many clinics," she says in front of dozens of people she has met only that morning or perhaps the night before. "I went to fourteen clinics." Again, many nod assent. The woman to her left says, "Adjè!"—meaning something along the lines of "You poor thing!"—and lifts a finger to her cheek. This crowd response seems to please Anite, who continues her narrative with gathering tempo. She still has not let me know how long she has been ill.

"Fourteen clinics," I respond. "What did they say was wrong with you? Did you have an operation or a biopsy?" The mass is now large and has completely destroyed the normal architecture of her breast; it is impossible to tell if she has had a procedure, as there is no skin left to scar.

"No," replies Anite. "Many told me I needed an operation, but the specialist who could do this was in the city, and it costs seven hundred dollars to see him. In any case, I had learned in a dream that it was not necessary to go to the city." ("The city" means Port-au-Prince, Haiti's capital.)

More of the crowd turns to listen; the shape of the line changes subtly, beginning to resemble more of a circle. I think uncomfortably of the privacy of a U.S. examination room and of the fact that in that country I have never seen a breast mass consume so much flesh without ever being biopsied. But I have seen many in Haiti, and almost all have proven malignant.

Anite continues her narrative. She repeats that on the day of the fall, she discovered the mass. It was "small and hard," she reports. "An abscess, I thought, for I was breastfeeding and had an infection while breastfeeding once before." This is about as clinical as the story is to get, for Anite returns to the real tale. She hurt her back in the fall. How was she to care for her children and for her mother, who was sick and lived with her? "They all depend on me. There was no time."

And so the mass grew slowly "and worked its way under my arm." I give up trying to establish chronology. I know it had to be months or even years ago that she first discovered this "small" mass. She had gone to clinic after clinic, she says, "spending our very last little money. No one told me what I had. I took many pills."

"What kind of pills?" I ask.

Anite continues. "Pills. I don't know what kind." She had given biomedicine its proper shot, she seems to say, but it had failed her. Perhaps her illness had more mysterious origins? "Maybe someone sent this my way," she suggests. "But I'm a poor woman—why would someone wish me ill?"

"Unlikely," an older man in line chimes in. "It's God's sickness." Anite had assumed as much—"God's sickness" being shorthand for natural illness rather than illness associated with sorcery—but she had gone to a local temple, a *houmfor*, to make sure. "The reason I went was because I'd had a dream. The mass was growing, and there were three other small masses growing under my arm. I had a dream in which a voice told me to stop taking medicines and to travel far away for treatment of this illness."

She had gone to a voodoo priest for help in interpreting this dream. Each of the lumps had significance, said the priest. They represented "the three mysteries," and to be cured she would have to travel to a clinic where doctors "worked with both hands" (this term suggesting that they would have to understand both natural and supernatural illness).

The story would have been absurd if it were not so painful. I know, and once knew more, about some of the cultural referents; I am familiar with the style of illness narrative dictating some of the contours of her story and the responses of those in line. But Anite has, I am almost sure, metastatic breast cancer. What she needs is surgery and chemotherapy if she is lucky (to my knowledge, there is no radiation therapy in Haiti at this time). She does not need, I think, to tell her story publicly for at least the fifteenth time.

But Anite seems to gather strength from the now-rapt crowd, all with their own stories to tell the harried doctors and nurses once they get into the clinic. The semicircle continues to grow. Some of the patients are straining, I can tell, for a chance to tell their own stories, but no one interrupts Anite. "In order to cure this illness, he told me, I would have to travel far north and east."

It has taken Anite over a week to reach our clinic. A diagnosis of metastatic breast cancer is later confirmed.

I am privileged to be presenting this lecture in honor of Sidney Mintz, someone whose work I very much admire. I will be talking about Haiti and about tuberculosis and AIDS. I'm not sure I would know how *not* to talk about these diseases, which each day claim almost fifteen thousand lives worldwide, most of them adults in their prime. I hope less to take on grand theory than to ask how the concept of *structural violence* might come to figure in work in anthropology and other disciplines seeking to understand modern social life. Standing on the shoulders of those who have studied slavery, racism, and other forms of institutionalized violence, a growing number of anthropologists now devote their attention to structural violence.

Just as everyone seems to have his or her own definitions of "structure" and "violence," so too does the term "structural violence" cause epistemological jitters in our ranks. It dates back at least to 1969, to Johan Galtung as well as the Latin American liberation theologians.[1] The latter used the term broadly to describe "sinful" social structures characterized by poverty and steep grades of social inequality, including racism and gender inequality. Structural violence is violence exerted systematically—that is, indirectly—by everyone who belongs to a certain social order: hence the discomfort these ideas provoke in a moral economy still geared to pinning praise or blame on individual actors. In short, the concept of structural violence is intended to inform the study of the social machinery of oppression. Oppression is a result of many conditions, not the least of which reside in consciousness. We will therefore need to examine, as well, the roles played by the erasure of historical memory and other forms of desocialization as enabling conditions of structures that are both "sinful" and ostensibly "nobody's fault."

The degree to which people can fight back against such infernal machinery—or its symbolic props—has been the subject of much discussion in anthropology. We have written about "the weapons of the weak," to use James Scott's term,[2] and many texts have celebrated various forms of "resistance" to the dominant social order and its supports, symbolic and material. Romanticism aside, the impact of extreme poverty and social marginalization is profound in many of the settings in which anthropologists work. These settings include not only the growing slums and shrinking villages of the Third World (or whatever it is called these days) but also, frequently, the cities of the United States. In some of these places, there really are social spaces of spirited resistance.

Often, however, the impact of such resistance is less than we make it out to be, especially when we contemplate the most desperate struggles and attempt in any serious way to keep a body count. One way of putting it is that the degree to which agency is constrained is correlated inversely, if not always neatly, with the ability to resist marginalization and other forms of oppression. We already have, for example, good ethnographic accounts of how young working-class "lads" in England resist, or do not resist, "learning to labor."[3] We have solid accounts of how women in industrialized countries—Japan and the United States—contest the meanings and experience of menopause.[4] We have in-depth reports on "social suffering" in France, India, the United States, Brazil, even highland Guatemala.[5] But because ethnographic work relies on conversations with the living—or on the records left by the literate—we are still not getting the entire picture. An anthropology that tallies the body count must of course look at the dead and those left for dead. Such inquiry seeks to understand how suffering is muted or elided altogether. It explores the complicity necessary to erase history and cover up the clear links between the dead and near-dead and those who are the winners in the struggle for survival.

Bringing these links—whether they are termed social, biological, or symbolic—into view is a key task for an anthropology of structural violence. I will argue here that keeping the material in focus is one way to avoid undue romanticism in accomplishing this task. An honest account of who wins, who loses, and what weapons are used is an important safeguard against the romantic illusions of those who, like us, are usually shielded from the sharp edges of structural violence. I find it helpful to think of the "materiality of the social," a term that underlines my conviction that social life in general and structural violence in particular will not be understood without a deeply materialist approach to whatever surfaces in the participant-observer's field of vision—the ethnographically visible.

By "materialist," I do not mean "economic" as if economic structures were not socially constructed. I do not mean "biological" as if biology were likewise somehow immune from social construction. I am not trying to establish a bedrock category of reality or engage worn-out or false debates—for example, trying to persuade old-school materialists that social life matters or to convince hard-line culturalists that the material (from the body to modes of economic production) is the very stuff of social construction. To push the metaphor, any social project requires construction materials, while the building process is itself inevitably social and thus cultural. The adverse outcomes associated with structural violence—death, injury, illness, subjugation, stigmatization, and even psychological terror—come to have their "final common pathway" in the material. Structural violence is embodied as adverse events if what we study, as anthropologists, is the experience of people who live in poverty or are marginalized by racism, gender inequality, or a noxious mix of all of the above.

The adverse events to be discussed here include epidemic disease, violations of human rights, and genocide.

Such an approach fits easily within the historically attested project of modern anthropology. This was true from the discipline's beginnings, and I will argue that it remains so today. In a chapter entitled "What Anthropology Is About," our clan ancestor Alfred Kroeber underlined the importance of "anthropology, biology, history." "In practice," he wrote in 1923, "anthropology is mostly classified as being both a biological science and a social science. . . . Such a situation of double participation is unusual among the sciences."[6] Unusual then, it is even more so now, when specialization and subspecialization have yielded great rewards in the biological sciences. The rewards are less evident, alas, within the social sciences, where increasing specialization has often brought with it the erasure of history and political economy. The erosion of social awareness is readily detected in modern psychology, epidemiology, and many branches of sociology. Desocialization is evident even in anthropology, held by many to be the most radically contextualizing of the social sciences.[7] Complex biosocial phenomena are the focus of most anthropological inquiries, and yet the integration of history, political economy, and biology remains lacking in contemporary anthropology or sociology.[8]

An anthropology of structural violence necessarily draws on history and biology, just as it necessarily draws on political economy. To tally body counts correctly requires epidemiology, forensic and clinical medicine, and demography. The erasure of these broad bodies of knowledge may be seen as the central problematic of a robust anthropology of structural violence. If we set for ourselves the cheerful task of coming to understand pestilence, death, and destruction, let us look at how the erasure of history—indeed, of temporality itself—and of biology comes to hobble an honest assessment of social life. I focus my attention on Haiti.

CREATING DESERTS, ERASING HISTORY

Tacitus is credited with the aphorism "They created a desert and called it peace."[9] Erasing history is perhaps the most common explanatory sleight-of-hand relied upon by the architects of structural violence. Erasure or distortion of history is part of the process of desocialization necessary for the emergence of hegemonic accounts of what happened and why. Haiti, as Sidney Mintz has shown, serves as the most painful example of this erasure and why it matters. And there are certain times, such as now, in which exploring the historical roots of a problem is not a popular process. There is not always much support for laying bare the fretwork of entrenched structures that promise more misery. Referring to the attitudes that prevailed after the events of September 11, 2001, English novelist John le Carré observed, "It's as if we have entered a new, Orwellian world . . .

Suggesting there is a historical context for the recent atrocities is by implication to make excuses for them. Anyone who is with us doesn't do that. Anyone who does, is against us."[10]

It is possible, of course, merely to deny history, but people are not that easily fooled—at least not all of them all of the time. The erasure of history is subtle and incremental and depends upon the erasure of links across time and space. We know, too, that forgetting is also a natural—indeed, biological—process. Time heals all wounds, including those which, never properly drained, are waiting to burst open again, to the "surprise" of those who have forgotten.

Getting a good accounting of an event is always a challenge for the ethnographer who remains committed to the quest for—let's say it—the truth. Anthropological inquiry often starts with current events and the ethnographically visible. When we study the social impact of a hydroelectric dam, of terrorism, or of a new epidemic, we run a great risk of partial blindness. Erasures, in these instances, prove expedient to the powerful, whose agency is usually unfettered. Imbalances of power cannot be erased without distortion of meaning. Without a historically deep and geographically broad analysis, one that takes into account political economy, we see only the residue of meaning. We see the puddles, perhaps, but not the rainstorms and certainly not the gathering thunderclouds.

Both parts of this explanatory duty—the geographically broad and the historically deep—are critical. Those who look only to the past to explain the ethnographically visible will miss the webs of living power that enmesh witnessed misery. Some of the links that must be made visible are the living links. The latter-day critique of the conduct of ethnographic fieldwork within the confines of the British Empire has served as the classic example in anthropology. The African anthropology of E. E. Evans-Pritchard and many others has been subjected to exercises that attempt to restore these elided links.[11] Indeed, Johannes Fabian has argued that "denial of coevalness" remains a major problem in anthropology.[12]

Those who look only to powerful present-day actors to explain misery will fail to see how inequality is structured and legitimated over time. Which construction materials were used, and when, and why, and how? Our attempts to freeze social process in an "ethnographic present" have in the end only complicated our task. "By some strange sleight of hand," Mintz has noted, "one anthropological monograph after another whisks out of view any signs of the present and how it came to be. This vanishing act imposes burdens on those who feel the need to perform it: those of us who do not ought to have been thinking much more soberly about what anthropologists should study."[13]

Richly socialized accounts take time and space. They are longer than sound bites, more than factoids. They still emerge in certain forms—books, say, or long documentary films—but are rare in the media that command popular attention.

Popular media adore the quick fix: best of all is a one-phrase explanation, such as "Islam made them do it" or "The clash of cultures is inevitable" or "They envy our good fortune." The works of anthropologists are long in part because the more we know about something, the less easy it is to dismiss any twist of interpretation, any ostensibly arcane historical detail, as irrelevant. How can we be sure of its irrelevance? If our epistemic sense of relevance filters something out, is that appropriate, or is it rather an occasion for critiquing our filters? Relevance depends on what we are looking for, and the richer our knowledge of the material, the more competing hypotheses we will derive from it. The burden of significance becomes overwhelming as links between apparently disparate acts and distant places are revealed. And the stakes are high, surely, when it is a matter of life and death.

Allow me to offer, through two vignettes from the 1780s, separated in space but not in time, an example of linked, coeval processes. The first concerns French cuisine and fashion—still celebrated—and the other a less well-known export item, French enslavement of Africans. I am quoting from a cultural history of the soon-to-be *ancien régime:*

> Hair powder (a mixture of starch and perfumed powders) had been in use through-out the century, but now you could not be in fashion unless you wore towers of hair piled up nearly three feet high and generously supplemented with cushions and hair pieces. This edifice was adorned with curls, a hat, ostrich feathers and jewels, but to be really modish you had to wear a headdress *de circonstance.* Thus, when Admiral d'Estaing won his battle over the English fleet, ladies wore an entire ship, almost a foot high and dangling a jeweled anchor in the back; they adorned themselves with flowers which drew water from flat bottles concealed deep within the structure, or with a mechanical jeweled bird which suddenly started to trill.[14]

This truly over-the-top haberdashery was to be found on the heads of the well-to-do, but even the growing upper middle class was able to partake in such excess well before France was said to have a middle class. "French cuisine," we read in the same book, by Olivier Bernier, "continued to progress in less exalted circles. The first modern cookbook was published in 1779. Entitled *La cuisinière bourgeoise,* it achieved instant and lasting popularity." Bernier reports that "if you were reasonably prosperous and wanted to give a dinner for fifteen in the summer, *La cuisinière bourgeoise* advised the following menu":

One large roast beef to be placed in the center of the table

FIRST SERVICE
　Two soups:
　　Cucumber soup
　　Green pea soup with croutons

Four appetizers:
  Fried mutton feet
  Veal roast in pastry
  Small pâtés
  Melons

SECOND SERVICE
  Boiled leg of mutton
  Roast veal marinated in cream
  Duckling with peas
  Squab with herbs
  Two chickens with little white onions
  Rabbit steaks with cucumbers

THIRD SERVICE
  Replace the roast beef in the center by a large brioche
  Four roasts:
    One small turkey
    One capon
    Four partridges
    Six squabs roasted like quails
  Two green salads

FOURTH SERVICE
  Apricot tartlets
  Scrambled eggs
  Vine-leaf fritters
  Cookies
  Small white beans in cream
  Artichokes with butter sauce

FIFTH SERVICE: DESSERT
  A large bowl of fresh fruit to be placed in the center of the table
  Four compotes:
    Peaches
    Prunes
    Pears
    Green grapes
  Four plates of ice cream
  One plate of cream cheese
  One plate of pastries

"Of course," continues Bernier, "not everybody ate every dish. Most people would choose one, or at most two, offerings from any given service, and the quantities eaten of anything were very small. Even so, fifteen *middle-class* people, who probably spent some three or four hours over their meal, could hardly have left the table hungry."[15]

Nor were they thirsty, not for spirits. If half the guests were women with miniature men-o'-war in their hair, the providential hostess would want to prevent shipwrecks around the table. So what of the drink? Bernier notes:

> No wines are mentioned in our menu because a variety of open bottles were set up on the sideboard. You would turn to one of the servants and ask for whatever you wanted to drink, white, red, or rosé, as often as your glass was empty. In great houses it was the custom for each guest to bring his own servant, who stood behind him throughout the meal and attended to his wants. *La cuisinière bourgeoise* aimed at a more modest milieu: it recommended having seven servants to pass the food and wine, six of whom were probably hired for the day.[16]

If the tone of Bernier's book is a bit flip, the ethnographic detail is meant to be accurate. The hairdos did have frigates in them, and the French had reason to incorporate ships into their adornment: much of their bounty and wealth then came from a special kind of naval trade.

It is hard to deny—with the subsequent French Revolution to prove it—that most people in eighteenth-century France lived in poverty; the less fortunate classes were also increasingly aware of the excesses of the *ancien régime*. But how could local agriculture have sustained such luxury? It didn't, of course. We need to travel back to France's most important colony. It is estimated that by the late eighteenth century two-thirds of all of Europe's tropical produce and a great deal of French wealth came from Haiti alone.[17] Indeed, although Bernier does not mention slavery until page 181 of the book I've just cited, he does spell out the cause-and-effect relationship between the accumulation of merchant capital through the triangular trade and the launch of powdered frigates into the salons of Paris, Bordeaux, and Versailles:

> French products went everywhere, but very few objects of foreign make came into France. The bulk of trade was in foodstuffs, tobacco and colonial products: sugar, spices, rice, tea, coffee. This allowed a number of businessmen, most from Bordeaux, to cash in on a highly profitable item of trade, referred to as *le bois d'ébène* (ebony wood): black slaves. Many French shipowners took part in the infamous triangular exchange of slaves, sugar and rum, and prospered. The city of Bordeaux was virtually rebuilt from scratch in the late eighteenth century and still looks glorious today. It was paid for in human flesh.[18]

Where, precisely, was all of this "ebony" going? According to Herbert Klein, approximately half of the slaves who crossed the Atlantic at this time were bound for a single slave colony, Saint-Domingue (as Haiti was then called):

By the late 1780s Saint-Domingue planters were recognized as the most efficient and productive sugar producers in the world. The slave population stood at 460,000 people, which was not only the largest of any island but represented close to half of the one million slaves then being held in all the Caribbean colonies. The exports of the island represented two-thirds of the total value of all French West Indian exports, and alone [were] greater than the combined exports from the British and Spanish Antilles. In any one year well over 600 vessels visited the ports of the island to carry its sugar, coffee, cotton, indigo, and cacao to European consumers.[19]

Six hundred vessels a year to take deliveries from that "efficient" colony— no wonder the ladies wore ships perched on their heads. This is significantly more harbor traffic than occurs today, even though the population of the island, descended from the slaves, is about twenty times as numerous. The colony's exemplary "efficiency" is, of course, disputed. Few of the slaves left accounts of their experience, but some European visitors wrote down their impressions. Among them was Médéric Louis Élie Moreau de Saint-Méry, who saw in the colony another face of the machinery of structural violence:

> In St. Domingue everything takes on an air of opulence that dazzles Europeans. That throng of slaves who await the orders and even the lifted finger of a lone individual, confers grandeur on him who commands them. To have four times as many servants as one needs marks the grandiloquence of a wealthy man. As for the ladies, their main talent is to surround themselves with a useless cohort of maidservants. Since the supreme happiness for a European is to be waited on, he even rents slaves until able to possess them in his own right.[20]

That the French slave colony was a hellish place was evident enough to French and other European visitors: few Frenchmen who had a choice left their comfortable European homes, though many were indirect beneficiaries of the colonial system. But justifications of slavery were well accepted by most Europeans, even at the height of the Enlightenment, and misgivings were not often expressed.[21] After the revolution that ended in 1803 made Haiti Latin America's first independent republic, some of the former slaves were able to commit their thoughts to paper. A fully socialized cultural history of fashion and cuisine in late-eighteenth-century France would benefit from cross-referencing a Haitian memoir from 1814. Speaking of his former French masters, Pompée-Valentin Vastey asks:

> Have they not hung up men with heads downward, drowned them in sacks, crucified them on planks, buried them alive, crushed them in mortars? Have they not forced them to eat shit? And, after having flayed them with the lash, have they not cast them alive to be devoured by worms, or onto anthills, or lashed them to stakes in the swamp to be devoured by mosquitoes? Have they not thrown them into boiling cauldrons of cane syrup? Have they not put men and women inside

barrels studded with spikes and rolled them down mountainsides into the abyss? Have they not consigned these miserable blacks to man-eating dogs until the latter, sated by human flesh, left the mangled victims to be finished off with bayonet and dagger?[22]

"MODERN" HAITI:
RESOCIALIZING HISTORY AND BIOLOGY

Two hundred years later, I had the good fortune to go to Haiti. There I learned a good deal about the selective erasure of history and the force, sometimes less readily hidden, of biology. though within Haiti these erasures had scarcely taken place. In Haiti, the past was present—in proverbs; in the very language spoken, itself a product of the slave colony; and in popular Haitian readings of its present-day misfortune. In Haiti, structural violence continues to play itself out in the daily lives and deaths of the part of the population living in poverty. People know about the body count because they bury their kin.

Mintz and others have pointed out that Haiti has long constituted a sort of living laboratory for the study of affliction, no matter how it is defined.[23] Helen Wiese observed a generation ago that "life for the Haitian peasant of today is abject misery and a rank familiarity with death."[24] The biggest problem, of course, is unimaginable poverty. While the dictatorships may be gone, the transnational political and economic structures that maintained them are still in place and still inflicting their harm.

An ethnographic study of modern Haiti may or may not discuss the ways in which West Africans were moved to Haiti. (Haiti's first victims, however, were the natives of the island, perhaps eight million strong in 1492 and completely gone by the time the French and Spanish struggled over the island in the late seventeenth century—eight million people, almost completely forgotten through the selective erasure of history and biology.) Such a study may or may not discuss tuberculosis, smallpox, measles, or yellow fever. A modern ethnographer may not mention that the former colony was forced to repay a "debt" to the French, supposedly incurred by the loss of the world's most profitable slave plantations. But these facts need to be included and their sequelae addressed: their absence makes a fully socialized accounting of the present nearly unthinkable. Allow me to sum up the post-independence history of Haiti.

The Haitian revolution began in 1791. France's refusal to accept the loss of so "efficient" and profitable a colony led, ultimately, to the expedition of the largest armada ever to cross the Atlantic. After the 1803 Battle of Vertières, in which Napoleon's troops were defeated, Haiti declared itself an independent nation. But its infrastructure lay in ruins: some estimate that more than half of the island's population perished in the war. The land was still fertile, if less so than when the

Europeans began monocropping it, and so the new republic's leadership, desperate to revive the economy, fought to restore the plantations without overt slavery. It was a losing battle, as Mintz has written: "An entire nation turned its back upon the system of large estates, worked by forced labor."[25]

Even if there were other ways of growing these products—and coffee, unlike sugar, was clearly a product that could be grown on small homesteads—who would buy them? The Europeans and the only other republic in the Western Hemisphere, the United States, were the only likely customers, and they mostly followed a French-led embargo on Haiti. How many people in France remember that in order to obtain diplomatic recognition, Haiti was required to indemnify France to the tune of 150 million francs, with payments to the government of Charles X beginning in 1825? One hundred fifty million francs in reparations to the slave owners—a social and economic fact redolent with meaning then and today and one with grave material consequences for the Haitians.[26] One scholarly history, written by Haitian anthropologist Jean Price-Mars, discusses these reparations in this way: "From a country whose expenditures and receipts were, until then, balanced, the incompetence and frivolity of the men in power had made a nation burdened with debts and entangled in a web of impossible financial obligations."[27]

This set the tone for the new century: trade concessions for European and U.S. partners and indirect taxes for the peasants who grew the produce, their backs bent under the weight of a hostile world. Especially hostile was the United States, the slave-owning republic to the north: "The United States blocked Haiti's invitation to the famous Western Hemisphere Panama Conference of 1825 and refused to recognize Haitian independence until 1862. This isolation was imposed on Haiti by a frightened white world, and Haiti became a test case, first for those arguing about emancipation and then, after the end of slavery, for those arguing about the capacity of blacks for self-government."[28]

In the years following independence, the United States and allied European powers helped France orchestrate a diplomatic quarantine of Haiti, and the new republic soon became the outcast of the international community. In 1824 Senator Robert Hayne of South Carolina declared, "Our policy with regard to Hayti is plain. We never can acknowledge her independence. . . . The peace and safety of a large portion of our union forbids us even to discuss [it]."[29]

But the isolation was largely diplomatic and rhetorical, as those who remember the broad outlines of gunboat diplomacy recall. The United States was increasingly present as a trading partner and policeman, leading to a number of famous run-ins with the Haitians—famous, I mean, in Haiti, though largely forgotten, of course, in the United States.[30] Continuous U.S. naval presence led, eventually, to an armed occupation of Haiti in 1915. This occupation, another chapter of U.S. history now almost completely forgotten by the occupiers, was to last twenty years. Although the rationale for our military occupation is debated, "control of the customs houses," observed President Woodrow Wilson, "constituted the essence of this whole affair."

Since 1915, at the latest, the United States has been the dominant force in Haitian politics. The modern Haitian army was created, in 1916, by an act of the U.S. Congress. From the time of troop withdrawal in 1934 until 1990, no Haitian administration has risen to power without the blessing of the U.S. government. This resulted in a string of military and paramilitary governments leading in 1957 to the Duvalier regime, which was, in terms of dollar support, a major recipient of U.S. largesse.[31] Indeed, there have been no major political discontinuities until perhaps 1990, with the result that the template of "colony"—a slave colony—continued to shape life in Haiti. Just as the wealthy were socialized for excess, the Haitian poor were socialized for scarcity. Management of time, affection, food, water, and family crises (including illness) all fit into this ancient framework of too much and too little.

This is the framework I had in mind when I began studying specific infectious diseases—one old, one new—in rural Haiti. In anthropology, a version of this framework has been called "world-systems theory,"[32] but it is not really theory-driven. It is an approach that is committed to ethnographically embedding evidence within the historically given social and economic structures that shape life so dramatically on the edge of life and death. These structures are transnational, and therefore not even their modern vestiges are really ethnographically visible. Many anthropologists have used this framework in an attempt to depict the social machinery of oppression by bringing connections into relief.[33]

Regardless of our specific research questions, we have struggled to define these social and economic structures, to understand how they work. For want of a better word, I have often used the term "neoliberal economics" to refer to the prevailing (at times contradictory) constellation of ideas about trade and development and governance that has been internalized by many in the affluent market societies. Neoliberalism is the ideology promoted by the victors of the struggles mentioned earlier. The dominance of a competition-driven market is said to be at the heart of this model, but in truth this ideology is indebted to and helps to replicate inequalities of power. It is an ideology that has little to say about the social and economic inequalities that distort real economies and instead reveals yet another means by which these economies can be further exploited. Neoliberal thought is central to modern development efforts, the goal of which is less to repair poverty and social inequalities than to manage them. Its opponents include some of those left behind by development, whose deep disaffection is rooted in the erased experience I have tried to summarize. Work throughout Latin America has convinced me that the disaffection is also associated with a set of ideas not too different, interestingly, from that expressed by the late Pierre Bourdieu:

> Scientific rationalism—the rationalism of the mathematical models which inspire the policy of the IMF or the World Bank, that of the great law firms, great juridical multinationals which impose the traditions of American law on the whole planet, that of rational-action theories, etc.—is both the expression and the justification of a Western arrogance, which leads [some] people to act as if they had the monopoly of reason and could set themselves up as world policemen, in other words as self-appointed holders of the monopoly of legitimate violence, capable of applying the force of arms in the service of universal justice.[34]

As someone who believes deeply in the promise and progress of science, I would point out that it is the ideology springing from market economies that is critiqued by most opponents of neoliberal thought. It is not affluence or modernity itself, still less a certain "way of life," that is under attack. Haitians living in poverty have ample reason to be wary of neoliberal nostrums, for theirs is an embodied understanding of modern inequality. Over the past decade, Haiti has undergone something of an economic devolution. Gross national product has declined; so has life expectancy. What are the causes of all this present-day misery? There is slavery, of course, and racism is central to slavery, and this is one reason that recent meetings in Durban, South Africa, focused on both. Allow me to quote from a draft of the document signed there by representatives of more than 150 countries:[35]

> The world conference acknowledges and profoundly regrets the massive human sufferings and the tragic plight of millions of men, women and children caused by slavery, slave trade, trans-Atlantic slave trade, apartheid, colonialism and genocide and calls upon states concerned to honor the memory of the victims of past tragedies and affirms that wherever and whenever these occurred they must be condemned and their reoccurrence prevented.
>
> The world conference regrets that these practices and structures, political, socioeconomic and cultural, have led to racism, racial discrimination, xenophobia and related intolerance.
>
> The world conference recognizes that these historical injustices have undeniably contributed to poverty, underdevelopment, marginalization, social exclusion, economic disparities, instability and insecurity that affect many people in different parts of the world, in particular in developing countries.
>
> The world conference recognizes the need to develop programs for the social and economic development of these societies and the diaspora within the framework of a new partnership based on the spirit of solidarity and mutual respect in the following areas: debt relief, poverty eradication, building or strengthening democratic institutions, promotion of foreign direct investment, market access.

Imagine what it is like for poor villagers to hear (I say "hear," because most cannot read) these words in Haiti, a country still stinging not only from the reparations paid to its former masters but from a series of sanctions that continue to this day. "Mutual respect" would be nice, but "solidarity" has rarely taken practical form. As Sidney Mintz once wrote, "If ever there were a society that ought to have ended up totally annihilated, materially and spiritually, by the trials of 'modernization,' it is Haiti."[36] If ever there were a society screaming out for precisely the sort of reparations recommended by "the international community," it is Haiti. Here war has created a desert, though no one can call it peace.

How on earth could one rebuild such a broken place? Haiti has no roads to speak of and poor telecommunications. Agriculture has faltered, perhaps irreparably, and no industry promises to replace it. There are, of course, great polemics regarding the methods of "grassroots" development and production for export and equally high sentiment regarding "foreign aid." The concept of "microcredit" has generated, fittingly enough, a cottage industry. But how does microcredit function in a failing economy? The poorest are those least likely to profit from credit in the odd event that it is extended to them.

The public health infrastructure is of special concern to me. In the past decade, I have witnessed two related processes in central Haiti: the collapse of the public health sector and the overwhelming of the hospital of which I am the medical director. Even if our hospital were uninterested in seeking foreign aid in the conventional sense, we would desperately be awaiting the rebuilding of the Haitian health system. The "international community" promised to help rebuild Haiti in 1994, when a $500 million aid package was proposed. But the international community is large enough—"diverse enough" would probably be the wording it would choose—to talk out of both sides of its mouth. We have read the Durban Declaration, which calls for reparations to postslavery societies. We agree that this hemisphere's poorest country is also and not coincidentally its largest postslavery society. Cuba would be the second-largest postslavery society. Guess which two Western Hemisphere republics are under an aid embargo? Does anyone think that Haitians, at least the ones I live among, do not see the continuity between the current and previous embargoes?

"What embargo?" one may well ask. "Imposed on Haiti? By whom?" Since the Haitian elections of 2000, the U.S. government has used its influence with international lending institutions such as the Inter-American Development Bank to withhold already approved loans earmarked for development and improving health, education, and water quality in Haiti. And direct aid from the U.S. government now bypasses the formal national structures (such as the Ministries of Health and Education) and is distributed solely to nongovernmental agencies.

What is the justification for such an embargo, given all our promises? Are there credible claims, for example, that Jean-Bertrand Aristide, as unpopular

in Washington, D.C., as he is popular in rural Haiti, did not win the presidential elections of November 2000 fair and square? No, the complaints this time
are about the legislative elections that took place in May 2000, months before
Aristide was reelected by the usual landslide, and in dispute were all of eight
senatorial seats. The argument is that since vote counting was supposedly not
done correctly, there should have been runoff elections. So, presto! official aid to
Haiti is frozen. Those of us who study the patterns of giving to other countries
may already be a bit suspicious as to the real motives behind such action. In
a recently published editorial, Larry Birns and Michael McCarthy put it well:
"Where else in the world does [Washington] deny sending crucial aid to a famished neighbor in spite of its underdeveloped political system? Haitians are well
aware of Washington's game and are likening its freezing of desperately needed
funds to the U.S. embargo imposed on Haiti after their 1804 revolution made the
island the world's first black republic."[37]

We seemed to have no trouble running hundreds of millions through the
Duvalier dictatorship. We were unstintingly generous to the post-Duvalier military, whose spectacular exploits included burning down Aristide's packed church
during mass. Looking elsewhere to see whether rigorous adherence to certain
electoral procedures, in general, determines the level of aid, we might consider
Pakistan, which until recently was under a similar embargo but with real justification, since General Pervez Musharraf came to power in a military coup.[38]
"My personal objective when I got here in August," U.S. ambassador Wendy
Chamberlin said in an interview, "was to work very hard to improve Pakistani-
American relations, with the aim that at the end of my three years here we could
lift American sanctions on Pakistan. I could never have dreamed that we'd have
accomplished so much of it in my first three months." Any U.S. reservations
about Pakistan's military government were quickly forgotten as of September 11.[39]

How does this hypocrisy play itself out among the poor? Take as an example
Inter-American Development Bank (IDB) Loan No. 1009/SF-HA, "Reorganiza-
tion of the National Health System." On July 21, 1998, the Haitian government
and the IDB signed a $22.5 million loan for phase 1 of a project to decentralize and
reorganize the Haitian health care system. The need to improve the health care
system was and remains urgent: there are 1.2 doctors, 1.3 nurses, and 0.04 dentists
per 10,000 Haitians; 40 percent of the population is without access to any form
of primary health care. HIV and tuberculosis rates are by far the highest in the
hemisphere, as are rates of infant, juvenile, and maternal mortality. To use the
bank's jargon, the project was to target 80 percent of the population for access
to primary health care through the construction of low-cost clinics and local
health dispensaries, the training of community health agents, and the purchase
of medical equipment and essential medicines.

To be judged successful by its own criteria, the project would need to produce a drop in the infant mortality rate from 74 to 50 deaths per 1,000 live births, a drop in the juvenile mortality rate from 131 to 110 deaths per 1,000 births, a drop in the birth rate from 4.6 to 4, and a drop in the general mortality rate attributable to the lack of proper health care from 10.7 to 9.7 per 1,000. These were not overly ambitious goals. Most who evaluated the project thought it feasible and well designed. The signing took place several years ago.

Ratification of the loan agreement was initially held up by Haiti's famously obstructionist 46th Legislature, whose goal was clear enough within Haiti—to paralyze all social services, including health care, in order to undermine every effort of the executive branch (even then associated with Aristide) to improve the living conditions of the poor majority that had elected him by a landslide in 1990 and in short order would do so again.

In October 2000, after the installation of the more representative 47th Legislature, the new parliament voted immediately to ratify the health project along with three other vital IDB loan agreements. Nevertheless, by early March 2001, the IDB had not yet disbursed the loan, though it announced that it fully intended to work with the new Aristide government and to finance projects already in the pipeline. It demanded, however, that a number of conditions be met, requiring the poorest nation in the hemisphere to pay back millions of dollars of outstanding debts racked up by the previous U.S.-supported dictatorships, as well as "credit commissions" and interest on undisbursed funds. For example, as of March 31, 2001, Haiti already owed the IDB $185,239.75 as a "commission fee" on a loan it had never received. The total amount of fees owed on five development loans from the IDB was $2,311,422. Whereas in the nineteenth century Haiti had had to pay "reparations" to slave owners, at the start of the twenty-first century a different sort of extortion is being practiced to ensure that Haiti will not become too independent.

The health loan has still not been disbursed, and thus the embargo on international aid to Haiti continues, even though the Haitian government has followed all the stipulations set down for resolving the disputed elections. In the meantime, the courtyard around our hospital remains overflowing—that is, the ethnographically visible part.

These details about loans and such may seem pedestrian to an academic audience. They certainly would hold no great interest for me were it not for their direct and profound impact on the bodies of the vulnerable.[40] Trust me, they are of life-and-death significance.

For those reluctant to trust a physician-anthropologist on this score, one has only to consider the case of Anite, dying of metastatic breast cancer. She inhabits a world in which it is possible to visit fourteen clinics without receiving a diagnosis or even palliative care. The contours of this world, a world in which her options and even her dreams are constrained sharply, have been shaped by the historical and economic processes described here. Bourdieu used the term "habitus" as a "structured and structuring" principle. Structural violence is structured and stricturing. It constricts the agency of its victims. It tightens a physical noose around their necks, and this garroting determines the way in which resources—food, medicine, even affection—are allocated and experienced. Socialization for scarcity is informed by a complex web of events and processes stretching far back in time and across continents. The Haitians have a proverb: *Grangou se mizè; vant plen se traka* (Hunger is misery; a full belly means trouble).

CREATING MIRAGES, ERASING BIOLOGY

Clearly, history and its erasure are often embodied as bad health outcomes. This is especially true among the vulnerable. The people who choke our clinic courtyard, instead of other, emptier clinics in which "users' fees" keep away the poor, may think of this as temporary. That will be up to decision makers in Washington, not in Port-au-Prince or in central Haiti. Structural violence takes on new forms in every era. As far as wages and work conditions go, we have heard of "the race to the bottom," and the stewards of the globalizing economy make sure that political compliance is rewarded with the table scraps of today's menu, a good deal less sumptuous than that described by *La cuisinière bourgeoise*.

If we cannot study structural violence without understanding history, the same can be said for understanding biology. How does structural violence take its toll? Sometimes with bombs or even airplanes turned into bombs or with bullets. However spectacular, terrorism and retaliatory bombardments are but minor players in terms of the body count. Structural violence, at the root of much terrorism and bombardment, is much more likely to wither bodies slowly, very often through infectious diseases.

There is a sense, within anthropology, that its medical subfield is somehow pedestrian. This is a mistake. I say this not because of wounded *amour propre* but because I am convinced that a robust medical anthropology could be critical to our understanding of how structural violence comes to harvest its victims. Tuberculosis and AIDS cause millions of premature deaths every year. These two pathogens are, in fact, the leading infectious causes of adult deaths in the world today. Everyone interested in structural violence should have a particular interest in these diseases and in the social structures that perpetuate them.

An anthropological understanding needs to be, as Kroeber suggests, both biological and social. Let me illustrate with the better-known of the two diseases. Tuberculosis was long called "the white plague," and it is widely believed that it arose with the Industrial Revolution and then faded. As historian Katherine Ott reminds us, however, "tuberculosis is not 'resurgent' to those who have been contending with and marginalized by it all their lives."[41] A third of the world's population is infected with the causative organism. We can expect eight to ten million cases a year, with two to three million deaths.

How would a critical anthropology look at tuberculosis? Unfortunately, much of the work to date has been focused on the "cultural beliefs," as they are termed, of the victims of tuberculosis. In Haiti, for example, anthropologists have hastened to note that the locals often regard tuberculosis as a disease sent by sorcery. I took up this question of folk belief some decades later and discovered that many of the terms used in late-twentieth-century Haiti came right out of the slave plantations.[42] In the Central Plateau, ethnographic research conducted in the 1980s revealed that the majority of those afflicted saw tuberculosis as "sent" to them by sorcery. A decade later, after an effective tuberculosis treatment program was put in place, Didi Bertrand and others reported that tuberculosis was increasingly seen as an airborne infectious disease. More to the point, it was seen as treatable, and the stigma associated with it was clearly on the wane.

This indissociable trio of anthropology, history, and biology is just as readily evident when we look closely at the world's most recent plague and the complex trajectory of its causative agent—a virus, in this case. Since the syndrome was first described, AIDS has also been termed a "social disease" and has been studied by social scientists, including anthropologists. Theses and books have been written. One scholar wrote, early on, of an "epidemic of signification."[43] When AIDS was first recognized, in the early 1980s, it was soon apparent that it was an infectious disease, even though other, more exotic interpretations abounded at the time. Well before Luc Montagnier discovered HIV in 1983, many believed that the etiologic agent was a never-before-described virus, and people wanted to know, as they so often do, where this new sickness came from. During those years, the hypotheses circulating in the United States suggested that HIV came to the United States from Haiti. Newspaper articles, television reports, and even scholarly publications confidently posited a scenario in which Haitian professionals who had fled the Duvalier regime ended up in western Africa and later brought the new virus back to Haiti, which introduced it to the Americas. AIDS was said to proliferate in Haiti because of strange practices involving voodoo blood rituals and animal sacrifice.

These theories are ethnographically absurd, but they are wrong in other ways, too. First, they happened to be incorrect epidemiologically. AIDS in Haiti had nothing to do with voodoo or Africa. Second, they had an adverse effect on Haiti—the tourism industry collapsed in the mid-1980s in large part as a result of rumors about HIV—and an adverse effect on Haitians living in North America and Europe. The perception in the minds of many Americans that "Haitian" was almost synonymous with "HIV-infected" has been well documented.[44]

How, then, was HIV introduced to the island nation of Haiti? An intracellular organism must necessarily cross water in a human host. It was clear from the outset that HIV did not come to Haiti from Africa. None of the first Haitians diagnosed with the new syndrome had ever been to Africa; most had never met an African. But many did have histories of sexual contact with North Americans. In a 1984 paper published in a scholarly journal, Haitian physician Jean Guérin and colleagues revealed that 17 percent of their patients reported a history of sexual contact with tourists from North America.[45] These exchanges involved the exchange of money, too, and so "sexual tourism"—which inevitably takes place across steep grades of economic inequality—was a critical first step in the introduction of HIV to Haiti. In fact, the viral subtype ("clade") seen in Haiti is a reflection of the fact that the Haitian AIDS epidemic is a subepidemic of the one already existing in the United States.[46]

There is more, of course, to the "hidden history" of AIDS in Haiti. By the time HIV was circulating in the Americas, Haiti was economically dependent not on France, as in previous centuries, but on the United States. From the time of the U.S. military occupation through the Duvalier dictatorships (1957–86), the United States had come to occupy the role of chief arbiter of Haitian affairs. After the withdrawal of troops in 1934, U.S. influence in Haiti grew rather than waned. U.S.-Haitian agribusiness projects may have failed, deepening social inequalities throughout Haiti as the rural peasantry became poorer, but U.S.-Haitian ties did not. Haiti became a leading recipient of U.S. "aid," and the United States and the "international financial institutions" were the Duvalier family's most reliable source of foreign currency. Haiti became, in turn, the ninth-largest assembler of U.S. goods in the world and bought almost all its imports from the United States. Tourism and offshore assembly replaced coffee and other agricultural products as the chief sources of foreign revenue in Haiti.

Haiti is the extreme example of a general pattern. If one uses trade data for Caribbean basin countries to assess the degree of their dependency on the United States at the time HIV appeared in the region, one sees that the five countries with the tightest ties to the United States were the five countries with the highest HIV prevalence. Cuba is the only country in the region not linked closely to the United States. Not coincidentally, Cuba was and remains the country with the lowest prevalence of HIV in the Americas. It was possible to conclude an earlier book on the subject by asserting that "AIDS in Haiti is about proximity rather than distance. AIDS in Haiti is a tale of ties to the United States, rather than to Africa; it is a story of unemployment rates greater than 70 percent. AIDS in Haiti has far more to do with the pursuit of trade and tourism in a dirt-poor country than with, to cite Alfred Métraux again, 'dark saturnalia celebrated by "blood-maddened, sex-maddened, god-maddened" negroes.'"[47]

But this was merely the beginning of a biosocial story of the virus. The Haitian men who had been the partners of North Americans were by and large poor men; they were trading sex for money. The Haitians in turn transmitted HIV to their wives and girlfriends. Through affective and economic connections, HIV rapidly became entrenched in Haiti's urban slums and then spread to smaller cities, towns, and, finally, villages like the one in which I work. Haiti is now the most HIV-affected country in the Americas, but the introduction and spread of the new virus have a history—a biosocial history that some would like to hide away.

Like many anthropologists, I was not always careful to avoid stripping away the social from the material. But HIV, though hastened forward by many social forces, is as material as any other microbe. Once in the body, its impact is profound both biologically and socially. As cell-mediated immunity is destroyed, poor people living with HIV are felled more often than not by tuberculosis. Last year, HIV was said to surpass tuberculosis as the leading infectious cause of adult deaths, but in truth these two epidemics are tightly linked. Further, merely looking at the impact of HIV on life expectancy in certain sub-Saharan African nations lets us know that this virus has had, in the span of a single generation, a profound effect on kinship structure.

All this is both interesting and horrible. What might have been done to avert the deaths caused by these two pathogens? What might be done right now? One would think that the tuberculosis question, at least, could be solved. Because there is no nonhuman host, simply detecting and treating promptly all active cases would eventually result in an end to deaths from this disease. Money and political will are what are missing—which brings us back to structural violence and its supporting hegemonies: the materiality of the social.

AIDS, one could argue, is thornier. There is no cure, but current therapies have had a profound impact on mortality among favored populations in the United States and Europe. The trick is to get therapy to those who need it most. Although this will require significant resources, the projected cost over the next few years is less than the monies allocated in a single day for rescuing the U.S. airline industry.[48] But the supporting hegemonies have already decreed AIDS an unmanageable problem. The justifications can be byzantine. For example, a high-ranking official within the U.S. Department of the Treasury (who wisely declined to be named) has argued that Africans have "a different concept of time" and would therefore be unable to take their medications on schedule; hence, no investment in AIDS therapy for Africa. The head of the U.S. Agency for International Development later identified a lack of wristwatches as the primary stumbling block.[49] Cheap wristwatches are not unheard of, but, as I have said, the primary problem is a matter of political will. Others have underlined, more honestly, the high costs of medications or the lack of health care infrastructure in the countries hit hardest by HIV. Still others point to fear of acquiring resistance to antiretroviral medications. The list is familiar to those interested in tuberculosis and other treatable, chronic diseases that disproportionately strike the poor.

The distribution of AIDS and tuberculosis—like that of slavery in earlier times—is historically given and economically driven. What common features underpin the afflictions of past and present centuries? Social inequalities are at the heart of structural violence. Racism of one form or another, gender inequality, and, above all, brute poverty in the face of affluence are linked to social plans and programs ranging from slavery to the current quest for unbridled growth. These conditions are the cause and result of displacements, wars both declared and undeclared, and the seething, submerged hatreds that make the irruption of *Schadenfreude* a shock to those who can afford to ignore, for the most part, the historical underpinnings of today's conflicts. Racism and related sentiments—disregard, even hatred, for the poor—underlie the current lack of resolve to address these and other problems squarely. It is not sufficient to change attitudes, but attitudes do make other things happen.

Structural violence is the natural expression of a political and economic order that seems as old as slavery. This social web of exploitation, in its many differing historical forms, has long been global, or almost so, in its reach. And this economic order has been crowned with success: more and more people can wear hairdos with frigates in them or the modern equivalent if they so choose. Indeed, one could argue that structural violence now comes with symbolic props far more powerful—indeed, far more convincing—than anything we might serve up to counter them; examples include the discounting of any divergent voice as "unrealistic" or "utopian," the dismal end of the socialist experiment in some (not all) of its homelands, the increasing centralization of command over finance capital, and what some see as the criminalization of poverty in economically advanced countries.

Exploring the anthropology of structural violence is a dour business. Our job is to document, as meticulously and as honestly as we can, the complex workings of a vast machinery rooted in a political economy that only a romantic would term fragile. What is fragile is rather our enterprise of creating a more truthful accounting and fighting amnesia. We will wait for the "glitch in the matrix" so that more can see clearly just what the cost is—not for us (for we who read the journals or engage in the social analyses are by definition shielded)—but for those who still set their backs to the impossible task of living on next to nothing while others wallow in surfeit.

NOTES

1. See Farmer, *Pathologies of Power*. See also Gilligan, *Violence*; Galtung, "Violence, Peace, and Peace Research."

2. See Scott, *The Moral Economy of the Peasant*; Scott, *Weapons of the Weak*; Scott, *Domination and the Arts of Resistance*.

3. Willis, *Learning to Labor*.

4. Lock, *Encounters with Aging*; Martin, *The Woman in the Body*.

5. See, for example, Bourdieu et al., *La misère du monde;* Bourdieu et al., *The Weight of the World;* Bourgois, "Confronting Anthropology, Education, and Inner-City Apartheid"; Bourgois, "Families and Children in the U.S. Inner City"; Cohen, *No Aging in India;* Green, *Fear as a Way of Life;* Scheper-Hughes, *Death without Weeping.*

6. Kroeber, *Anthropology,* p. 1.

7. I do not make much of a distinction between anthropology and sociology. This is not a polemical point but a humble one, also made by Alfred Kroeber: "Sociology and anthropology are hard to keep apart." He contrasted this with the troubled relationship between anthropology and psychology: "The relations of anthropology and psychology are not easy to deal with. Psychologists began by taking their own culture for granted, as if it were uniform and universal, and then studying psychic behavior within it" (ibid., p. 12).

8. It is no longer possible to argue that history and political economy are neglected within anthropology and sociology; reviews of the literature suggest a growing awareness within anthropology, at least, of these two disciplines. I am referring, rather, to the synthesis of the socializing disciplines and what I have termed "biological sciences"; these would include epidemiology and the natural history of disease. Medical and biological anthropologists Alan Goodman and Tom Leatherman (*Building a New Biocultural Synthesis*) have leveled a similar critique.

9. Tacitus, "Agricola," p. 30.

10. Le Carré, "A War We Cannot Win," p. 15.

11. See, for example, Rosaldo, "From the Door of His Tent."

12. Fabian, *Time and the Other.*

13. Mintz, *Sweetness and Power,* p. xxvii.

14. Bernier, *Pleasure and Privilege,* p. 77.

15. Ibid., pp. 97–98; emphasis added.

16. Ibid., p. 181.

17. For more details, see Farmer, *The Uses of Haiti,* pp. 54–55.

18. Bernier, *Pleasure and Privilege,* p. 181.

19. Klein, *African Slavery in Latin America and the Caribbean,* p. 57.

20. Moreau de Saint-Méry, *Description topographique, physique, civile, politique et historique de la partie française de l'isle Saint-Domingue,* pp. 9–10.

21. Vissière and Vissière, *La traite des noirs au siècle des Lumières.*

22. Vastey, *Notes à M. le Baron de V. P. Malouet,* p. 6.

23. Mintz, *Caribbean Transformations.* Mintz reminds us that many of the global phenomena under study today are not new. More specifically, the history of Haiti and much of the Caribbean presages current critiques concerning transnationalism: "Why, then, has the vocabulary of those events become so handy for today's transnationalists? Is one entitled to wonder whether this means that the world has now become a macrocosm of what the Caribbean region was, in the 16th century? If so, should we not ask what took the world so long to catch up especially since what is happening now is supposed to be qualitatively so different from the recent past? Or is it rather that the Caribbean experience was merely one chapter of a book being written, before the name of the book—world capitalism—became known to its authors?" (Mintz, "The Localization of Anthropological Practice," p. 120).

24. Wiese, "The Interaction of Western and Indigenous Medicine in Haiti in Regard to Tuberculosis," p. 38.

25. Mintz, "The Caribbean Region," p. 61.

26. During Jean-Bertrand Aristide's second presidency, Haiti sought restitution for the French debt. For more on the case for restitution, see Farmer, "Douze points en faveur de la restitution à Haïti de la dette française."

27. Price-Mars, *La République d'Haïti et la République Dominicaine*, pp. 169–70.

28. Lawless, *Haiti's Bad Press*, p. 56.

29. Hayne is quoted in Schmidt, *The United States Occupation of Haiti, 1915–1934*, p. 28.

30. For details, see Farmer, *The Uses of Haiti*, pp. 73–78.

31. For more on the dimensions of U.S. support for the Duvalier family dictatorship and for justifications proffered to explain it, see ibid., pp. 92–103, 290–91.

32. Wallerstein, *The Modern World-System*.

33. Mintz, "The So-Called World System"; see also Roseberry, "Political Economy."

34. Bourdieu, *Contre-feux*, p. 25.

35. "Durban Declaration and Programme of Action." Whether one calls this sociology or anthropology or political "science," let us stop and take a look at this "world conference." Who are these people? They are representatives of nations and of nongovernmental organizations. Many call them—they call themselves—the "international community." They went to major universities in the United States or Europe; they speak English in addition to other languages. They are us.

36. Mintz, "Introduction," in Métraux, *Voodoo in Haiti*, p. 7.

37. Birns and McCarthy, "Haiti Needs U.S. Aid, Not Ineffective Manipulation."

38. On August 21, 2002, Musharraf "unilaterally" amended Pakistan's constitution to expand his control of the country even further. In these amendments he claimed the right to dissolve the elected parliament and to make additional amendments at his own discretion (Rohde, "Musharraf Redraws Constitution, Blocking Prospects for Democracy").

39. Burns, "U.S. Envoy Sees Her Role Reverse."

40. Farmer, Smith Fawzi, and Nevil, "Unjust Embargo of Aid for Haiti."

41. Ott, *Fevered Lives*, p. 49.

42. Farmer, *AIDS and Accusation*, pp. 157–58, 203.

43. Treichler, "AIDS, Homophobia, and Biomedical Discourse."

44. Farmer, *AIDS and Accusation*. See also Farmer, *Pathologies of Power*, chap. 2.

45. Guérin et al., "Acquired Immune Deficiency Syndrome."

46. See Farmer, *AIDS and Accusation*, p. xii; Farmer, *Infections and Inequalities*, pp. 105, 124.

47. Farmer, *AIDS and Accusation*, p. 264.

48. See Swoboda and Hamilton, "Congress Passes $15 Billion Airline Bailout."

49. Andrew Natsios, at the time administrator of the U.S. Agency for International Development, who spent a decade in aid work in Africa, said that many Africans "don't know what Western time is. You have to take these AIDS drugs a certain number of hours each day, or they don't work. Many people in Africa have never seen a clock or a watch their entire lives. And if you say, one o'clock in the afternoon, they do not know what you are talking about. They know morning, they know noon, they know evening, they know the darkness at night. I'm sorry to be saying these things, but a lot of people like Jeffrey Sachs advocating these things have never worked in health care in rural areas in Africa or even in the cities" (Donnelly, "Prevention Urged in AIDS Fight").

18

Structural Violence
and Clinical Medicine

(2006)

Paul Farmer, Bruce Nizeye, Sara Stulac, and Salmaan Keshavjee

Because of our contact with patients, physicians readily appreciate that large-scale social forces—racism, gender inequality, poverty, political violence, and war, and sometimes the very policies that address them—often determine who falls ill and who has access to care. For practitioners of public health, the social determinants of disease are even harder to disregard.

Unfortunately, this awareness is seldom translated into formal analytic frameworks that link social analysis to everyday clinical practice. One reason for this gap is that the holy grail of modern medicine remains the search for the molecular basis of disease. While the practical yield of such circumscribed inquiry has been enormous, it has led to the increasing "desocialization" of scientific inquiry: a tendency to ask only biological questions about what are in fact *biosocial* phenomena.[1]

Biosocial understandings of medical phenomena are urgently needed. All those involved in public health sense this, especially when they serve populations living in poverty. Social analysis, however rudimentary, in fact occurs at the bedside, in the clinic, at field sites, and in the margins of the clinical literature. It is to be found, for example, in any significant survey of adherence to therapy for chronic diseases and in studies of what were once termed "social diseases," such as venereal disease and tuberculosis.[2] The emerging phenomenon of acquired resistance to antibiotics—including antibacterial, antiviral, and antiparasitic agents—is perforce a biosocial process, one that began less than a century ago as novel treatments were introduced. Social analysis is heard in discussion of illnesses for which a significant environmental component is believed to exist, such as asthma and lead poisoning.

Can we speak of the "natural history" of any of these diseases without addressing the social forces, including racism, pollution, poor housing, and poverty, that shape their course in both individuals and populations? When some of those who suffer from a disease have access to diagnosis and care and others do not, is it appropriate to speak of the disease's "natural history"? Does our clinical practice acknowledge what we already know—namely, that social and environmental forces will limit the effectiveness of our treatments? Asking these questions needs to be the beginning of a conversation within medicine and public health, rather than the end of one.

Indeed, the implications of a social analysis of disease extend all the way to the molecular level. Asthma, for example, is widely believed to be epidemic among children living in the urban United States. A survey of national data revealed that black non-Hispanic children had an asthma attack prevalence rate 44 percent higher than that of white non-Hispanic children in 2000;[3] other reviews have also confirmed that black children are more likely to be hospitalized and are more likely to die from asthma than their white counterparts.[4] Biology alone does not account for asthma's prevalence, and to speak of it in merely biological terms falsifies the problem: a comprehensive discussion cannot occur without reference to environmental allergens, air and housing quality, and access to clinical services. The course of this disease, like that of so many other chronic afflictions, is shaped by social forces well beyond the control of patients and their families. Pediatricians know this, even though they may lack the analytic frameworks (and the professional mandate) required to understand and alter the social determinants of the course of chronic asthma. They can see that housing and immigration policies, limited access to bank loans, and the lack of a national health insurance scheme are somehow related to the distribution and course of asthma in children.

A biosocial approach redefines many of our terms. Are our understandings of real estate and air pollution as sophisticated as our understanding of the molecular processes involved in an asthma exacerbation? Are certain children engaging in "high-risk behaviors" that place them at heightened risk of asthma? Does clinical discussion of the management of childhood asthma focus as much on the pertinent social determinants of disease course as on the efficacy of certain medications?

When a child comes into the world with heightened risk not readily ascribed to genetic predisposition, some would invoke the notion of injustice. If the burden of disease is found among children living in urban poverty, most of them African American or Latino, we should look to social arrangements rather than genetically determined risk for causes. "Structural violence" is one way of describing social arrangements marked by racism and other social inequalities.[5] In the influential view of sociologist Johan Galtung, structural violence is "the avoidable impairment of fundamental human needs," embedded in longstanding "ubiquitous social structures, normalized by stable institutions and regular experience."[6] Because they seem so ordinary in our ways of understanding the world, such violent structures are almost invisible. Disparate access to resources, political power, education, and health care as well as unequal legal standing are just a few examples. Such arrangements do violence to society's losers; the arrangements are structural because they are embedded in the economic organization of our social world. Those responsible for maintaining such inequalities are not the chief victims of structural violence, as the example of a childhood disease like asthma might suggest.

The concept of structural violence is intended to begin, or revive, discussions of social forces beyond the control of our patients. Like all concepts, it has sharp limitations. Nonetheless, we seek to apply the notion to those tasks that remain the primary goals of clinical medicine: preventing premature death and disability and improving the lives of those we care for. Many medical and public health interventions will be ineffective if we are unable to understand the social determinants of disease.

The good news is that such understandings are far more "actionable" than is widely recognized. There is already a vast and growing array of diagnostic and therapeutic tools born of scientific research; it is possible to use these tools in a manner informed by an understanding of structural violence and its impact both on disease distribution and on every step of the process leading from diagnosis to effective care. This means working at multiple levels, from "distal" interventions—performed late in the process, when patients are already sick—to "proximal" interventions—trying to prevent illness through efforts such as vaccination, a cleaner water supply, or improved housing.

DELIVERING AIDS CARE EQUITABLY IN THE UNITED STATES

The distribution and outcome of chronic infectious disease are so tightly linked to social arrangements that it is difficult for clinicians treating these diseases to ignore social factors. AIDS, a relatively new affliction, is considered a social disease, but clinicians often have radically different understandings of what makes AIDS "social." Although the illness was unknown three decades ago, complications of HIV infection have become a leading cause of young adult deaths in the United States.[7] Many doctors have focused on what are termed the "behaviors" or "lifestyles" that place some at risk for AIDS, while others are shielded.[8] Yet risk has never been determined solely by *individual* risk behaviors. Susceptibility to infection and poor outcomes is aggravated, instead, by *social* factors, including poverty, gender inequality, and racism.[9] In less than a decade, AIDS became a disease afflicting America's poor, many of whom engaged in "risk behaviors" at a far lower rate than others who were not at heightened risk of infection with sexually transmitted diseases.[10]

Although a more social—and less psychological and behaviorist—reading of AIDS risk affords a deeper understanding of the dynamics of the U.S. epidemic, no single model captures the complexity of risk for HIV infection and poor outcomes. As with childhood asthma, every step of the process occurs in a social context and is socially determined. HIV attacks the immune system in only one way, but its course and outcome are shaped by social forces having little to do with the universal pathophysiology of the disease. From the outset of acute HIV infection to the endgame of recurrent opportunistic infections, disease course is determined by whether or not post-exposure prophylaxis is available, whether or not the steady decline in immune function is hastened by concurrent illness or malnutrition, whether or not multiple HIV infections occur, whether or not tuberculosis is prevalent in the surrounding environment, whether or not prophylaxis for opportunistic infections is reliably available,[11] and whether or not antiretroviral therapy (ART) is offered to all those needing it. Throughout this usually decade-long process, structural violence has a profound influence on effective diagnosis, staging, and treatment of the disease and its associated pathologies. Each of these determinants of course and outcome is itself shaped by the very social forces that determine variable risk.

Although the variability of outcomes has been especially obvious in the era of antiretroviral therapy, it was so even before effective ART became available. Leaving aside disease distribution, some might expect that an untreatable disease would run the same course in all patients once infection occurs. But diagnosing and treating the chief opportunistic infections that were the cause of death among people living with AIDS did not wait for the development of specific antiretroviral therapy and specific serologic tests. In the United States, the ranking opportunistic infection was *Pneumocystis carinii* pneumonia, for which delays in diagnosis and initiation of therapy proved fatal to many, as did interruptions in the lifelong suppressive therapies required to control this and other opportunistic infections. In Baltimore in the early 1990s, data showed that race was associated with the timely receipt of therapeutics: among patients infected with HIV, blacks were significantly less likely than whites to have received antiretroviral therapy or *Pneumocystis* prophylaxis when they were first referred to an HIV clinic, regardless of disease stage at the time of presentation.[12] The timeline from HIV infection to death was further shortened in situations where the far more virulent tuberculosis was the leading opportunistic infection, as it is in much of the poor world.[13] The "natural history" of AIDS is a mirage. It must be replaced with biosocial understanding.

This was clear to researchers and clinicians in Baltimore, who described what they termed "excess mortality" among African Americans without insurance. Although such terminology was not used in the studies reviewed here, it is possible to argue that racism and other forms of structural violence were embodied as excess mortality.[14] What else accounted for racial disparities in clinical outcomes? Regardless of semantics, few epidemiologists seeking to understand the U.S. epidemic were able to ignore the social determinants of both distribution and outcome of this disease. Some argued for intrinsic "racial" susceptibility to poor outcomes. For others, this was merely a hypothesis to be explored.

As epidemiology, a focus on the standard "risk factors," which did not consider structural violence, did not lead far. But after documenting racial disparities in survival rates, the clinicians and researchers in Baltimore asked what would happen if race and insurance status no longer determined who had access to the standard of care (even before treatment routinely included three-drug ART). Their subsequent intervention was more proximal than previous ones, as it involved removing barriers to care. They sought to remove the obvious economic barriers at the point of care, and they also considered transportation costs and other incentives, as well as co-morbid conditions ranging from drug addiction to major mental illness. Improvements in community-based care, designed to make AIDS care more convenient and socially acceptable for patients, were implemented. The goal was to make sure that nothing within the medical system or the surrounding community prevented poor and otherwise marginalized patients from receiving the standard of care.

The results registered just a few years later were dramatic: disparities in outcome tied to race, gender, injection drug use, and socioeconomic status disappeared within the study population.[15] In other words, these program improvements may not have dealt with the lack of national health insurance, and still less with the persistent problems of racism and urban poverty, but they did lessen the embodiment of social inequalities as premature death from AIDS. Similarly ambitious (if smaller) studies have demonstrated that providers can indeed lessen the impact of social inequalities on AIDS outcomes among the homeless, the addicted, the mentally ill, and prisoners.[16] Making sure that these advances are preserved will require a great deal of vigilance, continued investment in proximal as well as distal interventions, and, eventually, the equitable use of any new therapeutic agents. Preserving these gains will also require increased emphasis on community-based care.

The Baltimore experience has implications for the future course of the U.S. AIDS epidemic; it has implications for all those concerned with structural violence in the United States. Eventually, such interventions, or the lack of them, will affect the virus at the molecular level. The program was improved in part by linking an understanding of social context to clinical services, but we argue that a properly biosocial analysis must embrace an understanding of social inequalities and also molecular-level complexities, in part because we are now witnessing the emergence of what might as well be called "MDR-HIV," or multidrug-resistant HIV. Acquired resistance to antibiotics, including antiretrovirals, is necessarily a biosocial phenomenon, one that has occurred only since the middle of the twentieth century, when effective antibiotics were first introduced. It is worth remembering that almost all isolates of *Staphylococcus aureus* were once susceptible to penicillin. Today, in the United States and elsewhere, drug-resistant strains predominate: rates of resistance range upward of 99 percent of strains.[17]

Most bacteria, and many viruses and parasites, mutate when challenged with antibiotics; the rate at which pathogens acquire resistance may be hastened by inadequate or interrupted therapy and by imprudent use of antibiotics.[18] Structural violence lessens access to effective therapy but is a rarely discussed contributor to epidemics of MDR-HIV. This is a major gap in our understanding of AIDS. Consider the implications of an important study by Carlos del Rio and colleagues in Atlanta, where Emory University and the public health service have established a state-of-the-art HIV clinic in an area close to the epicenter of the city's AIDS epidemic. Like most U.S. clinical care, however, the services offered are largely within clinic walls: patients have to reach the clinic and remain in care in order to enjoy long-term benefit. As elsewhere, the dominant model is one in which patients are prescribed ART by physicians and then seen in follow-up by physicians, nurses, and even social workers within the facility, rather than in their homes or neighborhoods. Among a largely African American patient population with high rates of addiction, housing instability, and co-morbid disease, it proved difficult to promote adherence. In one survey, fewer than 15 percent of all patients offered ART could be shown to have suppressed viral loads only a year after the initiation of therapy.[19]

Irregular ART will shape the epidemic in novel ways, as intermittent therapy, often attributed by clinicians to patient noncompliance and almost never to structural violence, is closely associated with rapidly acquired resistance to antiretrovirals. In a study of ten urban centers in the United States, the frequency of transmitted high-level resistance to one or more antiretroviral drugs was 12.4 percent during the period from 1999 to 2000.[20] As we've argued elsewhere, it is not possible to understand the dynamics of drug-resistant epidemics of AIDS, tuberculosis, or malaria without understanding structural violence.[21] Although epidemics of treatable infectious disease are perhaps uniquely susceptible to this particular complication of erratic care, structural violence can ensure poor outcomes for virtually all chronic illnesses for which there is a deliverable: seizure disorders, diabetes, hypertension, major mental illness, and several other chronic pathologies are managed effectively only when patients are able to adhere to daily therapies.

It makes sense to argue that structural violence exacts a new sort of toll as more effective therapies become available to some but not to all. A growing "outcome gap"[22] is registered even as the fruits of basic and clinical research lead to novel and increasingly effective interventions—the darker side of scientific progress.

PREVENTING PEDIATRIC AIDS IN RWANDA: LESSONS FROM RURAL HAITI

The impact of structural violence is even more obvious in the world's poorest countries, as is the impact of conventionally defined violence. Yet the mechanisms by which poverty and social inequalities come to take their toll among the destitute sick are no less numerous; the quality of analysis required to understand the dynamics of epidemic disease is no less, and no less biosocial in nature, than in affluent, inegalitarian societies. Such analysis has profound implications for all those seeking to provide clinical services in what are these days termed "resource-poor settings."

Over the past year, we have sought to address AIDS and tuberculosis (among other pathologies) in Africa, the world's poorest and most heavily burdened continent. Specifically, we have transplanted and adapted the "Haiti model" of care, which was designed to prevent the embodiment of poverty and social inequalities as excess mortality due to AIDS, tuberculosis, malaria, and other diseases of poverty.[23] In some senses, the model is simple: barriers to care, whether found in the clinic or in surrounding communities, are removed as diagnosis and treatment are declared a public good and made available free of charge to patients living in poverty. Furthermore, AIDS care is delivered not only at the clinic, in the conventional way, but also within the villages in which our patients work and live. Each patient offered ART or antituberculous therapy is paired with an *accompagnateur,* usually a neighbor trained to deliver ART and other supportive care in the patient's home. Using this model, we have offered ART to more than 2,100 patients in rural Haiti. Since conventional clinic-based (distal) services are complemented with daily, home-based care, this model is deemed by some to be the world's most effective way of removing structural barriers to quality care for AIDS and other chronic disease. It is also a way of creating jobs in rural regions in great need of them. We have used a similar model in urban Peru and in Boston, Massachusetts.[24]

Rwanda presents unique challenges, but many barriers to care are quite similar to those confronted in Haiti and other settings where social upheaval, poverty, and gender inequality decrease the effectiveness of distal services and prevention efforts. The parallels between the two countries are striking: both are densely populated, with over eight million inhabitants in a mountainous area roughly the size of the state of Maryland; both are agrarian societies in which the majority still live in rural regions. Although both countries have endured large-scale political violence, that registered in Rwanda was unprecedented in scale. Little over a decade ago, Rwanda was rent by war and genocide, itself the result of structural violence and also a contributor to the structural violence that persists even after the cessation of hostilities.

In the two rural districts of Rwanda in which the Haiti model was introduced in May 2005, an estimated 60 percent of inhabitants are refugees, returning exiles, or recent settlers; not a single physician was present to serve 350,000 people. AIDS has recently worsened this tableau, as violence and displacement inevitably promote HIV. Although Rwanda is less affected than southern Africa, AIDS has become a leading cause of young adult deaths. In spite of significant resources allocated to treat complications of HIV infection in Rwanda, almost all patients enrolled on ART live in cities or towns. But less than a year after our program began in 2005, more than 1,000 rural Rwandans with AIDS were enrolled in care using the Haiti model.

To deepen our discussion of interventions designed to counter structural violence, consider the prevention of mother-to-child transmission of HIV in rural Rwanda. Our experience in Haiti led us to conclude that it was possible to use the international standard of care—combination ART during pregnancy, followed by formula feeding and close follow-up of infants, complemented by sanitation projects within the catchment area—in even the most difficult regions, where electricity is scarce, food insecurity widespread, and health and sanitation infrastructure rudimentary at best. Another priority is to interrupt, when possible, HIV transmission through breastfeeding by offering similar services not only during pregnancy but during lactation. The impact of such an intervention would appear to be as effective in rural Haiti as it has been in the United States, reducing rates of transmission from as high as 25 to 40 percent to as low as 2 percent. Infant mortality from gastroenteritis is higher in bottle-fed infants (usually stemming from a lack of clean water to use in preparing formula), but it is lessened by the proximal interventions mentioned earlier, reducing mortality among infants born to HIV-positive mothers to a level far below the national level among all Haitian women, regardless of HIV status.[25]

At the outset of our project in rural Rwanda, we believed that mother-to-child transmission could be prevented only if our program was linked to efforts to intervene more proximally to improve water supplies and food security, enabling women living in dire poverty to comply with our recommendations. That is, prevention of mother-to-child transmission is possible if barriers to compliance—a lack of clean water and infant formula, users' fees for ART and other medical services—are removed.

Implementing this approach has not been easy in rural Africa, where policymakers, influenced by international regulatory bodies, have continued to advocate universal breastfeeding, a policy that made eminent sense prior to the advent of HIV. (Indeed, an understanding of the outsized influence of international policymakers in Africa is part of a proper biosocial analysis.) Both proximal and distal interventions require substantial funding if we are to launch novel projects in response to novel challenges such as a lethal infectious disease transmitted in utero and through breast milk. In the world's poorest countries, most of which are in Africa, public and foundation support for proposed health interventions is unlikely if the interventions are not deemed "cost-effective." At this writing, there is substantial opposition to programs that deviate from promoting universal breastfeeding, on the grounds that more infants will die from gastroenteritis than from AIDS; and this opposition has diminished support for Rwandan efforts to replicate the Haiti model. Formula feeding for rural Rwandan infants is not feasible, some claim. Others argue that HIV-related stigma will prevent Rwandan women from enrolling in such projects, since failing to breastfeed and receiving regular visits from *accompagnateurs* and clinic staff would signal to family and neighbors the serostatus of participating women.

That said, opposition to the Haiti model did not come from rural Rwandan women living with HIV disease. Since the project is being piloted now and is only a few months old, it is too early to declare success. But its feasibility is almost certain. In the first six months of operation, more than 31,000 persons were screened in the two districts in which we work. With no exceptions, pregnant women who were found to be infected with HIV expressed interest in ART to prevent transmission, and all of them requested assistance in procuring not only infant formula but also the means to boil water and to store the formula safely. To refer again to the anatomic metaphor, the distal intervention was to provide ART (when possible, a three-drug regimen) to all women in the catchment area, with the help of *accompagnateurs*. Proximal interventions included supplying kerosene stoves, kerosene, bottles, and infant formula; food aid was also offered, as was, in certain cases, housing assistance.

More than four hundred infants were enrolled in the formula program between August 2005 and January 2006. The mean age at enrollment was just over ten months, which means that most of the infants in this initial cohort had been born before this project was initiated, and therefore neither they nor their mothers benefited from the full package of care, which includes diagnosis of maternal HIV infection during pregnancy, ART for mothers, and substantial assistance to mothers seeking to prevent transmission through alternatives to breastfeeding. Thus some of these infants were infected with HIV prior to enrollment. Yet even when these services were offered tardily, this first group of children appear to have HIV infection rates of around 10 percent, less than half that expected without the intervention. As the program becomes well established, and services become available before the third trimester of pregnancy, rates of transmission will continue to decline. In fact, the mean age of enrollment in the infant formula program continues to drop precipitously, with a current mean age around four months.

To date, there is little reason to believe such interventions will fail. Any failure is more likely the result of problems in the program (for example, stockouts of drugs or supplies) than the result of stigma or noncompliance by the women enrolled in the program. This is because structural interventions of this sort remove the onus of adherence from vulnerable patients and place it squarely on the providers.

Interventions of a far more proximal character are readily imagined. Poverty-stricken, post-conflict rural Rwanda is a setting in which the majority of the adult population consists of refugees, widows, and genocide survivors; women-headed households are common and, in eastern Rwanda at least, food insecurity is the rule. These are precisely the settings in which projects such as ours are rendered more effective by efforts to improve housing, create jobs, and promote literacy. Even more important are efforts to increase agricultural productivity and to distribute land to women-headed households. Along with many partners, including the Rwandan government, we now seek to address structural violence in precisely this manner in these two districts.

Where ART is offered but universal breastfeeding is encouraged, a larger fraction of HIV transmission to children occurs through breastfeeding than was the case previously. Where clean water is unavailable and HIV prevalence is high, the policy of universal breastfeeding may be associated with lower rates of infant mortality, but infants infected with HIV will later develop AIDS, and the cost of pediatric HIV care or lifetime access to ART does not figure prominently in the cost-effectiveness analyses now in vogue.[26]

In middle-income countries with significant gaps between the rich and the poor, cost-effectiveness analyses and other metrics are often applied selectively. South Africa is one such country. In some ways more like the United States than Rwanda, South Africa is a country in which racial identity determined social standing for much of its history as a colony or state. Over the past two decades, it has become the country with the world's largest burden of HIV, leading some to say that HIV is not tightly associated with poverty, since many far poorer countries have lower rates of infection. But HIV transmission is more closely linked to social inequalities than to absolute poverty.[27] As HIV claimed more and more black lives, sparing the white and "colored" minorities, more was made of purported "behavioral" or "cultural" risk factors than of structural considerations, such as labor migration and land appropriation.

Structural violence is difficult to eradicate, even when political will is abundant. Post-apartheid South Africa is a case in point. The country is well known for its high-end medical services: the standard of care available in South African cities is the same as that in Europe and North America. But longstanding policies excluded the black majority from access to the goods and services taken for granted by more privileged citizens, and the end of apartheid has not yet erased these inequalities. Still, the 1994 constitution forbids racial discrimination, and more recent policies have in fact pushed for the highest standard of care for all. Over the past year, South Africa enrolled more patients on ART than any other African country; in several programs, infant formula was to be made available free of charge to women who had received ART during pregnancy. But the quality of these services has lagged far behind the policies. "Vertical," or free-standing, services were established to prevent mother-to-child transmission and distribute infant formula, but even for those fortunate enough to receive these services, drug stockouts were common, and the quality of counseling and other services was often poor. Mixed feeding is common, with many infants receiving both infant formula and breast milk.[28]

As a result of recent changes, South Africa is now registering precisely the sort of shift in transmission pattern mentioned earlier: a smaller fraction of all mother-to-child transmission occurs during the third trimester of pregnancy and a larger fraction through breastfeeding. As long as women remain on ART during breastfeeding, an overall decline in transmission to children will ensue. But there is an urgent need for improving the quality of services and increasing community-based accompaniment to support poor women seeking to keep their children free of both HIV and waterborne disease. Emerging data suggest that, over the past decade and, most significantly, among blacks, infant mortality has continued to rise.[29]

In response to these disturbing developments, some policymakers, not all of them South African (and fewer still black South Africans), have counseled a return to universal breastfeeding, even though the country is still in the midst of an expanding AIDS epidemic and already has the world's largest burden of HIV among women of childbearing age.[30] Since this is not the standard of care internationally or for South African whites, it is resisted by those seeking to erase the legacy of apartheid. As a compromise, these experts suggest that women who are diagnosed with HIV infection while pregnant be assessed for their "likeliness to comply" with recommendations regarding infant formula.[31] Those deemed likely to comply are counseled against breastfeeding; those deemed unlikely to comply are counseled to breastfeed. When pressed about what such an assessment might entail, researchers and policymakers describe a process that seeks to determine who is most able to procure clean water (or the fuel required to boil it) on a daily basis. Such an approach means that the poorest women, already those most likely to become infected with HIV, will be those least likely to receive the tools known to prevent HIV transmission to their infants. Thus the pediatric HIV epidemic will persist there, even if mortality during the first year of life is reduced by the immunological benefits of breast milk.

South Africa is frequently described as the continent's wealthiest country, but really it is better seen as a country damaged by a special kind of structural violence. Any comprehensive analysis seeking to understand the dynamics of the epidemic among children there will necessarily be biosocial, linking the history and political economy of southern Africa, including labor migration, to the feast-or-famine medical services available in the continent's wealthiest, though inegalitarian, country. Among the African poor, whether they live in South Africa or in Rwanda, success in preventing HIV transmission from mother to child will likely depend on implementing more proximal interventions.

INCORPORATING STRUCTURAL INTERVENTIONS
IN MEDICINE AND PUBLIC HEALTH

If structural violence is often a major determinant of both the distribution and outcome of chronic disease, why is this or a similar concept not in wider use in medicine and public health, especially when our interventions can radically alter clinical outcomes? One reason is that medical professionals are not trained to make structural interventions. Physicians can rightly note that such interventions are "not our job." Yet since structural interventions might arguably have a greater impact on disease control than conventional clinical interventions, we would do well not to confuse our own quests for personal efficacy with the needs of the poor.

Just as it is a mistake to focus solely on distal interventions, so too is it a mistake to focus solely on structural ones. For decades, those who study the determinants of disease have known that social or structural forces account for most epidemic disease. But truisms such as "poverty is the root cause of tuberculosis" have not led us very far. First, we don't yet have a curative prescription for poverty. But we do know how to cure tuberculosis. Second, those who argue that focusing solely on economic development will in time wipe out tuberculosis may be correct, but en route toward this utopia the body count will remain high if care is not taken to diagnose and treat the sick. The same holds true for other diseases of poverty. Clean water and sanitation will prevent cases of typhoid fever, but those who fall ill need antibiotics; clean water comes too late for them.

Similar debates about how best to use scarce resources are as old as medicine itself. It is in resource-poor settings especially that we must seek to avoid the "Luddite trap" that would have us focus solely on prevention, especially now that we have effective therapies for almost all the diseases of poverty.[32] Prevention and care are best seen not as competing priorities but as complementary, even synergistic, endeavors. Yet international public health is today rife with false debates along precisely these lines; many of its practitioners have fallen into the Luddite trap. For decades, we have seen subtle discussion of the chief social determinants of disease give way to bitter struggles over resource allocation. During recent years, these struggles have become even more acrimonious.

How many times have we heard, for example, that AIDS prevention alone must suffice in settings of poverty?[33] Or that we need not bother with drug-resistant or extrapulmonary tuberculosis, forms that are difficult to diagnose and treat? Or that passive case-finding, rather than more costly efforts to go and find the sick in their homes, is all that we can afford? Or that surgical services are not cost-effective in rural areas of Africa? The list of impossible choices facing those who work among the destitute sick seems endless. There is no good way to tackle the health crisis in Africa with the scant resources previously available, and thus is structural violence perpetuated at a time when science and medicine continue to yield truly miraculous tools. Without an equity plan to bring these tools to bear on the health problems of the destitute, these debates will continue to waste precious time.[34]

Returning to our case studies, what might constitute appropriate structural interventions offering the promise of decreasing premature morbidity and mortality? Several were mentioned here, but there are many others. In the United States and in South Africa, it is possible to decrease the extent to which racism and poverty become embodied as health disparities. Some interventions are straightforward enough, as this discussion has shown. To consider the problem in the broadest terms, there is an enormous flaw in the dominant model of medical care: as long as medical services are sold as commodities, they will remain available only to those who can purchase them. Insurance schemes based on helping those in greatest need or at heightened risk help to prevent structural violence from taking its toll among the poor. National health insurance and other social safety nets, including those that guarantee primary education and food security and clean water, are important because they promise rights, rather than commodities, to citizens. A lack of these social and economic rights is fundamental to the perpetuation of structural violence.[35]

Other, more proximal interventions, though deemed quite remote from the practice of clinical medicine, also promise to lessen premature morbidity and mortality. For example, at least one study, focusing on African American women in Los Angeles, has found less condom use—and thus a greater risk of transmitting HIV—among couples in which the woman is dependent on her male partner for rent money.[36] How might a right to housing or job security affect the HIV epidemic among U.S. women living in poverty? To put this in sociological terms, interventions that increase the agency (the ability to choose) of the poor will lessen the risk of HIV. Similarly, it is not possible to have an honest discussion of alcoholism among Native Americans,[37] or crack cocaine addiction among African Americans,[38] without discussing the history of genocide and slavery in North America. Again, such commentary is seen as altogether extraneous in medical and public health circles, where discussions of substance abuse are curiously desocialized, viewed as personal and psychological problems rather than societal ones. Here, too, structural violence is perpetuated through analytic omission.

Structural interventions would certainly have enormous impact in rural Rwanda. Certain interventions are already under way—provision of ART, infant formula, bottles, clean water, containers, fuel, and a cooker—and it is still possible to improve access to each component of the project: legislation to promote the use of generic medications; better distribution networks for ART and infant formula; clean-water campaigns; and the development of alternative fuels. More proximally still, additional interventions would include enhancing agricultural production, creating new jobs outside the agricultural sector, addressing gender inequality through legislation that concerns not only land tenure but also political representation (Rwanda has become a leader in this arena by mandating gender equity in parliament),[39] and promoting adult literacy.

Although these are not the tasks for which clinicians were trained, such projects are nonetheless central to the struggle to reduce premature suffering and death. The importance of such societal projects to the future of health care means that practitioners of medicine and public health must make common cause with others who *are* trained to intervene more proximally. Settings as disparate as inner-city America and rural Rwanda are similar in the need for basic social and economic rights, including national health insurance, improved public education, and gender equity in political representation; those who live there need more and better jobs, and fair trade policies.

Sometimes public health crises, such as the AIDS pandemic in Africa, can lead to bold and specific interventions, such as the campaign to provide AIDS prevention and care as a public good.[40] When linked to more structural interventions, such ostensibly specific campaigns can help to trigger a "virtuous social cycle" that promises to lessen the burden of pathology borne by children and young adults—a major victory in the struggle to decrease structural violence.

CONCLUSIONS

During the nineteenth century, pioneers of modern public health such as Rudolf Virchow understood that epidemic disease and dismal life expectancies were tied tightly to social conditions. Such leaders did not employ the term "structural violence," but they were well aware of its toll and argued compellingly for proximal interventions—land reform, education, basic sanitation, sovereignty, and an end to political oppression. These interventions are no less needed now that we have better distal tools, including vaccines, more accurate diagnostics, and a large armamentarium of effective therapeutics. Soon, medicine and public health will boast many of the tools that could conceivably help to prevent structural violence, in all its forms, from becoming embodied as adverse health outcomes. Although it is true that equitable use of distal interventions does not address social inequalities directly, the push for health equity remains a worthy goal for all practitioners of medicine and public health.

As increasingly effective interventions are developed, there is great danger in failing to consider what occurs when we do not adopt a rights-based approach to epidemic disease. Wherever our goods and services remain commodities to be purchased, there are always some who are unable to buy them. The poor are the natural constituency of public health; physicians, as Virchow argued, are the natural attorneys of the poor. In the twenty-first century, the greatest human rights struggles will include the right to health care.

In conclusion, it does not matter what we call it: structural violence remains a ranking cause of premature death and disability. We can begin by "resocializing" our understanding of disease distribution and outcome. Even new diseases such as AIDS have quickly become diseases of the poor, and even the development of effective therapies may have a perverse effect if we are unable to use them where they are needed most. By insisting that our services be delivered equitably, even physicians who work on the distal interventions characteristic of clinical medicine have much to contribute to reducing the toll of structural violence. Although we may reasonably observe that the structural interventions described here are not our responsibility, equity in health care *is* our responsibility. Only when we link our efforts to those of others committed to initiating virtuous social cycles can we expect a future in which medicine attains its noblest goals.

NOTES

1. See Farmer, "Social Medicine and the Challenge of Biosocial Research" (included in this volume as chapter 11).

2. See Osterberg and Blaschke, "Adherence to Medication"; Sumartojo, "When Tuberculosis Treatment Fails"; Brandt, *No Magic Bullet*; Dubos and Dubos, *The White Plague*; Packard, *White Plague, Black Labor*; Feldberg, *Disease and Class*.

3. Akinbami and Schoendorf, "Trends in Childhood Asthma."

4. McConnochie et al., "Socioeconomic Variation in Asthma Hospitalization"; Gottlieb, Beiser, and O'Connor, "Poverty, Race, and Medication Use Are Correlates of Asthma Hospitalization Rates."

5. Farmer, "An Anthropology of Structural Violence" (included in this volume as chapter 17).

6. Winter and Leighton, "Structural Violence, Introduction," p. 99, paraphrasing Galtung, "Violence, Peace, and Peace Research." See also Galtung, "Cultural Violence"; Gilligan, *Violence*. Galtung formulates the issue as follows:

Violence is present when human beings are being influenced so that their actual somatic and mental realizations are below their potential realizations. . . . Violence is here defined as the cause of the difference between the potential and the actual. . . . Thus, if a person died from tuberculosis in the eighteenth century it would be hard to conceive of this as violence since it might have been quite unavoidable, but if he dies from it today, despite all the medical resources in the world, then violence is present according to our definition. . . .

. . . We shall refer to the type of violence where there is an actor that commits the violence as personal or direct, and to violence where there is no such actor as structural or indirect. . . . There may not be any person who directly harms another person in the structure. The violence is built into the structure and shows up as unequal power and consequently as unequal life chances. ("Violence, Peace, and Peace Research," pp. 168, 170–71)

7. National Center for Health Statistics, "Annual Summary of Births, Marriages, Divorces, and Deaths: United States, 1993," pp. 18–20, table 8.

8. Treichler, "AIDS, Homophobia, and Biomedical Discourse."

9. See Farmer, *AIDS and Accusation;* Farmer, Connors, and Simmons, *Women, Poverty, and AIDS;* National Research Council, Panel on Monitoring the Social Impact of the AIDS Epidemic, *The Social Impact of AIDS in the United States.*

10. Toltzis et al., "Human Immunodeficiency Virus (HIV)-Related Risk-Taking Behaviors in Women Attending Inner-City Prenatal Clinics in the Mid-West"; Gottlieb et al., "Seroprevalence and Correlates of Herpes Simplex Virus Type 2 Infection in Five Sexually-Transmitted-Disease Clinics."

11. Wiktor et al., "Efficacy of Trimethoprim-Sulphamethoxazole Prophylaxis to Decrease Morbidity and Mortality in HIV-1-Infected Patients with Tuberculosis in Abidjan, Côte d'Ivoire."

12. Moore et al., "Racial Differences in the Use of Drug Therapy for HIV Disease in an Urban Community."

13. Lucas et al., "The Mortality and Pathology of HIV Infection in a West African City."

14. Scheper-Hughes and Lock, "The Mindful Body."

15. Chaisson, Keruly, and Moore, "Race, Sex, Drug Use, and Progression of Human Immunodeficiency Virus Disease."

16. See Bangsberg et al., "Protease Inhibitors in the Homeless"; Behforouz, Farmer, and Mukherjee, "From Directly Observed Therapy to *Accompagnateurs*"; Mitty et al., "The Use of Community-Based Modified Directly Observed Therapy for the Treatment of HIV-Infected Persons."

17. Fridkin et al., "Methicillin-Resistant Staphylococcus Aureus Disease in Three Communities"; Rajaduraipandi et al., "Prevalence and Antimicrobial Susceptibility Pattern of Methicillin Resistant Staphylococcus Aureus."

18. Neu, "The Crisis in Antibiotic Resistance."

19. Del Rio et al., "From Diagnosis to Undetectable."

20. Little et al., "Antiretroviral-Drug Resistance among Patients Recently Infected with HIV."

21. Farmer and Becerra, "Biosocial Research and the TDR Agenda"; Walton, Farmer, and Dillingham, "Social and Cultural Factors in Tropical Medicine."

22. Wise, "Confronting Racial Disparities in Infant Mortality."

23. Farmer, Léandre, Mukherjee, Claude, et al., "Community-Based Approaches to HIV Treatment in Resource-Poor Settings"; Walton et al., "Integrated HIV Prevention and Care Strengthens Primary Health Care" (included in this volume as chapter 13).

24. Mitnick et al., "Community-Based Therapy for Multidrug-Resistant Tuberculosis in Lima, Peru"; Shin et al., "Community-Based Treatment of Multidrug-Resistant Tuberculosis in Lima, Peru"; Behforouz, Farmer, and Mukherjee, "From Directly Observed Therapy to *Accompagnateurs*."

25. Raymonville et al., "Prevention of Mother-to-Child Transmission of HIV in Rural Haiti."

26. As Dr. Peter Piot, executive director of UNAIDS, commented in an interview: "This orphan crisis is a major reason for introducing treatment for adults on a wider scale. . . . I have never seen that in these simplistic cost-effectiveness analyses [of whether drugs are affordable in the developing

world]. . . . They haven't even thought that there are orphans left behind when adults die" (Boseley, "13.4M Children Are AIDS Orphans, Says Report").

27. Gakidou and King, "Measuring Total Health Inequality."

28. Bobat et al., "Breastfeeding by HIV-1-Infected Women and Outcome in Their Infants"; Bland et al., "Breastfeeding Practices in an Area of High HIV Prevalence in Rural South Africa"; Sibeko et al., "Beliefs, Attitudes, and Practices of Breastfeeding Mothers from a Periurban Community in South Africa."

29. Burgard and Treiman, "Trends and Racial Differences in Infant Mortality in South Africa."

30. Coutsoudis, "Infant Feeding Dilemmas Created by HIV."

31. "Given these dilemmas, recent consultations held by the UN Interagency Task Team concluded that an HIV-positive mother should be counselled on the risks and benefits of different infant feeding options and should be guided in selecting the most suitable option for her situation. The ideal option is the one that is most acceptable, feasible, affordable, sustainable and safe in her particular context. If one of these conditions is not met with regard to formula feeding, the woman should be counselled to practice exclusive breastfeeding for the first few months. The final decision should be the woman's, and she should be supported in her choice" (Joint United Nations Programme on HIV/AIDS, "Selected Issues," p. 22).

32. Farmer, *Infections and Inequalities*, pp. 217, 225, 264, 286.

33. Donnelly, "Prevention Urged in AIDS Fight."

34. Farmer, "The Major Infectious Diseases in the World—To Treat or Not to Treat?" (included in this volume as chapter 12).

35. Farmer, *Pathologies of Power*, pp. 162, 175.

36. Wyatt, "Transaction Sex and HIV Risks."

37. Shkilnyk, *A Poison Stronger Than Love.*

38. Chien, Connors, and Fox, "The Drug War in Perspective."

39. Lacey, "Women's Voices Rise as Rwanda Reinvents Itself."

40. Kim and Gilks, "Scaling Up Treatment—Why We Can't Wait."

19

Mother Courage and the Costs of War

(2008)

I won't let you spoil my war for me. Destroys the weak, does it?
Well, what does peace do for 'em, huh? War feeds its people better.
BERTOLT BRECHT, *MOTHER COURAGE AND HER CHILDREN*

WHAT IS IT GOOD FOR?

War is good for something, or someone, or it would not have persisted for mil-
lennia as a major staple of human interaction. War pays, goes the old saw. But
what are the wages of war? Whom does it pay, and who pays for it? How does
it pay? Most important, what are the real costs of war and conflict? My guess is
that Bertolt Brecht wrote his famous play *Mother Courage* in order to ask and
answer some of these questions. And the answers are revealed, over time, to his
unlikely protagonist, a Swedish market woman and mother seeking to keep her
head above water in the course of a seventeenth-century conflict whose purposes
were unclear then and were even more so by 1939, when Brecht created *Mother
Courage*. (The play was provoked, say his biographers, by the German invasion
of Poland in September of that year.) Mother Courage's ability to answer these
and other questions comes only as she loses her three children in quick succession. The lines cited above, in which she claims that war pays more than peace,
are uttered just as she, a shrewd businesswoman even in the worst of times, has
reaped a few of the meager and transient spoils of war. But the play is called
Mother Courage and Her Children because, by the end, the audience or reader
knows that the affective costs of losing one's children—and all victims of war are
someone's children—are simply too high to calculate.

Today, when we ask questions about the costs of war, we are offered disparate
quantitative answers. Were I to access a website regarding the cost of war, I could
read that the war in Iraq has cost the United States, to date, $503,336,825,602 or

393

$275 million per day, as compared to an estimated inflation-adjusted $549 billion for the twelve-year-long war in Vietnam and $5 trillion for what some have termed "the good war," the Second World War.[1] But Nobel laureate Joseph Stiglitz and Linda Bilmes have recently called Iraq the "Three Trillion Dollar War," after mining information not readily available to the public:

> From the unhealthy brew of emergency funding, multiple sets of books, and chronic underestimates of the resources required to prosecute the war, we have attempted to identify how much we have been spending—and how much we will, in the end, likely have to spend. The figure we arrive at is more than $3 trillion. Our calculations are based on conservative assumptions. They are conceptually simple, even if occasionally technically complicated. A $3 trillion figure for the total cost strikes us as judicious, and probably errs on the low side. Needless to say, this number represents the cost only to the United States. It does not reflect the enormous cost to the rest of the world, or to Iraq.[2]

They go on to note that "even in the best case scenario," the U.S. government will spend in Iraq twice what it spent during the course of the First World War, ten times what was disbursed during the first Gulf War, and a third more than was spent in prosecuting the war in Vietnam.

But what do these figures mean, really? Brecht wrote at least nine plays as contributions to the combat—the war—against fascism and Nazism. Following his vision, it would seem that the challenge of "costing" a war is far more complex than might be indicated by whatever procedures were used to offer the figures just cited. After all, these assessments are of costs to one nation, already a very powerful and wealthy one by the time of the First World War. Imagine what cost the Second World War represented to, say, the Russians, who lost an estimated twenty-seven million people and had a far weaker economic base; imagine the costs to European Jews. Anthropologists know that the true cost of armed conflict emerges from qualitative methodologies and locally relevant yardsticks. War also wreaks, to use modern parlance, "collateral damage" upon civilians and their institutions, including health care, education, housing, telecommunications, and transport. War is costly in personal, affective terms; physical and psychological damage is done to combatants, families, communities; harm is done even to a sense of where one fits in the world after peace treaties are signed and reconstruction begins. War spoils meanings in complex and enduring ways for which we have few metrics.

In short, although the experts can offer only crude measures of the cost of war, everyone who has thought about it knows that war costs too much. That is no doubt why the rhetoric of war always ennobles sacrifice.

Economists can help lead the way to estimating the social costs of war, but, as Mother Courage's travails suggest, the misery provoked by armed conflict has no end. Hers was called "the Thirty Years' War," but do wars ever really have a clear beginning and an end? As Beatriz Manz reports from Guatemala, costs continue to mount long after overt hostilities draw to a close.[3] This is what Carolyn Nordstrom means when she reminds us that "violence has a tomorrow."[4]

Improving metrics is not a self-sufficient goal. As a physician-anthropologist (and parent) concerned with the hopelessly utopian project of ensuring that more of us humans reach our full potential and full life expectancy, I am interested less in current discussions about how war might become less brutal in the third millennium and more in steps that might be taken to abolish it. (This in spite of sympathy for and even gratitude to those who fight back, sometimes with force, against genocide and atrocity and against the unjust economic and social arrangements that almost always underlie armed conflict; this in spite of understanding that not all wars are similar.)

It is not easy to say something new about war. I began with three modest goals. The first was to draw on my experience as a physician-anthropologist and offer glimpses of the myriad means by which war not only ends lives—one of the primary goals of war—but also damages them in slow-burning ways, ones that, as in the case of Mother Courage, reach from one generation into the next. The second goal was to reveal some of the mechanisms by which conflicts of all sorts are described in misleading terms. The third goal was to speak to my peers about the ways in which anthropology, like other resocializing disciplines, might help to curb dishonesty and lessen the damage of war in both the short and the long term.

I recommend *Mother Courage and Her Children* as a text offering great insight into war. But I will here introduce a courageous mother, a Haitian detained at Guantánamo, whose oldest son is now in Iraq. There's a gruesome symmetry in this circumstance: if Iraq is the current U.S. administration's best-known failure, its policies in Haiti—also disastrous—are perhaps its least well-known failure.

FROM HAITI TO IRAQ:
MOTHER COURAGE AND HER HAITIAN SON

Most historians of war report that conflicts involving armies are built in part on lies. At this late date, the lie regarding weapons of mass destruction in Iraq has been exposed in a raft of articles and books,[5] some of them written by scholars. For comparison's sake, I note that it was not until 1981 that we could read the first scholarly assessment of the CIA's involvement in the 1954 coup in Guatemala, the event that sparked another thirty years' war.[6] As Beatriz Manz and others have shown, that disastrous and unequal civil war, which included genocidal sprees against indigenous people, continues to damage lives over a decade after peace was declared.[7]

Let me return to the costs of war as calculated on the eve of the invasion of Iraq. This story is well documented, if less well known: when one of President George W. Bush's chief economic advisors, then head of the National Economic Council, hazarded an estimate of $200 billion to prosecute the war in Iraq, the riposte from then secretary of defense Donald Rumsfeld was swift: "Baloney."[8] Rumsfeld's own estimate, supported by the director of the Office of Management and Budget, was $50 to $60 billion, costs that would be shared by other members of "the Coalition of the Willing." Rumsfeld's deputy Paul Wolfowitz went further: the costs of postwar reconstruction in Iraq would be "self-financed," he claimed, through oil revenues from a more efficient post-Saddam Iraq.[9] "The tone of the entire administration was cavalier," observe Stiglitz and Bilmes crisply, "as if the sums involved were minimal."[10]

How did the administration get away with such errors? (Whether they resulted from chicanery or misjudgment matters little now.) Why is the true cost of this war still no more clearly recognized by the U.S. public than it was by Rumsfeld and Wolfowitz in 2003? Stiglitz and Bilmes hazard a guess: "Most Americans have yet to feel these costs. The price in blood has been paid by our voluntary military and by hired contractors. The price in treasure has, in a sense, been financed entirely by borrowing. Taxes have not been raised to pay for it—in fact, taxes on the rich have actually fallen."[11]

As of 2008, "most Americans" may not have begun to feel the costs, but others, not all Americans, have felt them directly. As always in war, the numbers are contested. We know how many U.S. troops have lost their lives—some four thousand so far—and we have less exact estimates of how many have been otherwise damaged physically or psychologically. Even less clear are the numbers of Iraqi dead. When a team from a U.S. research university published, in a prestigious medical journal, a community-based study of "excess" civilian mortality in Iraq a year into the war,[12] the number of deaths they reported—more than one hundred thousand between March 2003 and September 2004—caused a huge stir in the press. The study and its authors were denounced by the architects of the war, who claimed that the large figure should be taken with a grain of salt because of "concerns about the methodology."[13] Yet subsequent inquiry suggests that the study was sound,[14] while the responses from the powerful were not.[15] The popular press is diverse enough to include some critical and even self-critical voices, although it took the debacle of the missing weapons of mass destruction to instill a sense of shame in a cheerleading, war-happy press.[16]

In its time, Vietnam generated no small number of disputes regarding civilian deaths, and excellent studies of mainstream press reporting on the first Gulf War have recently been published.[17] But if sorting through discrepant accounts is the analytic task, few places prepare an anthropologist (or U.S. citizen) better than does Haiti, which gave me the interpretive grid that I've used to contemplate not only the rest of the world, including my own country, but also war and violence, regardless of the scale. And Haiti is tied as surely to my own country as it is to Iraq, as the experiences of Yolande Jean and her son reveal.

I'll start with Yolande's son, whom I'll call "Joe" since he's still in Iraq.

I met Joe because of the aftereffects of a 1991 military coup d'état in Haiti, where I'd been working since graduating from college less than a decade previously. Joe was ten years old in 1991. His parents were poor, but they were able to read and write and were interested in teaching others to do so (an estimated 60 percent of Haitian adults do not know how to read). They became deeply involved in a mass literacy movement that had taken root in Haiti around the time of that country's first democratic elections in December 1990. Seven months after a landslide victory raised a liberation theologian to the presidency and brought more resources to bear on Haiti's stubborn poverty, a violent military coup interrupted democratic rule in Haiti. I have elsewhere detailed the ways in which the U.S. government was involved in this coup, a pattern that was to be repeated in 2004.[18] The ensuing repression was fearsome. Refugees streamed out of the cities and into the hills; over the border into the Dominican Republic, where they were unwelcome; and onto the high seas.

Fleeing was not an obvious option for a young couple with two small boys. But on April 27, 1992, Yolande, Joe's mother, was arrested and taken to Recherches Criminelles, the police station that served as the headquarters of Colonel Michel François, the alleged boss of Haiti's death squads. During the course of her "interview" (to use the official euphemism for torture), Yolande, who was visibly pregnant with her third child, began to bleed. On her second day in prison, she miscarried. She did not receive medical attention.

As Yolande later told me, she decided at that moment that if she survived detention, she would leave Haiti. She was released from prison the following day. Shortly thereafter, she entrusted her sons to a kinswoman and headed for northern Haiti. Her husband remained in hiding. She would not see him again.

> I took the boat on May twelfth, and on the fourteenth [the U.S. Coast Guard] came to get us. They did not say where they were taking us. We were still in Haitian waters at the time.... We hadn't even reached the Windward Passage when American soldiers came for us. But we thought they might be coming to help us ... there were sick children on board. On the fourteenth, we reached the base at Guantánamo.[19]

Yolande's initial instinct—that the U.S. soldiers "might be coming to help us"—was soon corrected: "They burned all of our clothes, everything we had, the boat, our luggage, all the documents we were carrying." U.S. television had displayed images of Haitian boats burning, but both the Coast Guard and the media described the fires as the destruction of unseaworthy vessels—with no mention of personal items. When asked what reasons the U.S. soldiers gave for burning the refugees' effects, Yolande replied,

> They gave us none. They just started towing our belongings, and the next thing we know, the boat was in flames. Photos, documents. If you didn't have pockets in which to put things, you lost them. The reason that I came through with some of my documents is because I had a backpack and was wearing pants with pockets. They went through my bag and took some of my documents. Even my important papers they took. American soldiers did this. Fortunately, I had hidden some papers in my pockets.[20]

Haiti was full to overflowing with people just like Yolande Jean. Soon the U.S. military base on Guantánamo was full to overflowing as well. On May 24, 1992, President George H. W. Bush issued Executive Order 12,807 from his summer home in Kennebunkport, Maine. Referring to the Haitian boats, he ordered the Coast Guard "to return the vessel and its passengers to the country from which it came . . . provided, however, that the Attorney General, in his unreviewable discretion, may decide that a person who is a refugee will not be returned without his consent." As attorney Andrew Schoenholtz of the Lawyers Committee for Human Rights wryly observed, "Grace did not abound; all Haitians have been returned under the new order."[21]

I won't go through Yolande's whole story, which I've recounted elsewhere.[22] But she clearly had her sons on her mind every day. Because of her arrest and torture in Haiti and the documents she had managed to save to prove this, she was one of the tiny number of those on Guantánamo deemed to be a political refugee; U.S. law should therefore have provided her with asylum and a safe haven in the United States. But she was not processed through to the United States because she was found to be infected with HIV. The authorities had invoked U.S. immigration law, which barred immigrants testing positive for HIV from entering the country.

Yolande learned that she would not be sent back to Haiti, but neither would she be released to the United States. "Where will I go?" she asked. The answer came in the form of no answer: she, and hundreds of others, would simply linger in detention in the legal limbo that is Guantánamo, established as a U.S. military base in the early twentieth century and subject, clearly, to neither Cuban nor U.S. laws. Thus Guantánamo had a meaning for Haitians long before the enclave became synonymous with arbitrary and indeed illegal detention.

Many "boat people" from Haiti were lost at sea, but all were welcome nowhere, it seemed. In the same edition that announced, "Boat with 396 Haitians Missing; Cuba Reports 8 Survivors," the *Orlando Sentinel* wrote of "what could be a huge problem for the state: An explosion of Haitian migrants to South Florida." The story, which ran on the front page, continued by noting, "Many fear that tens of thousands of refugees could sail for Miami around Inauguration Day, Jan. 20, because of President-elect Bill Clinton's pledge to give Haitians a fair hearing for political asylum in the United States."[23] The plight of Haitian refugees had become enough of a cause célèbre during the 1992 U.S. elections to spur candidates Clinton and Gore, in their official platform, to call for an end to forced repatriation of Haitian boat people and to the detention of HIV-positive refugees on Guantánamo.[24] On January 28, however, Clinton began backpedaling, stating that he would continue his predecessor's policies.

On learning of this, a number of Guantánamo detainees began a hunger strike. Yolande, unlike Brecht's fictitious Mother Courage, decided to act on principle. Distrustful of the U.S. military doctors and even her own lawyers, she encouraged the other detainees to refuse to eat. This is what she said happened next:

> Before the strike, I'd been in prison, a tiny little cell, but crammed in with many others, men, women, and children. There was no privacy. Snakes would come in; we were lying on the ground, and lizards were climbing over us. One of us was bitten by a scorpion . . . there were spiders. Bees were stinging the children, and there were flies everywhere: whenever you tried to eat something, flies would fly into your mouth. Because of all this, I just got to the point, sometime in January, [that] I said to myself, come what may, I might well die, but we can't continue in this fashion.
>
> We called together the committee and decided to have a hunger strike. Children, pregnant women, everyone was lying outside, rain or shine, day and night. After fifteen days without food, people began to faint. The colonel called us together and warned us, and me particularly, to call off the strike. We said no.
>
> At four in the morning, as we were lying on the ground, the colonel came with many soldiers. They began to beat us—I still bear a scar from this—and to strike us with nightsticks. . . . True, we threw rocks back at them, but they outnumbered us, and they were armed. Then they used big tractors to back us against the shelter, and they barred our escape with barbed wire.[25]

Yolande was arrested and placed in solitary confinement in a place called Camp Bulkeley. Her version of the story did not make it into the *New York Times,* which reported only that "at least seven Haitian refugees protesting their detention here by refusing food have lost consciousness."[26] No mention was made of any retribution by the strikers' wardens.

Even the lawyers for the Haitian detainees, who reached the base in the middle of the strike, seemed a bit annoyed by their clients' actions: "The hunger strike took us all by surprise," said one, "especially given the fact that the litigation team is in the middle of settlement negotiations with the Department of Justice."[27] The Haitians, it seems, were no longer impressed by bureaucratic efforts to have them released. On March 11, 1993, eleven prisoners attempted to escape to Cuba but were recaptured. Two of the detainees tried to commit suicide, one by hanging. (The similarities with recent hunger strikes and suicides on Guantánamo, during what has been dubbed "the Global War on Terror," are striking but not supernatural.)

Brecht's Mother Courage was confident that she was a survivor; Yolande, less sure, had already decided to pursue her hunger strike until her release from Guantánamo. Her letter to her sons was widely circulated in the community of concern taking shape in response to the situation there. It was read out loud at a New York demonstration by American actress Susan Sarandon.

To my family:

Don't count on me anymore, because I have lost in the struggle for life. Thus, there is nothing left of me. Take care of my children, so they have strength to continue my struggle, because it is our duty.

As for me, my obligation ends here. [Joe] and Jeff, you have to continue with the struggle so that you may become men of the future. I have lost hope; I am alone in my distress. I know you will understand my situation, but do not worry about me because I have made my own decision. I am alone in life and will remain so. Life is no longer worth living to me.

[Joe] and Jeff, you no longer have a mother. Understand that you don't have a bad mother, it is simply that circumstances have taken me to where I am at this moment. I am sending you two pictures so you could look at me for a last time. Goodbye my children. Goodbye my family. We will meet again in another world.[28]

The Haitians' advocates, including a handful of celebrities like Sarandon, several human rights organizations, and Haitian refugee groups in the eastern United States, stepped up pressure on the U.S. government. And then something surprising happened: Judge Sterling Johnson of New York, though a Bush appointee to the federal bench, heard the case and ruled *against* the administration. The more depositions he heard, the more convinced he became that the detention of the HIV-positive Haitians represented "cruel and unusual punishment" in violation of the Eighth Amendment of the U.S. Constitution. In his 1993 ruling on the case, he described Haitians detained in Camp Bulkeley in these words:

> They live in camps surrounded by razor barbed wire. They tie plastic garbage bags to the sides of the building to keep the rain out. They sleep on cots and hang sheets to create some semblance of privacy. They are guarded by the military and are not permitted to leave the camp, except under military escort. The Haitian detainees have been subjected to pre-dawn military sweeps as they sleep by as many as 400 soldiers dressed in full riot gear. They are confined like prisoners and are subject to detention in the brig without hearing for camp rule infractions.[29]

On March 26, 1993, he ordered that all detainees "with fewer than 200 total T-lymphocytes" be transferred to the United States. It was the first time that such laboratory tests had ever been mentioned in a judicial order. A Justice Department spokesman complained that "there are aspects of Judge Johnson's decision that we would find it difficult to live with." The first of these, noted the spokesman, "would be the judge's very expansive view of the rights of aliens, who came into American hands purely out of our own humanitarian impulses to rescue them at sea."[30] Decades earlier, Judge Johnson had been a JAG officer, a military lawyer, on Gitmo, as the base is termed in military argot. Perhaps this gave him perspective on the way humanitarian impulses are expressed in an extralegal environment.

Although I was never permitted to go to Gitmo, I later got to know Yolande fairly well and visited her and other Haitian refugees in New York and Boston. When I first met Joe, he was about twelve; his brother, ten. They were, to me, the children of a courageous mother I wished to interview. I wanted to get her story out, and I did my best. Yolande's story was carried in the *Boston Globe*. But then a decade went by, and I confess I didn't think much about Yolande or Joe. I continued to work in Haiti and elsewhere and to argue on behalf of sick or afflicted Haitians in the United States who were being threatened with deportation.

After the events of September 11, 2001, Gitmo once again exploded in the world's conscience. Now everyone knows that Gitmo is the place where prisoners are held at the pleasure of the U.S. government, with no jurisdiction to which they can appeal. But the earlier use of Gitmo as a staging area for Haitians not deemed to deserve refugee status had been forgotten. It was as if the travails of Yolande Jean had been erased from the public memory. I noted this erasure, but did nothing. Having written about Gitmo, and having seen my account, like others, flushed down the public *oubliette,* I didn't see what I could add.

Toward the end of 2005, I received a message from Joe, Yolande's oldest son. It was in fact more than a message: he sent me, via a close friend of his, a check in the amount of $250. Joe said he wished to support our work in Haiti and to help us serve the destitute sick there.

I was grateful for the contribution, for we certainly needed the help in Haiti. What struck me most, though, was that it came from Fallujah. Joe had joined the U.S. Marines and been sent to Iraq.

I wrote back to him at once, and we stayed in touch through email and, once in a while, by phone. For a year, we corresponded regularly, at least once a week, but we didn't talk much about the war or his daily reality. By the time I began inquiring anxiously about his safety, he took great pains to let me know that he no longer went out on missions "beyond the wire" but instead was responsible for supplying another group of marines out on patrol. He didn't say much, over email, about his activities, noting only how relieved he felt when his "guys" returned safely to the forward operating base in Fallujah. More often than not, he'd tell me that I was the one who needed to be careful, since he knew about the violence and instability in Haiti.

But I guessed that being in Iraq was both a great outward and internal struggle for him. I guessed that Joe was distressed by what he was hearing about Gitmo, and I had to assume he was thinking about his own mother's experience there. Once, when I sent him a care package, I weighed carefully what sorts of books to include: something light, I thought; some videos and escapist novels. No, he responded by email, "send me things about Haiti. Like I told you, I want to go back to Haiti one day and work with you." And so I sent him one of my own books about Haiti, with some concern that he might find my detailed description of his mother's stay at Gitmo harrowing or upsetting. He didn't say one way or another, but after he read it, he asked me to send a copy to a friend of his. "He's Native American," wrote Joe. "He'll like it." I sent the book.

After a year of brief but regular emails, our connection deepened. We made plans to meet for a meal when Joe was next on leave. I was in Haiti when Joe wrote me one Monday in 2007. It was nighttime in Fallujah, and he was leaving just then for the States; he'd call me as soon as he landed, he wrote. I forgot to ask when, exactly, that would be and so started to worry right away. The most dangerous part, I thought, would be getting in and out of Baghdad. My phone rang on Saturday, and shortly thereafter I got to enjoy a lengthy reunion with Joe and to see his brother briefly. Joe allowed, during the course of a long meal that included what I reckoned to be the first red wine he'd had in a while, that the main reasons he was planning to stay in Iraq and complete his military tour were to ensure that he would have the resources to be able to look after his mother, who he knew might fall gravely ill at any time; to send his brother to a proper college; and eventually to buy a home and have a family. "I want to look forward, not back," said the irrepressibly optimistic Joe.

Some things we didn't discuss, including the fact that Joe, like many others serving in Iraq, is not yet a U.S. citizen. I felt too uneasy to ask what he thought about the war in Iraq. We never discussed U.S. policies in Haiti, nor did we discuss his mother's harrowing experience on Gitmo. But we did discuss his younger brother's plans. Whenever money was tight, Jeff thought about joining the military, too. "Do that only as a last resort," advised Joe. "I'll find the money for you to finish college." Yet in spite of the many things we left unspoken, there was so much remaining to talk about that we called each other often during Joe's leave, and I found his departure more distressing than I'd expected. As of this writing, Joe is still in Fallujah.

So what, exactly, is this story about and what might it reveal about the causes and consequences of war and conflict? Obviously enough, it's a story about connections. I let Joe and his family fall out of my life for a decade. Joe's generosity brought us back together. Returning to the theme of *Mother Courage and Her Children,* it is evident that Joe's mother made a very different set of choices than did Brecht's character. Following the 1991 coup and during her illegal internment on Guantánamo, Yolande's leadership and convictions led directly to the release of the detainees and to the reunification of what was left of her family. She never believed that war paid better than peace, and she was willing to take risks to make her point.

Next come other connections, of the kind best revealed by linking personal narrative to the study of history and political economy. Such connections seem at first glance impersonal, since they are invariably about the use or misuse of power, including the ability to wage war. The intimate links between my country and Haiti, the Western Hemisphere's two oldest republics, over the past two centuries make a shameful story, from an American point of view. And the connection between our country and Iraq will cause us grief, I fear, for generations. Fallujah, where Joe is based, is already a proverb for brutality. Just a year ago, one U.S. colonel deployed in Anbar province explained his approach to counter-insurgency: "Fix Ramadi, but don't destroy it. Don't do a Fallujah."[31] Fallujah, a city of roughly 435,000 people, was reduced to rubble in offensives launched after the Republicans decided that the 2004 U.S. presidential elections had filled their accounts with "political capital," and it is to this bloodbath that the U.S. officer refers.

But what about our military base so peculiarly located in Cuba? That must be a story about connection, too. Jonathan Hansen recently gave a talk about Gitmo at Harvard and described the place thus:

> A bay, a harbor, a hideout, a home, a military base, a sanctuary, a prison, an outpost on the threshold of nations where neither Cuban, nor U.S., nor international law applies. Guantánamo blurs the categories of modern political representation. Paradoxically, by doing so, it brings them into sharp relief. The history of Guantánamo illuminates the artificial and yet necessary distinctions that construct and sustain the modern world. This project is a tale of that world: on the one hand, of the interaction of nation-states and of national interest with international law; on the other hand, of individuals caught up in the system of states, trying to negotiate the tangle of allegiances and affiliations which that system imposes. Guantánamo Bay has been there all along—when the Taino Indians met Columbus, when Caribbean pirates preyed on the shipping of newly consolidated states, when Spain clashed with Britain, when the U.S. defeated Spain, when Kennedy confronted Castro, when George W. Bush set out to vanquish terror. To know Guantánamo is to know ourselves—as citizens, as a country, as individuals in a world of states.[32]

Gitmo is a place outside the reach of American constitutional protections, so you might think of it as a place of disconnection. But that very disconnection connects us to that place and to what is done there now, in 2008, when Guantánamo continues to serve as a detention center for men captured in Iraq, Afghanistan, and other places from which we "render" our enemies to unlimited detention. Guantánamo is a place where responsibility can be denied. Like all such denials—about the fate of Haitian refugees, about the price tag on war, about the reasons for prosecuting it in Iraq—this act won't hold up forever. Americans should be shamed and disquieted by the things done in their name in this place outside the law.

To reiterate: if Iraq is the best known of the current U.S. administration's foreign-policy blunders, Haiti is its best-kept dirty secret.

Between 2000 and 2004, the U.S. administration orchestrated an aid embargo against Haiti. Certain kinds of aid continued, however, as groups like the International Republican Institute funneled funds to various sectors of what is called "civil society"—in the eyes of the people I serve in Haiti and elsewhere in Latin America, this phrase invariably designates the minority of those who are not poor—in order to weaken the democratically elected government. Similar tactics were being used in Venezuela, but the government there was better defended than Haiti's. Mainstream U.S. news sources paid almost no attention to the sabotage in Haiti until its aims—which culminated in the kidnapping of a sitting head of state—were accomplished. Finally, in January 2006, investigative reporters at the *New York Times* released a long and devastating report about the precise mechanisms by which the government had been overthrown in late February 2004.[33] After the coup came a long interregnum of lawlessness, just as in postinvasion Iraq. One news report in December 2005 named Port-au-Prince the kidnapping capital of the world.[34]

The kidnapping of Haiti's president, Jean-Bertrand Aristide, has recently been the subject of two informative books.[35] Reading them is a good antidote to the effrontery of American officials. Donald Rumsfeld, soon to be replaced as secretary of defense, dismissed allegations of kidnapping as "ridiculous" (recalling, in tone and in credibility, his previous dismissal of a colleague's estimate of the Iraq war's cost as "baloney"). Our former secretary of state insisted that the Haitian president had been flown "to a destination of his choice. . . . So this was not a kidnapping."[36] Regardless of your views on the individual probity of the Bush administration's cabinet members, it seems unlikely that the Haitian president would choose as his destination the Central African Republic, a country he had never visited, one that had had its own coup d'état a few months earlier and was known for general lawlessness.

Haitians know a lot about kidnapping, of course. Almost all of them are descendants of people kidnapped from Africa. Toussaint L'Ouverture, the Haitian general who led the world's first successful slave revolt, was invited at the dawn of the nineteenth century to a parley with French forces and was given the assurances usual in a negotiation between the heads of opposed armies. Instead of a parley, what occurred was a kidnapping: he was chained and put on a boat bound for France, where he later died, apparently of tuberculosis, in an Alpine prison.

"Extraordinary rendition," the latest term for kidnapping, fits well with an age that has seen habeas corpus treated as an option, not a constitutional right.[37] When the president of our nation's oldest neighbor, Haiti, is "rendered" all the way to central Africa, the justifications offered by those responsible amount to no more than dismissals and character assassination.[38] The same sense of justice, accountability, and respect for public opinion ushered us into an apparently unending war in Iraq ("weapons of mass destruction," "links with Al Qaeda," "greeted as liberators"). The arrogance of power underwrites the connection between Joe's Haiti and his Iraq.

Finally, Joe's story, like his mother's and that of the country in which both of them were born, raises questions about the kind of world we want to live in, the kind of world we want to leave to our children. Does honest analysis of war and conflict make any difference at all? Pierre Bourdieu thought so: "To subject to scrutiny the mechanisms which render life painful, even untenable," he wrote, "is not to neutralize them; to bring to light contradictions is not to resolve them. But, as skeptical as one might be about the efficacy of the sociological message, we cannot dismiss the effect it can have by allowing sufferers to discover the possible social causes of their suffering and, thus, to be relieved of blame."[39] To the end, Bourdieu believed, despite all he had witnessed and written, in what is essentially an Enlightenment ideal: that we can lessen social suffering if we understand how it is generated and sustained over time, across generations.

MOTHER-COURAGE AND THE FIGHT TO ABOLISH WAR

As a physician, teacher, anthropologist, and parent, I meet almost no one—it may be true that I meet no one, period—who favors war. And yet war remains a major interest of societies rich and poor; war remains a major source not only of death and conquest but of profit; fifty years after the beginning of the nuclear era of "mutually assured destruction," war remains a growth industry. I began work on this essay with the hope that it might make a difference: that the efforts of academics and journalists might improve U.S. foreign policy (whether toward Haiti or in the Middle East); that they might help to shut down Guantánamo and other extralegal limbos; that they might stop practices such as extraordinary rendition; that they might even contribute to the utopian goal of abolishing war.

But there is of course cause for pessimism. Although the stories of Joe and his mother are singular in their detail, the underlying wish—to abolish war—is as old as war itself. It is as old as the grief of a parent who buries her children.

There is cause for pessimism, too, if the goal of our writing is suasion through enlightenment, through offering details about the causes and consequences, the true costs, of war. After all, arguments against war have been laid out persuasively enough before. Take, for example, what is often called the Russell-Einstein Manifesto (1955), in which two of the greatest minds of the last century insisted:

"We have to learn to ask ourselves, not what steps can be taken to give military victory to whatever group we prefer, for there no longer are such steps; the question we have to ask ourselves is: what steps can be taken to prevent a military contest of which the issue must be disastrous to all parties?" Albert Einstein and Bertrand Russell had nuclear weapons in mind, of course. The "overkill" such weapons promised was insane, they wrote (again and again). And they spoke of bonds between families and generations as a force that might rein in the ambitions of bellicose statesmen:

> The abolition of war will demand distasteful limitations of national sovereignty. But what perhaps impedes understanding of the situation more than anything else is that the term "mankind" feels vague and abstract. People scarcely realize in imagination that the danger is to themselves and their children and their grandchildren, and not only to a dimly apprehended humanity. They can scarcely bring themselves to grasp that they, individually, and those whom they love are in imminent danger of perishing agonizingly. And so they hope that perhaps war may be allowed to continue provided modern weapons are prohibited.[40]

Modern weapons, that is, "weapons of mass destruction." The threat of such weapons was brandished to justify the most recent invasion of Iraq, of course: a false pretext that was only prelude to a bloody war with more or less conventional weapons, and one of hundreds of rash decisions made through arrogance and incompetence.[41]

The testimonies of those who prosecute, participate in, or survive wars are countless, a rich literature. The title of Ernst Friedrich's 1924 work is inspiring: *War against War.*[42] Many are stirred, as Bertolt Brecht was, to give war an artistic form so as to reveal to a broad audience its stupidity and cruelty.

Brecht's Mother Courage was a Swedish woman caught up in the informal economy of the war—selling food, articles of daily use, and just about anything, in the mad optimistic belief that "war feeds its people better." But war is a machine that invariably devours its young. Toward the end, a peasant woman assures Mother Courage's doomed daughter, "There's nothing we can do. Pray, poor thing, pray! There's nothing we can do to stop this bloodshed, so even if you can't talk, at least pray. He hears, if no one else does."[43]

Who knows what God hears?

Nonetheless, there are certainly some things we can do, as scholars, physicians, parents, and kin. There is a nascent movement among scholars and ordinary citizens to fight back against war and injustice. It took just such a movement to end the slave trade in the nineteenth century; it took similar movements to achieve universal enfranchisement in the United States and abolish apartheid in South Africa. Sometimes movements such as these are founded on mother-courage in the best sense of the term. I have never had much opportunity to follow blogs, but it happens that there is one called "Mother Courage: Musings of a Marine Mother." Allow me to cite a recent posting by this mother:

> George W. Bush's Fourth of July speech to the usual hand-picked audience, this time the West Virginia National Guard, plumbed new depths of inanity, propaganda and the dumbing-down of U.S. history. I fired off several angry letters to the usual suspects—none were published though plenty of sentiments similar to mine were—then saw this riposte written by Marty Kaplan in Thursday's *Huffington Post*.
>
>> ... *"There are many ways for our fellow citizens to say thanks to the men and women who wear the uniform and their families. You can send a care package. You can reach out to a military family in your neighborhood... You can car pool."* [—A quotation from President George Bush]
>>   Instead of sending them a care package, how about sending them home? Instead of car pooling, how about an energy policy that prevents our country from financing the very nations who hold our economy hostage, let alone the terrorists they quietly harbor?

Not surprisingly, my favorite line: "Instead of sending [the troops] a care package, how about sending them home?" Pass it on.[44]

I don't know that we can stop war. I can't be sure that the best analysis in the world, the best plays imaginable or even a painting as beautiful as *Guernica* will stop the insanity, profitable to some few but devastating to the majority, that is war. I don't know how much I can do as a physician, either. Certainly, I can patch up some of the wounds, stanch the bleeding, make sure that blood is stocked and safe for transfusion.

But I do know this: we can marshal the evidence against war and we can pass it on.

NOTES

This essay is dedicated to the memory and gentle pacifism of Roz Zinn.

1. National Priorities Project, "Bringing the Federal Budget Home"; Weisman, "Projected Iraq War Costs Soar—Total Spending Is Likely to More Than Double, Analysis Finds"; Stiglitz and Bilmes, "The Three Trillion Dollar War."

2. Stiglitz and Bilmes, "The Three Trillion Dollar War."

3. Manz, *Paradise in Ashes*.

4. Nordstrom, "The Tomorrow of Violence."

5. See Hersh, *Chain of Command*; Massing, *Now They Tell Us*; Danner, *The Secret Way to War*.

6. Immerman, *The CIA in Guatemala*.

7. Manz, *Paradise in Ashes*.

8. Bilmes and Stiglitz, "The Iraq War Will Cost Us $3 Trillion, and Much More."

9. Alden, Dinmore, and Swann, "Wolfowitz Nomination a Shock for Europe."

10. Stiglitz and Bilmes, "The Three Trillion Dollar War."

11. Ibid.

12. Roberts et al., "Mortality before and after the 2003 Invasion of Iraq."

13. Prime Minister's Office, United Kingdom, "Prime Minister's Official Spokesperson Morning Briefing."

14. Al-Rubeyi, "Mortality before and after the Invasion of Iraq in 2003."

15. Two years later, Gilbert Burnham and colleagues published a figure of over 650,000 Iraqi civilian deaths from the start of the war until July 2006 ("Mortality after the 2003 Invasion of Iraq"). The most recent figures from the Iraq Family Health Survey Study Group estimate 151,000 civilian deaths in the same time period ("Violence-Related Mortality in Iraq from 2002 to 2006"). Clearly, the epidemiological debate rages on. See also the recent report by Amnesty International, *Carnage and Despair*.

16. Börjesson, *Feet to the Fire*.

17. See, for example, MacArthur, *Second Front*.

18. Farmer, *The Uses of Haiti*.

19. Ibid., p. 224.

20. Ibid.

21. Schoenholtz, "Aiding and Abetting Persecutors," p. 71.

22. Farmer, *Pathologies of Power*, chap. 2, pp. 51–90.

23. "South Florida Braces for Haitian Time Bomb," *Orlando Sentinel*.

24. Clinton and Gore, *Putting People First*.

25. Farmer, *The Uses of Haiti*, p. 233.

26. Hilts, "7 Haitians Held at Guantanamo Unconscious in a Hunger Strike."

27. Powell, "'Life' at Guantánamo," p. 60.

28. Farmer, *The Uses of Haiti*, p. 234.

29. Judge Johnson's description is cited in Annas, "Detention of HIV-Positive Haitians at Guantánamo," p. 590.

30. Friedman, "U.S. to Release 158 Haitian Detainees."

31. Michaels, "Behind Success in Ramadi."

32. Hansen, "Guantánamo Bay."

33. See Farmer and Smith Fawzi, "Unjust Embargo Deepens Haiti's Health Crisis"; Farmer, "Political Violence and Public Health in Haiti"; Farmer, "Who Removed Aristide?"; Farmer, Smith Fawzi, and Nevil, "Unjust Embargo of Aid for Haiti"; Kidder, "The Trials of Haiti"; Bogdanich and Nordberg, "Mixed U.S. Signals Helped Tilt Haiti toward Chaos."

34. Montesquiou, "Missionaries, Schoolkids, and Bystanders—No One Is Safe from Haiti's Kidnappers."

35. See Robinson, *An Unbroken Agony*; Hallward, *Damming the Flood*.

36. Williams, "Powell Defends U.S. Stance on Haiti."

37. See Sadat, "Ghost Prisoners and Black Sites."

38. See Hallward, *Damming the Flood*; "Did He Go or Was He Pushed?" *Economist*.

39. Bourdieu et al., *La misère du monde*, pp. 1453–54; translation mine.

40. Einstein and Russell, "The Russell-Einstein Manifesto."

41. As Michael Gordon reported in the *New York Times*: "'Anyone who is experienced in the ways of Washington knows the difference between an open, transparent policy process and slamming something through the system,' said Franklin C. Miller, the senior director for Defense Policy and Arms Control, who played an important role on the National Security Council in overseeing plans for the postwar phase. 'The most portentous decision of the occupation was carried out stealthily and without giving the president's principal advisers an opportunity to consider it and give the president their views'" ("Fateful Choice on Iraq Army Bypassed Debate").

42. Friedrich, *Krieg dem Kriege!*

43. Brecht, *Mother Courage and Her Children*, p. 105.

44. Anton, "Mother Courage" (blog), "Codependence Day," posted July 7, 2007.

"Landmine Boy"
and Stupid Deaths

(2008)

Even if our own approach to things is conditioned necessarily by the view
that things have no meanings apart from those that human transactions,
attributions, and motivations endow them with, the anthropological
problem is that this formal truth does not illuminate the concrete,
historical circulation of things. For that we have to follow the things
themselves, for their meanings are inscribed in their forms, their uses,
their trajectories. It is only through the analysis of these trajectories that
we can interpret the human transactions and calculations that enliven
things.

ARJUN APPADURAI, *THE SOCIAL LIFE OF THINGS*

I have been working in Haiti all of my adult life and in Rwanda since 2005. In Rwanda, I work predominantly as a physician rather than as an anthropologist conducting ethnographic fieldwork. Ethnographers of this region know the language, culture, and history of Rwanda far better than I do. If I spoke Kinyarwanda fluently and had spent many years in Rwanda, perhaps I might claim the ethnographer's privilege of systematic knowledge or offer to decipher, as many of my colleagues do, the symbolics or poetics of violence.[1] But work in Haiti and elsewhere in Latin America has given me rough-and-ready interpretive frameworks for understanding violence, both the "event"-centered kind, including war and political violence, and the structural kind, including racism and other forms of social inequalities.[2] In Rwanda, as part of a team reintroducing health and social services to a rural region devastated by the 1994 genocide, I write as an outsider looking at violence in a place that I am getting to know.

The history of war and genocide in Rwanda will be contested terrain for generations, but some conclusions are inescapable: that European notions of race and ethnicity, some of them inspired by colonial-era eugenics, helped to harden the precolonial social categories of Hutu and Tutsi; that the biased bestowal of colonial-era privileges in a social field of scarcity laid the framework for inter-group violence that began in 1959, at the close of the colonial era; and that control over the state apparatus, and the economic and social privileges associated with proximity to political power, was the chief goal of the government leaders who were the architects of the Rwandan genocide. Equally inescapable, for Rwandans, are the consequences of that damage. As Carolyn Nordstrom notes, "violence is not only enacted in the present—the immediacy of an act of harm—but violence has a tomorrow."[3] The tomorrow of violence is usually more violence, and it is this cycle that has been interrupted in Rwanda, as is the case in much of Western Europe over the past half century.

But violence has its tomorrow even in situations in which war and genocide have given way to peace and security and the promise of a more hopeful future. To better understand violence, and how it is dampened or fanned, we need to call not only on history and broad social context but also on personal narra-tive, on experience. To reflect on the causes and consequences of the Rwandan genocide, we might begin with a series of events that occurred in rural Rwanda on March 22, 2006, when two children picked up a landmine. This incident was just one of many brutal remainders of the genocide, itself the upshot of a complex series of precolonial, colonial, and postcolonial processes that laid the ground-work for what was to happen in 1994.

EVENT AND STRUCTURE:
ANTHROPOLOGIES OF VIOLENCE

Violence is a frequent theme in anthropological research nowadays.[4] It seems obvious that it should be—what human society is free of violence?—but it was far more rarely the focus of attention during the first century of the discipline, as Talal Asad, Orin Starn, and many others have observed.[5] *Event violence* is ethno-graphically visible—sometimes spectacularly grisly, as was the case in Rwanda in 1994. There are dozens of journalistic accounts of Africa's most devastating mass violence, which occurred during the course of a hundred days. However, its causes and consequences are complex and too often invisible to those who wit-ness or chronicle violent events. But it is not enough to understand violence done by and to human beings in specific places and times; we must also seek to throw light on *structural violence,* the kind of violence done on a collective and even impersonal scale, topics best analyzed using the complementary frameworks of history and political economy.

Anthropology aside, there is a vast literature on violence. For centuries, mili-tary planners and historians have written about how wars of all sorts are prosecuted. Victims of violence and their kin have also left behind a rich literature, to which anthropologists have contributed as well. Some unite scholarly and personal investments in the study of violence. For example, Philippe Bourgois, like Barbara Rylko-Bauer, is the child of a Holocaust survivor. In recent writings, the personal experiences and commentaries of their parents are worked into a resocializing analysis in which comments and even silences serve as clues, hinting at this or that less visible event, force, or process.[6]

Like the genocides of Europe, the Rwandan genocide will one day spawn such a literature and, as in the European case, we can expect it to span widely discrepant perspectives and explanatory frameworks. One problem with discrepant accounts—and violence engenders them inevitably—is that it takes time and careful research to weigh their veracity. In the case of genocide, there are victims and there are aggressors, but the victims of genocide are (with rare exceptions) no longer present and are thus unable to offer first-person narratives, even if their relatives can.[7] Some scholars, including Jean Hatzfeld,[8] have contributed to our understanding of the events of 1994 by interviewing survivors and perpetrators alike; these eyewitness interviews are necessarily structured in predictable ways, but they offer important first-order data.

In reading interviews with people who are the perpetrators or targets of genocide, interpretive grids of one sort or another both help and hinder attempts to reconstruct what happened and how. This necessary sifting and discernment of human perspectives and motives can be usefully complemented by a focus on *things*. Things, at least, don't manipulate their observers—or is that true? Take the case of so commonplace an object (alas) as a landmine. While in graduate school, I read Arjun Appadurai's edited volume *The Social Life of Things*.[9] A focus on the material—on things—need not detract from the everyday business of both physicians and anthropologists, which is a focus on what people say, on what they do, and on the ways they construct meaning. On the contrary, the "materiality of the social" has long been a source of illumination in anthropology.[10]

Ever since Bronislaw Malinowski's report on the kula ring, the meanings associated with certain things have been the focus of significant empirical research. Anthropologists agree that things take on meaning through exchange (sale, trade, other transactions), through rituals banal and freighted, and through other processes that confer value on things in the minds of those engaged in their circulation. Landmines and other ordnance, though expendable, are no exception. In the case of Rwanda, they force us to cast our net well beyond the immediate country or culture, since, unlike the cases seen in ritual transactions, the path leading from arms dealers to hapless children and other civilians (and even, at times, to combatants) involves little commonality, but rather a riven diversity, of agency and intent.

PICKING UP A LANDMINE

On a Wednesday morning in March 2006, while herding cows, two boys picked up a landmine. In Rwanda, this is an increasingly rare event, as many efforts have been made to find and disarm such weapons.[11] (Time will tell whether Rwanda has been successful in lessening the tomorrow of violence.) Unfortunately, it is an exceedingly common event elsewhere: in the past decade, it was estimated that there are 110 million landmines in the ground worldwide, and more than twice as many stockpiled. Today, thirteen countries continue to manufacture antiperson-nel devices, though as little as fifteen years ago that number was more than fifty countries[12] and almost a hundred private companies, forty-seven of which were based in the United States.[13] Of those who detonate the landmines unintention-ally, 80 percent are civilians, one in five of them children; about half die, virtually all the rest are injured, and many of them are permanently maimed.[14]

Both of the Rwandan boys survived. I came to know quite well the one who was injured more seriously, as he spent more time in the hospital and needed physical therapy, home visits, and social assistance. Around the hospital, reopened less than a year earlier, he was termed, affectionately enough, "Landmine Boy," but his real name is Faustin. I met him at ten in the morning on that Wednesday, as I was headed out of the hospital to a clinic a couple of hours away. The hos-pital had been built and was once owned by a Belgian mining company, which left Rwanda decades ago. After the war and genocide, the facility fell into dis-use, essentially abandoned until May of 2005, when we (Partners In Health, the Clinton Foundation, and the Rwandan Ministry of Health) rebuilt and opened it as the sole hospital serving more than two hundred thousand people, most of them resettled refugees, internally displaced persons, with almost all of them living in poverty.

By March 2006, we had cobbled together a medical and nursing staff consisting mostly of Rwandan professionals and a handful of expatriate volunteers. One of my colleagues, a physician from Cameroon, stopped me that morning, saying, "Come quickly to the emergency room. Two children have picked up a grenade." At that moment, I did not think it unlikely that someone in the region would have picked up a grenade and pulled the pin: after all, the boys live (and we practice medicine) in a region hit hard by the war and genocide. The boys said that they merely picked the thing up and threw it toward the cows they were herding; the cows took the full force of the explosion, and two were killed. It was an hour or so after seeing the boys before I began to think about the object itself, what it was, and where it had come from. In the meantime, neither I nor my colleagues were thinking about anything other than trauma care, which is of course precisely what trauma victims need most. In this case, it meant splinting fractures, debrid-ing wounds, and applying dressings. We worked attentively and in near silence.

Of the two boys, one, Grégoire, was not seriously injured. The other, Faustin, sustained multiple fractures, and many fragments had been blown into his skin. I had the privilege of splinting him, pulling the plastic fragments out of him, and preparing him for transport. Although we had just rebuilt the operating room, we did not have an orthopedic surgeon on staff, and Faustin needed to have his fractures set in the operating room with what is called an external fixator.

That was the first hour. The boys, who were alert but very quiet, were not sure of their age. (Faustin was in pain, he allowed, but he complained as little as the other boy.) One way to assess age when children do not know how old they are is to ask, "Were you alive during X or Y or Z?" I learned this in Haiti, where children and adults alike remembered certain political events, such as who was president at the time. In Rwanda, the major defining moment is 1994. I was pretty sure that 1994, or the year before, was when the "grenade" was placed and that 1994 was also about when these boys were born. But during the first hour of attending to these injuries, no one discussed any of this. It was afterward, before the police arrived, that I started to ask whether this really was a grenade. Grenades do not explode when you step on them or touch them; as anyone who watches movies knows, you pull a pin and then it explodes a few seconds later. So another kind of explosive device had to be at issue.

Injured by one thing, an explosive device, Faustin, said to be an orphan, according to one of the Rwandan nurses, needed another thing: a piece of metal to keep his tibia and fibula in place so that the bones would heal in line. It just so happens that this device is readily available in most hospitals in the United States. Such hardware is hard to come by in Rwanda, but the device that would soon be placed in Faustin's leg was actually invented there. It is called a "Byumba fix," named after a town in the northern part of the country, where tens of thousands of landmines, none of them manufactured in Rwanda, were placed in 1993 and 1994. A Rwandan doctor trained in orthopedics in Belgium was finishing his thesis in 1994 when the genocide erupted. Against the advice of his professors, he decided to return to his country to care for the wounded, many of whom needed precisely the sort of services he had been trained to provide. When in 1994 Dr. Innocent Nyaruhirira, who would later become a leading figure in public health, tried to acquire the necessary orthopedic materials from Belgium, he found that the hardware was simply too expensive. So he and colleagues in Byumba decided to manufacture the much-needed external fixators on their own; one of them, a dozen years later, would end up in Faustin's left leg.

Once Faustin was en route to the operating room in Kigali, the capital city, I checked on the other child, Grégoire, who had been admitted to the pediatric ward. I finally had a chance to ask him, "What happened? What was it that you picked up?" "Well, we were herding cattle . . . ," he began, trailing off once again into silence. Herding cattle in the middle of the morning meant that these boys were not in school. I sketched Grégoire a grenade and a landmine on a piece of paper—we looked up these images on the Internet—and he pointed immediately to the latter: "This is what it looked like."

Grégoire did not have much to say about the incident during his brief hospitalization, and Faustin, even in the course of interviews conducted at home, did not wish to add much more. "What I'd most like to do," he said only a few days after surgery, "is to go to school." It turned out that he was not an orphan after all, but that his mother, poor and bereft after the genocide, had struggled for years with mental illness and had finally placed him with another family in 2004. "My mother is not well," he told me later. "She can't take care of me, so she brought me to a relative, and I live here now. I would like to go to school, but [my adoptive family] has no money. So I herd cows every day, make sure they eat, move them to new grass."

When I asked him about the landmine, he was, to my astonishment, apologetic: "I didn't mean to pick up the grenade. I'm sorry I did it. I didn't mean to kill the cows. I'm sorry. It was an accident. We didn't know what we were doing; it was not our intention to kill the cows." Even after I reassured him that it was not his fault and sought to focus on his recovery and return to school, he sounded the same note: "My leg hurts, but I can walk well. I am happy that I can go to school and that they are not angry about the cows. If we had known that it was a grenade, we would not have touched it or thrown it. We didn't mean to throw it at the cows. We didn't know it was a grenade."

RWANDA AND THE POLITICAL ECONOMY OF GENOCIDE

Dramatic enough in itself, the event—two boys pick up a landmine on a sunny day in March 2006—demands to be resocialized, linked up to a wider world and a longer period of the calendar. How to do this? We begin by noting that not a single one of these landmines was produced in Rwanda. The cause of the explosion that nearly killed Faustin is to be found in the transnational political economy of armaments, in which there are many willing participants, as Carolyn Nordstrom explains: "Should any quaint notions exist that mercenaries and human rights violators only get weapons from 'sources in non-democratic locations,' anyone who has walked in warzones, myself included, can easily attest to the wide range of supplies available from all the major sellers in the world. In one square kilometer of land in central Angola I visited with Halo Trust (the British de-mining NGO), they removed land mines manufactured in thirty-one countries."[15]

About 150,000 landmines were placed in Rwanda, mostly during 1993. Rwanda is a tiny country with a population, before the genocide, of perhaps 8.5 million people. Yet in 1993 it was the third largest importer of arms in all of Africa, coming in behind Egypt and South Africa (still under apartheid). On the Rwandan government's 1993 shopping list were 2,000 plastic MAT-79 antipersonnel mines, copies of an Italian model purchased in bulk. Experts from the United Nations have found thirty-nine types of mines in Rwanda, mostly plastic. Some, it's said, were designed to look like toys. Their provenance: Belgium, the United States, Czechoslovakia, Pakistan, China, and all over the former Soviet Union. It's also known that the *génocidaire* government mined the area around Akagera National Park, which is where we live and work—and where these boys were herding cattle instead of attending school.

Who funded this appetite for arms? Not the local peasant farmers, who would later be the hapless recipients of the shrapnel (as, twelve years earlier, some had been the people who had carried out much of the killing: between 14 and 17 percent of the adult male Hutu population participated in the genocide).[16] It was the government of Rwanda that shaped the postcolonial army. France, as the predominant power in the region, also supplied much of the "aid" to Rwanda and influenced other donor nations' priorities in foreign assistance. Peter Uvin has argued persuasively that the aid itself helped to set the stage for the genocide.[17]

The Rwandan genocide resulted in the deaths of up to a million people in a few months and later sparked a war in the Congo—a huge part of the tomorrow of the genocide. A lot of us remember the machetes; that's the classic impression for anyone who has seen the film *Hotel Rwanda* or read about the genocide in the popular press. But Rwanda's macabre 1993 ranking as the third-largest importer of arms in Africa was not earned by purchase of machetes alone: the government that ordered the genocide had procured surface-to-air missiles, rockets and other large armaments, automatic weapons—and, of course, landmines. The intimate detail of structural violence extends so far that, according to some, even the machetes were procured in part with structural adjustment loans.[18]

The blast that injured Faustin and Grégoire in 2006 was a long-delayed repercussion of the violence of 1994; that much is hardly controversial. Many know the story of the Hutu and Tutsi, and some understand that 1994 was not, despite quick-release journalistic analyses, either ethnic fratricide or tribal war. Rwanda does not have different tribes, and the categories of ethnicity and race are not really apt, either. The term "ethnicity," to say nothing of "race," did not arrive until long after whichever century saw the evolution of such categories. The ethnic categories are not exactly a "native" product, as historians of the colonial period in Rwanda have argued. Jean-Pierre Chrétien allows that the distinction between Hutu and Tutsi arose within a "civilization," but he and many others agree that it is hazardous to guess *when* certain groups may have "migrated" in.[19] We are speaking, rather, about centuries and waves of population movements, unrecorded and largely unknowable. Certainly, there is no evidence of genetic differences, and yet the idea of alien immigration was all too useful, later, to the Belgians and *génocidaires*. When the Batutsi are said to have migrated into what is now Rwanda, the region was already inhabited by people who called themselves Batwa and Bahutu (following convention, I've shortened these terms).

The dates are contested, but for centuries Tutsis and Hutus, both ethnically Banyarwanda, shared a common language, diet, and cultural heritage. Many scholars agree that the so-called tribal categorizations represented, in important ways, social distinctions between those who owned cattle and those who farmed the land—perhaps initially a division of labor between agriculturalists and pastoralists. Intermarriage was common, and a Hutu could become a Tutsi by owning cattle. This is well known—no longer the exclusive affair of specialists—but the myth of tribalism dies hard, probably because it is so convenient for people to attribute the causes of genocide to an alien mode of thought.

It was convenient for the Europeans, certainly. Unlike much of the rest of East Africa, Rwanda was never penetrated, to use the local word, by slave traders or others seeking bounty. Rwanda's integration into the time of empire is essentially a twentieth-century tale. It is increasingly the fashion, among some commentators both in Africa and beyond, to describe precolonial central Africa as existing in a golden era when the social groupings just described coexisted without conflict.[20] Historian Catharine Newbury, however, contends that significant social stratification began to take shape well before the arrival of the Europeans, which is not surprising: can one imagine an agrarian society without social stratification?[21]

Chrétien argues that, aside from a tiny Tutsi aristocracy, the original difference was largely one of professions, but that the Belgians promoted it into something much larger, and fatal.[22] What the colonials focused on when they arrived was the tiny Tutsi aristocracy, as Chrétien points out. The vast majority of Tutsis—like the Hutus, peasants who worked the land—were invisible to them. Most Tutsis were subject to the same taxes and forced labor as the other inhabitants of the colony. The Belgians imagined that Rwanda and Burundi were like European feudal states and then shaped these societies to resemble them. Chrétien is at pains to say that the Hamitic myth, the notion that Tutsis were alien overlords from the north, Europeans in black skin, essentially, is colonial fantasy. Europeans (first Germans and then Belgians) helped to rigidify these distinctions as part of their obsessions with race and eugenics.[23]

Colonial Rwanda, mountainous and lush, soon became a major producer of tropical commodities, especially coffee and tea. As in the neighboring Congo and in the region surrounding the hospital we have rebuilt, mines were dug; although these would not prove as important as agriculture, the basic thrust of Belgian colonization was, in keeping with tradition, extractive. Who was to do the extracting was a problem, and the Belgians followed, fairly religiously, the divide-and-conquer approach then *à la mode:* they used the Tutsi elite, a minority, to control the "peasant majority," the Hutus. (The Twa, the smallest group in all senses, mostly stayed out of the way.) The enforced *corvée* labor contributions of Hutus originated in precolonial times but, scholars report, were increased significantly—from one day of labor per week to up to three—once Belgian administration was established. But the Belgians seemed to grapple with a problem: who was Tutsi, who was Hutu? The notion that it was possible to answer this question with a glance was just that, a notion. And so the Belgian colonial regime did what colonial regimes often did: it issued ethnic identity cards. Soon, one's ethnic affiliation and social aspirations became a matter of public record and much more immutable.

Even during the colonial period, Rwanda was crowded, from the point of view of farmers and pastoralists; it is now one of the most crowded countries on the face of the earth. Jared Diamond made much of this demographic pressure in his book *Collapse,* describing struggle in a field of great scarcity.[24] But the 1994 genocide was in essence a political process, and planned to the very last detail. Most Rwandans I know start the countdown to genocide in 1959. The short version: as decolonization swept Africa, the Belgians switched allegiances and began favoring the Hutu majority. Decades of preferential treatment for the Tutsi elites had engendered deep resentment, again in a field of material scarcity and a lack of access to education and other social services. From the moment that it was clear that the Belgians would leave and that Rwanda, like the rest of Africa, would become nominally independent, struggle for control of the state apparatus, the cash cow, began. It was really this—the struggle for control of power and wealth—and not any other ideology (ideologies were a means to an end) that laid the foundation for what would come to pass three decades later. "Ethnic" convulsions—unknown before 1959—were registered regularly in the decades that followed.[25]

France replaced Belgium as the major neocolonial power in Rwanda and had, it would seem, no problem aligning itself with the Hutu military governments that increasingly controlled not only the state but most commerce. The recipe for staying in power was straight from the latter days of colonialism: whip up anti-Tutsi sentiment among the Hutu majority, and count on French support. Most Rwandans relied on radio communications for news and even orders, and this became an instrument for fomenting hatred and violence. Backed by Hutu-Power extremists, proponents of a virulent Hutu-supremacist philosophy used officially sanctioned radio stations to spew forth not only anti-Tutsi (and anti-moderate Hutu) songs but also more explicit directions to the militias, including the *interahamwe* gangs charged with carrying out the genocide, along with the military. These gangs were growing as fast as the ranks of disaffected youth of the country, who faced grim prospects as the Rwandan economy continued to decline.

Some analyses have suggested that externally imposed structural adjustment programs—advocated by the International Monetary Fund (IMF) and other development experts who had become increasingly prominent in Kigali—served to deepen social inequalities within Rwanda, dumping fuel on the fire of alienation and enmity. Economist Michel Chossudovsky notes that postindependence Rwanda, while still mired in poverty, demographic pressures, and environmental stresses, was in fact registering economic and social progress during the 1970s and 1980s.[26] The situation began to deteriorate in the 1980s, and the international financial institutions intervened, in particular to review Rwanda's public expenditure programs. Inflation and outstanding external debt skyrocketed following the devaluation of the Rwandan franc; state administrative apparatus and public services, including health and education, began to collapse. The incidence of severe child malnutrition increased dramatically, and the number of recorded cases of malaria increased by 21 percent in the year following the adoption of the IMF program.[27]

Chossudovsky concludes that the restructuring of Rwanda's agricultural system, as directed by the IMF and the World Bank, precipitated the population's decline into abject poverty and destitution: "This deterioration of the economic environment, which immediately followed the collapse of the international coffee market and the imposition of sweeping macro-economic reforms by the Bretton Woods institutions, exacerbated simmering ethnic tensions and accelerated the process of political collapse."[28] Johan Pottier makes a similar point: "The coffee crash of 1989 created massive despair among poor farmers . . . the World Bank/ International Monetary Fund failed to bail Rwanda out (whereas Mexico and South Korea fared much better when their economies crashed)."[29]

The aid experts in Rwanda, by and large, turned a blind eye to the growing chorus of hate songs, the radio propaganda, and the burgeoning ranks of the *interahamwe* gangs. They were there to do development, as one insightful report from their ranks later confessed.[30] The aid experts may have failed to see the looming catastrophe, but others, including many of those exiled in and after 1959, saw it coming. A group of exiled Rwandans, including current president Paul Kagame, launched a rebel movement, the Rwandese Patriotic Front, from Uganda. Still a tiny force, they struck from the north in 1991. It was the position of the RPF that "genocide ideology" was of recent origin and that once-insignificant differences had been fanned into importance during the preceding century—the century of colonial rule. The French had taken up right where the Belgians left off, providing military training and matériel to the government. In spite of French military support for the government, the rebels gained ground and, as pogroms against Tutsis continued, they also gained new recruits.

In early August 1993, a year-long process of hammering out a regional peace plan was completed with the signing of the Arusha Accords in Arusha, Tanzania. Eight months later, while en route from Tanzania to Kigali, the French jet of the Rwandan dictator Juvénal Habyarimana was brought down by a missile launched from within the military base near the airport.

The spark that lit the fuse was the downing of that plane in April 1994. The Rwandan government immediately blamed the assassination of Habyarimana on the RPF, an accusation echoed in the French press. More independent observers, however, and much public speculation laid the blame on Hutu extremists—many of them members of the dictator's own entourage—who ardently opposed the Arusha Accords. Within an hour of the plane's destruction, the *interahamwe*, as if waiting for this very signal, swung into action. They clearly had a plan, but confusion reigned among others in Kigali.

This was especially true among representatives of the countries implicated in the crisis or those living in Rwanda. The U.S. government dithered (to learn how much, read the damning assessment by General Roméo Dallaire, the commander of the United Nations force stationed in Rwanda),[31] although the U.S. ambassador did suggest that ethnic identity cards be suppressed—a suggestion rebuffed by the French, who held the greatest sway there. The French government, furthermore, continued to back the Hutu interim government to the dreadful end, even though some of the troops later dispatched in Opération Turquoise—billed to the soldiers as a humanitarian intervention—would voice great bitterness upon discovering that things were not as promised by Paris. "'We have been deceived,' Sergeant Major Thierry Prungnaud told a reporter at a collection site for emaciated and machete-scarred Tutsi survivors in early July of 1994. 'This is not what we were led to believe. We were told that Tutsis were killing Hutus. We thought the Hutus were the good guys and the victims.'"[32] The UN peacekeeping force, led by Dallaire, played an especially painful role: that of impotent spectator to mass slaughter of civilians.[33]

The genocide was halted when the RPF, growing every day and including more and more Hutus who did not wish to follow orders to kill their neighbors, swept across Rwanda in the summer of 1994. It might be argued that the entire sordid mess was over, but the French had one more card to play: Opération Turquoise became an operation to protect the *génocidaire* government as it fled Rwanda to refugee camps in Goma, Zaïre. From across Lake Kivu, an almost intact *génocidaire* government clearly intended to attack again and again, until their genocidal project was complete. Scores of nongovernmental organizations (NGOs) had materialized to take care of the refugees, most of them probably Hutus chivvied along with threats and dire warnings; many had not in fact taken part in the killings. The new administration in Kigali, receiving precious little in the way of any international support, threatened to take out the camps if they could not be controlled by the UN and the NGOs.[34] Then cholera broke out in the camps, and all attention was turned to Goma, and away from Rwanda.

Even though Hutu-generated attacks did come from these camps, the UN claimed that it was powerless to stop them. The genocide ended in 1994, but the violence did not, for the genocide's architects were allowed to flee west (some VIP génocidaires made it to France, the United States, and several African nations; warrants for their arrest from the International Criminal Court still exist).

A million or so civilians were in a sense held hostage in the camps by the interahamwe and a government in exile. Cross-border attacks continued. In 1996, the Rwandan transitional government did just what it had threatened to do and broke up the camps, encouraging those not involved as architects of the genocide to return. It will take a long time for this story to come out, and it is clear that many innocents died in the breaking up of the camps, but primary sources are already publishing damning accounts. Fiona Terry of Médecins Sans Frontières, a group that was working in the Goma camps, made no bones about it: the génocidaires, not the humanitarians, ran the camps. As an appendix to her book, Terry included materials from the detritus found in the camps.[35] She published facsimiles of bills and receipts for large arms orders addressed to the Minister of Defense, Republic of Rwanda, Bukavu, Zaïre (another site of Hutu-controlled refugee camps). The new government in Kigali was proven right: the camps were being used as military bases from which to attack Rwanda with sophisticated armaments purchased from Russian, European, and U.S. arms merchants. The social life of things can be revealed, it transpires, by airway bills and receipts.

In other words, if Rwandans of the 1990s were struggling with manufactured categories, they were also struggling with manufactured things: armaments, for example, things with a highly active social life. They get around. Italy, the United States, and Russia were the major producers of the antipersonnel and landmine instruments used in Rwanda,[36] while France, Egypt, and apartheid South Africa were the Rwandan government's primary suppliers.[37] In short, a violent event in rural Rwanda in March 2006 reveals links to at least a dozen other countries far from central Africa, links that reach far back in time. This is a lesson that anthropology cannot forget, as Eric Wolf reminded us years ago.[38]

WHAT IS TO BE DONE ABOUT "STUPID DEATHS"?

They say your whole life flashes before you when you are about to die, but I'm pretty sure that is not true. When I think of all the dying people I've attended— many of them, happily, stopped dying—I can think of none who have described to me a flashing montage of key events in their lives. Some, like the two boys discussed in this chapter, said very little, at least to me. Of course, many of the dying cannot speak at all; some are mercifully obtunded. But some do talk and even *sing,* often through great pain. In country after country, I've seen dying people, young and old, who call for their mothers, who worry about unkept promises and loose ends, who are frightened, even if resigned (though most are not resigned to death itself, in my experience).

When I was a young man, between college and medical school, I had the great good fortune to go to Haiti. A country, rather than a person or a book, became my teacher. Back then, just about everything seemed instructive: interviews, surveys, books, reports, songs, everyday speech, customs, and certainly history, the most important resocializing discipline. But for someone on my trajectory, a physician-anthropologist in training, it may have been inevitable that I would find the most incisive those lessons learned the hard way, by witnessing other people's pain and learning about how they made sense of suffering. The Haitians with whom I lived were world experts on the topic. Everyone had a story, and almost no one, it seemed, was reluctant to share it.

I learned a lot about death, and in particular about a special type that the Haitians termed, simply enough, "stupid deaths." By this, they did not mean deaths by gunshot (there were plenty of these) or in road accidents (as vehicles crammed full went teetering down mountain "roads" with no guardrails). A drowning death in the nearby reservoir was not emblematic of a stupid death, nor was going down in one of the overstuffed wooden boats leaving Haiti for Florida. Rather, these were tragedies and seen by all around me as unfair.

What, then, were examples of stupid deaths in the eyes of those living in central Haiti? Dying in childbirth because obstetric care costs too much was dying a stupid death; worldwide, there are five hundred thousand of these each year. Dying of malaria was stupid, as were deaths from tetanus, rabies, pneumonia. Death from a road accident because of poor medical attention later: stupid. Being hauled out of the nearby reservoir by your kin, only to die two weeks later of pneumonia in a filthy hospital room: stupid.

Fascinated, horrified, with this typology, I developed my own nosology of stupid death and included many others that I knew, from my training in an American medical school, to be tragic and unnecessary: malignancies that could have been cured with timely diagnosis; third-trimester obstetric catastrophes; vaccine-preventable illnesses; and a host of afflictions that our patients would have survived had they been born in a country such as the one in which I was born. Almost all of these deaths occur among the poor.

But the stupidest of all, I thought, was the industrial-strength murder that could come only from bombs, firearms, landmines, and other "modern" ordnance of war, with the casualties occurring disproportionately among civilians, in particular children like Faustin. So, what is to be done to change this state of affairs, in Haiti, in Rwanda, in many other places of today's world?

It is possible to discuss "distal" and "proximal" responses to the sort of violence endured by Faustin and Grégoire. These terms are contested, in part because in anthropology (and in epidemiology and other fields) we use these words in a fashion quite contrary to the way they are used in anatomy and medicine. If you think about an artery, the large end of the vessel is termed "proximal"; the small end, the capillaries, is called "distal." Some colleagues and I recently wrote an essay titled "Structural Violence and Clinical Medicine" and spoke about distal and proximal problems and responses to a number of pressing health issues, from asthma in American cities to AIDS in Africa.[39] Perhaps in part because the meanings of the words are reversed in different fields of inquiry, Nancy Krieger has recently suggested that these terms be banned from discussions of causality.[40]

But in the case of Faustin, our distal responses meant debriding the wounds and splinting the fractures; Faustin now walks with the slightest limp. And moving backward, or proximally, our response means getting children in school—Faustin is now regularly attending classes. It means providing basic health care, as we seek to do in rural Rwanda. It means demining all of Rwanda, a process nearly complete, in spite of the misfortune of these boys.[41] Finally, it requires approaches to the big questions, such as how we might prevent people from planting landmines in the first place.

In closing, then, what is to be done? As a doctor, I have to admit that it is not so easy to place an external fixator. A surgeon in the capital city did this for Faustin. But with the right medical equipment, which in this case included orthopedic hardware, it is possible to do a good job in this very distal effort. And that is really what Rwandans ask of us in the event of trauma. They are unlikely to say, "Please, do the ethnography or political economy of brutality; come and study the political economy of landmines." They quite reasonably want action in the present, addressing immediate needs such as food, clean water, shelter, schooling, decent employment, and accessible health care. Retracing the causal links, we are faced with the situation that created Faustin's injury: a countryside once littered with landmines. For that, the remedy is demining. I thought it must be some sophisticated procedure, but the process is rather crude: you sandbag the area around the landmines and then detonate them. These children were demining, in their own way and without the sandbags. Innocently, they mistook a landmine for a toy or a trinket.

Gino Strada, a trauma surgeon from Italy, has written eloquently about landmines after caring for hundreds of people injured by them. Most were civilians; many were children. His book is called *Green Parrots*, the nickname for what may well be the very landmine that Faustin picked up. Made of plastic, they're in fact designed to look like toys. Let me cite Strada's conclusion:

We had thought that war was an old, primitive instrument, a cancer that mankind did not know how to eradicate; on this point we were mistaken. Tragically, we—and not only we—had failed to see that war, rather than being a burdensome inheritance from the past, was becoming a fearful prospect for our future and for generations to come. In the operating theatre we saw the devastation produced in human bodies by bombs and mines, by projectiles and rockets. Yet we did not succeed in grasping the effects of other weapons, "unconventional" ones: finance and international loans, trade agreements, the "structural adjustments" imposed on the policies of many poor countries, the new arms races in richer countries.[42]

For a trauma surgeon, this is going surprisingly far up the causal river from the injured person. But his thought-journey toward the source of the problem is inspired by his experience of the problem's effects. It is startling and welcome to hear a surgeon speak in such terms, because Afghanistan, Iraq, Haiti, Rwanda, and other places riven by violence demand such thinking. There is always going to be distal work, the work of patching up children and anyone else who happens to be injured in this manner. Clinicians should be proud to do this work. But we also need to move closer to the roots of the problem for the sake of prevention, and this will be done only by examining the political economy of brutality. The global health community, which includes physicians, certainly has a very pragmatic role to play in this process.[43] However, anthropology and other resocializing disciplines are uniquely poised to reveal the complexity of these problems and to lay out the challenges faced by all those who seek to lessen the violence that maims and kills so many.

Of course, the threat of renewed violence must be there somewhere, even if it is not easy to see on the spotless streets of Kigali or in the hills and valleys in which we work. None of us knows what lies beneath the impassive faces of our hosts, unless they choose to tell us; no one can be sure if reconciliation is possible here. But the entire process—from demining to offering alternatives to prison for *génocidaires* willing to atone publicly, as well as the collective refusal to sweep the events of 1994 under the carpet but rather to put memories on full display—seems more hopeful than in the other strife-torn places in which I have served. The social life of ordnance continues, but each year such reminders grow less frequent in Rwanda. Certainly there are days when we wonder if stability is going to last. There are countless reminders of war and genocide: there are landmines, and there are the museums and memorial sites—even the small towns in which we work have them, and they are usually located over mass graves. A huge building perched on the top of one of Kigali's hills is still pocked with mortar rounds fired in 1994. But this year, as cranes and metal scaffolding surround the building, the message, if that's what it is, seems clear enough:

Rwandans are moving forward, even if they know, as we do, that some wounds never heal completely.

The government of Rwanda and its citizenry have done much to lessen the tomorrow of violence within that country's boundaries. To study the "social life of things" is to examine the ways in which commodities of one sort or another take on meaning through social transactions and through their "concrete, historical circulation," as Appadurai noted two decades ago.[44] Thus are things, even instruments of death, "enlivened." But much more can be said, using other frameworks.

Rwanda will emerge from mass violence by seeking to ensure that social inequalities—in the recent past, Hutu versus Tutsi, and in the present *and* past, the poor versus the nonpoor—are lessened, re-creating a social field in which such distinctions are muted by improving access to the very services that Faustin mentioned repeatedly in his brief commentaries on his own experience. He spoke of school, cows, and medical care. These are things, too—but should they remain commodities only? Should access to school, health care (including, in Faustin's case, orthopedic surgery), and a livelihood be considered mere commodities, to be bought and sold? Or does the framework of basic rights have something to add as postgenocidal Rwanda seeks to lessen the tomorrow of violence?

Elsewhere, I have argued that the framework of social and economic rights— the right to health care, education, and freedom from want—will help us to imagine a future in which poverty alone does not determine who has access to such services.[45] That Faustin was not maimed permanently by poverty and misfortune, not to be confused with accident or happenstance, is the result of his access to modern medical care. By rebuilding a hospital abandoned since the genocide, we were able to take care of him a dozen years after the cessation of "event violence." By insisting that education be a right, rather than a commodity, we were able to alter his trajectory and allow him to participate in a future in which he, a Rwandan citizen, is guaranteed certain rights.

The precise formula by which any of us may participate in a tomorrow with less violence is, granted, uncertain. But asking if basic services might be reimagined as rights rather than commodities is precisely the question we must raise if we seek formulas that will end, or at least lessen, the status quo in which some people are shielded from risk while others, like Faustin, are assured a future in which violence plays a major and determinant role. Stopping "stupid deaths" may play a larger role in lessening the tomorrow of violence than we, shielded from such insults, imagine.

NOTES

1. See Taylor, "King Sacrifice, President Habyarimana, and the Iconography of Pregenocidal Rwandan Political Literature."

2. Farmer, *Pathologies of Power;* Farmer, "An Anthropology of Structural Violence" (included in this volume as chapter 17).

3. Nordstrom, "The Tomorrow of Violence," p. 224.

4. See, for example, Das, *Violence and Subjectivity;* Scheper-Hughes and Bourgois, *Violence in War and Peace;* Whitehead, *Violence;* Das, *Life and Words.*

5. Asad, *Anthropology and the Colonial Encounter;* Starn, "Missing the Revolution."

6. See Bourgois, "Missing the Holocaust"; Farmer, "The Banality of Agency"; Rylko-Bauer, "Lessons about Humanity and Survival from My Mother and from the Holocaust"; Waterston and Rylko-Bauer, "Out of the Shadows of History and Memory."

7. For one moving account from Rwanda, see Mushikiwabo and Kramer, *Rwanda Means the Universe.*

8. Hatzfeld, *Machete Season;* Hatzfeld, *Life Laid Bare.*

9. Appadurai, *The Social Life of Things.*

10. Farmer, "La violence structurelle et la matérialité du social."

11. International Campaign to Ban Landmines, "Rwanda" (1999, 2007).

12. International Campaign to Ban Landmines, *Landmine Monitor Report 1999* and *Landmine Monitor Report 2007.*

13. Human Rights Watch/The Arms Project and Physicians for Human Rights, *Landmines;* Human Rights Watch, "Exposing the Source."

14. Landmine Action, *Explosive Remnants of War;* UNICEF, "Saving Children from the Tragedy of Landmines."

15. Nordstrom, *Shadows of War,* p. 95.

16. Straus, *The Order of Genocide.*

17. Uvin, *Aiding Violence.*

18. Chossudovsky, *The Globalization of Poverty and the New World Order.*

19. Chrétien, *The Great Lakes of Africa.*

20. Pottier, *Re-Imagining Rwanda.*

21. Newbury, *The Cohesion of Oppression.*

22. Chrétien, *The Great Lakes of Africa.*

23. Mamdani, *When Victims Become Killers.*

24. Diamond, *Collapse.*

25. Gourevitch, *We Wish to Inform You That Tomorrow We Will Be Killed with Our Families.*

26. Chossudovsky, *The Globalization of Poverty and the New World Order.*

27. Gervais, "Étude de la pratique des ajustements au Niger et au Rwanda."

28. Chossudovsky, *The Globalization of Poverty and the New World Order,* p. 103.

29. Pottier, *Re-Imagining Rwanda,* p. 2.

30. Uvin, *Aiding Violence.*

31. Dallaire and Beardsley, *Shake Hands with the Devil.*

32. Cited in Gourevitch, *We Wish to Inform You That Tomorrow We Will Be Killed with Our Families,* p. 160.

33. Dallaire and Beardsley, *Shake Hands with the Devil.*

34. Terry, *Condemned to Repeat?*

35. Ibid.

36. International Campaign to Ban Landmines, "Rwanda" (1999, 2007).

37. Goose and Smyth, "Arming Genocide in Rwanda—The High Cost of Small Arms Transfers."

38. Wolf, *Europe and the People without History.*

39. Farmer, Nizeye, et al., "Structural Violence and Clinical Medicine" (included in this volume as chapter 18).

40. Krieger, "Proximal, Distal, and the Politics of Causation."

41. Integrated Regional Information Network, "Rwanda."

42. Strada, *Green Parrots,* p. 132.

43. Zwi, "How Should the Health Community Respond to Violent Political Conflict?"

44. Appadurai, *The Social Life of Things,* p. 5.

45. Farmer, Nizeye, et al., "Structural Violence and Clinical Medicine" (included in this volume as chapter 18).

Human Rights and
a Critique of Medical Ethics

Introduction to Part 4

Paul Farmer

The bloody massacre in Bangladesh quickly covered the memory of the Russian invasion of Czechoslovakia, the assassination of Allende drowned out the groans of Bangladesh, the war in the Sinai desert made people forget Allende, the Cambodian massacre made people forget Sinai, and so on and so forth until ultimately everyone lets everything be forgotten.

MILAN KUNDERA, *THE BOOK OF LAUGHTER AND FORGETTING*

The fourth part of this book offers critical reflections on human rights regimes and on narrowly defined bioethics. To say "regimes" (or even "narrowly defined") is to invoke, again, a sociology-of-knowledge perspective like that of Peter Berger and Thomas Luckmann (quoted at the opening of chapter 11).[1] For years, I failed to apply this perspective to human rights and medical ethics. To be frank, I simply assumed such topics to be above reproach. As a student and as a young physician, I spent many years unaware that there were competing rights agendas. Human rights struck me as a generally decent thing to push for, but the Haitians with whom I lived and worked taught me that, yet again, such concepts could be distorted in predictable ways. My friends and patients in village Haiti were not slow to condemn certain human rights groups as "fronts" for antidemocratic agendas—and, sure enough, events proved them right. I spent a lot of time cultivating contacts inside rights organizations I trusted and trying to untangle a confused, and highly political, swirl of extravagant claims, many of them, as in the case of epidemics, completely discrepant.

Along the way, I learned in Haiti that the right to vote, the right to a fair and speedy trial, and other political rights were only part of the picture. What about the right to education, health care, and freedom from want? my neighbors and coworkers asked. So I began, a decade ago, to seek to reflect these views in writing about human rights. Some of my early work in this vein is published here.

For a while, it seemed like a lonely agenda to push, at least in bibliographical terms. Much later, I discovered an essay by Chidi Anselm Odinkalu, who wrote that although "in Africa, the realization of human rights is a very serious business indeed," many Africans "feel that their realities and aspirations are not adequately captured by human rights organizations and their language."[2]

In these essays, and in my book *Pathologies of Power*, I've sought to avoid pitting civil and political rights against social and economic rights. (Such a competitive exercise reminds me of the ill-considered practice of pitting prevention against care, too commonly encountered among public health experts.) I've sought instead to underline the importance—especially to the poor—of social and economic rights and also to acknowledge that, while those of us working through nongovernmental organizations can offer pragmatic solidarity to the poor, we cannot confer rights: only governments can do that. This reality was driven home in Haiti, where thousands of NGOs and missionary groups inadvertently undermine the public sector by allowing (and sometimes cheering for) the privatization of health, education, and even water.

A couple of these chapters examine the desocialization of medical ethics—a discipline that seems fated to be desocialized the more it aspires to shape itself into a calculus or set of rules. In expressing my doubts about medical ethics, I am relieved to be in good company. Jonathan Glover, observing rather drily that ethics "could be more empirical than it is," opens a daunting interrogation of ethics by the twentieth century's history, in turn letting that history be interrogated by ethics. "The aim of using ethics to interrogate history is to help understand a side of human nature often left in darkness. It will also be argued that, in understanding the history, philosophical questions about ethics cannot be ignored. Poor answers to these questions have contributed to a climate in which some of the disasters were made possible."[3] Glover, a bioethicist, takes a huge step back from the arcane issues usually treated by bioethicists (organ transplantation, brain death, and so on) and offers a sweeping critique of ethics and philosophy.

This historical critique is valuable, but it still leaves us with the mundane problems of medical ethics, which include, in my view, the near invisibility of the poor in this field. Take the example of our introduction of cancer care into rural Rwanda. One of our pediatricians, after giving a talk in a Harvard teaching hospital about our work, was upbraided about "ethical concerns regarding the delivery of cancer care by people not trained in oncology." This critique, I might point out, was addressed to one of the two practicing pediatricians in rural Rwanda; although there is plenty of cancer in such regions, there are no oncologists.

As further examples of the perversion of medical ethics, of its blindness, consider these incidents from the past few months. I was recently at a conference on multidrug-resistant tuberculosis, which belatedly acknowledged the occurrence of up to five hundred thousand incident cases annually. Since so very few of those newly announced cases from previous years were ever treated properly, imagine how many prevalent cases remain in the world today, with most of these individuals still breathing and still suffering and still infecting others. When speaking of the lack of treatment for children with this disease, some mentioned "ethical concerns" about using some of the drugs not yet approved for children by the Food and Drug Administration or similar regulatory bodies. (One of the key classes of drugs, we heard, seemed to cause cartilage damage in beagle puppies; it might then retard proper development in human children.) These essentially litigious concerns were miscategorized as ethical ones, since of course the primary ethical challenge is millions of people not receiving treatment for a deadly (and airborne) disease rather than the hypothetical challenge of using old drugs in new ways.

AIDS, a "new disease," offers in so many instances the best example of the failure and promise of ethics—failure because, as described throughout this book, so many experts were willing to declare the disease "untreatable" in settings of poverty; promise because so many others (led by AIDS activists and people living with AIDS and followed, however timidly, by their caregivers) rejected this surrender by proxy. There are many ways to move from premature surrender to mounting a defense against premature deaths. I recently wrote a foreword to a book about an excellent AIDS program in an East African city in which the book's protagonist, an American physician, observes that "it is easy to sit in a conference room and say it is not wise to provide treatment here."[4] He meant this as a critique of those who argued that it was not feasible or cost-effective to treat AIDS in Africa. But think about this physician's assertion and ask the unposed question: why on earth would it be *easy* to sit in a conference room, anywhere in the world, and argue that it is "not wise" to provide treatment for the leading infectious killer of young people? As both an anthropologist and a physician, one is supposed to listen carefully to one's interlocutors, and I assure you that it was never easy for me to sit in a conference room or anywhere and argue against treatment for AIDS or any other illness on the grounds that patients are too poor. Similar sentiments—empathy? sympathy? pity? outrage?—led to the required change in the program described in the book: the turning point for this American medical professor, we learn, was seeing one of his own students dying from AIDS and tuberculosis.

Though empathy served to reveal the untenable nature of such double standards, it's important to understand that the work described in that book and this one is not built only on the foundation of empathy. It is built on other sentiments, too: solidarity (perhaps the noblest of human sentiments); commitment; pity and mercy (sentiments not to be scorned in this age); curiosity about problems new and old; the desire to be effective as a clinician and teacher (or student); and even love (of learning, of using the tools that science gives us, of others).

The longest chapter in this book, "Never Again? Reflections on Human Values and Human Rights" (chapter 23), was part of the series of Tanner Lectures on Human Values. It is published in full here, as it seeks to tie together a number of themes central to all the work included in this volume. Starting with the aim of casting light on ways of generating empathy (and less volatile sentiments and programs) for those suffering far away and moving on to the relationship between different forms of violence and then to the salutary aspects of humble service to the poor, this chapter is guided by the words of Emmanuel Levinas on the foundational significance of ethical comportment, what he called "the establishing of [the] primacy of the ethical, that is, of the relationship of man to man—signification, teaching, and justice—a primacy of an irreducible structure upon which all the other structures rest."[5]

A moment ago I described empathy as an emotion, a volatile reaction, and implied that such emotions are different in kind from programs, institutions, and vocations. That would scant the intensity of emotions and their motivating power. I might add that one thing that scarcely appears in this book is the deep emotion that accompanies the work of solidarity. On any given day, one can plumb the depths and peaks of emotion simply by working in a maternity ward in rural Africa (if it is not properly stocked and staffed, get ready for the depths). When I was a child, I lived not far from towns such as Selma, where the police set dogs on peaceful protestors. Going to a museum in Soweto with one's children reawakens the moral shock (my oldest daughter, then eight, asked me: "Now tell me, step by step, how apartheid could happen?"). I now sometimes walk through the last section of the genocide memorial in Kigali, where one looks at simple, life-size photographs of happy kids only to learn, by gazing at the bottom of the posters, not only what their favorite hobbies were but how they died—by murder, all of them.

Reconciliation has earned a bad name among many in Haiti, since it was a code word for impunity. The Haitians taught me that only the aggrieved may offer forgiveness. Jean Hatzfeld has just written his third book based on interviews with Rwanda genocide survivors and perpetrators, which considers the official efforts to hasten this process along. Here's my chance to say that, as a physician working in Rwanda (and working, even, in the prisons), I have gratitude and admiration for these official efforts. But I understand that my own views are hardly the most important ones, and so I am grateful for Hatzfeld's yeoman's efforts to bring the key (often discrepant) views into focus. He cites one man, a formally pardoned génocidaire whom he knows well, who opines that "reconciliation is a very beneficial political policy." Survivors have a different view. "Yes," remarks one, "we're enduring this cohabitation, we're striving to rise above ourselves so as not to load another burden on a head that is already bowed down.

Reconciliation? I can't give you a precise definition of that word. Cohabitation is one form of reconciliation, though. Still, trust is unthinkable in the future."[6]

It's not honest, I've argued throughout all these chapters, to erase history and political economy; it's not wise, even if it's expedient. To underscore this point, Hatzfeld cites a poet, writing of her experience in Auschwitz and Ravensbrück:

> *Leaving history behind*
> *To enter life*
> *Try it you lot and you'll see.*[7]

There come times when writing and social theory fail us all. I've lived through moments like these, and some of them are noted, if obliquely, in this book. There are the patients who die "stupid deaths," to use the Haitian expression; there is the violence one sees coming from miles away and is powerless to stop; there is the misunderstanding of one's peers who have bought into the brightly packaged myths and mystifications, however briefly. During these bad times—and times are always bad for people somewhere—there is solace to be found in returning to first principles and simply remaining at one's post as a servant attending to the needs of the sick and the poor. This is what the theologian Jennie Block calls "the ministry of showing up." Sometimes, I have argued in more than one of these chapters, the links between such humble service and more ambitious efforts to lessen structural violence come back into view. Decades ago, sociologist Robert Merton wrote about the unintended consequences of purposive social action: "with the complex interaction which constitutes society, action ramifies, its consequences are not restricted to the specific area in which they were initially intended to center, they occur in interrelated fields explicitly ignored at the time of action. Yet it is because these fields are in fact interrelated that the further consequences in adjacent areas tend to react upon the fundamental value-system."[8] The intended consequence of tending to the sick, or visiting prisoners, or clothing the naked, or burying the dead (to name a few of the corporal works of mercy) is to help the person at hand or, in the case of burying the dead, to demonstrate a belief not only in mercy but in human dignity. The unintended ramifications of such efforts, when they are ambitious enough, may be significant, reaching far beyond our immediate understanding.

Engaged in such corporal works as tending to the sick or preventing illness or assuaging suffering, why write books like this one? Orwell speaks for me: "My starting point is always a feeling of partisanship, a sense of injustice." My first editor, Stan Holwitz of University of California Press, encouraged me to incorporate some of the indignation that any physician feels when people die of readily treatable afflictions; Naomi Schneider (my editor with the same press) has encouraged the same candor; and Haun Saussy has been with me throughout these long decades of work and reflection. What place is there, in scholarship, for passion? Is it truly "neutral" to remain dispassionate before unnecessary suffering? Is it always advisable to make a show of neutrality? What if one is hoping, as a writer, to "push the world in a different direction," as Orwell put it?[9]

The best medical journals routinely (and often correctly, in my view) strip affect from even the discussion sections of papers chosen for publication. But I could not contemplate the terrible things I witnessed, in Haiti and later elsewhere, and strip affect from the less technical part of my writing. I don't know that I'm more emotional, in the face of needless misery, than anyone else, or that exceptional bravery and sacrifice move me to tears more than they move others. I don't know if reading about the struggles of those who made difficult, even impossible choices—the leaders of doomed popular movements in Latin America (such as Oscar Romero), or Dietrich Bonhoeffer, or the nameless (to me) monks in Burma—is a more powerful experience for me than for other readers. I don't think so; and while emotion may, in this age of spectacle and virtuality, lead nowhere, I am hoping it will strike a spark of activism in some, maybe many, readers of this book.

NOTES

1. Berger and Luckmann, *The Social Construction of Reality.*
2. Odinkalu, "Why More Africans Don't Use Human Rights Language."
3. Glover, *Humanity,* pp. 5, 4.
4. Quigley, *Walking Together, Walking Far,* p. 3.
5. Levinas, *Totality and Infinity,* p. 79.
6. Hatzfeld, *The Antelope's Strategy,* pp. 206, 207.
7. The poet is Charlotte Delbo, cited in ibid., pp. 206–7.
8. Merton, "The Unanticipated Consequences of Purposive Social Action," p. 903.
9. Orwell, "Why I Write," in Orwell, *The Collected Essays, Journalism, and Letters of George Orwell,* vol. 4, p. 2. I've also discussed Orwell's influence in the introduction to part 1 of this volume.

21

Rethinking Health
and Human Rights

Time for a Paradigm Shift

(1999, 2003)

As the global market economy pulverized traditional societies and moralities and drew every corner of the planet into a single economic machine, human rights emerged as the secular creed that the new global middle class needed in order to justify their domination of the new cosmopolitan order.

KENNETH ANDERSON, FORMERLY OF HUMAN RIGHTS WATCH

From the perspective of a preferential option for the poor, the right to health care, housing, decent work, protection against hunger, and other economic, social, and cultural necessities are as important as civil and political rights and more so.

LEIGH BINFORD, *THE EL MOZOTE MASSACRE*

Medicine and its allied health sciences have for too long been only peripherally involved in work on human rights. Fifty years ago, the door to greater involvement was opened by Article 25 of the Universal Declaration of Human Rights, which underlined social and economic rights: "Everyone has the right to a standard of living adequate for the health and well-being of himself and of his family, including food, clothing, housing, and medical care and necessary social services, and the right to security in the event of unemployment, sickness, disability, widowhood, old age or other lack of livelihood in circumstances beyond his control."[1]

But the intervening decades have seen little progress in the efforts to secure social and economic rights, even though we can point with some pride to gains in civil or political rights. These distinctions are crucial, as a visit to a Russian prison makes clear.

In the cramped, crammed detention centers where hundreds of thousands of Russian detainees await due process, many fall ill with tuberculosis. Convicted prisoners who are diagnosed with tuberculosis are sent to one of more than fifty "TB colonies." I bring up these colonies in order to illustrate the difference between civil rights and social and economic rights. Imagine a Siberian prison in which the cells are as cramped as cattle cars, the fetid air thick with tubercle bacilli. Imagine a cell in which most of the prisoners are coughing and all are said to have active tuberculosis. Let the mean age of the inmates be less than thirty years. Finally, imagine that many of these young men are receiving ineffective treatment for their disease—which, given drug toxicity, is worse than receiving a placebo—even though they are the beneficiaries of directly observed therapy with first-line antituberculous agents, delivered (however ambivalently) by European humanitarian organizations and their Russian colleagues.

If this seems hard to imagine, it shouldn't be; I have seen this situation in several prisons. At this writing, most of these prisoners are still receiving directly observed doses of medications that cannot cure them. For many of these prisoners, the therapy is ineffective because the strains of tuberculosis that are epidemic within the prisons are resistant to the drugs being administered. Various observers, including some from international human rights organizations, aver that these prisoners have "untreatable forms" of tuberculosis, and few challenge this claim, even though treatment based on the standard of care used elsewhere in Europe and North America can in fact cure the great majority of such cases.[2] "Untreatable," in these debates, really means "expensive to treat." For this and other reasons, tuberculosis has again become the leading cause of death among Russian prisoners, even among those receiving treatment. One can find similar situations throughout the former Soviet Union.

Are human rights violated in this dismal scenario? Conventional views of human rights would lead one to focus on a single violation: prolonged pre-trial detention. Individuals who are arrested are routinely detained for up to a year before making a court appearance. In many documented cases, young detainees have died of prison-acquired tuberculosis before their cases ever went to trial. Such detention clearly violates not only Russian law but also several human rights charters to which the country is signatory. Russian and international human rights activists have focused on this problem, demanding that all detainees be rapidly brought to trial. But an impasse is quickly reached when the underfunded Russian courts wearily respond that they are working as fast as they can. The Ministry of Justice agrees with the human rights activists and is interested in amnesty for prisoners and alternatives to imprisonment. These measures may prove helpful, but they will not save those who are already sick.

What of other, complementary approaches, those invoking the rights of prisoners? Has agitation for shorter pre-trial detention, in the form of letters and other protests, proven adequate to solve the problem of prison tuberculosis? If laws were not being violated, but prisoners or former convicts continued to die of tuberculosis, would this suggest that the law is sufficient to protect the health of the vulnerable? I suggest that the answer to both these questions is no. In fact, from the perspective of the poor—and most of these prisoners are poor—neither legal nor conventional human rights approaches have even begun to understand the nature of the problem.

Let us reconsider tuberculosis in Russian prisons as a question of social and economic rights. Such an exercise yields a far longer list of violations—but also a longer list of possible interventions. First, pre-trial detention is illegally prolonged and conditions are deplorable. The directors of the former gulag do not dispute this point. The head of the federal penitentiary system, speaking to Amnesty International, described the prisoners as living in "conditions amounting to torture."[3] Some of the more astute prison administrators remind their critics that the dismantling of the Soviet economy has led to a sharp rise in petty crime—"People now have to steal for food," in the words of one official[4]—which has swamped the prison system even as "economic restructuring," planned with the help of Western economic advisors, has gutted budgets for prison health care.[5]

Second, detainees are subjected to conditions that guarantee increased exposure to drug-resistant strains of *M. tuberculosis*. In other words, excess tuberculosis risks within prisons and jails should be seen as a violation of rights, a violation further compounded by a lack of commitment on the part of many—including some in the humanitarian assistance community—to providing truly effective treatment.

Third, the prisoners are denied not only adequate food but also medical care. Again, where does the blame lie? Interview medical staff in these prisons, and you will find them distraught about the funding cuts that have followed the restructuring and collapse of the Russian economy. In the words of one physician: "I have spent my entire medical career caring for prisoners with tuberculosis. And although we complained about shortages in the eighties, we had no idea how good we had it then. Now it's a daily struggle for food, drugs, lab supplies, even heat and electricity."[6]

Fourth, prisoners are dying of ineffectively treated multidrug-resistant tuberculosis. Article 27 of the Universal Declaration of Human Rights, which insists that everyone has a right "to share in scientific advancement and its benefits," leads us to raise questions of why representatives of wealthy donor nations—relief workers—are giving prisoners drugs to which their infecting tuberculosis strains have documented resistance. Thus the rights of prisoners are violated by the logic of cost-effectiveness, which argues that the appropriate drugs are too expensive for use in "the developing world," to which post-perestroika Russia has been demoted. All the prison rights activism in the world will come to naught if prisoners are guaranteed the right to treatment but given the wrong prescriptions. All the penal reform in the world will come to naught if prisoners with tuberculosis are granted amnesty only to find the civilian TB service demolished in the name of "health care reform." In short, conventional legal and human rights views on recrudescent tuberculosis in Russian prisons fail to recognize the true dimensions of the problem.

QUESTIONING "IMMODEST CLAIMS OF CAUSALITY"

This picture is further complicated by the competing explanations offered by various actors on the scene. Some international health experts insist that the heart of the problem lies with Russian physicians, who have failed to adopt modern approaches to tuberculosis control.[7] Others, basing their arguments on technical considerations or issues of cost-effectiveness, argue that multidrug-resistant tuberculosis (MDRTB) is untreatable in such settings. Experts from the international public health community have argued that it is not necessary to treat MDRTB—the "untreatable form" in question—in this region, contending that all patients should be treated with identical doses of the same drugs and that MDRTB will somehow disappear if such strategies are adopted.[8] Other experts, both Russian and international, claim that the fault for poor treatment outcomes lies with the prisoners, who are said to refuse treatment.[9]

How many of these claims are true? First, it seems absurd to lay the blame for a burgeoning tuberculosis epidemic on Russia's hapless tuberculosis specialists, given that economic restructuring (and not ill-advised clinical management strategies) has brought the nation's public health infrastructure to its knees. Second, cost-efficacy arguments against treating drug-resistant tuberculosis almost always fail to note that most of the drugs necessary for such treatment have been off-patent for years. As to assertions that MDRTB is untreatable, they are simply not true. Partners In Health has done work in Peru and Haiti showing that MDRTB can be cured in resource-poor settings.[10] By constituting a coalition of international groups able to lobby for lower prices for these drugs, we were able to drop prices of many second-line drugs by more than 90 percent in less than two years.[11] We also know from painful experience in New York prisons that failure to identify and treat MDRTB will lead to outbreaks of disease throughout a prison system, and thence on to the public hospitals and beyond. Claims that low-cost, short-course chemotherapy can eliminate the problem are thus dangerously incorrect.[12]

There is reason to suspect that the other assertion, that prisoners refuse treatment, is also false. How might this claim be assessed? One option would be to ask the concerned parties. During visits to Siberia, I have often asked prisoners with tuberculosis, "How many of you want to be treated?" All hands go up. "Why, then, is it so widely rumored that you refuse treatment?" "Hearsay," according to some. "Just not true," another will remark, "but we want treatment that will cure us." In prison after prison, it's the same story. That conventional therapy was failing to cure them was as obvious to the prisoners as it was to the medical technologists who, during each month of treatment, documented the presence of tubercle bacilli in the prisoners' sputum.

Clearly, the veracity of competing claims about a matter as complicated as epidemic MDRTB cannot be assessed by a show of hands. MDRTB in Russian prisons is an example of a complex human rights problem that requires the application of epidemiology, subspecialty clinical medicine, and a critical sociology of knowledge. Social science can also help to unmask the immodest claims of causality filling the explanatory void. Facile claims about the nature of excess deaths among prisoners are patterned and predictable. They serve recognizable (though hardly honorable) purposes. The analysis also calls for an international political economy of relief work—that is, a critical look at how humanitarian work is conducted in the global, inegalitarian era.[13]

But what, more specifically, does a focus on health bring to the struggle for human rights? I have argued that a narrow legal approach to health and human rights can obscure the nature of violations, thereby enfeebling our best responses to them. Casting prison-based tuberculosis epidemics in terms of social and economic rights offers an entrée for public health and medicine, an important step in the process that could halt these epidemics. Conversely, failure to consider social and economic rights can prevent the allied health professions and the social sciences from making their fullest contribution to the struggle for human rights.

One of the central points in my argument is that public health and access to medical care are social and economic rights; they are at least as critical as civil rights. An irony of this global era is that while public health has increasingly sacrificed equity for efficiency, the poor have become well informed enough to reject separate standards of care. In our professional journals, these subaltern voices have been well-nigh blotted out. But we heard snatches of their rebuke recently with regard to access to antiretroviral therapy for HIV disease. For over a decade, those living with both poverty and HIV (they are tens of millions strong, even if they have no acronym) have been demanding access to effective therapy. In the past several years, these demands have become increasingly specific, as a group of rural Haitians living with HIV made clear in a declaration made public in August 2001. The patients traced the links between the right to treatment and other social and economic rights:

It is we who are sick; it is therefore we who take the responsibility to declare our suffering, our misery, and our pain, as well as our hope. We hear many poignant statements about our circumstances, but feel compelled to say something clearer and more resounding than what we've heard from others.

[We] are fortunate to have access to medications and health care even though we do not have money to buy them. Many of our health problems have been resolved with [antiretroviral] medications. Given how dire our situation was prior to treatment, we have benefited greatly. But while we feel fortunate to have access to these services, we feel great sadness for others who don't receive the same treatment we do.

And in addition to our health problems, we have other tribulations. Although less preoccupied with our illness, we still have problems paying for housing. We have trouble finding employment. We remain concerned about sending our children to school. Each day we face the distressing reality that we cannot find the means to support them. Not being able to feed our children is the greatest challenge faced by mothers and fathers across the country of Haiti. We have learned that such calamities also occur in other countries. As we reflect on all these tragedies we must ask: is every human being not a person?

Yes, all human beings are people. It is we, the afflicted, who speak now. We have come together ... to discuss the great difficulties facing the sick. We've also brought some ideas of our own in our knapsacks; we would like to share them with you, the authorities, in the hope that you might do something to help resolve the health problems of the poor.

When we the sick, living with AIDS, speak to the subject of "health and human rights," we are aware of two rights that ought to be indivisible and inalienable. Those who are sick should have the right to health care. We who are already infected believe in prevention too. But prevention will not save those who are already ill. All people need treatment when we are sick, but for the poor there are no clinics, no doctors, no nurses, no health care.

Furthermore, the medications now available are too expensive. For HIV treatment, for example, we read in the newspapers that treatment costs less than $600 per year [in developing countries]. Although that is what is quoted in press releases, here in a poor, small country like Haiti, it costs more than twice that much.

The right to health is the right to life. Everyone has a right to live. If we were not living in misery, but rather in decent poverty, many of us would not be in this predicament today ...

We have a message for the people who are here and for all those able to hear our plea. We are asking for your solidarity. The battle we're fighting—to find adequate care for those with AIDS, tuberculosis, and other illnesses—is the same as the combat that's long been waged by other oppressed people so that everyone can live as human beings.[14]

Whether or not we continue to ignore them, the destitute sick are increasingly clear on one point: making social and economic rights a reality is the key goal for health and human rights in the twenty-first century.

Although trained in anthropology, I do not embrace the rigidly particularist and relativist tendencies popularly associated with the discipline.[15] (Nor do most anthropologists.) That is, I believe that violations of human dignity are not to be accepted merely because they are buttressed by local ideology or longstanding tradition. But anthropology—in common with sociological and historical perspectives in general—allows us to place in broader contexts both human rights abuses and the discourses (and other responses) they generate. Furthermore, these disciplines permit us to ground our understanding of human rights violations in broader analyses of power and social inequality. Whereas a purely legal view of human rights tends to obscure the dynamics of human rights violations, the contextualizing disciplines reveal them to be pathologies of power. Social inequalities based on race or ethnicity, gender, religious creed, and—above all—social class are the motor force behind most human rights violations. In other words, violence against individuals is usually embedded in entrenched structural violence.

In exploring the relationships between structural violence and human rights, I have drawn on my own experience serving the destitute sick in settings such as Haiti and Chiapas and Russia, where human rights violations are a daily concern (even if structural violence is not always seen as a human rights issue). I cite this experience not to make overmuch of my personal acquaintance with other people's suffering, but rather to ground a theoretical discussion in the reality that has shaped my views on health and human rights. Each of these situations calls for us not only to recognize the relationship between structural violence and human rights violations but also to implement what we have termed pragmatic solidarity: the rapid deployment of our tools and resources to improve the health and well-being of those who suffer this violence.

Rather than examining in detail the covenants and conventions that constitute the key documents of the human rights movement, my goals here are to raise, and to answer, some questions relevant to health and human rights; to explore the promise of pragmatic solidarity as a response to structural violence; and to identify promising directions for future work in this field. These, I believe, are the most important issues raised in this discussion, and the conclusions that follow are the most important challenges before those who concern themselves with health and human rights.

HOW FAR HAS THE HUMAN RIGHTS MOVEMENT COME?

The field of health and human rights, most would agree, is in its infancy. Attempting to define a new field is necessarily a treacherous enterprise. Sometimes we appear to step on the toes of those who have long been at work when we mean instead to stand on their shoulders. Human rights law, which focuses on civil and political rights, is much older than human rights medicine. And if vigor is assessed in the typical academic style—by length of bibliography—human rights law is also the more robust field. That legal documents and scholarship dominate the human rights literature is not surprising, Henry Steiner and Philip Alston point out, given that the human rights movement has "struggled to assume so lawlike a character."[16]

But even in legal terms, the international human rights movement is essentially a modern phenomenon, beginning, some argue, with the Nuremberg trials.[17] It is this movement that has led, most recently, to the creation of international tribunals to judge war crimes in the Balkans and in Rwanda.[18] Some fifty years after the Universal Declaration of Human Rights, and fifty years after the four Geneva Conventions, what do we have to show for these efforts? Do we have some sense of outcomes? When Aryeh Neier, former executive director of Human Rights Watch, reviewed the history of various treaties and covenants from Nuremberg to the Convention Against Torture and Other Cruel, Inhuman or Degrading Treatment or Punishment, he concluded, "Nations have honored these obligations largely in the breach."[19]

Although few could argue against Neier's dour assessment, the past few years have been marked by a certain amount of human rights triumphalism. The fiftieth anniversary of the Universal Declaration has led to many celebrations but to few careful assessments of current realities. For some, including many in the liberation theology movement, human rights discourse is at times so divorced from reality that an "alternative language" is necessary if we are to speak of the "rights of the poor," as Gustavo Gutiérrez puts it. The basic problem, in his view, is that "liberal doctrines" about human rights presuppose "that our society enjoys an equality that in fact does not exist."[20] Jon Sobrino agrees that this lack of connection to reality is one of the reasons that liberal human rights discourses are sometimes regarded with suspicion by advocates of the poor:

> A major characterization of our era is the formulation and doctrine of human rights. And it is of no small merit for our age to have succeeded in conceptualizing and universalizing such rights—to have come to be able to speak of the right to life, to liberty, to dignity, and to so many other blessings accompanying these. But this accomplishment does not yet bring us down to basics. Reality is, after all, antecedent to doctrine, and to the philosophical or theological founding of doctrine. The concrete is antecedent to the universal.[21]

Even those within the legal community acknowledge that it would be difficult to correlate a steep rise in the publication of human rights documents with a statistically significant drop in the number of human rights abuses. Rosalyn Higgins says pointedly:

No one doubts that there exists a norm prohibiting torture. No state denies the existence of such a norm; and, indeed, it is widely recognized as a customary rule of international law by national courts. But it is equally clear from, for example, the reports of Amnesty International, that the *great majority* of states systematically engage in torture. If one takes the view that noncompliance is relevant to the retention of normative quality, are we to conclude that there is not really any prohibition of torture under customary international law?[22]

Whether these laws are binding or largely hortatory constitutes a substantial debate in the legal literature, but such debates seem academic in the face of overwhelming evidence of persistent abuses.

When we expand the concept of rights to include social and economic rights, the gap between ideal and reality is even wider. Local and global inequalities mean that the fruits of medical and scientific advances are stockpiled for some and denied to others. The dimensions of this inequality are staggering, and the trends are bad. To cite just a few examples: By 1995, the total wealth of the top 358 "global billionaires" equaled the combined income of the world's 2.3 billion poorest people.[23] In 1998, Michael Jordan earned from Nike the equivalent of 60,000 years' salary for an Indonesian footwear assembly worker. Haitian factory workers, most of them women, make 28 cents per hour sewing Pocahontas pajamas, while Disney's U.S.-based chief executive officer makes $97,000 for each hour he toils.[24]

Although the pathogenic effects of such inequality per se are now recognized,[25] many governments, including that of the United States, refuse to redress inequalities in health, while others are largely powerless to address such inequity.[26] The reasons for failure are many and varied, but even optimists allow that human rights charters and covenants have not brought an end to—and may not even have slowed—egregious abuses, however they are defined. States large and small—but especially large ones, since their reach is transnational—violate civil, economic, and social rights; and inequality both prompts and covers these violations.

There are, of course, exceptions; victories have been declared. But not many of them are very encouraging on close scrutiny. Haiti, the case I know best, offers a humbling example. In that country, the struggle for social and economic rights—food, medical care, education, housing, decent jobs—has been dealt crippling blows. Such basic entitlements, the centerpiece of the popular movement that in 1990 brought the country's first democratically elected president to power, were buried under an avalanche of human rights violations after the military coup of 1991. And although human rights groups were among those credited with helping to restore constitutional rule in Haiti, this was accomplished, to a large extent, by sacrificing the struggle for social and economic rights.[27] In recent years, it has sometimes seemed as if the movement to bring to justice those responsible for the murder and mayhem that have made Haiti such a difficult place to live has simply run out of steam. Despite a few notable exceptions—such as the sentencing of military officials responsible for the 1994 civilian massacre at Raboteau—both the legal and socioeconomic campaigns are slowed almost to a standstill.[28] Although wildly discrepant theories are advanced to explain how this struggle has been stymied, it is important to underscore the ongoing sabotage by the most powerful. Most of the most powerful are not to be found within the borders of Haiti.

Or take Argentina, a far less dependent and immiserated country by all accounts. The gruesome details of the "dirty war" are familiar to many.[29] Seeking what Neier has chillingly termed "a better mousetrap of repression," the Argentine military government began "disappearing" (as Latin Americans said in the special syntax crafted for the occasion) people it identified as leftists.[30] Many people know, now, about the death flights that took place every Wednesday for two years. Thousands of citizens the government deemed subversive, many of them students and most of them having barely survived torture, were flown from a military installation out over the Atlantic, stripped, and shoved out of the plane. A better mousetrap, indeed.

What happened next in Argentina is well documented, although it is a classic instance of the half-empty, half-full glass. Those who say the glass is half full note that an elected civilian government subsequently tried and convicted high-ranking military figures, including the generals who shared, in the fashion of runners in a relay, the presidential office. Those who say the glass is half empty note that the prompt pardoning and release of the criminals meant that, once again, no one has been held accountable for thousands of murders.[31] Similar stories abound in Guatemala, El Salvador, the state of Chiapas in Mexico, and elsewhere in Latin America.[32]

These painful experiences are, of course, no reason to declare legal proceedings ineffective. On the contrary, they remind us that some of what was previously hidden away is now out in the open. Disclosure is often the first step in the struggle against impunity, and human rights organizations—almost all of them nongovernmental—have at times forced unwilling governments to acknowledge what really happened. These efforts should serve as a rallying cry for those who now look to constitute international criminal tribunals.

Still, the results to date suggest that we would be unwise to place all our hopes on an approach that emphasizes legal battles. Complementary strategies and new openings are critically needed. The health and human rights "angle" can provide new opportunities and new strategies at the same time that it lends strength and purpose to a movement sorely in need of buttressing. Pragmatic solidarity with those who seem to have suffered human rights abuses—or with those most likely to suffer—is one such strategy, as discussed later in this essay.

CAN ONE MERELY STUDY HUMAN RIGHTS ABUSES?

A few years ago, French sociologist Pierre Bourdieu and his colleagues pulled together a compendium of testimonies from those the French term "the excluded" in order to bring into relief *la misère du monde*. Bourdieu and colleagues qualify their claims for the role of scholarship in addressing this misery: "To subject to scrutiny the mechanisms which render life painful, even untenable, is not to neutralize them; to bring to light contradictions is not to resolve them."[33] It is precisely such humility that is needed, and rarely exhibited, in academic commentary on human rights. Indeed, Michael Ignatieff has underlined, in *Human Rights as Politics and Idolatry*, both the lack of humility and the hypocrisy that far too often pervade the statements and actions of a "human rights community" tied closely to power:

> As the West intervenes ever more frequently but ever more inconsistently in the affairs of other societies, the legitimacy of its rights standards is put into question. Human rights is increasingly seen as the language of a moral imperialism just as ruthless and just as self-deceived as the colonial hubris of yesteryear. . . . .
>
> From being the insurgent creed of activists during the Cold War, human rights has become "mainstreamed" into the policy framework of states, multilateral lending institutions like the World Bank, and the United Nations itself. The foreign policy rhetoric of most Western liberal states now repeats the mantra that national interests must be balanced by due respect for values, chief of which is human rights. But human rights is not just an additional item in the policy priorities of states. If taken seriously, human rights values put interests into question, interests such as sustaining a large export sector in a nation's defense industry, for example. It becomes incoherent for states like Britain and the United States to condemn Indonesia or Turkey for their human rights performance while providing their military with vehicles or weapons that can be used for the repression of civilian dissent. When values do not actually constrain interests, an "ethical foreign policy"—the self-proclaimed goal of Britain's Labour government—becomes a contradiction in terms.[34]

It is difficult merely to study human rights abuses. We know with certainty that rights are being abused at this moment. That we can study, rather than endure, these abuses is a reminder that we too are implicated in and benefit from the increasingly global structures that determine, to an important extent, the nature and distribution of assaults on dignity.

Ivory-tower engagement with health and human rights can reduce us to seminar-room warriors. At worst, we stand revealed as the hypocrites that our critics in many parts of the world have not hesitated to call us. Anthropologists have long been familiar with these critiques; specialists in international health, including AIDS researchers, have recently had a crash course.[35] It is possible, usually, to drown out the voices of those demanding that we stop studying them, even when they go to great lengths to make sure we get the message. But social scientists with more acute hearing have documented a rich trove of graffiti, songs, demonstrations, tracts, and broadsides on the subject. A hit record album in Haiti called *International Organizations* has a title cut that includes the following lines: "International organizations are not on our side. They're there to help the thieves rob and devour . . . International health stays on the sidelines of our struggle."[36]

In the context of longstanding international support for sundry Haitian dictatorships, one could readily see the gripe with international organizations in general. But *international health?* The international community's extraordinary largesse to the Duvalier regime has certainly been well documented.[37] Subsequent patterns of giving, addressed as they were to the various Duvalierist military juntas, did nothing to improve the reputation of U.S. foreign aid or the international organizations; such "aid" helped to arm murderous bands and line the pockets of their leaders. Haitians saw international health "aid" either as originating from within institutions such as the U.S. Agency for International Development (USAID) or as part of the same bureaucracy that shored up dictators. Now that there is at long last a democratically elected government, however, the U.S. government has decided to pass its aid (and influence) through nongovernmental channels. The Bush administration has exercised its authority to veto already approved aid loans from the Inter-American Development Bank. Although few outside Haiti seem to be paying attention—notably, human rights organizations have had nothing to say about the hypocrisy and disregard for rights apparent in such decisions—there is widespread awareness within Haiti of what it means to be so generous to dictators and military juntas and to subsequently block a series of loans for clean water, education, and health care. Such critiques are not specific to Haiti, although Haitians have pronounced them with exceptional frankness and richness of detail. Their accusations have been echoed and amplified throughout what some are beginning to call the global geoculture.[38] A full decade before the recent various debates over AIDS research, it was possible to collect a bookful of such commentary.[39]

It is in this context of globalization, growing inequality, and pervasive transnational media influence (which both exposes and exacerbates such inequality) that the new field of health and human rights emerges. Context is particularly salient when we think about social and economic rights, as Steiner and Alston point out: "An examination of the concept of the right to development and its implications in the 1990s cannot avoid consideration of the effects of the globalization of the economy and the consequences of the near-universal embrace of the market economy."[40] This context defines our research agenda and directs our praxis. We are leaving behind the terra firma of double-blinded, placebo-controlled studies, of cost-effectiveness, and of sustainability. Indeed, many of these concepts end up looking more like strategies for managing, rather than challenging, inequality.

What, then, should be the role of the First World university, of researchers and health care professionals? What should be the role of students and others lucky enough to be among the "winners" in the global era? We can agree, perhaps, that these centers are fine places from which to conduct research, to document, and to teach. A university does not have the same entanglements or constraints as an international institution such as the United Nations or an organization such as Amnesty International or Physicians for Human Rights. Universities could, in theory, provide a unique and privileged space for conducting research and engaging in critical assessment.

In human rights work, however, research and critical assessment are insufficient. No more adequate, for all their virtues, are denunciation and exhortation, whether in the form of press conferences or reports or harangues directed at students. To confront, as an observer, ongoing abuses of human rights is to be faced with a moral dilemma: does one's action help the sufferers or the system? The increasingly baroque codes of research ethics generated by institutional review boards will not help us out of this dilemma, nor will medical ethics, so often restricted to the quandary ethics of the individual. But certain models of engagement are relevant. If the university-based human rights worker is in a peculiar position, it is not entirely unlike that of the clinician researcher. Both study suffering; both are bound to relieve it; neither is in possession of a tried-and-true remedy. Both the human rights specialist and the clinician researcher have blind spots, too.

To push the analogy further, one could argue that both lines of work carry obligations regarding the standard of care. What if we are in possession of tried-and-true remedies? Returning again to the treatment of AIDS and drug-resistant tuberculosis, we already have a great deal of knowledge regarding how best to manage both diseases. Once a reasonably effective intervention has been identified, it—and not a placebo—is considered the standard against which a new remedy must be tested. In the global era, is it wise to set, as *policy goals,* double standards for the rich world and the poor world, when we know that these are not different worlds but in fact the same one? Are the acrid complaints of the vulnerable necessary to remind us that they invariably see the world as one world, riven by terrible inequality and injustice? A placebo is a placebo is a placebo.

As an even sterner rebuke to the self-described pragmatism of those pushing for relaxed ethical practices in settings of great poverty, we once again hear the voice from liberation theology. This voice does not call for equally good treatment of the poor; it demands *preferential treatment* for the poor. And to look at many of its central documents, one would swear that the human rights movement was once headed in the same direction: fighting to protect the rights

of the vulnerable, over and above the rights of the powerful. Of course, pushing for higher standards for the victims is always a utopian enterprise. Many
factors might limit feasibility, but that didn't stop the authors of the Universal
Declaration from setting high goals. That we have failed to meet them does not
imply that the next step is to lower our sights, although this has been the default
logic in many instances. Rather, the next step is to try new approaches and to
hedge our bets with indisputably effective interventions.

How do we best hedge our bets? Providing pragmatic services to the afflicted
is one obvious form of intervention. In other words, we cannot exclude social and
economic rights from the campaign for health and human rights. But the spirit
in which these services are delivered makes all the difference. Service delivery
can be just that—or it can be pragmatic solidarity, linked to the broader goals
of equality and justice for the poor. Again, my own experience in Haiti, which
began in 1983, made this clear. The Duvalier dictatorship was then in power,
seemingly immovable. Its chief source of external financial aid was the United
States and various international institutions, many of them ostensibly charitable
in nature. The local director of USAID at the time had frequently expressed the
view that if Haiti was underdeveloped, one could find the causes in Haitian culture.[41] The World Bank and the International Monetary Fund seemed to be part
of the same giant blur of international aid organizations that Haitians associated,
accurately enough, with U.S. foreign policy.

Popular cynicism regarding these transnational institutions was at its peak
when my colleagues and I began working in Haiti, and that is why we chose to
work through nascent community-based organizations and for a group of rural
peasants who had been dispossessed of their land by the construction of a hydroelectric dam. Although we conducted research and published it, research did not
figure on the wish list of the people we were trying to serve. Services were what
they asked for, and as people who had been displaced by political and economic
violence, they regarded these services as a rightful remedy for what they had
suffered. In other words, the Haitian poor themselves believed that social and
economic rights were central to the struggle for human rights. As the struggle
against the dictatorship gathered strength in the mid-1980s, the language was
explicitly couched in broad human rights terms. *Pa gen lapè nan tèt si pa gen lapè
nan vant* (there can be no peace of mind if there is no peace in the belly). Health
and education figured high on the list of demands as the Haitian popular movement began to swell.

The same has been true of the struggle in Chiapas. The Zapatista rebellion
was launched on the day the North American Free Trade Agreement was signed,
and the initial statement of the rebellion's leaders put their demands in terms of
social and economic rights: "We have been denied the most elemental education
so that others can use us as cannon fodder and pillage the wealth of our country.

They don't care that we have nothing, absolutely nothing, not even a roof over our heads, no land, no work, no health care, no food, and no education. Nor are we able freely and democratically to elect our political representatives, nor is there independence from foreigners, nor is there peace or justice for ourselves and our children."[42]

In settings such as these, we are afforded a rare clarity about choices that are in fact choices for all of us, everywhere. There's little doubt that discernment is a daily struggle. We must decide how health professionals (from providers to researchers) might best make common cause with the destitute sick, whose rights are violated daily. Helping governments shore up failing public health systems may or may not be wise. Pragmatic solidarity on behalf of Russian prisoners with tuberculosis, for example, includes working with their jailers. But sometimes we are warned against consorting with governments. In Haiti in the 1980s, it made all the difference that we formed our own nongovernmental organization far from the reach of the governments of both Haiti and the United States. In 1991, after Haiti's first-ever democratic elections brought to power the leader of the country's popular movement, we immediately began to work with the Ministry of Health. But seven months later, a military coup brought an abrupt end to that collaboration, a divorce that was to last for three long years.

In Chiapas, the situation was even more dramatic. Many poor communities simply refuse to use government health services. In village after village, we heard the same story. In some "autonomous zones," the Mexican army entered these villages and destroyed local health records and what meager independent infrastructure had been developed.[43] To quote one health worker: "The government uses health services against us. They persecute us if they think we are on the side of the rebels." Our own investigations have been amply confirmed by others, including Physicians for Human Rights: "At best, [Mexican] Government health and other services are subordinate to Government counterinsurgency efforts. At worst, these services are themselves components of repression, manipulated to reward supporters and to penalize and demoralize dissenters. In either case, Government health services in the zone are discriminatory, exacerbate political divisions, and fail utterly to address the real health needs of the population."[44]

It's not acceptable for those of us fortunate enough to have ties to universities and other "resource-rich" institutions to throw up our hands and bemoan the place-to-place complexity. Underlying this complexity is a series of very simple first principles regarding human rights, as the liberation theologians remind us. Our commitments, our loyalties, must be *primarily* to the poor and vulnerable. As a reminder of how unique this commitment is, remember that the international agencies affiliated with the United Nations, including the World Health Organization, are called to work with governments. Think, once again, of Chiapas. An individual member of any one of these international institutions may have loyalties to the Zapatistas, but no choice in his or her agency's primary interlocutor: this will be the Mexican government. That membership in a university (or hospital or local church) permits us more flexibility in making allegiances is a gift that we should not squander by mindlessly mimicking the choices of the parastatal international organizations. Close allegiance with suffering communities reminds us that it is not possible to merely study human rights abuses. But part of pragmatic solidarity is bringing to light the real story.

WHAT IS THE DIFFERENCE, IN HUMAN RIGHTS WORK, BETWEEN ANALYSIS AND STRATEGY?

If we accept the need to think both theoretically and instrumentally, we find there is a difference, in human rights work, between analysis and strategy. Failure to recognize this difference can hobble interventions designed to prevent or allay human rights violations. In this arena, analysis means bringing out the truth, no matter how clumsy or embarrassing or inexpedient. It means documenting, as Neier recently put it, "Who did what to whom, and when?"[45] Strategy asks a different question: What is to be done?

What is to be done? It's the oldest question around. Sometimes it's posed in a way calculated to discourage discussion, the subtext being that misery and unfairness are so ubiquitous that only hopeless romantics would discern opportunities for effective intervention. But even more frequently, the question is asked by people of goodwill. I know, for example, that many students seek opportunities to play a part in diminishing structural violence or its symptoms. Too often, their contributions are diluted when they become ensnarled in institutions—foundations, aid agencies, government-affiliated groups, universities, political parties, even organized labor—that put sharp limits on activism. On the other side of the ledger are the purists, who recognize the fundamentally conservative nature of such institutions and see themselves as too good, really, to rub shoulders with those who are engaged in providing services.

How can we build an agenda for action that moves beyond good analysis? If solidarity is among the most noble of human sentiments, then surely its more tangible forms are better still. Adding the material dimension to the equation—pragmatic solidarity—responds to the needs expressed by the people and communities who are living, and sometimes dying, on the edge. When we move beyond sentiments to action, we of course incur risks, and these deter many. But it is possible, clearly, to link lofty ideals to sound analysis.

This linkage does not always occur in human rights work, in part because of a reluctance to examine the political economy of suffering and brutality.

For example, high-minded charters are utopian strategies that may become laws to be flouted or obeyed; they are not analysis. The notion that everyone shares the risk of having his or her rights violated is reminiscent of catchy public health slogans such as "AIDS is for everyone." These slogans may be useful for social marketing, but they are redolent of the most soft-headed thinking. The distribution of AIDS is strikingly localized and nonrandom; so is that of human rights abuses. Both HIV transmission and human rights abuses are social processes and are embedded, most commonly, in the inegalitarian social structures I have called structural violence. Whether one examines these steep grades of inequality as an epidemiologist or as a social scientist, one comes to discern the context of risk by restoring the history and political economy of these precarious situations. There is considerable overlap between "groups at risk": if you are likely to be tortured or otherwise abused, you are also likely to be in the AIDS risk group composed of the poor and the defenseless.

Human rights can and should be declared universal, but the risk of having one's rights violated is not universal. Moreover, not every offense should be automatically classified as a human rights violation. Sticks and stones, we know, may break bones; and although it is not entirely true that "names will never hurt me," it is usually unwise to take verbal violations as seriously as bodily ones.

Identity politics in the United States have indeed sought to extend the reach of rights language. But identity politics have remained parochial and national (indeed subnational) in this global era, and in a nation as affluent as our own, turning a human rights struggle into a bitter competition for a bigger slice of the pie results in the erasure of many linked to our affluence. It makes sense to distinguish between a struggle for access to power—breaking the gendered "glass ceiling" of transnational corporations, say—and a struggle for access to a basic good such as primary health care, especially if the same corporations that reluctantly open their boardrooms to a few women and minorities are involved in causing the deepening inequality between rich and poor. Should the frenzied quest for access to power and wealth be regarded as serving a social good simply because those who were historically underrepresented are now filling roles that involve replicating inequality?

At the other end of the scale, moral relativism is similarly pernicious. Not all forms of suffering are equivalent. The public health and medical communities are accustomed to triage, to assessment of gravity, followed by action to address the problem at hand. It makes sense, in my view, to distinguish between the harm done by six lashes for vandalism—a tremendous cause célèbre when meted out to a U.S. citizen abroad, to judge by inches of newspaper copy—and the harm done to millions by a lifetime of institutionalized racism.[46] To make distinctions between committing genocide and censoring intellectuals is not to declare the latter trivial. But our job of telling the truth as best we can compels us to weight those wrongs differently.

The risk of stretching the concept of rights to cover every possible case is that obscene inequalities of risk will be drowned in a rising tide of petty complaint.[47] Only careful comparative analysis gives us a sense of scale; only careful analysis brings causal mechanisms into the light. We have seen brisk debate about a hierarchy of human rights abuses and about whether it makes sense to consider some rights "fundamental." The struggle for recognition of social and economic rights has engendered even more acrimony.[48] But this debate has been legal in nature—centered in and destined toward law, where it is customary to speak of inalienable rights and to wait decades or centuries to see them vindicated.

Merely telling the truth, of course, often calls for exhaustive research. In the current era, human rights violations are usually both local and global. Telling who did what to whom and when becomes a complicated affair. Take the case of Chouchou Louis, a young man tortured to death in Haiti in early 1992. I have told his story in more detail elsewhere;[49] here I will merely state that I was called to see him after he was cast out of police headquarters to die in the dirt. He did just that. I was too late, too unequipped, medically, to save his life. Documenting what had happened to him was the least I could do.[50]

Was I to document only the "distal" events? Although all present were terrified, it was possible—in fact, quite easy—to obtain the names of those who had arrested and tortured Chouchou Louis. But the chain of complicity, I learned, kept reaching higher. At the time, U.S. officialdom's explanation of human rights abuses in Haiti, including the torture and murder of people like Chouchou Louis, focused almost exclusively on local actors and local factors. One heard of the "culture of violence" that rendered this and other similarly grisly deaths comprehensible. Such official analyses, constructed by conflating structural violence and cultural difference, were distancing tactics.

Innumerable immodest claims of causality—such as attributing a sudden upsurge in the number of persons tortured while in police custody to longstanding local custom—play into the convenient alibi that refuses to follow the chain of events to their source, that keeps all the trouble local. Such alibis obscure the fact that the modern Haitian military was created by an act of the U.S. Congress during the twenty-year U.S. occupation of Haiti, from 1915 to 1934. Most official analyses around the time of Chouchou's death did not discuss generous U.S. assistance to the post-Duvalier military: more than $200 million in aid passed through the hands of the Haitian military in the eighteen months after Jean-Claude Duvalier left Haiti on a U.S. cargo plane in 1986. Bush administration statements, and their faithful echoes in the establishment press, failed to mention that many of the commanders who issued the orders to detain and torture civilians had been trained by the U.S. military in Fort Benning, Georgia.[51] At this writing, human rights groups in the United States and Haiti have filed suit against the U.S. government in order to force the return of more than one hundred thousand pages of documents (taken away during the U.S. invasion of Haiti in the fall of 1994) revealing links between Washington and the paramilitary groups that held sway in Haiti between 1991 and 1994.[52]

Elsewhere too the mechanisms of human rights violations have been masked. In El Salvador, the massacres of entire villages could not in good conscience be considered unrelated to U.S. foreign policy, since the U.S. government was the primary funder, advisor, and supporter of the Salvadoran government's war against its own people. Yet officialdom maintained precisely that fiction of deniability, even though the United States was also the primary purveyor of armaments, as physical evidence later showed.[53] It was years before we could read accounts such as that by Mark Danner, who, on investigating the slaughter of every man, woman, and child in one village, concluded: "Of the two hundred and forty-five cartridge cases that were studied—all but one from American M16 rifles—'184 had discernable headstamps, identifying the ammunition as having been manufactured for the United States Government at Lake City, Missouri.'"[54] The fiction of local struggles ("ethnic," "religious," "historical," or otherwise picturesque) is exploded by any honest attempt to understand. Paramilitary groups linked tightly with the Mexican government were and are responsible for the bulk of intimidation and violence in the villages of Chiapas.[55] But federal authorities have insisted that such violence results from "local intercommunity and interparty tension" or ethnic rivalries.[56]

Similarly inaccurate were claims that the U.S. military base on Guantánamo had become "an oasis" for Haitian refugees in the early 1990s and that Cuba's AIDS sanatoriums were "prison camps." Immodest claims of causality are not always so flagrantly self-serving as those proffered to explain Haiti's agony, the violence in El Salvador or Chiapas, or the contrasting AIDS dramas on the island of Cuba. But only careful analysis allows us to rebut them with any confidence. We cannot *merely* study human rights abuses, but we must not fail to study them.

WHAT CAN A FOCUS ON HEALTH BRING TO THE STRUGGLE FOR HUMAN RIGHTS?

Medicine and public health, and also the social sciences relevant to these disciplines, have much to contribute to the great, often rancorous debates on human rights. But what might be our greatest contribution? Rudolf Virchow saw doctors as "the natural attorneys of the poor."[57] A "health angle" can promote a broader human rights agenda in unique ways. In fact, the health part of the formula may prove critical to the success of the human rights movement. The esteem in which public health and medicine are held affords us openings—again, a space of privilege—enjoyed by few other professions. For example, it is unlikely that my colleagues and I would have been welcomed so warmly into Russian prisons if we had presented ourselves as social scientists or human rights investigators. We went, instead, as TB specialists, with the expectation that a visiting group of doctors might be able to do more for the rights of these prisoners than a delegation from a conventional human rights organization. It is important to get the story straight: the leading cause of death among young Russian detainees is tuberculosis, not torture or starvation. Prison officials were opening their facilities to us and asking for pragmatic solidarity. (In Haiti and Chiapas, by contrast, we were asked to leave when we openly espoused the cause of the oppressed.)

Medicine and public health benefit from an extraordinary symbolic capital that is, so far, sadly underutilized in human rights work. No one made this point more clearly and persistently than the late Jonathan Mann. In an essay written with Daniel Tarantola, Mann noted that AIDS "has helped catalyze the modern health and human rights movement, which leads far beyond AIDS, for it considers that promoting and protecting health and promoting and protecting human rights are inextricably connected."[58]

But have we gone far beyond AIDS? Is it not a human rights issue that Russian prisoners are exposed, often during illegally prolonged pre-trial detention, to epidemic MDRTB and then denied effective treatment? Is it not a human rights issue that international expert opinion has mistakenly informed Russian prison officials that treatment with second-line drugs is not cost-effective or is just plain unnecessary? Is it not a human rights issue that in relatively wealthy South Africa (where a glossy program reminded participants at the thirteenth annual AIDS meetings that "medical care is readily available in South Africa") the antiretroviral therapy that could prolong millions of (black) lives is declared "cost-ineffective"? Is it not a human rights issue that villagers in Chiapas lack access to the most basic medical services, even as government medical facilities stand idly by? Is it not a human rights issue that thousands of Haitian peasants displaced by a hydroelectric dam end up sick with HIV disease after working as servants in Port-au-Prince?

Standing on the shoulders of giants—from the authors of the Universal Declaration to Jonathan Mann—we can recognize the human rights abuses in each of these situations, including epidemic tuberculosis within prisons. But what, precisely, is to be done? Russian penal codes already prohibit overcrowding, long pre-trial detention, and undue risk from malnutrition and communicable disease. Prison officials already regard the tuberculosis problem as a top priority; that's why they let TB specialists in. In a 1998 interview, one high-ranking prison official told me that the ministry saw their chief problems as lack of resources, overcrowding, and tuberculosis.[59] And the pièce de résistance might be that Boris Yeltsin had already declared 1998 "the year of human rights."

Passing more human rights legislation is not a sufficient response to these human rights challenges, because those in charge already disregard many of those (clearly nonbinding) instruments. The Haitian military coup leaders were beyond the pale. But how about Chiapas? Instruments to which Mexico is already signatory include the Geneva Conventions of 1949; the International Covenant on Civil and Political Rights; the International Covenant on Economic, Social and Cultural Rights; the International Labor Organization Convention 169; the American Convention on Human Rights; the Maastricht Guidelines on Violations of Economic, Social and Cultural Rights; and the Convention on the Elimination of All Forms of Discrimination against Women. Each one of these is flouted every day in Chiapas.

As the Haitians say, "Laws are made of paper; bayonets are made of steel." Law alone is not up to the task of relieving such immense suffering. Louis Henkin has reminded us that international law is fundamentally a set of rules and norms designed to protect the interests of states, not their citizens. "Until recently," he observed in 1989, "international law took no note of individual human beings."[60] And states, as we have seen, honor human rights law largely in the breach—sometimes intentionally and sometimes through sheer impotence. This chief irony of human rights work—that states will not or cannot obey the treaties they sign—can lead to despair or to cynicism, if all of one's eggs are in the international-law basket.

Laws are not science; they are normative ideology and are thus tightly tied to power.[61] Biomedicine and public health, though also vulnerable to being deformed by ideology, serve different imperatives, ask different questions. They do not ask whether an event or a process violates an existing rule; they ask whether that event or process has ill effects on a patient or a population. They ask whether such events can be prevented or remediated. A change of approach in that direction would have, I believe, a salutary effect on many human rights debates. And when medicine and public health are explicitly placed at the service of the poor, it provides even greater insurance against their perversion.

To return to the case of prisoners with MDRTB, the best way to protect their rights is to cure them of their disease. And the best way to protect the rights of other prisoners, and those who take care of them, is to prevent transmission by treating the sick. Thus, after years of hemming and hawing, all parties involved are being forced to admit that the right thing to do in Russia's prisons is also the human rights thing to do. A variety of strategies, from human rights arguments to epidemiologic scare tactics, have been used to make headway in raising the funds necessary to treat these and other prisoners. In the end, then, the health angle on human rights may prove more pragmatic than approaching the problem as one of penal reform alone. Previously closed institutions have opened their doors to international collaboration designed to halt prison epidemics. This approach—pragmatic solidarity—is, in the end, leading to penal reform as well. Similarly pragmatic approaches to addressing treatment and prevention of HIV also promise to reverse scandalous inequalities of risk and access.

In 1998, working in central Haiti, Partners In Health launched the "HIV Equity Initiative" in order to complement prevention efforts with antiretroviral treatment for those for whom prevention had failed. The care component includes an uninterrupted supply of antiretroviral agents, but only modest lab infrastructure. Use of these drugs is supervised, preferably by community-based health workers, called *accompagnateurs,* who visit patients each day. Between 10 and 12 percent—too small a proportion—of the more than fifteen hundred HIV-positive patients followed in the affiliated clinic receive such therapy. A clinical algorithm, described elsewhere, is used to identify those patients in greatest need.[62]

This project has been limited by an inability to find significant donor support for an integrated HIV prevention and care project in a setting as poor as rural Haiti. Though we felt we had no choice but to move forward—years ago, HIV surpassed tuberculosis as the leading infectious cause of adult deaths in Haiti—we had to rely on private donations, support from patients in the United States, and the largesse of a major donor who has long supported our work in Haiti. In short, we would have much more to report in 2002 if we had been able to find pragmatic solidarity in the donor community. Instead, we encountered the argument that such projects were neither cost-effective nor feasible in a setting of such profound poverty.

All this could change: through the newly established Global Fund to Fight AIDS, Tuberculosis, and Malaria, the United Nations has promised Haiti significant funds for HIV prevention and care. As we and other groups based in regions where poverty and HIV are the ranking threats to health contemplate the advent of new resources, we need to ask hard questions of ourselves and also of those who will evaluate their use. In seeking to promote accountability, will we develop yet another set of burdensome reporting requirements that will force us to hire expensive consultants from far beyond the boundaries of afflicted communities? Or will we seek innovative and realistic means of evaluating the impact of long-overdue investments? The point of bringing new funding to allay the suffering caused by AIDS, tuberculosis, and malaria is not merely to mimic existing transnational research projects, already struggling with serious ethical dilemmas, but rather to remediate inequalities of access to proven therapies. This goal should be embraced without apology.

Embracing this goal, and embedding such actions in the rights framework, helps us to answer the question, What is the purpose of the research and evaluation that must certainly accompany such disbursements? Not merely to please skeptics, one hopes, since accountability should be to the afflicted rather than to the privileged. The purpose of this research should be to do a better job of bringing the fruits of science and public health to the poorest communities. If the purpose of the new funds is also to help us better promote access to health care as a fundamental human right, we will of course be called to address, in addition to nascent HIV projects, not only tuberculosis and malaria but also eclampsia, cervical cancer, and the long list of maladies transmitted by unsafe drinking water. This will mean making common cause with community health workers and others in the trenches. In the end, the burden of proof should lie on the shoulders of those who argue against making the elimination of inequalities of access to prevention and care our top priority in international public health.

I will return to the strategy of pragmatic solidarity in proposing a new agenda for health and human rights but will proceed under the assumption that any approach to human rights that regards research as an end in itself contains many pitfalls—moral, strategic, and analytic.[63]

A NEW AGENDA FOR HEALTH AND HUMAN RIGHTS

As I've argued thus far, we have a long way to go in the struggle for health and human rights. We cannot merely study this topic without proposing meaningful and pragmatic interventions; but to succeed, we must distinguish between our best analyses and our best strategies. The focus on health offers a critical new dimension to human rights work and is a largely untapped vein of resources, passion, and goodwill.

Is it grandiose to seek to define a new agenda? When one reads the powerfully worded statutes, conventions, treaties, and charters stemming from international revulsion over the crimes of the Third Reich, it might seem pointless to call for better instruments of this sort. Yet events in the former Yugoslavia and in Rwanda serve as a powerful rebuke to undue confidence in these approaches: "That it should nevertheless be possible for Nazi-like crimes to be repeated half a century later in full view of the whole world," remarks Neier, "points up the weakness of that system—and the need for fresh approaches."[64] Steiner and Alston, similarly, call for "heightened attention to the problems of implementation and enforcement of the new ideal norms. The old techniques," they conclude, "simply won't work."[65]

A corollary question is whether a coherent agenda springs from the critique inherent in the answers to the questions presented here. If so, is this agenda compatible with existing approaches and documents, including the Universal Declaration of Human Rights? To those who believe that social and economic rights must be central to the health and human rights agenda, the answers to these questions are yes. This agenda, inspired by the notion of a preferential option for the poor, is coherent, pragmatic, and informed by careful scholarship. Largely because it focuses on social and economic rights, this agenda, though novel, builds on five decades of work within the traditional human rights framework: Articles 25 and 27 of the Universal Declaration inspire the vision of this emerging agenda, which could rely on tighter links between universities, medical providers, and both nongovernmental and community-based organizations. The truly novel part of these alliances comes in subjugating these networks to the aspirations of oppressed and abused people.

How might we proceed with this effort, if most reviews of the effects of international laws and treaties designed to protect human rights raise serious questions of efficacy (to say the least)? What can we do to advance a new agenda of health and human rights? In concluding, I offer six suggestions, which are intended to complement ongoing efforts.

Make Health and Healing the Symbolic Core of the Agenda

If health and healing are the symbolic core of our new agenda, we tap into something truly universal—concern for the sick—and, at the same time, engage medicine, public health, and the allied health professions, including the basic sciences. Put another way, we need to throw the full weight of the medical and scientific communities behind a noble cause. Physicians and health researchers are not hostile to this cause; quite the contrary. What we lack, with some notable exceptions, are concerted efforts to engage health professionals in human rights work, broadly conceived. One of those notable exceptions is the recent AIDS initiative advanced by Physicians for Human Rights and partner organizations, which argues that access to care should be construed as a basic right.[66] It is tragic, surely, that such initiatives remain unusual within the mainstream human rights community.

Although many global health indicators show significant improvement, we still have endless work to do before we can claim to have made the slightest headway in ensuring the highest possible level of health for all. In fact, several studies suggest that inequalities in health outcomes are growing in many places.[67] From the human rights perspective advanced in this essay, this growing outcome gap constitutes both a human rights violation and a means of tracking the efficacy of our interventions. That is, reduction of the outcome gap is the goal of our pragmatic solidarity with the destitute sick.

Make Provision of Services Central to the Agenda

We need to listen to the sick and abused and to those most likely to have their rights violated. Whether they are nearby or far away, we know, often enough, who they are. The abused offer, to those willing to listen, critiques far sharper than my own. They are not asking for new centers of study and reflection. They have not commissioned new studies of their suffering. That means we need new programs in addition to the traditional ventures of a university or a research center (the journals, books, articles, courses, conferences, research). Law schools have clinics, and so do medical schools. Not only should programs promoting health and human rights have legal clinics; in addition, a broad range of health professionals should help to establish, in every major medical center, referral clinics for those subjected to torture and other human rights abuses as classically defined.

But a far larger group calls for our pragmatic solidarity. We need programs designed to remediate inequalities of access to services that can help all humans to lead free and healthy lives. If everyone has a right "to share in scientific advancement and its benefits," where are our pragmatic efforts to improve the spread of these advances? Such efforts exist, but, again, the widening outcome gap stands as the sharpest rebuke to the health and human rights community. Even as our biomedical interventions become more effective, our capacity to distribute them equitably is further eroded. The world's poor and otherwise marginalized people currently constitute a vast control group of the untreated, and even cursory examination of the annual tally of victims reminds us that this sector also constitutes the group most likely to have their rights violated.

How can we make the rapid deployment of services to improve health—pragmatic solidarity—central to the work of health and human rights programs? Our own group, Partners In Health, has worked largely with community-based organizations in Haiti and Peru and Mexico whose expressed goal has been to remediate inequalities of access. This community of providers and scholars believes that "the vitality of practice" lends a corrective strength to our research and writing.[68] The possibilities for programmatic collaboration range, we have learned, from Russian prison officials to peasant collectives in the autonomous zones of Chiapas. Novel collaborations of this sort are certainly necessary if we are to address the increasing inequalities of access here in wealthy, inegalitarian countries such as the United States. Relying exclusively on nation-states' compliance with a social justice agenda is naïve at best. At the same time, it is important to respect the sovereignty of states, for experience shows that states, not "Western" human rights groups, are best placed to protect the basic social and economic rights of populations living in poverty. Ignatieff emphasizes precisely this point. "We are rediscovering," he notes, "the necessity of state order as a guarantee of rights. It can be said with certainty that the liberties of citizens are better protected by their own institutions than by the well-meaning interventions of outsiders. . . . State failure cannot be rectified by human rights activism on the part of NGOs."[69] We will not be excused from discernment.

These questions of new collaborations are raised at a time that is filled with contradiction: despite increasing globalization, our action agenda has remained parochial. We lag behind trade and finance, since we are still at the first steps in the press for universal rights while the Masters of the Universe are already "harmonizing" their own standards and practices. Fifteen years of work in the most difficult field conditions have taught our group that it is hard, perhaps impossible, to meet the highest standards of health care in every situation. But it is imperative that we try to do so. Projects striving for excellence and inclusiveness—rather than, say, "cost-effectiveness" or "sustainability," which are often at odds with social justice approaches to medicine and public health—are not merely misguided quests for personal efficacy. Such projects respond to widespread demands for equity in health care. The din around AIDS research in the Third World is merely the latest insistence that we reject low standards as official policy. That such standards are widely seen as violating human rights is no surprise for those interested in social and economic rights. Efficiency cannot trump equity in the field of health and human rights.

Establish New Research Agendas

We need to make room in the academy for serious scholarly work on the multiple dynamics of health and human rights, on the health effects of war and political-economic disruption, and on the pathogenic effects of social inequalities, including racism, gender inequality, and the growing gap between rich and poor. By what mechanisms do such noxious events and processes become embodied as adverse health outcomes? Why are some at risk and others spared?

Here again, we lag far behind. As Nancy Krieger observes, "epidemiologic research explicitly focused on discrimination as a determinant of population health is in its infancy."[70] To answer the questions posed earlier, we require a new level of cooperation between disciplines ranging from social anthropology to molecular epidemiology. We need a new sociology of knowledge that can pick apart a wide body of commentary and scholarship: complex international law; the claims and disclaimers of officialdom; postmodern relativist readings of suffering; clinical and epidemiological studies of the long-term effects of, say, torture and racism.[71] But remember that none of the victims of these events or processes are asking us to conduct research. For this reason alone, research in the arena of health and human rights is necessarily fraught with pitfalls: "Imperiled populations in developing countries include extraordinarily vulnerable individuals ripped from their cultures and communities and victimized by myriad forms of abuse and violence. Public health research on violence and victimization among these groups must vigilantly guard against contributing to emotional and social harm."[72]

That research is and should remain a secondary concern does not mean that careful documentation is not critical to both our understanding of suffering and our ability to prevent or allay it. And because of its link to service, we need operational research by which we can gauge the efficacy of interventions that are quite different from those measured in the past.

Assume a Broader Educational Mandate

Human rights work usually has a suasive component. If the primary objective is to set things right, education is central to our task. But the educational mandate should not make two conventional mistakes: we must not limit ourselves to teaching only a select group of students who have an avowed interest in health and human rights, nor should we focus on trying to teach lessons to recalcitrant governments and international financial institutions. Jonathan Mann signaled the limitations of the latter approach: "Support for human rights–based action to promote health . . . at the level of declarations and speeches is welcome, and useful in some ways, but the limits of official organizational support for the call for societal transformation inherent in human rights promotion must be recognized."[73] A broader educational mandate would mean engaging students from all faculties—but also engaging the members of these faculties. Beyond the university and various governmental bodies lies the broader public, for whom the connections between health and human rights have not even been traced. It is doubtful that the destitute sick have much to learn from us about health and human rights, but there is little doubt that, as their students, we can learn to better convey the complexity and historicity of their messages.

Achieve Independence
from Powerful Governments and Bureaucracies

We need to be untrammeled by obligations to powerful states and international bureaucracies. A central irony of human rights law is that it consists largely of appeals to the perpetrators. After all, most crimes against humanity are committed by powerful states, not by rogue factions or gangs or cults or terrorists. That makes it difficult for institutions accountable to states to take their constituents to task. When in 1994 the United Nations created the post of High Commissioner for Human Rights, the $700,000 annual budget was paltry even by the standards of a nongovernmental organization. The results were predictable: "With denunciation of those responsible for abuses the only means available for carrying out his mission," the first commissioner "managed to go through his first year in his post without publicly criticizing a single government anywhere in the world."[74] It is not merely a problem of budgetary constraints. Many of the chief donor nations are themselves major violators of one or another of the international covenants discussed here. The United States and China are the world leaders in capital punishment, and the United States is implacably opposed, it would seem, to the creation of the International Criminal Court. And what about Mexico, partner with Canada and the United States in the world's largest "free trade" agreement? In Chiapas, numerous observers have documented the displacement and massacre of presumed Zapatista supporters by paramilitary groups tightly tied to the government: "State and federal authorities have permitted these groups to act with impunity, and state Public Security Police have not only failed to protect victims, but have sometimes participated in the evictions."[75]

None of this is to say that international organizations have little to offer to those seeking to prevent or assuage human rights abuses. It is rather to remind us that their supposed "neutrality" comes at a great cost, and that cost is usually paid by people who are not represented by ambassadors in places like New York, Paris, Geneva, Washington, London, or Tokyo. Along with nongovernmental organizations, university- and hospital-based programs have the potential to be independent, well designed, pragmatic, and feasible. The imprimatur of medicine and public health would afford even more weight and independence. And only a failure of imagination has led us to ignore the potential of collaboration with community-based organizations and with communities in resistance to ongoing violations of human rights.

Secure More Resources for Health and Human Rights

In our own era, "growth is wildly uneven, inequality is immense, anxiety is endemic," says Todd Gitlin. "The state, as a result, is continually urged to do more but deprived of the means to do so."[76] The halting but ineluctable spread of the global economy is linked to an evolving human rights irony: states become less able to help their citizens attain social and economic rights, even though they often retain their ability to violate human rights. Even where reforms have led to the enjoyment of basic political rights, the implementation of neoliberal economic policies can erode the right to freedom from want. This is particularly true of many developing countries, as Steiner and Alston explain: "Civil and political rights have been greatly strengthened in many countries. Nonetheless, related contemporary phenomena—including privatization, deregulation, the expanded provision of incentives to entrepreneurial behavior, and structural adjustment programs and related pressures from international financial institutions and developed countries—have had mixed, and sometimes seriously adverse, effects on the enjoyment of economic and social rights."[77]

Of course, it's easy to demand more resources; what's hard is to produce them. But if social and economic rights are acknowledged as such, then foundations, governments, businesses, and international financial institutions—many of them now awash in resources—may be called on to prioritize human rights endeavors that reflect the paradigm shift advocated here.

Regardless of where one stands on the process of globalization and its multiple engines, these processes have important implications for efforts to promote health and human rights. As states weaken, it's easy to discern an increasing role for nongovernmental institutions, including universities and medical centers. But it's also easy to discern a trap: *the withdrawal of states from the basic business*

of providing housing, education, and medical services usually means further ero-
sion of the social and economic rights of the poor. Our independent involvement
must be quite different from current trends, which have nongovernmental organizations relieving the state of its duty to provide basic services. We must avoid
becoming witting or unwitting abettors of neoliberal policies that declare every
service and every thing to be for sale.

How will we live up to the challenge to promote the highest possible level of
health for all? Universities and medical centers, I have argued, should conduct
research, but the subject—health and human rights—demands complementary
services. These services need to be provided urgently but must also be tied tightly
to demands for social and economic rights for the poor. Linking research to
service—and to social justice—costs money. An ambitious plan to redress injustice is what we need. "We could do more than we do," argues Ignatieff, "to stop
unmerited suffering and gross physical cruelty. That I take to be the elemental
priority of all human rights activism: to stop torture, beatings, killings, rape,
and assault and to improve, as best we can, the security of ordinary people."[78]
"Unmerited suffering" is what we encounter each day in clinics in Haiti, Chiapas,
Siberia, the slums of Peru. This suffering can be prevented or, at the very least,
alleviated. But if we lack ambition, we should expect the next fifty years to yield
a harvest of shame.

The experience of Partners In Health suggests that ambitious goals can be
met even without a large springboard. Over the past decade and more, against
a steady current of nay-saying, we have channeled significant resources to the
destitute sick in Haiti, Peru, Mexico, and Boston. We didn't argue that it was
"cost-effective," nor did we promise that such efforts would be replicable. We
argued that it was the right thing to do. It was also the human rights thing to do.

Some of the problems born of structural violence are so large that they have
paralyzed many who want to do the right thing. But we can find more resources,
and we can find them without sacrificing our independence and discernment.
We will not do this by adopting defensive postures that are tantamount to simply managing inequality with the latest tools from economists and technocrats.
Utopian ideals are the bedrock of human rights. By arguing that we must set
standards high, we must also argue for redistribution of some of the world's vast
wealth.

Claims that we live in an era of limited resources fail to mention that these
resources happen to be less limited now than ever before in human history.
Arguing that it is too expensive to treat MDRTB among prisoners in Russia, say,
sounds nothing short of ludicrous when this world contains individuals worth
more than $100 billion.[79] Arguments against treating HIV disease in precisely
those areas in which it exacts its greatest toll warn us that misguided notions of
cost-effectiveness have already trumped equity. Arguing that nominal legal and

political rights are the best we can hope for means that members of the healing professions will have their hands tied, forced to stand by as the rights and dignity of the poor and marginalized undergo further sustained and deadly assault.

NOTES

1. United Nations, "Universal Declaration of Human Rights."

2. Telzak et al., "Multidrug-Resistant Tuberculosis in Patients without HIV Infection," p. 911. For papers reporting MDRTB cure rates greater than 80 percent, see these reports of preliminary outcomes in urban Peru: Farmer, Bayona, Shin, et al., "Preliminary Outcomes of Community-Based MDRTB Treatment in Lima, Peru"; Farmer, Kim, et al., "Responding to Outbreaks of Multidrug-Resistant Tuberculosis"; Mitnick et al., "Community-Based Therapy for Multidrug-Resistant Tuberculosis in Lima, Peru." For a more recent report of high cure rates in Turkey, see Tahaoğlu et al., "The Treatment of Multidrug-Resistant Tuberculosis in Turkey." In an editorial originally written to present this last article in the *New England Journal of Medicine*, I argue that such efforts should be seen in a human rights framework; see Farmer, "The Major Infectious Diseases in the World—To Treat or Not to Treat?" (included in this volume as chapter 12).

3. Amnesty International, *Torture in Russia*, p. 31.

4. Ivan Nikitovich Simonov, former chief inspector of prisons and now with the Chief Board of Punishment Execution, Ministry of Internal Affairs, Russian Federation, Moscow, interview with the author, June 4, 1998.

5. Wedel, *Collision and Collusion*, p. 5. Another way of phrasing this, of course, is that structural violence has become more extreme in the post-Soviet era and that, as elsewhere, high levels of structural violence are associated with criminality. To the extent that Western advisors have been architects of many of these changes in Russia, they share responsibility for the prison-seated tuberculosis epidemic.

6. Dr. Natalya Vezhina, medical director, TB Colony 33, Mariinsk, Kemerovo, Russian Federation, interview with the author, September 1998.

7. For example, see Dlugy, "The Prisoners' Plague—Overcrowded Jails Are Fueling a Frightening New Epidemic of Drug-Resistant Tuberculosis." Anti-Russian prejudices are subtle but widespread in international TB circles.

8. See, for example, Alexander, "Money Isn't the Issue; It's (Still) Political Will." At about the same time, however, forces within the WHO Global Tuberculosis Programme began supporting the search for alternative forms of therapy for patients with MDRTB. For more on this process, see Farmer and Kim, "Community-Based Approaches to the Control of Multidrug-Resistant Tuberculosis"; World Health Organization, "Coordination of DOTS-Plus Pilot Projects for the Management of MDR-TB"; World Health Organization, *Report, Multidrug Resistant Tuberculosis (MDRTB)*.

9. This topic is discussed in Reyes and Coninx, "Pitfalls of Tuberculosis Programmes in Prisons." See also the exchange in Coker, "'Extrapolitis'"; as well as Farmer and Kim, "Resurgent TB in Russia."

10. Farmer, Bayona, Shin, et al., "Preliminary Outcomes of Community-Based MDRTB Treatment in Lima, Peru"; Mitnick et al., "Community-Based Therapy for Multidrug-Resistant Tuberculosis in Lima, Peru."

11. See Gupta et al., "Responding to Market Failures in Tuberculosis Control."

12. For a rebuttal of these claims, see Farmer, Bayona, Becerra, et al., "The Dilemma of MDR-TB in the Global Era." A WHO-led review more recently came to the same conclusion; see Espinal et al., "Standard Short-Course Chemotherapy for Drug-Resistant Tuberculosis."

13. Michael Ignatieff points out that, despite the possible improvements brought about by human rights groups, their actions do not always fully coincide with the wishes of those for whom they purport to speak: "[Human rights activists] are not elected by the victim groups they represent, and in the nature of things they cannot be. But this leaves unresolved their right to speak for and on behalf of the people whose rights they defend. . . . Few mechanisms of genuine accountability connect NGOs and the communities in civil society whose interests they seek to advance" (*Human Rights as Politics and Idolatry*, p. 10).

14. My translation from Haitian Creole. The original declaration—with translations into French and Spanish and another English translation—may be found at the Partners In Health website, www.pih.org/inforesources/essays/Cange_declaration.html (accessed October 7, 2009).

15. Cultural relativism as a "metaethical theory" has its role and, contrary to popular belief, is not incompatible with universal values. Although I cannot review the topic here, my thinking on these matters has been informed by my fieldwork in Haiti as well as by others in and outside anthropology. See, for example, Campbell, "Herskovits, Cultural Relativism, and Metascience"; Geertz, "Anti Anti-Relativism"; Hatch, *Culture and Morality*; Renteln, "Relativism and the Search for Human Rights"; Schmidt, "Some Criticisms of Cultural Relativism." Also see Talal Asad's discussion of torture: "Although the phrase 'torture or cruel, inhuman, or degrading treatment' serves today as a cross-cultural criterion for making moral and legal judgments about pain and suffering, it nevertheless derives much of its operative sense historically and culturally" ("On Torture, or Cruel, Inhuman, and Degrading Treatment," p. 285). For an exploration of cultural relativism and bioethics, see Macklin, *Against Relativism*.

16. Steiner and Alston, *International Human Rights in Context*, p. vi.

17. A notable precedent can be found in the multinational mobilization against King Leopold's brutal exploitation of the Congo; see the gripping account of "the first great international human rights movement of the twentieth century" in Hochschild, *King Leopold's Ghost*. Ignatieff correctly observes that "all human rights activism in the modern world properly traces its origins back to the campaigns to abolish the slave trade and then slavery itself" (*Human Rights as Politics and Idolatry*, p. 10).

18. For an examination of the search for justice in the aftermath of the genocides in Rwanda and Bosnia, both at the international level of the war crimes tribunals and at the personal level through the struggles of individual victims, see Neuffer, *The Key to My Neighbor's House*.

19. Neier, *War Crimes*, p. 75. Leigh Binford makes a similar point: "The fact that human rights organizations key their analyses to international laws that provide substantial protection to civilians who live in the midst of civil war makes little difference, because the laws are not obeyed" (*The El Mozote Massacre*, p. 6). Why do states sign human rights accords that they do not intend to respect? In 1989, Louis Henkin wrote: "One can only speculate as to why States accepted these norms and agreements, but it may be reasonable to doubt whether those developments authentically reflected sensitivity to human rights generally. States attended to what occurred inside another State when such happenings impinged upon their political-economic interests" (quoted in Steiner and Alston, *International Human Rights in Context*, p. 114).

20. Gutiérrez, *The Power of the Poor in History*, p. 87.

21. Sobrino, *Spirituality of Liberation*, p. 105.

22. Higgins is cited in Steiner and Alston, *International Human Rights in Context*, p. 141; emphasis in the original.

23. Keegan, "Second Front." These disparities have only grown since the mid-1990s. By the end of the decade, the United Nations Development Programme estimated that the fifteen richest individuals on earth controlled more assets than the combined annual gross domestic product (GDP) of all of sub-Saharan Africa (United Nations Development Programme, *Human Develop-*

ment Report 1998). Furthermore, the wealth of the three richest people in the world exceeded the total annual GDP of the forty-eight least developed countries (United Nations Development Programme, *Human Development Report 1999*).

24. Millen and Holtz, "Dying for Growth, Part I."

25. On the pathogenic effects of inequality, see Farmer, "Cruel and Unusual" (included in this volume as chapter 9). See also Wilkinson, *Unhealthy Societies*; Kawachi et al., "Social Capital, Income Inequality, and Mortality"; Fassin, *L'espace politique de la santé*; Dozon and Fassin, *Critique de la santé publique*; Leclerc et al., *Les inégalités sociales de santé*. This literature is of recent vintage, but the 1946 constitution of the World Health Organization underscores a similar point: "Unequal development in different countries in the promotion of health and control of disease, especially communicable disease, is a common danger" ("Constitution of the World Health Organization").

26. A growing number of public health practitioners and physicians have been pushing for a concerted effort to reduce inequalities in health; for a review, see Whitehead, Scott-Samuel, and Dahlgren, "Setting Targets to Address Inequalities in Health." One of the trends emerging from this literature is that, despite improvement in absolute health indicators for both rich and poor populations, the outcome gap is widening, and this rising inequity has its own pathogenic impact. For case studies from Brazil, see Victora et al., "Explaining Trends in Inequities." One of the pioneers in U.S. efforts to set goals for reducing inequalities of health outcomes was Dr. Julius Richmond, who not coincidentally was the U.S. representative to the famous 1978 meeting in Almaty (formerly Alma-Ata), Kazakhstan, which issued a call for "health for all by the year 2000" ("Declaration of Alma-Ata"). Many were surprised that the U.S. delegation did not attempt to prevent the ratification of a document that designated access to health care as a fundamental human right.

27. I am, of course, glossing a very complicated process in simple terms. The defeat of the social justice agenda of the Aristide government, which explicitly endorsed the "right to development," seemed almost complete by the time the Haitian government signed on to a structural adjustment project endorsed by the World Bank and the U.S. government; for a more in-depth discussion of this process, see Farmer, "The Significance of Haiti." But the movement remains alive within Haiti. The concept of development as a new human right, most eloquently endorsed by Judge Mohammed Bedjaoui, president of the International Court of Justice, has been hotly contested by the United States, described by Henry Steiner and Philip Alston as "an implacable opponent of the right to development" (*International Human Rights in Context*, p. 1113). For a more detailed examination of the relationship between human rights and structural adjustment projects, see Skogly, "Structural Adjustment and Development."

28. For a consideration of obstacles that hinder efforts to punish crimes against humanity in Haiti, see Hayner, *Unspeakable Truths*. Brian Concannon is able to end his own overview on a positive note: "After this Article's submission, the Raboteau Massacre trial reached its conclusion. The jury convicted sixteen of the twenty-two defendants in custody, most of whom received life sentences. The judge convicted all thirty-seven in absentia defendants, including the leaders of the dictatorship, all members of the military high command, and leaders of FRAPH, the main paramilitary organization. The court awarded $150 million in compensatory damages. The trial's principal lesson to the international community is that a poor country with an underdeveloped judiciary making a difficult democratic transition can still provide high-quality justice for its victims" ("Beyond Complementarity," pp. 248–49).

29. The report of the Alfonsín-appointed Sábato Commission remains the best text on the subject; see Comisión Nacional Sobre la Desaparición de Personas, *Nunca más*. Its English translation is introduced by Ronald Dworkin, who writes of a "system of licensed sadism." See also Dussel, Finocchio, and Gojman, *Haciendo memoria en el país de nunca más*; Steadman, "Struggling for a 'Never Again'"; Ciancaglini and Granovsky, *Nada más que la verdad*. Martin Andersen's *Dossier*

secreto is close to a definitive treatment of the Argentine case. On El Salvador, the official report was published in *Estudios Centroamericanos;* see Comisión de la Verdad para El Salvador, "De la locura a la esperanza." Priscilla Hayner, in *Unspeakable Truths,* has recently reviewed the fate of some twenty truth commissions, including all those mentioned here.

30. Neier, *War Crimes,* p. 33.

31. This view is compellingly defended by Aryeh Neier, who wonders "why the Argentine prosecution of crimes against human rights started so promisingly and why it ended so badly" ("What Should Be Done about the Guilty?" p. 34). See also Neier, *War Crimes.* The later rearrest of General Massera may augur a resurgence of official interest in ending impunity in Argentina.

32. For overviews, see Guillermoprieto, *The Heart That Bleeds;* Chomsky, *Turning the Tide;* LaFeber, *Inevitable Revolutions.* For a case study from El Salvador, see Binford, *The El Mozote Massacre;* Danner, "The Truth at El Mozote"; Danner, *The Massacre at El Mozote.*

33. Bourdieu et al., *La misère du monde,* p. 944; my translation.

34. Ignatieff, *Human Rights as Politics and Idolatry,* pp. 19–20, 22–23.

35. For an overview of critiques of anthropology as a colonial project, see Asad, *Anthropology and the Colonial Encounter.* See also the classic essays by Dell Hymes ("The Uses of Anthropology") and Gerald Berreman ("'Bringing It All Back Home'").

These debates resonate with recent critiques of U.S.-funded AIDS research in the developing world. For her comparison of placebo studies of HIV-infected mothers in Africa with the Tuskegee syphilis experiments on African Americans, *New England Journal of Medicine* editor Marcia Angell was taken to task by prominent figures in the scientific community (see, for example, Varmus and Satcher, "Ethical Complexities of Conducting Research in Developing Countries"), and two influential AIDS specialists resigned from the editorial board of the journal in protest (Saltus, "Journal Departures Reflect AIDS Dispute"). The debate continued with a *New York Times* front-page exploration of the ironies of U.S.-funded AIDS research in the Ivory Coast (French, "AIDS Research in Africa"). Angell justified her analogy by making a point-by-point comparison between the AIDS trials and the infamous syphilis study ("Tuskegee Revisited").

36. From the album *Manno Charlemagne;* my translation, with the help of the songwriter, Manno Charlemagne.

37. For overviews of the type and extent of international aid to these regimes, see Farmer, *The Uses of Haiti;* Hancock, *Lords of Poverty.*

38. See Wallerstein, "The Insurmountable Contradictions of Liberalism."

39. Farmer, *AIDS and Accusation.*

40. Steiner and Alston, *International Human Rights in Context,* p. 1110.

41. Harrison, "Voodoo Politics," p. 102. For a discussion of this position, see Farmer, *The Uses of Haiti,* p. 57. Lawrence Harrison subsequently became director of the entire agency.

42. Comandancia General del EZLN, "Primera declaración de la Selva Lacandona"; my translation.

43. Compare the situation in Chiapas to the impact of militarization in the Philippines, as described by Lynn Kwiatkowski in *Struggling with Development.*

44. Physicians for Human Rights, *Health Care Held Hostage,* p. 4.

45. Neier, *War Crimes,* p. 50.

46. I refer here to the case of Michael Fay, an eighteen-year-old U.S. citizen convicted of vandalizing cars and tearing down traffic signs in Singapore. According to the *Fort Worth Star-Telegram,* "Amnesty International sees the Fay case as one more reason to refocus international attention on the inhumaneness of flogging." But "many Americans," according to the article, were "surprisingly unsympathetic to the plight of the Ohio youth" (DeWitt, "Many Americans Back Singapore's Decision to Flog Teen"). The piece went on to claim that letters to the editor of the *Dayton Daily*

News, Fay's hometown newspaper, were "running against the youth," and the Singapore embassy in Washington, D.C., asserted that the majority of mail it received supported Singapore's position.

47. This trend has already occasioned much commentary in the popular and scholarly literature. See, for example, Gitlin, *The Twilight of Common Dreams;* Glendon, *Rights Talk;* Hughes, *Culture of Complaint;* Jacoby, *Dogmatic Wisdom.* Todd Gitlin notes trenchantly that "the politics of identity is silent on the deepest sources of social misery: the devastation of the cities, the draining of resources away from the public and into the private hands of the few. It does not organize to reduce the sickening inequality between rich and poor" (*The Twilight of Common Dreams,* p. 236).

48. For an overview of the legal controversy over a hierarchy of rights, see Steiner and Alston, *International Human Rights in Context,* pp. 128–31. See also Alston's 1984 discussion of the proliferation of proposed rights, which have ranged from the "right to sleep" to the "right to tourism" ("Conjuring Up New Human Rights").

49. The passion of Chouchou Louis is recounted in Farmer, *The Uses of Haiti,* pp. 244–62; and in chapter 16 of this volume.

50. With the help of courageous colleagues in Haiti, it was possible for North Americans to work in solidarity on several levels following this killing. For example, an account of the murder of Chouchou Louis appeared under David Nyhan's name in the *Boston Globe* (Nyhan, "Murder in Haiti"). Subsequent accounts appeared in a political magazine and in my book *The Uses of Haiti.* Pax Christi visited central Haiti in the spring of 1992 and interviewed torture victims and the families of the disappeared, including the widow of Chouchou Louis; see Pax Christi International, *Pax Christi Newsletter.*

51. Precisely the same pattern has been well documented in El Salvador and Guatemala; for a comparison of these two countries and Haiti, see Farmer, *The Uses of Haiti,* pp. 197–213.

The effects of the 1991 coup d'état on the health of the local population are explored in Farmer, "Haiti's Lost Years," and discussed in Farmer and Bertrand, "Hypocrisies of Development and the Health of the Haitian Poor." For a penetrating view of "Operation Uphold Democracy," as the 1994 U.S.-led restoration of Aristide was termed, see Shacochis, *The Immaculate Invasion.* In the 2000 elections, the Haitian people again turned out in force (in contrast to the spurious reporting in the official press and the U.S. media) to hand an overwhelming majority to Aristide and other members of Fanmi Lavalas, the party he founded. To the majority of Haitians, Aristide is still associated with the primary goals of the Haitian popular movement—social and economic rights for the poor.

52. For more on these events and related topics, see Concannon, "Beyond Complementarity."

53. Even after the Salvadoran army's murderous rampages against unarmed civilians were confirmed by indisputable evidence—in the form of eyewitness reports from survivor Rufina Amaya, forensic data, and front-page stories in the *New York Times* and the *Washington Post*—the Reagan administration had little trouble "recertifying" El Salvador as a country that respected human rights: "In the United States, the free press was not to be denied: El Mozote was reported; Rufina's story was told; the angry debate in Congress intensified. But then the Republican Administration, burdened as it was with the heavy duties of national security, denied that any credible evidence existed that a massacre had taken place; and the Democratic Congress, after denouncing, yet again, the murderous abuses of the Salvadoran regime, in the end accepted the Administration's 'certification' that its ally was nonetheless making a 'significant effort to comply with internationally recognized human rights.' The flow of aid went on, and soon increased" (Danner, "The Truth at El Mozote," p. 53). Meanwhile, the sole Latin American country that is not a U.S. client state has endured repeated U.S. attempts to discredit it on human rights grounds. This is in large part because the United States has used human rights arguments as a means of advancing its own foreign policy but also because, as Peter Schwab notes, "economic and social rights are fundamental in Cuba" (*Cuba,* p. 9).

54. Danner, "The Truth at El Mozote," p: 132. Mark Danner quotes from the Truth Commission's report (Comisión de la Verdad para El Salvador, "De la locura a la esperanza"). See also Danner, *The Massacre at El Mozote*.

55. At the time of this writing, Chiapas remains wracked by officially tolerated—perhaps sanctioned—paramilitary violence.

56. Physicians for Human Rights, *Health Care Held Hostage*, p. 4.

57. Virchow, *Die Einheitsbestrebungen in der Wissenschaftlichen Medicin*, p. 48. See also Eisenberg, "Rudolf Ludwig Karl Virchow, Where Are You Now That We Need You?"

58. Mann and Tarantola, "Responding to HIV/AIDS," p. 8. See also the collection of articles in Mann et al., *Health and Human Rights*. For a review of documents that provide the basis for an international human right to health, as established through international conventions and laws as well as in the constitutions of various nations (but not that of the United States), see Kinney, "The International Human Right to Health."

59. Simonov interview.

60. Henkin, *International Law, Politics, Values, and Functions*, p. 208.

61. Oscar Schachter has observed: "International law must also be seen as the product of historical experience in which power and the 'relation of forces' are determinants. Those States with power (i.e., the ability to control the outcomes contested by others) will have a disproportionate and often decisive influence in determining the content of rules and their application in practice. Because this is the case, international law, in a broad sense, both reflects and sustains the existing political order and distribution of power" (*International Law in Theory and Practice*, p. 6).

Furthermore, legal commentary often reminds us of the power of normative, procedural thinking. During and after the Nuremberg trials, there was debate—again, cast in legal terms—over whether the trials themselves were legal or merely reflected "victors' justice." The *American Journal of International Law* published some key trial documents in 1947: "It was urged on behalf of the defendants that a fundamental principle of all law—international and domestic—is that there can be no punishment of crime without a pre-existing law. . . . It was submitted that ex post facto punishment is abhorrent to the law of all civilized nations" (International Military Tribunal [Nuremberg], "Judgment and Sentences," p. 173). In other words, the defense argued that if there had been no law against genocide or "aggressive war" on the books before the fact, it would therefore have been illegitimate to prosecute the Nazis for these actions. Those arguing the illegality of the Nuremberg trials were not fringe elements. Citing such concerns, U.S. Chief Justice Harlan Fiske Stone referred to the "high-grade lynching party in Nuremberg" (quoted in Mason, *Harlan Fiske Stone*, p. 746). Justice Radhabinod Pal's similar dissent from the Tokyo War Crimes Tribunal is well known.

62. Farmer, Léandre, Mukherjee, Claude, et al., "Community-Based Approaches to HIV Treatment in Resource-Poor Settings."

63. I do not refer here to historical investigation, which is crucial to an understanding of the dynamics of structural violence. But the study of human rights abuses in the slave trade, for example, or in the silver mines of fifth-century B.C. Greece, is quite different from an investigation of ongoing, documentable suffering.

64. Neier, *War Crimes*, p. xiii.

65. Steiner and Alston, *International Human Rights in Context*, p. viii.

66. For more on this initiative, see Physicians for Human Rights, "Health Action AIDS Campaign."

67. For a review of widening outcome gaps and their relationship to economic policy, see Kim, Millen, et al., *Dying for Growth*.

68. For an overview of this group and its "vitality of practice," see Farmer, *Infections and Inequalities*, chap. 1.

69. Ignatieff, *Human Rights as Politics and Idolatry*, p. 35; paragraphing altered.

70. Krieger, "Embodying Inequality," p. 295.

71. An example of this approach can be found in Asad's recent discussion of torture and modern human rights discourse. He notes: "If cruelty is increasingly represented in the language of rights (and especially of human rights), this is because *perpetual legal struggle* has now become the dominant mode of moral engagement in an interconnected, uncertain, and rapidly changing world" ("On Torture, or Cruel, Inhuman, and Degrading Treatment," pp. 304–5).

72. Neugebauer, "Research on Violence in Developing Countries," p. 1474.

73. Mann, "AIDS and Human Rights," pp. 145–46.

74. Neier, *War Crimes,* pp. 23–24.

75. Physicians for Human Rights, *Health Care Held Hostage,* p. 12.

76. Gitlin, *The Twilight of Common Dreams,* p. 224.

77. Steiner and Alston, *International Human Rights in Context,* p. 1140.

78. Ignatieff, *Human Rights as Politics and Idolatry,* p. 172.

79. See, for example, the website entitled "Bill Gates's Personal Wealth Clock," http://philip.greenspun.com/WealthClock (accessed July 28, 2009).

22

Rethinking Medical Ethics

A View from Below

(2004)

Paul Farmer and Nicole Gastineau Campos

Bioethics and medical ethics are necessarily contentious enterprises. These fields have the potential to embrace not only empiric research but philosophical commentary, informed opinion, and essay as well. The best scholarship in these related fields often addresses "unresolved issues" of moral conflict. Some issues are unresolved because they stem from novel developments, such as xenotransplantation or the latest in stem cell research; other issues are unresolved because too little attention has been paid to them in recent decades, in part because the discipline of medical ethics has arisen in certain social contexts and not in others. We argue here that lack of access to the fruits of modern medicine and the science that informs it is an important and neglected topic within bioethics and medical ethics. This is especially clear to those working in what are now termed "resource-poor settings," or, to put it in plain language, among populations living in dire poverty.

AIDS research has been a case in point. In a commentary on the ethics of HIV vaccine trials, physician Joia Mukherjee voiced in print what many who do not read or write are saying about the ethics of AIDS research conducted in settings in which AIDS is now the leading infectious cause of adult death:

> When asked, "Have you no morals?" Alfred Doolittle, in George Bernard Shaw's *Pygmalion*, answered, "Can't afford them, governor. Neither could you if you was as poor as me." The modern concept of human rights underpins a moral society and holds government responsible for fulfilling those rights. From informed consent to the right to privacy, civil and political rights have dominated the human rights focus of the HIV-1 epidemic. Yet the economic and social rights of people with HIV-1 infection, in particular the rights to health care and to share in scientific advances, are glaringly disparate between rich and poor countries. This disparity has become the focus of debate in transnational HIV-1 vaccine research.[1]

Mukherjee's commentary will resonate with some and rankle others. But many who would find her views compelling will never read a medical journal because they do not read; others read but do not have access to journals. These are the people whose views we seek to transmit in offering a view of medical ethics "from below."

What is meant by "a view from below"? What is not intended by this expression? We have offered elsewhere a critique of the scholarship on suffering from the perspective of people living in great poverty.[2] Imbalances of power are present in all medical exchanges: between well and sick, expert and nonexpert, white and black—the list goes on. But the language of academic medicine and public health can mask these asymmetries. In a 1992 book, Howard Brody asserted that "the word *power* is essentially absent from the vocabulary that scholars of medical ethics have constructed for their discipline and that has been accepted by almost everyone who does work in the field or tries to apply medical-ethics insights to the clinical context."[3] Now consider this statement's meaning when taken beyond the boundaries of the world's most affluent nations, the birthplace of professional societies of medical ethicists and bioethicists. Since the topic of medical rationing, which implies scarcity, is a staple of the medical ethics literature,[4] it would seem essential to consider the effects of rationing on the world's poor, especially the poor of the poorest countries. But when the question "Who shall live?" is posed, these people do not figure in the discussion.

Subaltern populations within rich and middle-income countries have long been involved in key dramas of medical ethics: witness the withholding of treatment in the Tuskegee syphilis study, which followed six hundred African American men in Alabama from 1932 to 1972 and continues to have its echoes even today.[5] Similar experiences have been documented in Europe, South Africa, and Brazil.[6] But to this day, the poorest people in the poorest countries are likely to appear only in the margins of the bioethics literature, if they appear at all. We have seen their critiques of research ethics dismissed as confused and ill-informed commentary or as "conspiracy theories." But in-depth and sympathetic explorations suggest that much is to be gleaned from such critiques.[7]

The point of view of people living in great poverty anticipates many of the perspectives advanced by the "socializing disciplines," including anthropology, history, political economy, and the sociology of knowledge. Resocializing medical ethics is a necessary move in our globalized, market-driven world, as a rejoinder to the dominant psychological or individualist readings of social problems ranging from addiction to AIDS to "noncompliance" with medical regimens: such readings are in effect a means of blaming the victims and serve to keep much-needed resources out of reach.[8] Our experience in Haiti and the United States suggests that both medical ethics and the human rights discourse that supports much of the thinking in medical ethics would profit from a change in perspective. One of us being a physician-anthropologist and the other a special-ist in health policy, we are equipped to offer divergent views; but we start from critiques internal to medical ethics.

WHAT'S WRONG WITH MEDICAL ETHICS?

In the social field in which bioethics and medical ethics have emerged—affluent industrialized countries, by and large, and within the past few decades—prac-titioners of these disciplines are seen, by themselves and by others, as liberal reformers. Among them, we can discern three major and overlapping groups. Within clinical settings, ethicists are the guardians of morally sound practice and a safeguard against abuses. By the close of the twentieth century, most major teaching hospitals had ethics committees; many boast in-house ethicists who are active in addressing the quandary ethics of individual patients. As often as not, ethics consultations in such hospitals address discord between patients' families and medical staff or withdrawal of care for those deemed unlikely to be saved by "heroic interventions." The salutary impact of these developments is not disputed.

A second major stream of medical ethics is constituted by the everyday practice of ethics within modern biomedical research. The research arena has been home to an explosive growth of institutional review boards (IRBs); human subjects committees abound. Disclaimers regarding potential personal gain are required when one publishes data, and it is not possible to publish even photographs or comments of patients without "ethical clearance." In the university with which we are affiliated, students cannot undertake research involving human subjects without going through an ethics course and filling out an application. These are positive developments, coherent with a philosophy of individual autonomy and respect for the patient. But the proliferation of such committees and regulations does not correlate with a more ethical treatment of the destitute sick. To observe this discrepancy, let us take a global perspective.

It is possible to read, for example, front-page exposés of research projects in Africa conducted by First World universities and learn that, although research subjects have signed informed-consent forms, they have no clear notion about what the research explores or how they figure in the endeavor.[9] Other research projects, duly blessed by multiple review boards in both the research university and the host country, call up memories of Tuskegee. Consider studies involving placebo controls in AZT trials attempting to develop a cheaper drug regimen to prevent mother-to-child transmission (MTCT) of HIV.[10] Research subjects found to be infected with HIV received no therapy for their disease if they were assigned to the control group. Even though the U.S. Public Health Service had begun recommending the use of zidovudine to prevent MTCT in 1994, a review by Peter Lurie and Sidney Wolfe in 1997 counted fifteen studies taking place in developing countries in which some or all of the participants were not receiving antiretroviral therapy to prevent MTCT.[11]

Marcia Angell, editor of the *New England Journal of Medicine,* drew the comparison to Tuskegee and chastised the National Institutes of Health and the Centers for Disease Control and Prevention for funding several such projects: "Many studies are done in the Third World that simply could not be done in the countries sponsoring the work. Clinical trials have become a big business, with many of the same imperatives. To survive, it is necessary to get the work done as quickly as possible, with a minimum of obstacles. When these considerations prevail, it seems as if we have not come very far from Tuskegee after all."[12] This is not simply a matter of seeking lower costs or larger markets abroad, as businesses are wont to do. The majority of such international biomedical research has inequality as its foundation, and ethical codes developed in affluent countries are quickly ditched as soon as affluent universities undertake research in poor countries. Then come a series of efforts to develop alternative (that is, less stringent) codes "appropriate" to settings of destitution.

A third strand of work, less closely tied to clinical care or research endeavors, is teaching and scholarship on bioethics and medical ethics. Again, the explosive growth of these fields is easy to gauge simply by looking at journals, publications, and the number of faculty appointments within schools of medicine, nursing, and public health. Many of these scholars have formal training in both medicine and philosophy.

Critique internal to this discipline focuses on the technicality or triviality of professional commentary, and the gulf between specialist hair-splitting and the dilemmas of choice facing patients, families, and caregivers. In this spirit, Larry Churchill observes: "Bioethical disputes—as measured by the debates in journals and conferences in the United States—often seem to be remote from the values of ordinary people and largely irrelevant to the decisions they encounter in health care. In this sense, philosophical theorizing might be considered harmless entertainment, which if taken too seriously would look ridiculous, as several Monty Python skits have successfully demonstrated."[13] Churchill's critique of philosophical theorizing is even more poignant when applied to "ordinary people" who do not have access to modern health care—to people whose desperation might lead them to agree to take part in a Tuskegee-style clinical trial in Kenya or Uganda today.

If medical ethics is about decision and informed consent, what of the decisions made by the world's poorest, who are also, by any honest accounting, the globe's sickest? We have found it useful to go directly to the destitute sick and interview them about what they regard as their ranking problems and thus to elicit their views on the ethics of research.

In so doing, we emulate certain principles of John Rawls's theory of justice. Rawls is, of course, famous for his difference principle, which requires preferential treatment for the most disadvantaged, regardless of the social costs this principle can entail.[14] Critics have rightly noted the principle's underemphasis on health,[15] but one can read Rawls as making a broader point about how we should view social practices, including the practice of evaluating the common good.

We draw on our experience with infectious diseases in some of the poorest communities in the world to interrogate the central imperatives of bioethics and medical ethics. AIDS, tuberculosis, and malaria are the three leading infectious killers of adults in the world today. Because each disease is treatable with already available therapies, the lack of access to medical care is widely perceived in heavily disease-burdened areas as constituting an ethical and moral scandal.[16] To quote a woman who had returned to central Haiti, dying of AIDS, after years in the city, "We're good enough to study but not good enough to care for." This woman, who later received therapy for her disease and stopped dying, did not lose her passion for the topic after her own lack of care was addressed and she began to respond to antiretroviral therapy. In another interview, conducted in her home, she expounded at some length:[17]

> I was diagnosed [with HIV infection] because of a research project that [a U.S. research university] was doing. That was ten years ago. This was in [a slum in Port-au-Prince]. I went back a lot to have my blood drawn, but I never got any treatment. And I knew from the radio that other people received treatment. These were people who could pay two hundred dollars a month. They were people who could go and make a deposit at a bank and then they'd get their medicines for a month. I came home [to central Haiti] to die, but even now that I'm better, I'm still angry about it. Ten years of them sucking my blood and nothing! I was a skeleton sitting on the bench waiting for them to call my name. It's when I got to be a skeleton that the nurse told me that I didn't have to come any more. It's as if poor people were animals. But we won't serve as their guinea pigs [*Men nou p'ap sevi kom kobay yo*].[18]

Although the expression "First World diagnostics and Third World therapeutics" may not be the term commonly used in Haiti, the idea behind the expression has wide currency among patients and nonpatients there. This is because, for many infectious diseases, the research enterprise is fundamentally a transnational one. It is also a fundamentally inegalitarian exercise in the sense that medicine and science are expanding rapidly, but in a social context of growing global inequality, which ensures that the fruits of medicine and science are not available to many who need them most.[19]

Medicine, public health, and research are all caught up in a web of unequal relations. The link between research on AIDS and access to therapy for HIV has been the most scrutinized. But other startling examples abound. Organ transplantation is a disturbing case in point. In countries as poor as Haiti, organ transplantation is altogether unknown, but it is common in wealthier but inegalitarian countries and regions throughout the developing world. Trafficking in organs occurs in predictable ways—predictable, that is, to those who look at social inequalities across borders. To quote one anthropologist who works on this topic, "the flow of organs follows the modern routes of capital: from South to North, from Third to First World, from poor to rich, from black and brown to white, and from female to male."[20]

The unbalanced dynamic of organ donation in the poor world has been noted by other anthropologists[21] and by adventurous ethicists as well. Although egregious violations of rights are easily discerned—the literature is rife with stories of organs, from kidneys to corneas, quite literally stolen—the greater problem is the legal and "ethically approved" transfer of organs across social gradients. The ethical codes currently in place, in other words, have not prevented but rather have worked to justify abuses grounded, however subtly, in growing inequalities.

When someone living in destitution "opts" to sell a kidney and signs all informed-consent forms in front of multiple witnesses, is the term "informed consent" really meaningful? What degree of "information" grounds the consent? One expects that the donor will have been informed about the medical risks inherent in the operation, but has there been a discussion about the donor's chances of survival without the money disbursed upon donation?

So it is with much AIDS research. If individuals living in slums in African cities, unable to read and write, are to participate in clinical trials, what sort of process must they go through in order to provide informed consent? Or is there a darker possibility, that research conducted across such deep gradients of inequality is itself fundamentally coercive unless special measures are taken? And what would those special measures be?

These questions get at one of the oldest and most fraught debates within social theory: the reticulated relationship between structure and agency. A "view from below" would ask how poverty, racism, and gender inequality come to constrain agency, the ability to make choices. If one believes—as we do—in the ability of research to lessen misery and suffering, what ethical measures might compensate for the pursuit of research in settings of great poverty? How might we ensure that the measures are not in and of themselves coercive, as many incentives are deemed to be?

To answer these and related questions, it is necessary to reframe the problems at hand—the quest for vaccines, say, or novel therapeutics or organ transplantation—as social action in order to have a broader view of the inequalities in which such endeavors are grounded, whether or not researchers see them. Efforts to resocialize problems allow all concerned to have a more meaningful understanding of what the research subjects (or organ donors) hope to gain from participating in what are, often enough, their only encounters with modern biomedicine. Even a preliminary attempt to consider these topics in their broader social contexts allows us to come to a preliminary conclusion: the more desperate the poverty of sample populations (research subjects or organ donors who live in poverty, sick prisoners), the greater the constraint on their agency. In other words, the steeper the gradient of social inequality across which such transactions occur, the greater the risk of abuse without the "special measures" we discuss later in this essay.

One of the ways of rethinking medical ethics is to make the "outcome gap" a central ethical issue. The term "outcome gap" admits of many meanings, but here we follow the example of pediatrician Paul Wise, who some years ago interrogated conventional wisdom regarding low birth weights in the urban United States, where race and class are strongly associated with rates of premature delivery, with weight at birth, and with rates of infant mortality. In the last quarter of the twentieth century, these oft-noted disparities of outcome led to a movement to divert money from neonatal intensive care units (NICUs) to improving social conditions for African American women. But Wise argued that such a diversion would not get to the heart of the matter: "Too often, those who elevate the role of social determinants indict clinical technologies as failed strategies. But devaluing clinical intervention diverts attention from the essential goal that it be provided equitably to all those in need. Belittling the role of clinical care tends to unburden policy of the requirement to provide equitable access to such care."[22]

Arguments about resource allocation—a perennial staple of commentary within medical ethics—are not really "socialized," since they do not include an honest accounting of how an affluent society, or even a city, chooses to spend available resources. Resocializing the problem of low birth rate would require frank discussion of racism, the juxtaposition of subsidies for private enterprise and shrinking resources for public facilities, military expenditures, and the growing gap between rich and poor. It would also require careful consideration of equitable access to clinical care. These topics are rarely encountered in professional journals devoted to medical ethics. Perhaps they are deemed "too political." Indeed.

And so it is with each of the problems mentioned in this essay: AIDS, chronic renal failure, prison-seated epidemics of tuberculosis, and racial disparities in infant mortality. Each problem has generated debates within medical ethics, and new technologies to address them may generate debates within bioethics. But it is possible to discern in scholarly discourse what might be termed a "Luddite approach" to the problem: the position that we should halt AIDS research in resource-poor settings, we should stop performing kidney transplants, we should focus exclusively on prison reform rather than treating epidemic tuberculosis within prisons, and we should stop building NICUs. We might assume that such unwelcome conclusions would emerge only as a reductio ad absurdum retort to the charge that modern medicine practices and manages inequality ("if you insist on treating everyone equally, then you must be against providing excellent services to anyone"). But such a position, far from being a mere rhetorical dodge, is expressed not only within the medical ethics scholarship but also in its applied echoes in clinical medicine, medical education, and public health.

We oppose the Luddite trap. Each of the dilemmas discussed here calls for new and better technologies, whether they are for managing renal failure or for developing a vaccine for AIDS. To argue, as we do, that the primary ethical issue of modern medicine and public health is the outcome gap, itself rooted in transnational and growing social inequalities, is not to argue for merely shuffling around research and service priorities with decisions based on primitive notions of cost-effectiveness, the latest fashion in policymaking. The problem is much deeper. Indeed, we have argued elsewhere that the growing outcome gap constitutes the chief human rights challenge of the twenty-first century.[23] This assertion will seem odd to many who consider themselves experts in the field of human rights, accustomed as they are to exhorting governments to respect civil and political rights. But social and economic rights are of paramount importance in settings of poverty, which are also settings of excess morbidity and mortality.

What does it mean, for both bioethics and human rights, when a person living in poverty is able to vote, is protected from torture or imprisonment without due process, but dies of untreated AIDS? What does it mean when a person with renal failure experiences no abuse of his or her civil and political rights, but dies without ever having been offered access to dialysis, to say nothing of transplants? What does it mean when an African American neonate does not have ready access to the care afforded only in a NICU?

The concept of the "Third World" is a clog on the imagination. The world's poor do not live on another planet, nor do they live in countries where such technologies are unavailable. Surveys have shown that even in the world's poorest countries, wealthy people have ready access to both antiretroviral agents and therapy for renal insufficiency; NICUs are close at hand for infants born to affluent families. At the same time, even in wealthy nations, the poor do not have reliable access to good medical care or to the fruits of medical science. To give the Luddites their due, the ethical problem thus delineated grows more pressing with the development of every innovative and more effective therapy. The problem is new because some of the diseases and all of the technologies are new. In the absence of an equity plan, improvements in care add to a growing outcome gap—the unmentioned elephant in the room of medical ethics.

LINKING BIOETHICS TO SOCIAL ANALYSIS:
RETHINKING THE CASE OF TUBERCULOSIS IN PRISONS

We have underlined two steps that would make medical ethics more credible in settings of great poverty: using the socializing disciplines to frame the ethical dilemmas faced by people without resources or broad agency; and, in a related gambit, using them to see the destitute sick not just as reservoirs of antibodies or organs but as agents facing economic, social, and political predicaments. A third step is to link research across steep gradients with the interventions that are demanded by the poor or otherwise marginalized. In the cases cited earlier, understanding the ethics of AIDS research in Africa or Haiti would rely heavily on interviewing people living with both poverty and this disease. But what is true for AIDS is true for most other maladies afflicting the poor disproportionately.

The example of prisoners in Russia who are sick with drug-resistant tuberculosis helps to underline the shortcomings of current approaches to these problems.[24] To summarize a complex biosocial process in a few words: A doubling of incarceration rates occurred after the collapse of the Soviet Union. In "democratic" Russia, the number of prisoners in the infamous gulag more than tripled, with Siberian incarceration rates exceeding, at one point, 1,000 per 100,000 population (only the United States rivals this ratio). Overcrowding, poor ventilation, interruption of medical supplies and salaries for overworked prison staff, and malnutrition led to explosive epidemics of tuberculosis within Russia's prisons. But theirs was not the tuberculosis seen in Haiti or sub-Saharan Africa. In some senses, the Russian epidemics were more reminiscent of the prison-seated outbreaks documented in New York beginning in the late 1980s: although HIV was not a factor in the Russian epidemics, they involved strains of highly drug-resistant *Mycobacterium tuberculosis* in a tightly packed carceral population.[25]

Into this dramatic and novel situation came, for the first time, non-Russian aid agencies and nongovernmental organizations. To date, there have been few thorough studies of this stunning development.[26] By the mid-1990s, such organizations were prominent players in post-Soviet states, all of which had seen catastrophic deterioration in their social safety nets and medical systems. The nongovernmental organizations were mostly European and North American, and in the post-perestroika disarray they had something their Russian (and Azeri, Georgian, Kazakh, and so forth) partners did not then have: money and clout. The ability of these aid organizations to shape responses to epidemic tuberculosis in Siberia was significant. They insisted on what they termed the most "cost-effective" approach, the one endorsed by international tuberculosis experts, including the World Health Organization: directly observed therapy with "first-line" antituberculous drugs.

But some of the Russian prison physicians objected, as did members of Russia's large and crumbling tuberculosis treatment infrastructure: the prisoner-patients had drug-resistant tuberculosis and would not be cured by standard first-line regimens. Other legal and humanitarian objections were expressed as well. These voices were drowned in an undercurrent of officious opinion from the international experts and the nongovernmental agencies, which, flush with resources and backed by international expert opinion, insisted on giving all prisoners the same doses of the same first-line drugs.

In Siberia and in other pilot sites, treatment outcomes were nothing short of catastrophic: fewer than half of all patients were deemed cured (expected cure rates for supervised therapy of drug-susceptible tuberculosis exceed 95 percent).[27] Worse, prisoner-patients who were not cured by therapy with first-line drugs emerged from this treatment, if they survived, with "amplified" resistance. That is, their prognosis had worsened dramatically even if they were to be afforded care with the right drugs.[28] But the non-Russian groups, whether international tuberculosis experts or aid groups, did not concede that they had made an error. Instead, they pressed on, delivering precisely the same medications even to prisoner-patients with documented multidrug-resistant tuberculosis.

More delegations visited Siberia in 1998. Members of at least one delegation pointed out that drug resistance was not the *likely* cause of treatment failure; it was the cause *already documented*. Somewhat discreetly, it would seem, the lead nongovernmental organization had sent sputum samples for drug-susceptibility testing to at least two reference laboratories in Western Europe. Both laboratories confirmed that patients within Siberian prisons were sick from highly resistant strains of M. *tuberculosis*—strains resistant to precisely those drugs being administered, under direct supervision, by the nongovernmental organizations that had been chastising Russian experts for their lack of knowledge of modern tuberculosis control.

Well before 2000, tuberculosis had become the leading cause of death in Russian prisons. In Siberian facilities, surviving prisoners had become less and less treatable, and patients with multidrug-resistant tuberculosis were cohorted behind barbed wire and declared altogether "untreatable." But this was not the case: multidrug-resistant tuberculosis is treatable with other, more expensive drugs; data from a slum in Peru and rural Haiti have made it clear that such efforts can succeed in settings far poorer than Siberia.[29] The real debate was not about the efficacy of therapy but about its costs.

In 2001, the lead nongovernmental organization appeared to yield to growing pressure from prisoners, their guards, and expert opinion: it would work with its Russian partners to treat patients with multidrug-resistant tuberculosis using the drugs to which their strains had been shown to be susceptible. It took the organization well over a year to procure the drugs. Early in 2002, it announced that the treatment program was to commence right away. The need was great: a single oblast in western Siberia counted some two thousand prisoner-patients, warehoused with active multidrug-resistant tuberculosis. Drugs began to arrive in Siberia, but, unaccountably, no treatment occurred in the ensuing year. In September 2003, the lead organization issued a press release: they were pulling out of Siberia. As of today, not a single prisoner in Siberia has been treated for multidrug-resistant tuberculosis by nongovernmental organizations based there for a decade, although thousands, perhaps more, have died of this disease. The press release blames Russian officials, particularly those in the Ministry of Health, for their intransigence, but it is likely that careful study of what occurred will come to a somewhat different conclusion.[30]

The story is a sad one, but worse is yet to come. Circulating strains of multidrug-resistant *M. tuberculosis* will mean that prisoners and detainees are exposed to epidemic strains of highly drug-resistant tuberculosis and then do not receive care when they need it. The international authorities that presented themselves as the patients' advocates endorsed treatment regimens that, far from curing the disease, amplified it. They should have been the first to acknowledge their error and then pledge to help correct it. But no mea culpa has been issued by any of the decision makers involved.

All interested parties, including those willing to underline the ethical and technical lapses of such deficient care, must be part of a broader movement not merely to point to error, be it masked or acknowledged, but also to address it. In the case of multidrug-resistant tuberculosis in Russian prisons, that means staying there and seeing these patients through treatment that is effective, not simply "cost-effective." The practice of giving prisoners with drug-resistant tuberculosis drugs that had an effectiveness of zero, whatever their cost, reminds us that concepts such as "cost-effectiveness" are in fact ideological constructs. If we take Rawls seriously, we have to ask ourselves if we truly care about the most disadvantaged when we give prisoners therapy of this kind.[31] Cases like this one outline, in our view, the most pressing questions for medical ethics today.

ALTERNATIVE AND COMPLEMENTARY FRAMEWORKS: PRAXIS MAKES PERFECT?

Cases like those we have described have received scant attention in the medical ethics literature, and much of that attention has been inaccurate. To blame a lack of HIV care on beleaguered and cash-poor African governments is similar to blaming tuberculosis outbreaks in Siberia on prolonged pre-trial detention or the malfeasance of local prison officials. Such observations are superficial and also self-serving, since they deflect attention from the truly powerful forces that shape epidemics and the actors who declare which interventions are cost-effective and which are not. These decision makers are more likely to be found in New York, Washington, Geneva, or London than in Siberia, Port-au-Prince, or Pretoria. And those are precisely the people who need to be educated in the workings of social inequality, the context and driving force of the world's great epidemics.[32] One lesson of Tuskegee is that ethics may take decades to catch up with observations that come quite naturally to those marginalized by poverty and racism.

Here we quote another Haitian woman whose commentary easily spans the gulf from access to AIDS therapies to the right to employment. She made these comments in 2001 after gaining more than twenty pounds on antiretroviral medications:

> We're always sick here. If we're not dying of AIDS, we're dying of hunger, or both. Now that I am better, it's not as if my problems have disappeared. It's that I can wake up and fight them again. For two years I lay in bed, my children watching me die, bringing me sips of water. . . . [Their father] is gone—my sister has seven children of her own. All I could think about was what will happen to my children when I die? My sister had already purchased my coffin but then [the clinic] gave me these [antiretroviral] medicines. Someone comes to see me every day, to make sure I take them. The first thing that hit me was hunger. The medicines started killing the virus and then I became hungry. But we had no food in the house—how would that be possible, if [the father of her children] were gone and I was dying? Charity food does not allow you to regain your strength and to feed your children at the same time. That's why we always reach the same conclusions in our [support group meetings]. If you want to prevent AIDS among poor women, give them jobs. . . . I'm happy I'm better, and I'd rather be alive than dead. But all I do every day, still, is worry about how I'm going to feed my children. I don't want to become a thief.

This woman did not need to spend years in graduate school before she could link the biomedical, social, and economic constraints on human agency. Medical ethics extends to questions of basic equity.

Listening to the afflicted is not merely moral praxis, although it is that. It affords us rich insights into the sorts of problems that we have outlined in this essay. Because the poor quite literally embody many of the ethical dilemmas stemming from injustices within medicine and public health, they add insights that cannot be obtained through reference to philosophy, statistics, or policy papers. Ethical reflection is part of everyday life, and when the stakes are high— in a squatter settlement in Haiti, say, or a prison in western Siberia—soliciting these views is central to the quest for understanding. With the exception of sociopaths, as Churchill notes, the capacity to think critically about moral values and direct our actions in terms of such values "is common to all of us."[33]

Although ethics and philosophy have long been entangled in religious reflection, there is thus far very little synergy between medical ethics and the one branch of theology that concerns itself chiefly with the problem of poverty in the modern world. The conclusions of Marcio Fabri dos Anjos are worth citing here: "First, to what level of quality can medical ethics aspire, if it ignores callous discrimination in medical practice against large populations of the innocent poor? Second, how effective can such theories be in addressing the critical issues of medical and clinical ethics if they are unable to contribute to the closing of the gap of socio-medical disparity?"[34]

We anticipate that those who study ethical dilemmas will increasingly be called to have a hand in remediating them. These calls will come from "below," from the afflicted themselves. The concept of pragmatic solidarity is instructive as medicine, science, and public health stumble and fall in the very regions most in need of them. AIDS in Africa and tuberculosis in prisons are cases in point. Pragmatic solidarity is a cumbersome term, perhaps, and one that makes many academics uncomfortable. Anthropologists, for example, have long argued that their task is to observe rather than intervene, but this claim is undermined by the arguments that anthropology's supposed neutrality was in fact perceived by others, including those studied, as a small but at times integral part of the colonial project.[35] So, too, researchers from the modern university are invariably actors in a social field, and medical ethicists who work across steep gradients of inequality are, all objections to the contrary notwithstanding, powerful actors when compared to those they study.

Listening to the poorest will lead us back, inevitably, to the outcome gap. The "special measures" mentioned earlier will vary from place to place and from problem to problem, but medical ethicists should expect to become part of teams seeking to lessen the outcome gap by remediating access to effective medical care. And once that step is taken, we will have the option of trying to ignore what we are being told by the afflicted, or to take seriously the challenge of linking the struggle for social and economic rights—the right to food, housing, clean water, education, and jobs—to scholarly inquiry that breaches the frighteningly deep gap between the haves and the have-nots.

CONCLUSIONS OR NEW DIRECTIONS?

Like any established fields of scholarly inquiry, bioethics and medical ethics are broad and large enough to contain their own internal critics. And like many practitioners of an academic discipline, ethicists are not always eager to embrace critiques from beyond the field. But this essay is meant merely to complement ongoing research and reflection within bioethics and medical ethics.

Writing of AIDS, historian Allan Brandt astutely predicts that "in the years ahead we will, no doubt, learn a great deal more about AIDS and how to control it. We will also learn a great deal about the nature of our society from the manner in which we address the disease. AIDS will be a standard by which we may measure not only our medical and scientific skill but also our capacity for justice and compassion."[36]

When Brandt writes of "our society," he refers to the global village through which HIV has raced. HIV treatment, like "our capacity for justice and compassion," has not been so quick to follow.

Research in medical ethics has thus far been conducted largely in affluent and industrialized nations. Yet these "resource-rich" settings are tied, and intimately so, to the poorest parts of the world. As a matter of self-awareness on the part of bioscientists and social researchers, the central topics of bioethics and medical ethics need to be linked to questions of social justice and to consideration of how inequalities of all sorts are also linked. In almost all countries in which medical ethics and bioethics have taken root—which is to say in most countries, at this writing—access to care, even access to informed participation in clinical trials, is determined as much by social standing as by disease process. This basic epidemiological and social fact emboldens us to close with a warning: if social inequalities persist and grow, we will no longer be welcome to conduct research or even to comment on it. To cite Joia Mukherjee again, "If the medical community is to use data generated in high-burden and vulnerable populations to develop an HIV-1 vaccine, we must ensure that the global community will help governments fulfill the right to health and share the fruits of research with the world's poorest communities."[37]

NOTES

1. Mukherjee, "HIV-1 Care in Resource-Poor Settings," p. 994.

2. Farmer, "On Suffering and Structural Violence" (included in this volume as chapter 16).

3. Brody, *The Healer's Power*, p. 12.

4. Fuchs, *Who Shall Live?*

5. Roughly four hundred of these men had syphilis, and most lived in poverty. Despite the 1947 discovery of a cure for the disease—to this day, syphilis is treated with penicillin—subjects were never offered that very inexpensive drug, even though they had joined the study assuming that they would be treated. Nor were they informed of the study's real purpose. See Reverby, *Tuskegee's Truths;* Brandt, *No Magic Bullet.*

6. See, for example, Dos Reis, "Norplant in Brazil," for commentary on Norplant trials in Brazil.

7. Farmer, *AIDS and Accusation.*

8. Lipovetsky, *L'ère du vide.*

9. French, "AIDS Research in Africa."

10. Also consider the more recent example of a randomized-control trial conducted between November 1994 and October 1998, which examined the relationship between serum viral load, concurrent sexually transmitted diseases, and other known and putative HIV risk factors. The research team screened 15,127 individuals in a rural district of Uganda, of whom 415 were identified as HIV-positive with an initially HIV-negative partner. The researchers then tracked these serodiscordant couples for thirty months, following the viral load of the infected partner and the rate of seroconversion among the previously uninfected partners. The study concludes that "viral load is

the chief predictor of the risk of heterosexual transmission of HIV-1" (Quinn et al., "Viral Load and Heterosexual Transmission of Human Immunodeficiency Virus Type 1").

In an accompanying editorial, *New England Journal of Medicine* editor Marcia Angell voiced her hesitation about publishing the study and was quite pointed in her criticism: "It is important to be clear about what this study meant for the participants. It meant that for up to 30 months, several hundred people with HIV infection were observed but not treated." Furthermore, "the very condition that justified doing the study in Uganda in the first place—the lack of availability of antiretroviral treatment—will greatly limit the relevance of the results there" ("Investigators' Responsibilities for Human Subjects in Developing Countries").

Explicit comparisons to Tuskegee were made in the popular press; in the electronic magazine *Slate,* one writer asked: "The . . . volunteers in the sample were not offered treatment nor were their healthy sex partners informed that the research subjects were HIV positive. Excuse please, but why isn't this like the [*New England Journal of Medicine*] supporting the Tuskegee experiments?" (Shuger, "Supreme Court Cover-Up").

11. Lurie and Wolfe, "Unethical Trials of Interventions to Reduce Perinatal Transmission of the Human Immunodeficiency Virus in Developing Countries."

12. Angell, "The Ethics of Clinical Research in the Third World."

13. Churchill, "Are We Professionals?" p. 255.

14. Rawls, *A Theory of Justice,* pp. 130–39, sec. 26, and pp. 65–73, sec. 13. John Rawls's more precise definition of the difference, or maximin, principle is that society must choose the scheme of institutions that most advantages the least advantaged persons in society. In practice, this emphasis on the absolute position of the most disadvantaged in society may force society to forgo schemes that produce lesser aggregate wealth or utility. Other scholars have cited the tensions between distributive "injustice" and overconsumption by the wealthy, which may lead to such harms as environmental degradation and exploitation of the poor (Jameton and Pierce, "Environment and Health").

15. Brock, "Broadening the Bioethics Agenda." Philosopher Norman Daniels has also contributed to bioethical literature by applying Rawlsian principles to justify the right to health; see, for example, Daniels, "Justice, Health, and Health Care." Both Brock and Daniels discuss resource prioritization for the worst-off.

16. Ezekiel Emanuel, David Wendler, and Christine Grady have suggested guidelines for "what makes clinical research ethical." Among their criteria is "fair subject selection"—subjects should not be vulnerable individuals and must have the potential to experience the benefits of any ethical research project ("What Makes Clinical Research Ethical?").

17. Several patients being treated for HIV at the Clinique Bon Sauveur in rural Haiti are quoted in this article. These interviews were not part of a formal ethnographic study, but rather are an effort to convey patient stories in their own words.

18. The research project mentioned has, by report, since been terminated.

19. On the growth of global inequality since 1980, see Galbraith, "A Perfect Crime."

20. Scheper-Hughes, "The Global Traffic in Human Organs," p. 193.

21. See, for example, the work of Nancy Scheper-Hughes, including "The Global Traffic in Human Organs," and her forthcoming book *A World Cut in Two.*

22. Wise, "Confronting Racial Disparities in Infant Mortality," p. 9.

23. Farmer, *Pathologies of Power.*

24. Ibid., chap. 9 (included in this volume as chapter 21).

25. For a review, see Farmer, Kononets, et al., "Recrudescent Tuberculosis in the Russian Federation." See also Stern, *Sentenced to Die?*

26. For one such study, see Bukhman, "Reform and Resistance in Post-Soviet Tuberculosis Control."

27. Kimerling et al., "Inadequacy of the Current WHO Re-Treatment Regimen in a Central Siberian Prison."

28. Farmer, "Managerial Successes, Clinical Failures."

29. Farmer, Bayona, Shin, et al., "Preliminary Outcomes of Community-Based MDRTB Treatment in Lima, Peru"; Mitnick et al., "Community-Based Therapy for Multidrug-Resistant Tuberculosis in Lima, Peru."

30. Médecins Sans Frontières, "MSF Ends Tuberculosis Treatment in Kemerovo Region, Russia."

31. This attitude toward prisoners is also hard to square with an equally important, though largely forgotten, aspect of Rawls's theory of justice—the inviolability of each person. As Rawls himself elegantly puts it, "each person possesses an inviolability founded on justice that even the welfare of society as a whole cannot override" (A Theory of Justice, p. 3, sec. 1, n. 26).

32. Farmer, Infections and Inequalities.

33. Churchill, "Are We Professionals?" p. 259, n. 13.

34. Anjos, "Medical Ethics in the Developing World."

35. Asad, Anthropology and the Colonial Encounter.

36. Brandt, "AIDS," p. 168.

37. Mukherjee, "HIV-1 Care in Resource-Poor Settings," p. 995, n. 1.

Never Again? Reflections on Human Values and Human Rights

(2005)

To designate a hell is not, of course, to tell us anything about how to extract people from that hell, how to moderate hell's flames. Still, it seems a good in itself to acknowledge, to have enlarged, one's sense of how much suffering caused by human wickedness there is in the world we share with others. Someone who is perennially surprised that depravity exists, who continues to feel disillusioned (even incredulous) when confronted with evidence of what humans are capable of inflicting in the way of gruesome, hands-on cruelties upon other humans, has not reached moral or psychological adulthood. No one after a certain age has the right to this kind of innocence, of superficiality, to this degree of ignorance, or amnesia.

SUSAN SONTAG, *REGARDING THE PAIN OF OTHERS*

PRELIMINARIES

A lecture on human values? Since all humans have values, to claim expertise in the universal arena of value-making is necessarily a perilous activity. Arguments abound. Are some values truly universal, the products of growing up in a human body and within a human family of some sort or another? Or are all human values socially constructed, with no real bedrock but what we create through culture? Aren't all values by definition human? Many ethologists and sociobiologists dispute this last point fiercely.

I would like to consider a small aspect of these issues: how photographs and stories may be used to spark reflection on human, and humane, values. Chastened by Susan Sontag's admonition that "no 'we' should be taken for granted when the subject is looking at other people's pain,"[1] I note at the outset that the stories in question belong to other people, not to me; the photographs I will speak of were taken by me and by other physicians working with Partners In Health, a nongovernmental organization seeking to put into practice the belief that health care is a human right. Partners In Health has worked in rural Haiti for many years; we have also had the privilege of caring for patients in places as far-flung as Peru, Siberia, and Rwanda.

In the course of doing this work, we've learned a great deal about how best to deliver medical care to the very poorest, to prisoners, and to the victims of violence. This work has also taught us that those seeking to serve such patients must know something about human rights. We've learned, for example, that there is no single coherent "human rights movement"; rather, there are heterogeneous groups of people with very different conceptions of how rights are related to values and different conceptions of how human rights and values should come into play, particularly in the course of responding to the problems of persistent poverty and inequality, violence, and even epidemic disease.

This diversity of opinions and our own experience working among the destitute sick have also forced us to consider the following questions: Should access to health care be considered a human right? If so, what kind of right is it? What is the relationship between social conditions and human rights?

Answers to these questions are powerfully contested within various human rights movements. There are reasons why some who do not live in poverty—for example, people who give or read lectures such as this one, and those who write about rights—do not always wish to see an analysis of poverty and inequality figure centrally in debates about human values and human rights. One reason is that the affluent share a single world with the poorest, just as the violent share a world with victims of violence and the healthy share a world with the sick. In *Regarding the Pain of Others,* Sontag explores human values and human rights and also the role played by photographs, reminding us that viewer and victim share the same time and space: "Being a spectator of calamities taking place in another country," she warns, "is a quintessential modern experience."[2] But the notion that we belong to different worlds—the First and Third, for example—is a fiction that can be conjured or shattered by photographs and stories, depending upon the ways in which they are presented. Sontag exhorts us that "to set aside the sympathy we extend to others beset by war and murderous politics for a reflection on how our privileges are located on the same map as their suffering, and may—in ways we might prefer not to imagine—be linked to their suffering, as the wealth of some may imply the destitution of others, is a task for which the painful, stirring images supply only an initial spark."[3]

Proximity and connections are often the subtext of current-day discussions of "globalization," and these discussions, too, bring their own arcane debates. Here I will reflect on extreme suffering as it occurs in this global web of hidden connections. If we are located on the same map as the suffering of others, how do we describe the fact that some of us are shielded from violence and epidemic disease while others are faced, from birth forward, with enormous risks? One way to trace this geography of unequal risk is to consider how structural violence is meted out to the poor in myriad ways. This phrase, "structural violence," has been known to cause epistemological jitters among researchers into social process. Scholars I much admire—in particular, Loïc Wacquant and Philippe Bourgois—have taken me to task for relying on a concept that does too little to parse very different kinds of violence.[4]

There are, to be sure, many kinds of violence, and a term that attempts to bridge the social (including the historical and economic), the psychological, and the biological without making the necessary distinctions may both create an unwanted black box in the place of human motivations and leave us no way of measuring the degrees, assessing the kinds, and forecasting the consequences of violence and rights violations. Even if, descriptively, it makes sense to say that societies built on deep inequality consist of wall-to-wall structural violence, such an analysis leaves us at a loss for prescriptions and for ways to distinguish legitimate from illegitimate force.

For scholarly as well as practical reasons, I desire to do a better job of parsing the concept of structural violence and cataloging its many forms. That would also promote the human values that might lessen the toll taken by the violence and disease that are so tightly bound to poverty and social inequalities.

Part of my difficulty in making sense of violence stems, no doubt, from my experience working as a physician in settings of great poverty. The physician's task is to serve the sick; medicine is more a vocation than an analytic discipline. But many doctors know a great deal about structural violence. Violence in one form or another is frequently the force that propels people into our clinic waiting areas; violence, which we have little difficulty in tracking to its sources, can interrupt or frustrate the job of identifying and remedying disease.

Structural violence is embodied as epidemic disease, violations of human rights, and genocide; it becomes visible, I argue, through stories and images that convey its damaging effects. But we must be conscious of the often discouraging limitations of stories and images whenever we seek, to use Sontag's words, "to moderate hell's flames."[5]

EPIDEMIC DISEASE AS STRUCTURAL VIOLENCE

It was the philosopher Emmanuel Levinas who observed—and I'm just paraphrasing here—that ethics precedes epistemology. Our responsibility to each other precedes and grounds our duty to discover the truth. But where does ethics start? What makes a problem an ethical problem, as opposed to a merely technical or public relations one?[6] Can ethical thinking assume the willingness to act ethically? Do theory and rhetoric lead to action? Since these questions too have been argued for ages, I will start in what is, for me, an uncontentious arena: the medical and public health challenges before us right now.

The control of epidemic disease may seem an unlikely place to start in discussing human values, but the numbers are telling. Even if we consider only the big three infectious killers—AIDS, tuberculosis, and malaria—we are faced with tens of millions of preventable deaths slated to occur during our lifetimes. A recent document from the United Nations suggests, for example, that more than eighty million Africans might die from AIDS alone by 2025.[7] A similar toll will be taken on that continent by tuberculosis and malaria. Adding other infectious killers to the list, the butcher's bill totals hundreds of millions of premature deaths over the next century.

Sadly, these numbers have lost their ability to shock or even move us. What are the human values in question when we hear, and fail to react to, the news that each day thousands die of these maladies unattended? Where, in the midst of all these numbers, is the human face of suffering? Can the reader discern the human faces in these reports? A failure of imagination is one of the greatest failures registered in contemplating the fate of the world's poorest. Can photographs and personal narratives play a role, even as rhetorical tools, in promoting those human values that might lessen the magnitude of these disasters?

The strategy of countering a failure of imagination by having readers see the face of suffering is an old one in human rights struggles, as old at least as the eighteenth-century antislavery movement. Images, stories, and first-person testimony—rhetorical strategies or documentation or both?—remain the most relied-upon means of rendering these abstract struggles personal. Personalizing human suffering can help to make rights violations real to people who are unlikely to suffer them. Sometimes the challenge is to use narrative and imagery to shift the issue from "preserving my rights" to "defending the rights of the other person."

Sontag has written compellingly of the minefields one must traverse to use vivid images relating the pain and suffering of others. Writing of famine, genocide, and AIDS in Africa, she warns that the photographs "carry a double message. They show a suffering that is outrageous, unjust, and should be repaired. They confirm that this is the sort of thing which happens in that place. The ubiquity of those photographs, and those horrors, cannot help but nourish belief in the inevitability of tragedy in the benighted or backward—that is, poor—parts of the world."[8] I would endorse the first message and, of course, reject the second. But Sontag's point is that we cannot guarantee that the right message will be received, especially when predominant views and narrow interests tilt toward leaving the unfortunate to their fates. The same critique of inefficacy has been leveled at the use of personal narratives.

For me, too, the ethics of responding to the large-scale misery still rife in the modern world precedes the epistemological issues. And to prevent us from assuming that these tragedies are inevitable, I turn to the experience of a young Haitian man who lay dying of AIDS and tuberculosis only a year or two ago. The story of his illness, and also of his failure to die, offers us a chance to consider the role human values play in confronting what is surely one of the greatest moral challenges of our times: addressing, through medicine and public health, inequalities of risk and outcome that have grown as steadily as has the gap between the richest and the poorest.

On the afternoon of March 17, 2003, four men appeared at the public clinic in Lascahobas, a town in central Haiti; each carried one corner of a makeshift stretcher. On the stretcher lay a young man, eyes closed, seemingly unaware of the five-mile journey he had just taken on the shoulders of his neighbors. When they reached the clinic after the four-hour trip, the men placed their neighbor, Joseph, on an examination table. The physician tried to interview him, but Joseph was already stuporous. His brother recounted the dying man's story.

Joseph, twenty-six years old, had been sick for months. His illness had started with intermittent fevers, followed by a cough, weight loss, weakness, and diarrhea. His family, too poor, they thought, to take him to a hospital, brought Joseph to a traditional healer. Joseph would later explain: "My father sold nearly all that he had—our crops, our land, and our livestock—to pay the healer, but I kept getting worse. My family barely had enough to eat, but they sold everything to try to save me."

Joseph was bed-bound for two months after the onset of his symptoms. He became increasingly emaciated and soon lost all interest in food. As he later recalled, "My mother, who was caring for me, was taking care of skin and bones."

Faced with what they saw as Joseph's imminent death, his family purchased a coffin. Several days later, a community health worker, employed by Partners In Health, visited their hut. The health worker was trained to recognize the signs and symptoms of tuberculosis and HIV and immediately suspected that the barely responsive Joseph might have one or both of these diseases. Hearing that their son might have one last chance for survival, Joseph's parents pleaded with their neighbors to help carry him to the clinic, since he was too sick to travel on a donkey and too poor to afford a ride in a vehicle.

At the clinic, Joseph was indeed diagnosed with advanced AIDS and disseminated tuberculosis. He was hospitalized and treated with both antiretrovirals and antituberculous medications. Like his family, however, Joseph too had almost lost faith in the possibility of recovery. He remembers telling his physicians, early in the course of his treatment, "I'm dead already, and these medications can't save me." Contemplating a photograph taken by Dr. David Walton as Joseph began his treatment (figure 23.1), one can readily understand why he had given up hope.

Despite his doubts, Joseph dutifully took his medications each day, and he

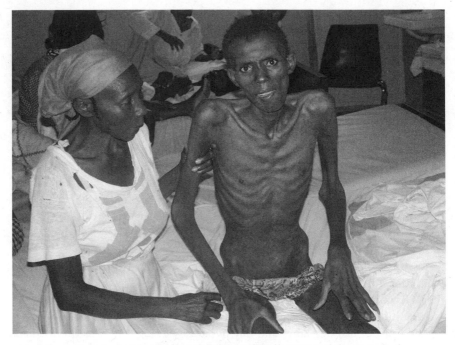

FIGURE 23.1. Joseph shortly after being diagnosed with AIDS and disseminated tuberculosis but prior to receiving therapy, with his mother. Photo by David A. Walton.

slowly began to improve. Several weeks later, he was able to walk. His fevers subsided, and his appetite returned. After discharge from the hospital, he received what is termed "directly observed therapy" for both AIDS and tuberculosis, visited each day by a neighbor serving as an *accompagnateur*. After several months of therapy, Joseph had gained more than thirty pounds (figure 23.2).

Now, a couple of years later, Joseph frequently speaks in front of large audiences about his experience. "When I was sick," he says, "I couldn't farm the land; I couldn't get up to use the latrine; I couldn't even walk. Now I can do any sort of work. I can walk to the clinic just like anyone else. I care as much about my medications as I do about myself. There may be other illnesses that can break you, but AIDS isn't one of them. If you take these pills, this disease doesn't have to break you."

What sort of human values might be necessary to save a young man's life? Compassion, pity, mercy, solidarity, and empathy come immediately to mind. But we also must have hope and imagination, not to mention know-how, in order to make sure that proper medical care reaches the destitute sick. Naysayers still argue that it is simply not possible, or even wise, to deliver complex medi-

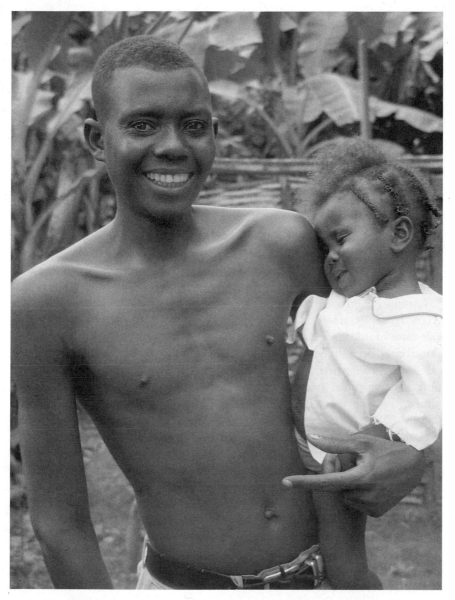

FIGURE 23.2. Joseph after six months of AIDS and tuberculosis therapy. Photo by David A. Walton.

cal services in settings as poor as rural Haiti, where prevention, they insist, should be the sole focus.[9] Joseph's story answers their misgivings, I feel, both in terms of fact (you can successfully treat advanced AIDS in this setting, and good treatment serves to strengthen prevention programs) and in terms of value (it is worthwhile to try to do so). Certainly Joseph and his family would agree, as would thousands of other Haitians who have benefited from these services.

But is the story over? Are the human values of compassion, pity, mercy, solidarity, and empathy all there is to it? How might the notion of rights reframe a question typically put as a matter of charity or compassion? Conversely, what happens when other, unfortunately undeniable, human values come into play in settings of epidemic disease? What happens when the human values in question are selfishness, greed, callousness, resignation, or just plain lack of imagination?

We know at least one answer to these questions. The director of Partners In Health and I were in Kenya in January 2004. Along the shores of Lake Victoria, we visited a number of communities seemingly bereft of young adults. We had not met any poor Kenyans receiving antiretroviral therapy—to date the only effective means of treating AIDS—and were anxious to learn more about efforts to introduce this therapy to the Lake Victoria region, one of the epicenters of the AIDS pandemic, where surveys of young adults over the past two decades indicate rates of infection that range upward of 30 percent.[10] Many of those people infected are dead or dying—even now, well over a decade after the introduction of effective antiretroviral therapy. In some areas, kinship networks have been nearly overwhelmed: in certain villages, children of those who die of AIDS are placed in orphanages almost as often as they are placed among their extended families. These days we hear a lot about the need for compassion for AIDS orphans, who number in the millions in Africa alone, but what arrangements might have prevented them from being orphaned?

The medications that saved Joseph's life are commodities available anywhere in the global economy to those who can pay for them, in Kenya just as elsewhere. The people who have died without a single dose of effective therapy over the past decade were, almost without exception, people who lived and died in poverty. In order to make sure that poor people dying from AIDS stop dying, it will be necessary to move beyond what Sontag referred to as the "unstable emotions" of compassion or pity,[11] to more stable arrangements for all those afflicted with this and other treatable diseases.

Translating compassion, pity, mercy, solidarity, or empathy into policy or rights is a difficult task. But it is not impossible. How might we draw on certain human values to promote the notion of a right to health care and spark the imagination? A subsequent visit to Kenya, a year after the first one and again in the company of the director of Partners In Health, reminded us of the power of photographs. This time, we were traveling with the head of missions of a large charity that had recently received a significant amount of funding for AIDS relief. "Treatment is important," he remarked after a day of home visits, adding that he'd recently seen before-and-after-treatment photographs of a man whom he assumed was Kenyan, since these images had appeared in a Kenyan newspaper. "The difference between the two photographs was extraordinary," he added. It was clear that he'd been moved, and it seemed, too, that he was in a position to do something about it—to translate his reaction to the photographs, however "unstable," into interventions designed to save the lives of those already sick. The photographs, it turns out, were the same ones you see here. Joseph's images had made it across the world from Haiti to Kenya.

Do the destitute sick of Haiti or Kenya ask for our pity and compassion? Often they do. But can't we offer something better? The human values required to save one person's life, or to prevent children in a single family from losing their parents, surely include pity and compassion, and those sentiments are not to be scorned. Sometimes it is possible to save a life, to save a family. But "scaling up" such efforts requires a modicum of stability and the cooperation of policymakers and funders who are themselves unlikely to suffer the indignities of structural violence.

Partners In Health has worked for a long time in a small number of settings, seeking to make common cause with local partners to establish long-term medical projects that strengthen, rather than weaken, public health. This means strengthening what is termed "the public sector" rather than, say, other nongovernmental organizations like ours or private clinics and hospitals. Against the reigning cult of private initiative, profits, and civil society, we hold that nongovernmental organizations can and should strengthen the faltering public sector.[12] We proceed in this manner because we've learned that the public sector, however weak in these places, is typically the sole guarantor of the *right* of the poor to health care. Our own efforts take seriously the notion of the right to health care and also to freedom from hunger, homelessness, illiteracy, and other problems encountered in settings of great poverty. Others involved in nongovernmental organizations are also learning these lessons when they seek to inspire projects by appealing to social justice and a rights framework rather than by appealing to what Rony Brauman of Médecins Sans Frontières has termed "the politics of pity."[13]

To move from pity and compassion for a sufferer like Joseph—a young man with a story, a face, and a name—to the universal values inherent in notions of human rights is a long leap. For many, especially those far removed from conditions such as those faced in rural Haiti or rural Kenya, the struggle for basic rights lacks immediacy. But sometimes we can entrap ourselves into becoming decent and humane people by advancing sound policies and laws. The road from unstable emotions to hard entitlements—rights—is one we must travel if we are to transform humane values into meaningful and effective programs that will serve precisely those who need our empathy and solidarity most. In other words, we at Partners In Health are not opposed to pity, but we're anxious to press for more: for policies that would protect vulnerable populations from structural violence and advance the cause of social and economic rights.

Social and economic rights, which include the right to health care, have been termed the "neglected stepchildren" of the human rights movements and have been held up in opposition to the political and civil rights now embraced, at least on paper, by many of the world's most powerful governments. So striking is this division within the rights movements that some have come to refer to social and economic rights as "the rights of the poor." Certain African voices, at least, have argued that human rights language is not widely used on that continent because so little attention is paid by the mainstream human rights organizations to health care, clean water, primary education, and other basic entitlements. This means that little attention is paid to the voices of those who do not enjoy these rights.[14] The language of political rights has become meaningless to many people living in the worst imaginable poverty. Conversely, the language of economic rights is sometimes viewed as exorbitant and irresponsible—a menacing blank check to be foisted on those lucky enough to live in the midst of plenty.

This growing rift, I would argue, is the most pressing human rights problem of our time. As long as mainstream human rights organizations do not understand poverty and inequality as human rights violations and view them simply as distracting background considerations, there is little hope of advancing the case for social and economic rights. Any doctor or public health specialist concerned with the health of the poor should agree. As long as certain fruits of modernity—in speaking of AIDS, certain diagnostic tests and medications—are considered commodities rather than rights, such sentiments as pity and compassion are not likely to be translated into meaningful changes for the millions who now need these resources to survive.

FROM EPIDEMICS TO MASS KILLINGS: ARGUING GENOCIDE

Photographs, as we have seen, can provide a glimpse of the scandal of untreated disease and trigger the need to make sense of a problem such as AIDS in Africa; stories such as Joseph's can "humanize" a colossal and impersonal catastrophe. But questions remain: When and where are such strategies effective? How does one measure efficacy?

Take the case of genocide, one of the defining human rights questions of our time. The term is of recent provenance: it was coined by Raphael Lemkin in the mid-twentieth century to describe the policies of the Nazis. Although a fairly precise definition was proposed originally for the term, it is not often invoked. The feeling, among many, is that we know genocide when we see it. But do we?

Visuals have always been an important part of the evidence advanced in arguing genocide. Again, we are leery of misusing images, because, as Sontag warns, "As one can become habituated to horror in real life, one can become habituated to the horror of certain images."[15] But we shouldn't have to apologize for reporting what is really occurring. On February 23, 2005, Nicholas Kristof published an article, "The Secret Genocide Archive," in the *New York Times,* noting that "photos don't normally appear with columns in this newspaper." Kristof continues:

> But it's time for all of us to look squarely at the victims of our indifference. These are just four photos in a secret archive of thousands of photos and reports that document the genocide underway in Darfur. The materials were gathered by African Union monitors, who are just about the only people able to travel widely in that part of Sudan. . . .
>
> I'm sorry for inflicting these horrific photos on you. But the real obscenity isn't in printing pictures of dead babies—it's in our passivity, which allows these people to be slaughtered.
>
> During past genocides against Armenians, Jews and Cambodians, it was possible to claim that we didn't fully know what was going on. This time, President Bush, Congress and the European Parliament have already declared genocide to be underway. And we have the photos. This time we have no excuse.[16]

In his column, as in my telling of Joseph's story and its echoes in Kenya, Kristof credits photographs with extraordinary evidentiary power—power that was not to be found, it would seem, in the equally graphic and far more detailed verbal testimony from Sudan that had been in heavy circulation for more than a year previous. The power of the photograph, in his view, brings something new, something inarguable, to the equation.

And yet, as Sontag observes, photographs have long been used in this manner: "For a long time some people believed that if the horror could be made vivid enough, most people would finally take in the outrageousness, the insanity of war."[17] Earlier she asks: "Who are the 'we' at whom such shock-pictures are aimed? That 'we' would include not just the sympathizers of a smallish nation or a stateless people fighting for its life, but—a far larger constituency—those only nominally concerned about some nasty war taking place in another country. The photographs are a means of making 'real' (or 'more real') matters that the privileged and the merely safe might prefer to ignore."[18]

Even during the course of the earlier genocides mentioned in Kristof's piece, photographs of the slaughter existed; though widely circulated, they failed to stop the violence from continuing. There are also omissions in Kristof's inventory of recent genocides. One that didn't make his list, at least not in the column cited, occurred in Rwanda, where I have the great privilege of working as a physician. During the 1994 Rwandan genocide, some eight hundred thousand people, perhaps more, were killed in a hundred days. Survivors continue to grapple with the legacy of the killing, and not the least of their problems is how to discuss or represent what happened during that year. For a long time, it was true that most people not from that region were simply unaware of the magnitude of the killing. A movie about the Rwandan genocide, which dramatizes the struggle of one middle-class Rwandan hotelier at a time when close to a million died, is far more likely to result in widespread awareness of events already well chronicled and well photographed in scores of books.

But such movies are not always honest about the history of such conflicts or why they happen. Do they, too, contribute to the belief that such tragedies are inevitable "in the benighted or backward—that is, poor—parts of the world"? Do images and films and personal narratives erase the political economy of suffering in Rwanda and Haiti and elsewhere? The film industry has little stomach for exposing the inner workings of structural violence.

What is most often left out of the story? An honest and unromantic look at that genocide would focus on the region's history and its relation to the rest of the world. This is what Sontag means when she asks us to reflect "on how our privi-leges are located on the same map as their suffering." Although much is made of the primitive agricultural implements used to do the killing, tiny Rwanda was in 1993 the continent's third largest arms importer, behind Egypt and apartheid South Africa: some of the killing was in fact executed with modern weapons acquired from arms dealers operating out of Europe and elsewhere, far from central Africa. And every honest exploration of the Rwandan genocide shows the key roles played by the government of France, which abetted the killers, and by the United Nations and the United States, which did little to stop them.[19] A geographically broad web of violence linked events in Rwanda, and later Zaïre, with the complicity, rather than the detachment, of the industrial powers and of that mysterious entity "the international community."

The roots of what was termed, somewhat misleadingly, "ethnic fratricide" reach deep into the bloody soil of the colonial era, during which first German and then Belgian authorities laid down in great anthropometric detail the real and imagined differences between the Hutu and Tutsi "races"—a term I place in quotation marks because it is technically incorrect and historically tendentious. Although social distinctions between these groups are real and long predate European penetration of central Africa, colonial regimes ascribed to the region's inhabitants immutable physical and social characteristics, buttressing and hard-ening hierarchies of human worth that had been less rigid in centuries prior to European contact.[20] Layered upon this political and ideological foundation for inequality was the more recent field of growing social scarcity that served as an incubator for a bitter struggle for power—a slow-motion social catastrophe that incited little interest among the powerful international actors who might have acted to avert what came to constitute the world's largest mass killing in the latter half of the twentieth century.

Certain international actors, however, were far from passive bystanders. After the Rwandan military officer Juvénal Habyarimana seized power from fellow Hutu Grégoire Kayibanda in 1973, the new dictator promised to ease growing tensions between the "Hutu Power Movement," with which he and his predecessor were associated, and the Tutsi minority once favored by the Belgian colonial administration. Instead, the Habyarimana government was "relentless in the task of discrimination [against] and scapegoating" of Tutsis,[21] all the while siphoning off vast sums of government funds and foreign aid on the side. This did not deter those sending aid to an increasingly *génocidaire* government.

Reminded by Sontag of our obligation to locate our privilege on the same map as the suffering of our contemporaries, consider Franco-Rwandan relations. Journalist Philip Gourevitch underlines the close ties between the governments of Habyarimana and François Mitterrand, ties that strengthened the Hutu-dominated military considerably. These ties were not focused exclusively on economic or development assistance:

> A military agreement signed in 1975 between France and Rwanda expressly forbade the involvement of French troops in Rwandan combat, combat training, or police operations. But President Mitterrand liked Habyarimana, and Mitterrand's son Jean-Christophe, an arms dealer and sometime commissar of African affairs in the French Foreign Ministry, liked him too. (As military expenditures drained Rwanda's treasury and the war [between the Habyarimana government and the Rwandan Patriotic Front] dragged on, an illegal drug trade developed in Rwanda; army officers set up marijuana plantations, and Jean-Christophe Mitterrand is widely rumored to have profited from the traffic.) France funneled huge shipments of armaments to Rwanda—right through the killings in 1994—and throughout the early 1990s, French officers and troops served as Rwandan auxiliaries, directing everything from air traffic control and the interrogation of RPF prisoners to frontline combat.[22]

The role played by France was dishonorable; the roles played by other powers were hardly glorious; United Nations efforts were, at best, wholly ineffectual. Others attempting to salve the suffering, including those working in nongovernmental organizations and human rights groups, were overwhelmed. In some instances, these organizations made things worse. It has been claimed that humanitarian aid to refugees of the Rwandan genocide served to prolong the conflict; some veteran humanitarian groups eventually conceded that they were doing more harm than good working in Rwandan refugee camps in Zaïre.[23]

As post-genocide Rwandans struggle to confront a burgeoning AIDS epidemic, itself accelerated by violence and poverty, the bloody residue of 1994 proves difficult to wipe away.[24] It even clings to health care providers concerned only to serve the sickest, regardless of their social or ethnic identities.

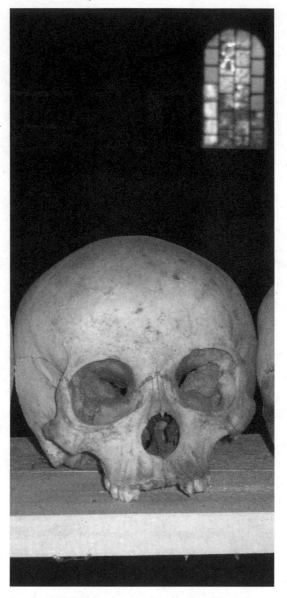

FIGURE 23.3. In the chapel of Ntarama, Rwanda, March 2005, nearly eleven years after the Rwandan genocide claimed eight hundred thousand lives. Photo by Paul Farmer.

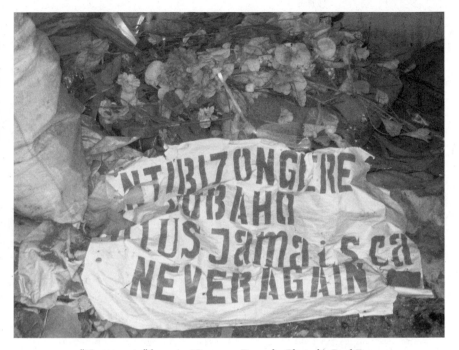

FIGURE 23.4. "Never again" banner, Ntarama, Rwanda. Photo by Paul Farmer.

Some in Rwanda believe it is unwise to try to wipe away the residue of genocide. Better to display it. There are many genocide memorials in Rwanda; survivors have their reasons for leaving the evidence intact. I took a photograph (figure
23.3) inside a church in the village of Ntarama, about an hour from the capital city
of Kigali. Not far from the church, a banner promising "Never again" was draped
over more bags of bones (figure 23.4). Since I do not work in that village, I am
relying on others brave enough to tell their stories and on those who translated
them from Kinyarwanda into English. Dancilla was born and raised in Ntarama;
she lives there still and helps to tend the church, which is now a genocide memorial. Here is her story:

> When the militia came in April 1994, I hid in the little church at Ntarama with my
> children. There were several thousand people crammed into the building—people
> who could not run into the hills. Our men had left us there as they thought we
> would be safe. In previous years when the government came to kill, they usually
> killed the men and left the women and children alone. We were very frightened but
> could not imagine what was going to happen.

The gendarmes arrived and broke some holes in the wall of the church—which you can still see today. They threw grenades into the crowds of people, then fired shots into the congregation. The noise of screaming and the mess was awful.

There were parts of bodies everywhere. I was covered by dying people, blood and filth. Some were still moving slowly, but most were dead. Then the doors were broken down so that the militia could come in and find anyone still alive—then they finished them off with machetes. I could hear the militia going about their "work" while my friends and neighbors groaned and breathed their last. I dared not move and thought I would suffocate under the bodies while I waited my turn to be butchered. There were so many people in there that they did not find me buried under the bodies.

After the militia left and everything was silent and dark, I crawled out from under the corpses. I learned later that my husband had been killed not far away from the church. My two children had been killed in the church also.

We survivors of Ntarama decided not to bury our loved ones. Why do we leave the bones of our families lying on the floor of the church? It would be easier and better for us to bury our loved ones and give them dignity. But that would also make it easy for everyone to forget. We do not want people to forget. Everyone must know what happened because of the extremists and because of the hatred. If people forget what happened when the UN left us, they will not learn. It might then happen again—maybe to somebody else. We owe it to our families to make the world remember. That is why we wait here like this. It makes me happy that people can come here and learn what happened, or that people far away can know about this place. For the sake of the future we must keep this memory alive.[25]

Dancilla's experience is far from unusual, except that, left for dead, she survived to recount her story. Psychological horrors aside, it was not difficult to meet her or to document her story. Her account also belies the claim that only machetes were used to kill eight hundred thousand people in a hundred days. The grenades and guns Dancilla mentions were not made in Rwanda, and following the paper trail will likely reveal that even the machetes were imported—some with the help of loans from aid agencies deeply implicated, some have argued, in setting the stage for what was to follow.[26] Once again, it wasn't a failure of intelligence, to use the jargon of our times, that allowed genocide to happen.

What human values might have stopped or at least slowed these mass killings? How might we have "moderated the flames" of the hell that was Rwanda in 1994? Indignation is not enough, we know; nor is the goodwill of people like you or me. Nor do "bearing witness" and providing documentation suffice; these were abundant at the time. Even United Nations officials ostensibly in a position to do something to save lives in Rwanda found themselves hobbled by forces much larger than they were.

Take the experience of Lt. General Roméo Dallaire, who led the UN peace-keeping force in Rwanda and survived the genocide, although some of his troops did not. The impotence of his office is evident in his memoir *Shake Hands with the Devil.* Dallaire watched as Rwanda went up in hell's flames and hundreds of thousands of people were murdered at close range, but he found his every move hampered by bureaucratic processes and worse. Dallaire couldn't get the extra troops he needed; nor could he get materials, armored vehicles, even water. The French government, as noted, helped to arm and train the *génocidaire* government and stymied peacekeeping in ways that will eventually come to light: long-overdue investigations of French complicity in the genocide are now under way in both France and Rwanda. The U.S. administration, still smarting from the killing of American soldiers in Somalia, pressed for a *reduction* in the size of the peacekeeping force in Rwanda and refused to commit any troops to the effort. African lives, it seems, just weren't worth it. A passage from Dallaire's memoir merits highlighting:

> As to the value of the 800,000 lives in the balance books of Washington, during those last weeks we received a shocking call from an American staffer, whose name I have long forgotten. He was engaged in some sort of planning exercise and wanted to know how many Rwandans had died, how many were refugees, and how many were internally-displaced. He told me that his estimates indicated that it would take the deaths of 85,000 Rwandans to justify the risking of the life of one American soldier. It was macabre, to say the least.[27]

A cost-effectiveness analysis, a price tag, applied to a peacekeeping effort in Africa. Macabre indeed. And how terrible it felt, we learned, to have survived when so many others died.[28] Dallaire does not mistake himself for a vulnerable Rwandan. He does not claim to be the victim. But he did not stand aside and let things take their course: he tried to act on his realization and, by his own account, failed.[29]

Dallaire has often said that what happened in Rwanda was made possible by the world's racism. The world's indifference to the fate of a large subset of humanity continues to haunt him. He wasn't able to stop the genocide, but he couldn't walk away from it. He wanted to make sure the lesson would not be forgotten, and so he spoke out about the genocide after he was relieved of his duties in Rwanda. This included testifying at tribunals to judge the guilty. For his pains, Dallaire was given a stern dressing-down by his superiors in the Canadian armed forces:

> Either Dallaire had to abandon the "Rwanda business" and stop testifying at the tribunal and publicly faulting the international community for not doing more, or he would have to leave his beloved military. For Dallaire, only one answer was possible: "I told them I would never give up on Rwanda.... I was the force commander and I would complete my duty, testifying and doing whatever it takes to bring these guys to justice." In April 2000 Dallaire was forced out of the Canadian armed services and given a medical discharge. Dallaire had always said, "The day I take off my uniform will be the day that I will also [answer for] my soul." But since becoming a civilian he has realized that his soul is not readily retrievable. "My soul is in Rwanda," he says. "It has never, ever come back, and I'm not sure it ever will."[30]

The list of human values that would be relevant to averting genocide, if we agree that values might avert genocide, grows long in considering even a few paragraphs from Dallaire's book or from the many others written about the Rwandan genocide. These values are, by and large, the same ones that might avert deaths from untreated infectious disease. But once again we must ask if values alone can prevent death on a massive scale.

A good lecturer shouldn't repeat himself, at least not too much. But the forms of violence, the epidemics killing the poor, and human rights abuses of all sorts make up a catalog of repetitions. The most massive and lethal upheavals, especially genocides, are inevitably followed by pledges "never again" to countenance genocide. "Never again"—again and again. As one journalist recently wrote in reporting from Darfur:

> There are mass graves and there is mass rape. Men and boys are taken away to be killed.
> Then the government denies the scale of the violence. It keeps journalists out, blocks aid workers.
> Many more die from hunger and disease. The world expresses concern but does too little, invariably too late.
> A handful of foreign troops are allowed to deploy, but they are too few and their mandate is too restrictive to allow them to intervene and fight the killers.
> Yes, we have been here before.
> Bosnia, Rwanda and those are only the ones that have happened in our own time.
> I gave up having any faith in the phrase "never again" after Rwanda.
> I now add another verbal formulation to the list of redundant phrases.
> It is the sentence "We must learn the lessons."
> It is of course invariably the precursor to the words "never again."
> "We must learn the lessons of the Holocaust, or of Cambodia, or of Bosnia, or of Rwanda . . . and make sure that things like this" . . . and you know how this sentence ends . . . "things like this never happen again."[31]

Staring at the "never again" banner in Ntarama, it occurred to me that although the photographs of Joseph and others had a certain persuasive power in promoting AIDS treatment in Haiti and in Africa, there is little reason to believe that even more graphic images might have moved those with power to avert genocide in Rwanda or Sudan. The Rwandan genocide was among the world's most reported and photographed of mass killings. But abundant documentation, visual or otherwise, had virtually no role in halting that genocide. It was in fact a Rwandan rebel force—a military action, performed by people wielding guns, not cameras—that halted the killing. This is one of those unpleasant facts that gall all those who hope that knowledge and documentation will sway the powerful and alter the course of history.

HUMAN SUFFERING AND
THE POLITICS OF REPRESENTATION

This is the world in which we live, the world in which we consider the meaning of human values. A world in which one is obliged to apologize for displeasing images, even in the print news media. A world in which certain images are dismissed as gratuitous or even pornographic, while the policies and arms sales that feed the killing depicted in those images are ignored, as are most of the political and economic mechanisms by which structural violence is perpetuated. A world in which we cannot, granted, be sure that such images will do anything to move the viewer beyond the unstable emotion of pity or revulsion to meaningful action.

Contemplating Darfur leads me back to Haiti. The UN undersecretary-general for peacekeeping, Jean-Marie Guéhenno, recently traveled from Darfur to Haiti, commenting that many Haitians endure conditions worse than those suffered by internally displaced Sudanese.[32] The situation is certainly dire some two centuries after Haiti, once France's most lucrative colony, became an independent republic. There should have been much to celebrate at Haiti's bicentennial in 2004: the country is in many senses the birthplace of values that we celebrate as modern, as it was the first nation in the world to outlaw slavery—the source of vast European profits—after the slave revolt that transformed the colony into Latin America's first sovereign nation. Haiti's second constitution, promulgated in 1805, declared that all citizens, regardless of skin color, were to be known as *nègres;* prohibited foreign ownership of land; and reclaimed as the country's name the term used by the island's indigenous people. Haiti meant "high country" to the original inhabitants, millions of Arawak who had almost all died out a century after Christopher Columbus established Europe's first New World settlement in 1492. The constitution declared "the Black Republic" a safe haven not only for escaped slaves from other colonies and from its only sovereign neighbor, the United States, but also for indigenous people lucky enough to have survived their first contact with the Europeans.[33]

Haiti in 1804 had few friends. The small country, in cinders after a decade of war waged successfully against Europe's greatest powers, was surrounded by the slave economies of Jamaica, Cuba, and the southern United States. Its leaders tried to make some friends by helping Simón Bolívar and others cast off colonial rule in the New World. One of the conditions of this assistance—imagine Haiti offering foreign aid to Bolívar!—was that slavery be abolished in the nascent republics of South America. And Haitian troops, former slaves, marched east to abolish slavery in what is now the Dominican Republic.

Haiti's first century as an independent nation was a difficult one. Bolívar did not keep his promise and in fact tried to block Haiti's formal participation in international affairs. The Dominican Republic, after independence, became and remains a country in which racism—and dislike of all things Haitian—is tolerated or condoned.[34] Throughout the nineteenth century, Haiti remained isolated by trade embargoes and the world's refusal to recognize the sovereignty of a country born of a slave revolt. The twentieth century was no better: gunboat diplomacy was followed, in 1915, by U.S. military occupation. Franklin Delano Roosevelt ended the occupation in 1934, but decades of military and paramilitary dictatorships ensued. Haiti's first democratic elections were not held until 1990.

What transpired over the next fourteen years is much disputed, but it needn't be: Haiti's brief experience with democracy is readily documented if one searches long and hard enough for the facts. Honest and careful historians will no doubt hash it out in scholarly texts to come, should the fate of democracy in Haiti ever prove worthy of impartial judgment. What we know is this: that in spite of a spectacular coup attempt (by Duvaliériste and paramilitary forces) between the elections and the installation of the elected president, the inauguration of liberation theologian Jean-Bertrand Aristide took place on February 7, 1991. Father Aristide's government's policies reflected liberation theology: ambitious programs to promote adult literacy, public health, and primary education were quickly launched, as were campaigns to raise the minimum wage (opposed vigorously by Haitian and U.S. factory owners) and to promote land reform (opposed by those with large and often fallow landholdings). Tensions were high, and in September 1991 the Aristide government was overthrown by yet another military coup, this one anything but bloodless. And another military dictatorship began.

Earlier I promised to focus on proximity and connections, to continue following Sontag's exhortation that we look hard at the ways in which our privileges are located on the same map as others' suffering—"in ways we might prefer not to imagine." This strategy is especially revealing, and painful, to Americans seeking the truth about Haiti. It is an incontrovertible fact that the modern Haitian military was supported by the foreign government that had created it during the U.S. occupation of Haiti. (Some will note a certain symmetry, here, with the recent history of Rwanda. But in the case of Haiti, as elsewhere in Latin America, it was the U.S. government and not France that gave assistance and training to the army.) The degree to which the first Bush administration secretly abetted the 1991 coup, its claims to the contrary aside, is much debated. But there is no doubt that a CIA asset in Haiti formed and led the vicious paramilitary group named FRAPH, credited with many of the murders committed during the years following the coup.[35]

By 1992, Haiti was like a burning building from which the only exit was over the border shared with the Dominican Republic or across the sea. Tens of thousands of refugees headed for the United States; the United Nations condemned the U.S. policy of forcibly returning Haitian refugees and declared post-coup Haiti "a human rights nightmare." Hundreds of thousands were internal refugees, partisans or suspected partisans of Aristide, fleeing their homes in the urban slums that had been targeted by the military and paramilitary forces to rural refuges or to the neighboring republic, famously hostile to Haitians.

Endless negotiations, orchestrated by the United Nations and the Organization of American States, seemed to lead nowhere—the military dictators refused to budge—until there was a change of administration in Washington, D.C. During his campaign, Bill Clinton had promised to stop the forced repatriation of Haitian refugees and to restore constitutional rule to Haiti. President Clinton did not find, in his own country, much support for his proposed sanctuary of Haitian asylum-seekers. The flood of unwelcome refugees to Florida played a role in forcing his administration to stanch the flow of new arrivals by stopping military and paramilitary terror in Haiti.

Given the topic of this lecture, I'd like to turn again to the role of photographs in shaping the policy that eventually led to the reestablishment of constitutional rule in Haiti. The insider's tale has recently been published by John Shattuck, a self-described "human rights hawk." A human rights lawyer and former vice chairman of Amnesty International who had taught at Harvard, Shattuck joined the Clinton administration in June 1993, as assistant secretary of state for democracy, human rights, and labor. "Soon after taking office," Shattuck recalls, "the administration of Bill Clinton was confronted by the post–Cold War forces of disintegration. Within 18 months, disaster had struck in Somalia, Rwanda, Haiti, Bosnia, and China. Human rights conflicts were erupting or escalating in virtually every part of the world."[36]

Conflagrations in Rwanda and Haiti came to occupy much of Shattuck's time, but since Haiti is a close neighbor with strong ties to the United States, it is not surprising that the crisis in "our backyard," then generating huge numbers of refugees, loomed larger than the catastrophe evolving in Rwanda (the government of France, malicious enough in Haiti, focused more on its own "sphere of influence"). Shattuck's account of how the United States came to intervene in Haiti is interesting for many reasons, but one of them is surely that we get a clearer view of how decisions about such grave matters are made.

Clinton himself favored using military force, if necessary, to restore democracy in Haiti: "the strategy had many opponents inside the Beltway, but the President knew it was time to reach over their heads and take it to the public."[37] How did Clinton come to feel so strongly about this matter when Washington's power elite saw little reason to waste time and energy or to jeopardize American lives on account of Haiti? How did his government manage to promote what was, in the United States, a fairly unpopular policy? Shattuck reports that he called the U.S. ambassador in Haiti, asking him for photographs of the atrocities taking place there. In the end, he reports, it was Amnesty International that proved more helpful on this score: there was, as I mentioned earlier, plenty of documentation about what was going on in Haiti. Shattuck's job was to brief the president on September 14, 1994, since Clinton himself planned to present his proposal to the U.S. public the very next day. Shattuck continues:

> Early in the afternoon of September 14, I spread my photos of the disfigured faces and bodies of Haitians who had recently been attacked by the FRAPH on a coffee table in the Oval Office. Examining them closely one at a time, the President swore quietly, "Those bastards," and vowed that Haiti's reign of terror would be brought to an end. The statistics I summarized for the President spoke for themselves—more than three thousand killed since the 1991 coup against Aristide, including nearly a thousand in the first eight months of 1994; mass graves found by human rights monitors; an estimated 300,000, or 5% of the population, driven into flight or hiding; and thousands of cases of mutilation, rape, and beating of Aristide supporters by the regime's network of gangs. As I talked, the President stared at the hacked and mutilated bodies of men, women, and children trapped on an island ruled by thugs.[38]

And so the deed was done: constitutional rule was restored to Haiti in 1994 with U.S. military force, a policy buttressed with photographic evidence of the butchery that had prevailed during the previous three years. Not a single American life was lost from hostile fire during the course of the operation. But there are many ways to undermine popular democracy, and what followed was a decade of "structural adjustment" programs forced on Haiti by the same international community which had declared that Haitian democracy should be restored. Aristide served out what little was left of his term and became, in 1996, the first Haitian president ever to hand over power to another elected president—on precisely the day such a transfer of power was slated to occur.

Aristide was reelected in 2000, the first year he could run again according to the Haitian constitution. A second Bush administration was installed at almost the same time that Aristide returned to office. The strength of the Haitian leader's mandate—Aristide won more than 90 percent of the votes cast—did not mean that he would have any economic strength, since the bulk of his political support came from the poor rather than from Haiti's wealthy elite, notoriously reluctant to pay taxes. And it is clear that the "new" U.S. policy gurus on Haiti were the same people who had disparaged the left-leaning Haitian populist during the Bush Senior administration.

What ensued is, again, readily documented: a virtual embargo on aid or credits to the cash-poor Aristide government. The impact of such policies in a country as poor as Haiti is readily imagined: facts and figures abound.[39] Haiti in 2004 was the most impoverished nation in the hemisphere and one of the poorest in the world. There was simply no way to ease poverty in Haiti without access to credits or the ability to recover the billions that had been extorted from Haiti in the preceding centuries. Every credible economist examining the case came to precisely this conclusion, that the aid embargo was strangling Haiti. Shortly after its bicentennial celebration, marked solemnly by post-apartheid South Africa but by precious few other nations, Haiti endured its thirty-third coup d'état and in the course of that spring lost tens of thousands to violence, floods, and epidemic disease.

Questions remain. In many ways, Haiti was the first state in the Western Hemisphere to put into practice the modern notion of rights: it was the first nation to proclaim universal equality among races, and the first to offer a sanctuary to oppressed refugees. Then why is Haiti so burdened with violence and degradation and disease? Why does every tropical storm lead to more loss of life and devastation in Haiti than in neighboring countries? Why is Haiti the hemisphere's most HIV-affected nation? Why was this the island on which polio, declared eradicated from the Western Hemisphere in 1989, reemerged? Why is Haiti, the source of much of eighteenth-century France's wealth, now one of the poorest and most volatile countries on the face of the earth? Why is political stability so elusive, and violence and rights violations so endemic? Why is it so difficult, even when the tools of the trade are made available, to practice good medicine and public health in the Western Hemisphere's neediest nation?

To answer each of these questions, it is less useful to examine the culture of the "natives" than to seek to understand Haiti's history and its place in the modern world economy. I have tried to do that elsewhere and stand by my conclusion that Haiti's poor majority is by no means to blame for the mess it finds itself in, today or at any point in the last two hundred years.[40]

Not all the news from Haiti is bad. We know from our own experience that it is possible to deliver high-quality health care in rural central Haiti, where there are neither paved roads nor electricity. Haiti can also claim to have led the charge against AIDS in the poor world, having launched some of its first integrated prevention and care programs; Joseph's experience is not rare in central Haiti. These public health efforts have not gone unnoticed. As the neighboring republic, with a gross national product several times that of Haiti, retreated from its goal of offering all poor Dominicans access to modern AIDS care,[41] some Haitian public health leaders pressed on.

A new funding mechanism, the Global Fund to Fight AIDS, Tuberculosis, and Malaria, allowed Haiti to ramp up longstanding efforts to prevent new infections and to improve care for the sick. Even as some poor nations seemed ready to concede defeat in the struggle against what had become the world's leading infectious cause of adult deaths, Haiti could point to real victories. Laurie Garrett, writing in the *New York Times* in July 2004, noted that "a new Global Fund report shows that of the 25 projects supported by the fund for more than a year, 80% have already either achieved or even surpassed their five-year goals. As chaotic as it is, Haiti surpassed its 2006 targets after only a year of Global Fund support."[42] Another article, even more detailed and based on reporting from central Haiti, was titled "Rural Haitians Are Vanguard in AIDS Battle."[43] People like Joseph, and those who cared for him, were leading a movement not only to make AIDS prevention and care a right but also to revitalize Haiti's shattered public health sector, often with assistance from the Global Fund. It seemed to be working.

It was optimism born of just such experiences—and a belief in the suasive power of photographs and narratives—that led friends and coworkers from Partners In Health to put together a photographic exhibit called Structural Violence: A View from Below. Most of the pictures were taken in Latin America. Many of these photographs were of my own patients, and all of them were taken by my colleagues, some of whom chose the photographs and the title of the exhibit; others did the work of hanging them in a public space in a Harvard University building and designing and mailing an invitation.

The response to the exhibit was largely positive, judging from comments in the guest book. One photograph, however, offended a visitor, who wrote in the guest book, "Not appropriate at all." This verdict was underlined twice and also telephoned to the building administration as a formal complaint. To avoid giving offense to this visitor and—presumably—others similarly affected, the organizers of the photography show took the picture down.

The offending photo (figure 23.5) is one in a series of informal portraits of a Haitian woman struggling to survive breast cancer and poverty. It was taken by her physician, once again Dr. David Walton, during the course of a home visit. Like most women living in dire poverty, Lorièze, who is from the same town as Joseph, had been diagnosed tardily. In her case, the tumor had already consumed much of her breast. She had a mastectomy at the Partners In Health hospital in central Haiti. Afterward, another physician carried some of the tissue to Boston in order to find out if Lorièze might benefit from chemotherapy. She would, and she did. These interventions were delivered with technical competence and hope and a great deal of love—some of the human values central to good medicine.

Surgery and chemotherapy—services hard to come by in rural Haiti and available to the rural poor, to my knowledge, only in our hospital—gave Lorièze a second lease on life. The photo was taken with the subject's blessing, as were the other photographs in the display. Indeed, many of our patients, including Joseph, have asked that their pictures be taken; many have asked for copies of these images. What about this photograph, I wonder, prompted such an extreme reaction? It can't be just the depiction of a breast (a spectacle to which the general public is no doubt as inured as I am, a medical professional). Is it the suggestion of disease, surgery, pain, and other things we prefer not to think about? Or is it the deeper history that the photograph expresses, if we only know how to decipher it?

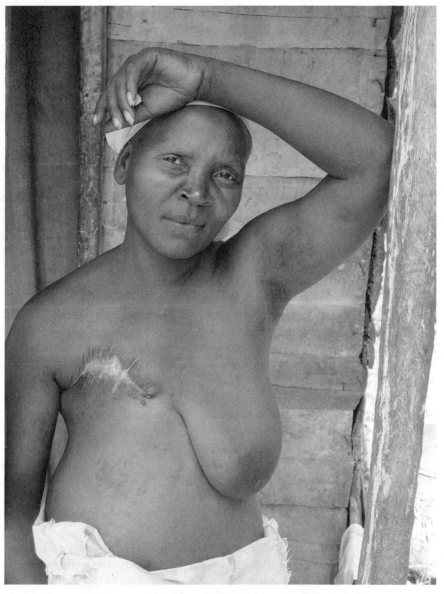

FIGURE 23.5. Lorièze after surgery and chemotherapy for breast cancer, Lascahobas, Haiti. Photo by David A. Walton.

Lorièze is doing much better, according to her doctors. But nothing will change the fact that she wandered around Haiti's towns for more than a year, looking for someone to diagnose and treat her illness, and found nobody. There is no right to health care for the Haitian poor. Breast cancer is awful anywhere; so are other malignancies, AIDS, drug-resistant tuberculosis, and a host of other diseases that afflict the poor disproportionately. But once afflicted, the victims of structural violence are in a very different situation than others diagnosed with the same illnesses. The destitute sick, if they are ever diagnosed, are unlikely to receive proper therapy for their afflictions. Again, there is no right to health care.

Surely the right to health care, like other social and economic rights, is important. It grows more so as modern medicine delivers increasingly effective therapies: just over a decade ago, there was no treatment for AIDS. But people living with AIDS face many other problems. Those we serve in Haiti, Rwanda, Peru, Boston, and Siberia have told us in no uncertain terms that food, housing, jobs, and shelter—freedom from want—are the rights they care most about. Yet these are not the rights commonly discussed in the affluent world, where civil and political rights have long dominated the agenda, when human rights are discussed at all.

Have we tried hard enough to push for the rights of the poor? Surely the answer to this question is a resounding no. As I noted earlier, there's a good deal of ambivalence within human rights circles about most social and economic rights. Is the right to health care somehow different? We've discovered that some people who don't think much about the right to food or housing or employment are sympathetic to the right to health care, perhaps because almost anyone, rich or poor, can imagine what it would be like to be sick and without medical care. When health services are for sale and the destitute are not, by definition, capable buyers, what happens to them? In Haiti, only an hour and a half from Miami, civil and political rights are important—nothing could be more clear from recent news as scores die each week, fighting to restore constitutional democracy there[44]—but the daily struggle is mostly for survival. And although Haitians do not enjoy the right to health care, they do, in my experience, have systematic and comprehensive notions about such rights.

An expanding notion of human rights (and I'm not just talking about the theory) is now emerging, but it is coming from the poor rather than from the mainstream human rights groups that receive their funding from the powerful.[45] Many of the patients we serve are articulate in asserting that *tout moun se moun*—everyone is human. The currency of this proverb is striking in Haiti, the very land in which human rights have so long had little practical reality. The subtext of *tout moun se moun* is usually that poor people deserve access to food, education, housing, and medical services. We hear this sort of commentary almost every day in our clinics in central Haiti.

The commodification of medical care is one of the biggest human rights issues facing the "modern" world today.[46] Why use quotation marks around the word "modern"? Scare quotes are typically a craven ploy, but I use them here because the woman whose picture offended the viewer, though undeniably our contemporary, lives in a low-medieval hut, with a dirt floor and a thatch roof. There is no running water. As in Kenya and even Rwanda, modern health care is available, for a price, in the private clinics of the city, but she received it for free in a rural squatter settlement only after a long time spent knocking fruitlessly on the doors of those modern clinics as a patient without money. Until she wandered into our clinic and hospital, she was effectively locked out of the modern world, with all its shiny laboratories and amazing medications.

The experience of a Haitian woman dying of breast cancer, her death delayed by desperate but effective measures, offers more lessons about structural violence, itself an effect of the dizzying social inequalities spanned by our lives and work. All those involved in her care agree that it is "not at all appropriate" that only a tiny fraction of the afflicted have access to proper medical care. We join our voices to those of our patients, who, not having visas to leave their countries, cannot be "empowered" to come and tell their stories in Boston or New York or Geneva or Salt Lake City.

Spanning the worlds of rich and poor is what human rights organizations, aid organizations, and universities do; so do rich-world governments. The images and narratives shown so far, and also the histories of Haiti and Rwanda, all remind us of proximity rather than distance. Wealthy and powerful institutions have certain obligations to the rest of the world. What are these obligations? Do wealthy and powerful people who do *not* support the noxious policies of their own governments have obligations to the victims? No good answers to these questions are forthcoming as long as those who can span these worlds do not understand the struggles of people facing poverty and disease.

Are photographs of awful suffering "not at all appropriate," are they cause for apology when printed in the *New York Times* because they break down boundaries erected in order to keep misery far away? Are disturbing images of ongoing suffering "inappropriate" because they undermine facile and fashionable notions of "empowerment"—facile because the concept lacks any meaning if not linked to social and economic rights, including the right to health? None of this is to say that representation of the sufferings of others is not fraught with danger. Sontag examines the photographic record of black victims of lynching in early twentieth-century America and asks: "What is the point of exhibiting these pictures? To awaken indignation? To make us feel 'bad'; that is, to appall and sadden? To help us mourn? Is looking at such pictures really necessary, given that these horrors lie in a past remote enough to be beyond punishment?"[47] But recall that the images and stories shown here, during this lecture, are those of our contemporaries, caught up in the same web of privilege and suffering as we are. Are these photographs and stories disturbing because they depict not people from another era but rather fellow beings who share our time and (in the era of globalization) space—people who really are destitute and sick and frightened, and would be so whether or not someone took their pictures or told their stories?

The list of questions, worrying this thin membrane separating the fortunate from the unfortunate, goes on and on.

The political and moral culture of affluent universities (or mainstream human rights or aid organizations) seems, at times, not to share a planet with rural Haiti or with Rwanda. Major campus and institutional struggles have often concerned issues of representation. Representing is inherently controversial: I can easily agree with the proposition that the photographer (even the physician-photographer) stands, through luck, privilege, education, and social status, in an unequal relationship to the person photographed. As a graduate student in anthropology, I heard frequent discussion of who has the right to take a photograph and display it. Academics and commentators such as Sontag have written tomes on photography, and anthropologists have a strange obsession with representation (in both artistic and political senses).

But the photographs in the Partners In Health exhibit and in this lecture were displayed not to exploit the suffering of others but to bring people whose lives are different and far less difficult—that is, people like us—into a human rights movement to which the fortunate would have a great deal to offer. The goal of these photographs and stories is to inspire, not offend; to alter the fates of people like Joseph, Dancilla, and Lorièze—and others who may not survive. When linked to other forms of analysis (in the case of the photographic exhibit, to books and articles and lectures—the traditional products of a university), these photographs do not simply move people to pity or indignation, useful though those feelings may be. The photographs are meant to take us beyond superficial analyses of longstanding ills. The point is to testify to deep questions of history and political economy and to offer us all a chance to think about health care as a right. Dismissing such images as "not at all appropriate" is an excellent way of stopping that conversation and of undermining our understanding of why, for example, the likeliest outcome for the poor in Haiti, Kenya, or Rwanda would be death without even a diagnosis, much less therapy.

An apology from a *New York Times* columnist serves, as no doubt intended, to draw our attention to an ongoing catastrophe. His apology is "strategically useful as a rhetorical tool," to echo Loïc Wacquant again. Our eyes are drawn to these images. But we are also often called to avert our gaze from suffering. An anonymous visitor's expression of anger cannot readily be glossed as "political correctness"—the blanket claim, typically heard from conservative corners, that such images have no place in public spaces. These sentiments bespeak, I believe, a very different malady: a desire to avert our gaze from things that should in all propriety make us uncomfortable. Of course, we should also try to approach this peremptory comment—"not at all appropriate"—as generously as we can. Personal experience is immediate and truthful as far as it goes; an avowal of discomfort can never be dismissed. But one might wish that such images would at least inspire pity and compassion, regardless of the viewers' personal experiences. Better still that they inspire more stable emotions, such as empathy, and result in solidarity—in some ways surely the most noble of human sentiments.

In reflecting on human values, wouldn't it be wonderful if the comment was meant to tell us that it is "not at all appropriate" that some die of treatable diseases while others are spared that risk? Or that photographs from Darfur or Rwanda should spark, among the millions who see them in print or broadcast or posted on the Internet, the desire to stand with the victims, to stop the killing? Because without such sentiments, we will not forge a movement to reverse the trends now registered, and we will live in a world divided, in an increasingly violent fashion, between haves and have-nots.

Such sentiments, of course, will not suffice. But the promise of social move ments based on solidarity and empathy remains alive, however tenuously. For "never again" to inspire something other than cynicism, nothing less than a movement will do.

HUMAN VALUES AND SOCIAL MOVEMENTS

Why do we need a movement to promote the "rights of the poor," and how might such a movement prevent events like those registered in Haiti, Rwanda, and Sudan? The relationship of poverty to human rights is no mystery to those who live in poverty, as we learned in rural Haiti; nor is the relationship of poverty to violence, including extreme violence and genocide. I've learned a great deal about rights by listening to people in rural Haiti. Every year for the past decade, our Haitian patients and coworkers have sponsored a conference on health and human rights. In 2004, as in previous years, the huge crowd included patients with AIDS who were actually receiving proper therapy for the disease at no cost to them. This was the only way they could receive such care, as a public good rather than as a commodity. Many more in the audience were dying of untreated or inappropriately treated AIDS, but these individuals—not yet patients, to their dismay—were from elsewhere in Haiti and were there to fight for their right to health care.

One of the speakers that year was none other than Joseph (figure 23.6). Since the time of his miraculous resuscitation, he has been involved in AIDS prevention efforts; he has become, as had many of those gathered together for the conference, an eloquent spokesperson on behalf of people living with AIDS

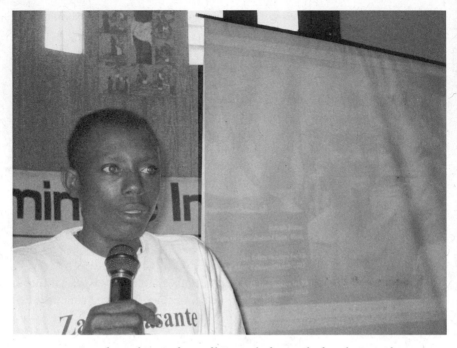

FIGURE 23.6. Joseph speaking in front of his own before-and-after photographs, Tenth International Seminar on Health and Social Justice, Cange, Haiti. Photo by Joia Mukherjee.

and in poverty. On that day, as he spoke, he projected photographs of himself before and after treatment—the very same photographs I've shown you, the same photographs that had made their way to Africa and beyond. As elsewhere, the photographs drew applause. In the hands of Joseph, the images were a witness not only to the miracles of modern medicine but also to the power of first-person testimony. He spoke with passion and with a certain humor about his own near-death experience and about his hopes for the future. "One of the things I'd like to do is to learn how to read," he said. "It's ridiculous that even today adults who are poor do not know how to read."

A number of questions were raised, largely for the sake of discussion. More likely, they were "rhetorical tools," aimed perhaps at members of the audience who were health professionals or policymakers, a distinct minority in rural Haiti. Should people dying of AIDS be spared only if they can pay for the antiretroviral therapies that will save them? Should people living in poverty have a right to primary education, to learn how to read? Should they have the right to food and shelter? Should poor women have the right to benefit from early detection of breast cancer? And when it is detected, should they have the right to chemo-therapy? The people who showed up to discuss health care in a church in rural Haiti knew that the answers were self-evident: yes, of course. But such questions would strike some of my colleagues in both the international health and human rights "communities" as absurd. This is because most external determinants of disease—poverty, inequalities of all sorts—are still considered off-topic by many human rights experts and policymakers.

The view of many of my academic colleagues seems to be that good scholar-ship and activism don't mix. The view of many of my human rights colleagues seems to be that social and economic rights—those violated in settings of poverty and disease—are "pie in the sky." We're having a hard enough time, I'm scolded by friends in large human rights organizations, getting civil and political rights respected. The view of many in both sectors seems to be that, if such rights are to be promoted, then the victims themselves should be "empowered" to start their own social movements. And yet it is not possible to argue that those gathered in central Haiti need to form a movement to promote human rights; they already have. The missing movement is the one that would occur among the privileged; it would be one based on solidarity and empathy, rather than some sort of shared experience.

The people living with HIV who spoke at the conference were aware of the long list of reasons marshaled by university-trained experts to show that we cannot provide "cost-effective" care for AIDS, for example, in the world's poor-est communities. Typically, the list of reasons is not overtly racist or sexist, nor does it include anything approaching frank contempt. Instead, the reasons (or excuses) for not addressing these complex diseases are framed more subtly: fairy tales about primitives who, lacking "a concept of time," are unable to take medicines on schedule, for instance. The Haitian AIDS sufferers had heard these stories and retorted, as they had done in previous conferences on health and human rights, "We may be poor, but we're not stupid."[48] They were familiar with the thousand other excuses we dish up to explain genocide, human rights abuses, the persistence of poverty, the growth of inequality, and the futility of trying to fight diseases as complex as breast cancer and AIDS in places as poor as Haiti.

Relativism is a part of the problem. Why is it impolitic in the groves of aca-deme to argue that dying of never-treated AIDS in a dirt-floor hut in Africa is worse than dying of AIDS in a comfortable hospice in Boston after having failed a decade of therapy? I've been present for both kinds of death—at matside and at bedside. No death of a young person can reasonably be called good. But I've seen almost nothing worse than dying of AIDS and poverty, incontinent and dirty and hungry and thirsty and in pain. I've experienced almost nothing worse than hearing that a Rwandan woman raped during the genocide and now dying of AIDS cannot be treated because she cannot afford the various laboratory tests and medications required to treat her disease. I've seen almost nothing worse than a poor Haitian woman dying of breast cancer without any care at all, leading to what's called, aptly enough, a fungating mass that completely replaces normal breast tissue and then consumes flesh and bones—an excruciatingly painful death uneased, in settings of poverty, by palliative care or even wound care. That is the fate that structural violence reserves for those living with both poverty and disease.

So it is with human rights violations as conventionally defined: the victims are disproportionately to be found among those living in poverty. Ask those who've invested their lives, their medical careers, in providing medical services to some of the most desperately endangered people in the world. Dr. Gino Strada, a successful Italian transplant surgeon, decided that he would try to help civilians—most of them children and the great majority of them poor—who had been injured by landmines and other man-made pathogens. After a decade of this grueling work, in Rwanda and Pakistan and many other places, Dr. Strada concludes that he was wrong not to have done all his homework on what might as well be termed structural violence: "In the operating theatre we saw the devastation produced in human bodies by bombs and mines, by projectiles and rockets. Yet we did not succeed in grasping the effects of other weapons, 'unconventional' ones: finance and international loans, trade agreements, the 'structural adjustments' imposed on the policies of many poor countries, the new arms races in richer countries."[49]

Whether or not we see these horrible deaths, whether or not we avert our gaze, they are happening. Those who must face structural violence every day encounter precious little in the way of support for the right to food, water, housing, or medical care. Even within the human rights movement, where civil and political rights are privileged, there is far too little support for social and economic rights. Maybe magical thinking persuades us that when political rights are granted, economic rights will follow. But that step-by-step attitude has not always been the orthodoxy: there are historical precedents for enshrining social and economic rights in official human rights declarations. One need only read the Universal Declaration of Human Rights: Articles 25 and 27 seem to speak directly to the issue of what "human values" might mean:

> Article 25: (1) Everyone has the right to a standard of living adequate for the health and well-being of himself and of his family, including food, clothing, housing and medical care and necessary social services, and the right to security in the event of unemployment, sickness, disability, widowhood, old age or other lack of livelihood in circumstances beyond his control. (2) Motherhood and childhood are entitled to special care and assistance. All children, whether born in or out of wedlock, shall enjoy the same social protection.

Article 27: (1) Everyone has the right freely to participate in the cultural life of the community, to enjoy the arts and to share in scientific advancement and its benefits.

And these articles are actionable, at least on a small scale and almost surely on a much larger one, if we can find the rhetorical tools necessary to bring the privileged on board as we build a movement to promote the rights of the poor. Indeed, following this mandate led Partners In Health from rural Haiti to shantytowns in Peru to prisons in Siberia and on to the former killing fields in Rwanda. But for these basic rights to be extended to all those who need them—a prescription that would prevent, in my view, much of the violence discussed here and much of the terrorism about which we read—we will need a movement based in nations like the United States, wealthy nations that now control the fates of billions who live far from their shores.

The tasks at hand in each of these places are overwhelming. A daunting to-do list serves as a reminder that only a social movement involving millions, most of us living far from these difficult settings, could allow us to change the course of history. But history also provides us examples of just how powerful broad-based social movements can be. Some have argued that the first great human rights struggle—to abolish the slave trade and slavery itself—got its start when the Englishman Thomas Clarkson, born in the late eighteenth century, submitted an essay in Latin just prior to graduating from Cambridge University. It was an essay about slavery, an enterprise in which his home country was deeply invested but of which he had no personal experience. In his memoirs, a source for an important new book by Adam Hochschild, Clarkson recalls his own inner debate as he rode back to London after graduation. He stopped by the side of the road, unable to ride on as his thoughts about slavery consumed him. "Are these things true?" he asked himself. "The answer followed as instantaneously. 'They are.'" His initial conclusion: "'Then surely some person should interfere.' Only gradually, it seems, did it dawn on him that he was that person."[50]

Clarkson asked a very "unpostmodern" question. *Yes, or no, are these things true?* And he came up with a very unpostmodern answer. *Yes.* Surely someone should interfere with this man-made abomination, slavery?

And interfere he did. Clarkson and his friends and consociates, some of them former slaves, spent decades building an antislavery movement, performing the hard chores of what we now call "community organizing." He and a dozen or so others, many of them Quakers and several of them influential in England, began a vast campaign. They went from town to town, traveling tens of thousands of miles on horseback, to collect signatures for petitions, to call town meetings, and to research the slave trade, gathering expert witnesses and amassing testimony. Photography did not yet exist, but those spearheading the movement relied heavily on stories and images, including the infamous floor plans of a slaving ship, as rhetorical tools and as documentation. Personal narratives were offered by, or written about, former slaves. Although the antislavery documents compiled for the lower house of Parliament were praised for their "dispassionate" tone, there was no doubt that the sugar boycotts and giant parchment petitions were fueled by indignation. These rhetorical tools proved effective.

If the antislavery movement sounds like an up-to-date organization, this is because it was. Imagine what these people were up against. They lived in a monarchy; very few British subjects could vote. England derived huge profits from the triangular trade; that was in part why it ruled the waves. Sugar, rum, tobacco, and other tropical produce had become everyday staples in Europe and the emerging "new world" on which we stand today—"necessities," if you asked the people lucky enough to enjoy them—and yet the movement attained its goal within a few decades of Clarkson's epiphany.

The story of the antislavery movement does not teach us, as blurb writers like to say, that one person can change the world. That may be argued, but the lesson to be gathered from the abolitionists is that *broad social movements* can have great force in the world. The human rights movements of today have too often been co-opted by powerful states, whose leaders have their own reasons for claiming to respect human rights. But powerful governments do not form movements. Their citizenry might.

VIOLENCE AND VALUES:
REHABILITATING COMPASSION, PITY, SOLIDARITY, EMPATHY?

It's a fact that abominable events and processes—from torture to slavery to genocide to unassuaged suffering from epidemic disease—are documented and recognized as such even as they are occurring. But recognition is not enough. Sontag says it best: "What does it mean to protest suffering, as distinct from acknowledging it?"[51] Even protest is not enough. If ever we are to say "never again" and mean it, we will need more than resolutions and more than photographs or stories or museums or Hollywood-style movies. We need another modern movement, a globalized movement that will use whatever facts, stories, and images it can to promote respect for human rights, especially the rights of the poor. For such a movement to come about, we need to rehabilitate a series of sentiments long out of fashion in academic and policy circles: indignation on behalf not of oneself but of the less fortunate; solidarity; empathy; and even pity, compassion, mercy, and remorse.

Sparking such emotions with testimony and photographs is one thing; linking them effectively, enduringly, to the broader project of promoting basic rights, including social and economic rights, is quite another. Stories and images need to be linked to the historically deeper and geographically wider analyses that can allow the listener or the observer to understand the ways in which AIDS, a new disease, is rooted in the historically defined conditions that promote its spread and deny its treatment; the ways in which genocide today, like slavery before it, is a fundamentally "transnational" event; the reasons why breast cancer is inevitably fatal for most affected women who live in poverty; the meaning of rights in an interconnected world riven by poverty and inequality. In short, serious social ills require in-depth analyses. We are living, it is true, at a time when movies and gossip are more likely to garner widespread attention than are scholarly books or lectures or long essays. And yet comparable troves of attention are required to reconfigure existing arrangements if we are to slow the steady movement of resources from poor to rich—transfers that have always been associated, as in Rwanda and Haiti, with violence and epidemic disease.

I entitled this Tanner Lecture "Never Again" because the human values I prize are those that would make such horrors—dying unattended from treatable disease, facing genocide—things of the past. The lecture was meant to be ambitious and humble. The lecture is ambitious because I promised to link poverty and inequality to epidemic disease and genocide and to argue that a broad-based movement founded on the values of solidarity and empathy could attack twenty-first-century poverty and inequality. In so doing, we would make a signal contribution to preventing violence, since it is almost always rooted in precisely those social arrangements I've termed structural violence. This is as true in Haiti as it is in Rwanda and Sudan; it is true elsewhere, too. The lecture is humble because it raises many questions, and I don't know the answers. It is often better simply to say so, as the Polish poet Wisława Szymborska has observed: "I just keep on not knowing, and I cling to that like a redemptive handrail."[52]

Szymborska's poem "Tortures" packs violence and its increasing interconnection with history into just a few lines:

> Nothing has changed.
> The body still trembles as it trembled
> before Rome was founded and after,
> in the twentieth century before and after Christ.
> Tortures are just what they were, only the earth has shrunk
> and whatever goes on sounds as if it's just a room away.[53]

We live in a world in which violence and epidemic disease, only a room away, are intimately linked to those who are spared. A world bound tightly together and yet held firmly apart. A world in which violence—the reflection, surely, of certain values—seems to be ineradicable. A world in which terror is met with more terror. We live in a nation and world in which there exists great and alarming confusion about the term "moral values."

I've tried to dissipate some of that confusion by making use here of stories and images while linking them to a deeper analysis that is not visible in either image or personal narrative. That is, I've tried to use the media that create an illusion of immediacy, to remind us of the very real closeness among people and places that our society keeps as far apart as it can. Our collective inattention is periodically broken by stories and arresting images. In such lucid and engaged moments, we can seek to understand the violence of our world system, which it is suddenly once again fashionable to call an "empire."[54] To claim, after all we have seen and heard, that such violence will never again occur is not only to ignore the lessons of history but to be willfully blind to structural violence.

Understanding the nexus of violence and disease is a discouraging enough endeavor. Whether or not this or other similarly sorrowful exercises prove useful to those seeking to improve the health and well-being of the world's poor— whether or not we can say "never again" with any conviction—will depend on our collective courage to examine and understand the roots of modern violence and the violation of a broad array of rights, including social and economic rights. To argue that such an undertaking leads to nothing "actionable" is to raise a white flag and to surrender our chance to lessen the heavy toll of both violence and disease.

NOTES

1. Sontag, *Regarding the Pain of Others*, p. 7.

2. Ibid., p. 18.

3. Ibid., pp. 102–3.

4. Loïc Wacquant and Philippe Bourgois were among a distinguished group invited to comment on my piece "An Anthropology of Structural Violence" (Bourgois et al., "Commentary on Farmer, Paul, 'An Anthropology of Structural Violence.'"). A helpful anthropological reader on violence has been assembled and edited by Nancy Scheper-Hughes and Philippe Bourgois, *Violence in War and Peace*. Arthur Kleinman, a previous Tanner lecturer, has devoted much of his career to exploring this topic; see Kleinman, "Experience and Its Moral Modes." I am of course deeply indebted to these colleagues, and especially to Arthur and Joan Kleinman's essay about the representation of suffering (Kleinman and Kleinman, "The Appeal of Experience; the Dismay of Images"). See also Kleinman, *What Really Matters*.

5. Sontag, *Regarding the Pain of Others*, p. 114.

6. Elsewhere we have argued that contemporary medical ethics focuses on certain challenges (defining brain death, say, or the ethics of stem cell research) while ignoring others (lack of access to care for those living in poverty). See Farmer and Gastineau Campos, "Rethinking Medical Ethics" (included in this volume as chapter 22).

7. Joint United Nations Programme on HIV/AIDS, *AIDS in Africa*. One hopes and expects, of course, that the toll will be much lower. But the report outlines three plausible scenarios for the African HIV/AIDS epidemic over the next twenty years based on the current actions of the global and African communities. All three scenarios—a "best-case situation," a "middle-case" condition, and a "doomsday scenario"—warn that "the worst . . . is still to come" (p. 20).

8. Sontag, *Regarding the Pain of Others*, p. 71.

9. These debates continue. See, to cite but one very recent example, the assertions by Harvard-trained economist Emily Oster, who seems to argue against providing antiretroviral therapy to patients such as Joseph, claiming that "antiretroviral treatment is around 100 times as expensive in preventing AIDS deaths as treating other sexually transmitted infections and around 25 times as expensive as education" ("Treating HIV Doesn't Pay"). But these inputs are changing rapidly with time: over the past few years, we have seen a decline of more than 90 percent in the cost of antiretrovirals, and there is little agreement about the efficacy of current prevention methods and educational campaigns among the very poor—the victims of structural violence.

While acknowledging that "it may be that we have an objective other than maximizing the efficiency of dollars spent," Oster nevertheless hews to static cost-effectiveness analyses, despite these changes and debates: "In my work I have assumed that our goal in the face of the epidemic is to maximize life. In other words, to save the most years of life with the funding available." But why is funding the constant in this life-or-death equation when funding and the cost of inputs are poorly studied and rapidly changing?

Nor is her analysis epidemiologically sound: while citing the importance of treating sexually transmitted infections in order to prevent HIV transmission, she fails to note the advantages of treating HIV infection in order to prevent HIV transmission. Our experience in rural Haiti has shown that demand for HIV screening, a cornerstone of prevention efforts, is low as long as effective care remains unavailable.

For more on the debate, see Farmer, "Prevention without Treatment Is Not Sustainable." My exchange with Edward Green explores some of these complexities; see Green, "New Challenges to the AIDS Prevention Paradigm"; Farmer, "AIDS." On other aspects of the African response to the epidemic, see Epstein, "God and the Fight against AIDS" and "The Lost Children of AIDS."

10. World Health Organization and UNAIDS, "UNAIDS/WHO Epidemiological Fact Sheets on HIV/AIDS and Sexually Transmitted Infections, 2004 Update."

11. Sontag, *Regarding the Pain of Others*, p. 101.

12. Walton et al., "Integrated HIV Prevention and Care Strengthens Primary Health Care" (included in this volume as chapter 13).

13. See Brauman, "L'assistance humanitaire internationale." Reflecting on his experience during the convoluted Cambodian refugee crisis of the late 1970s and early 1980s, Brauman notes that, for aid workers, "the choice was . . . not between a political position and a neutral position, but between two political positions: one active and the other by default" ("Refugee Camps, Population Transfers, and NGOs," p. 181).

14. Chidi Anselm Odinkalu, in critiquing conventional human rights work in Africa, hazards a guess as to why so many human rights groups mirror the inequalities of our world: "Local human rights groups exist to please the international agencies that fund or support them. Local problems are only defined as potential pots of project cash, not as human experiences to be resolved in just terms, thereby delegitimizing human rights language and robbing its ideas of popular appeal" ("Why More Africans Don't Use Human Rights Language").

15. Sontag, *Regarding the Pain of Others*, p. 82.

16. Kristof, "The Secret Genocide Archive." See also the continuation of these thoughts in his lucid essay "All Ears for Tom Cruise, All Eyes on Brad Pitt."

17. Sontag, *Regarding the Pain of Others*, p. 14.

18. Ibid., p. 7.

19. Meredith, *The Fate of Africa*. See especially the damning assessment of France's policies during the Rwandan genocide.

20. Many books treat this subject; see, for example, Gourevitch, *We Wish to Inform You That*

Tomorrow We Will Be Killed with Our Families; Prunier, *The Rwanda Crisis;* Lemarchand, "The Rwanda Genocide"; Mamdani, *When Victims Become Killers.*

21. Keane, *Season of Blood,* p. 21.

22. Gourevitch, *We Wish to Inform You That Tomorrow We Will Be Killed with Our Families,* p. 89.

23. Fiona Terry, reflecting on her experiences working with Médecins Sans Frontières in the Goma (Zaïre) refugee camp, writes of "the paradox of humanitarian action: it can contradict its fundamental purpose by prolonging the suffering it intends to alleviate" (*Condemned to Repeat?* pp. 1–2).

24. Even now in 2006 in rural Rwanda, as I edit proofs for the publication of this essay, I read or hear about the ongoing struggle for meaning, for a dominant narrative, that might "explain" what happened in 1994. Rwanda today is a safe and lawful nation, at least compared to the other countries in which I work and most of the countries that surround it. But the tensions persist. I sense them in the prisons, which are filled with *génocidaires;* in the sometimes uneasy relations between patients and doctors; in the impoverished villages we serve; and in the wild rumors and predictions one hears in working in this traumatized nation. I read it in the news.

25. Dancilla's story is told on the website of the Rwanda Fund (www.rwandafund.com/sections/survivors/dancill.htm [accessed October 8, 2009]), an organization dedicated to preserving the memory of the genocide and promoting educational and economic opportunities for Rwandan children. I thank Beth Collins for taking me to Ntarama and for finding Dancilla's testimony. I am, of course, deeply grateful to Dancilla for leading us through the memorial.

With *Machete Season* (first published as *Une saison de machettes* in 2003), Jean Hatzfeld has made a valuable contribution by interviewing, in prison, about a dozen low-level *génocidaires* and a couple of more notorious criminals, all of them Hutu. The entire book (and his previous one, *Life Laid Bare* [*Dans le nu de la vie,* published in 2000], which focuses on genocide survivors) merits careful reading, but here I'd just like to translate the comments of one of the killers who participated in the massacre in Ntarama. What were the killers thinking when they violated the church in order to kill everyone inside?

> Thursday, when we entered the church in Ntarama, the people were lying quietly in the shadows. The wounded were visible between the pews; the still unwounded scattered under the pews; the dead in the aisles at the foot of the altar.
>
> We were the ones making all the noise. They awaited death quietly in the church's tranquillity. For us, it was no longer important that we were in the house of God. We yelled, we joked, we gave orders, we insulted. We went person to person, checking everyone's face, to finish them off carefully. If we had any doubt regarding whether or not someone was dead or dying, we dragged the body outside to inspect it in the light of day.
>
> Myself, I'd been baptized sincerely as a Catholic, but I preferred not to pray in any traditional manner during these killings. There was nothing to be asked of God as regards these filthy acts. Nonetheless, to be able to sleep certain nights, I couldn't help kneeling in the dark to lessen, with timid apologies, my darkest fears. (Hatzfeld, *Une saison de machettes,* p. 160; translation mine; see Hatzfeld, *Machete Season,* for a more recent translation)

26. Peter Uvin's book *Aiding Violence,* which explores humanitarian and development aid in Rwanda just prior to the genocide, remains a classic and cautionary tale for all of us seeking to "manage inequality" through the conventional aid apparatus.

27. Dallaire and Beardsley, *Shake Hands with the Devil,* pp. 322–23.

28. Sontag's comments may remind us of how Dallaire felt about surviving the Rwandan genocide: "We can't imagine how dreadful, how terrifying war is; and how normal it becomes. Can't

understand, can't imagine. That's what every soldier, and every journalist and aid worker and independent observer who has put in time under fire, and had the luck to elude the death that struck down others nearby, stubbornly feels. And they are right" (*Regarding the Pain of Others*, pp. 125–26).

29. Dallaire, as Samantha Power remarks in her foreword to his book, "was of course not a Tutsi and thus not a member of the group that had been marked for extermination in Rwanda. . . . But . . . Dallaire warned of the horrors that lay ahead and described the massacres as they were happening" (Dallaire and Beardsley, *Shake Hands with the Devil*, p. ix).

30. Ibid., p. xvi; translation of Dallaire's remarks modified.

31. Keane, "Why 'Never Again' Keeps Happening."

32. Heinlein, "UN Peacekeeping Chief." In the wake of mounting evidence that UN forces may have killed up to two dozen civilians, Guéhenno admitted that the peacekeeping forces in Haiti had not been sufficiently trained and equipped to curb the mounting political violence (Buncombe, "UN Admits Haiti Force Is Not Up to the Job It Faces").

33. Haiti's early constitutions were based to some extent on France's brief experiment with *liberté, fraternité,* and *egalité;* but with Napoleon Bonaparte's reestablishment of slavery in France's other New World holdings, Haiti could claim rightly enough to constitute a better example of these Enlightenment ideals than its former colonizers.

34. There are no monuments to the Haitian Revolution in the Dominican Republic; in fact, the past century has been marked by a number of anti-Haitian pogroms. In 2003, it was clear enough that the Dominicans were turning a blind eye to former Haitian soldiers using that country as a base from which to conduct raids against Haitian government officials. The past two years have seen a marked resurgence of anti-Haitian violence in the Dominican Republic.

35. FRAPH's brutal methods have been well documented by watchdog groups since its inception in 1993; see, for example, Human Rights Watch's annual reports at http://hrw.org (accessed October 9, 2009). Regarding the ties between FRAPH's leadership and the CIA, see, for example, Nairn, "Behind Haiti's Paramilitaries," p. 458; and "The Eagle Is Landing," p. 346. This information was later reported in magazines such as *Newsweek* and *Time* as well as the major dailies.

36. Shattuck, *Freedom on Fire*, p. 13.

37. Ibid., p. 106.

38. Ibid., pp. 106–7. It's worth citing the rest of Shattuck's account of that day: "Later that afternoon I worked with Taylor Branch and the White House speechwriting team to hone Clinton's television message. The speech should apply equally to American values and American self-interest, pointing out that in a country near the coast of Florida human rights and refugee crises were also threats to U.S. security. Clinton's response should be measured, firm, and deliberate. 'The nations of the world have tried every possible way to restore Haiti's democratic government peacefully,' the President would say. 'The dictators have rejected every possible solution. The terror, the desperation, and the instability will not end until they leave.' Then would come the ultimatum: 'The message of the United States is clear. Your time is up. Leave now or we will force you from power.' On September 15, 1994, the President delivered this message in a televised address to the nation" (*Freedom on Fire*, p. 107).

39. We attempted to offer such documentation in reviewing the effects, over the years, of aid embargoes on Haiti (Farmer, Smith Fawzi, and Nevil, "Unjust Embargo of Aid for Haiti"), although the impact of such a review in the medical literature is probably negligible.

40. See Farmer, *The Uses of Haiti.*

41. Schiff, "Deadly Bureaucracy."

42. Garrett, "Bragging in Bangkok."

43. Dugger, "Rural Haitians Are Vanguard in AIDS Battle."

44. The current crisis in Haiti was precipitated by the overthrow of constitutional rule in Feb-

ruary 2004. For more on those events, see Farmer, "Who Removed Aristide?"; Hallward, "Option Zero in Haiti." A recent report from the University of Miami School of Law details the agonies of the Haitian pro-democracy movement, especially that part of it that is committed to respecting the rights of the poor majority. Photographs, often gruesome, lend great power to the report—as if such images are more difficult to gainsay than are other forms of documentation. See Griffin, *Haiti Human Rights Investigation, November 11–21, 2004.*

45. Although there are scores of human rights organizations in the United States, one in particular, the National Economic and Social Rights Initiative (www.nesri.org [accessed October 9, 2009]), focuses on social and economic rights.

46. Linking medical care to the ability to pay has had devastating consequences for the majority in a country as poor as Haiti. But commodification of care is also a significant problem in certain wealthier industrialized countries. The most obvious example is the United States, where access to health care is increasingly shaped by market forces rather than by need, and where an ever-growing number of people may go without care because they lack the means to purchase it. For more on the commodification of medical care, especially in the United States, see Rylko-Bauer and Farmer, "Managed Care or Managed Inequality?"

The Kaiser Commission on Medicaid and the Uninsured reports that more than forty-five million Americans went without health coverage during 2004 ("Health Insurance Coverage in America"). Even more are irregularly insured or underinsured. In a 2002 publication, the Institute of Medicine attempted to clarify, through a meta-review, what it means to have no reliable insurance (Institute of Medicine, Board on Health Care Services, Committee on the Consequences of Uninsurance, *Care without Coverage*). One study, for example, followed forty-seven hundred Americans for at least thirteen years and found that death rates were 18.4 percent for those without insurance and 9.6 percent for the insured. Another study found more than eighteen thousand "excess deaths" among uninsured Americans, compared with those with health insurance. Mary Sue Coleman, president of the Iowa Health System and the University of Iowa, who cochaired the IOM committee, summarized: "Because we don't see many people dying in the streets in this country, we assume that the uninsured manage to get the care they need, but the evidence refutes that assumption. . . . The fact is that the quality and length of life are distinctly different for insured and uninsured populations" (quoted in Connolly, "Study"). If this is the case within the borders of the richest, most powerful nation in human history, you can imagine the situation in countries where people are indeed "dying in the streets."

47. Sontag, *Regarding the Pain of Others,* pp. 91–92.

48. For a conference statement in which a group of people living with HIV pressed for the right to health care (including antiretroviral therapy), see www.pih.org/inforesources/essays/Cange_declaration.html (accessed October 7, 2009).

49. Strada, *Green Parrots,* p. 132.

50. Hochschild, *Bury the Chains,* p. 90.

51. Sontag, *Regarding the Pain of Others,* p. 40.

52. Szymborska, "Some People Like Poetry," in *Poems, New and Collected, 1957–1997,* p. 227.

53. Szymborska, *View with a Grain of Sand,* pp. 151–52.

54. Hardt and Negri, *Empire.* It is impossible to close an essay about violence and suffering without reference to Iraq. David Rieff, who has been one of the few reliable observers of the human rights debates mentioned in this lecture, has recently reviewed two books about Iraq: *Squandered Victory,* by Larry Diamond; and *Losing Iraq,* by David L. Phillips. In both books, we see the myth of "never again" raised as a reason to reflect on what some of us would term the misadventures of our imperial ambitions, even though neither author has any real gripe with the idea of invading a sovereign nation. Diamond asserts that "if we learn from our mistakes, our next engagement to help

rebuild a collapsed state might have a more successful outcome" (Rieff, "No Exit Strategy," p. 33). Phillips seeks to lay out the U.S. administration's "mistakes in Iraq so that it does not repeat them elsewhere" (ibid., p. 34).

Rieff concludes: "Both books illustrate and exemplify the extraordinary consensus about the duty to intervene that has arisen over the course of the post–cold war world. We have not yet *begun* to pay the price for this not because we do it ineptly but rather because it rarely seems possible except on the far fringes of the political right and left, what with the 'historical compromise' between the Bush Administration and the human rights movement over humanitarian intervention, if not over torture, rendition, the Patriot Act and myriad other issues, to have a serious conversation about whether the United States has any business trying to create democracy by force of arms. Instead, the consensus not just of two writers and activists but of the great and the good from the Kennedy School of Government, to 1600 Pennsylvania Avenue, to the thirty-eighth floor of the UN, to 10 Downing Street seems to be that we—whether the 'we' in question proves to be the United States, the UN or that mythical entity, the international community—must learn to do this sort of thing better, more effectively, perhaps more humanely" (ibid., p. 36).

Rich World, Poor World

Medical Ethics and Global Inequality

(2006)

Allow me to begin, as philosophers so often have, by considering an altogether hypothetical situation. Let's say we're in a First World medical school. Let's add, merely for the sake of argument, of course, that it's a very large medical school in the Northeast of the United States—in fact, the world's largest medical school, in terms of wealth and prestige; pronouncements from its faculty have considerable weight. Allow me to proceed as if I myself were on the faculty of said school and perhaps even, to round out the argument, an alumnus who for years has been able to move between a city in the Northeast and, say, a small and very poor island nation, one hard by the United States, with a big AIDS problem. Let's pretend, again for the sake of argument, that it's Haiti.

As a grateful member of the university community, I would want to be of service to the next generation of students. One way to do that would be to serve on what's termed "the international committee," which oversees student research and training abroad. Now say it's 2000, and an increasing fraction of students are interested in studying in Africa and working on AIDS, the world's leading infectious cause of young adult deaths. To further complicate the situation, imagine that students and some faculty members are pushing for consensus regarding the necessity of AIDS treatment in the African setting, or in Haiti, where the university has research and training partners. Imagine that this consensus would later come to pass but is not forthcoming initially, in part because treatment with antiretrovirals, or ARVs, is not deemed "cost-effective" in poor societies.

Let us say that, at the very time it's proving difficult to get most faculty to agree with the proposition that it is feasible to treat AIDS there, the university continues to send students off to Africa to participate in research on AIDS. The students end up, in this hypothetical scenario, in African research settings in which no therapy is available to patients with AIDS. Yet when students receive funding to do their research projects, let's imagine that they are dispatched south with a month's supply of ARVs on the off chance that they, the students, might somehow be exposed to HIV infection.

Here are some of the ethical questions that might arise: What obligation do those students and researchers and faculty have to insist that the African patients in question receive proper AIDS therapy? How are cost and effectiveness—the key words of the regnant paradigm in what's now termed "global health"— calculated? Are the students, researchers, and African nonpatients really from different "societies"? How do ethical dilemmas so described fit into a broader rights framework?

I suspect that certain ethicists and moral philosophers (whether writing from utilitarian, Kantian, or Rawlsian perspectives) would discuss such a scenario in terms of the ongoing debate about "the moral significance of distance." In this emerging literature, the African nonpatients, some of them research subjects, would be termed "the distant needy." To draw on a recently published book on the topic, *The Ethics of Assistance,* edited by Deen Chatterjee, the terms of the debate are as follows: "If we have duties and obligations toward each other in everyday moral contexts, should these duties be extended to the distant needy? If so, what should be the nature and role of institutions implementing such duties beyond our own borders of special ties and communities? Though moral philosophers have pondered these questions in the past, such issues have become the focus of especially intense debate."[1]

These philosophers' awareness of "the distant needy" is most welcome, just as the medical students' ARVs would have been most welcome in Africa. But the notion of the "moral significance of distance" generates as many questions as it answers. Would our neighbors in equally poor Haiti be classed as the distant needy, or would they be "the nearby needy"? What if we were speaking of those Haitians (or Africans or Dominicans) who work to keep our universities sparkling, Haitians who live right around the corner from here? Are they suddenly members of a newly discovered and remote society? Also, what sparked this "especially intense debate," and what are its contours?

Chatterjee offers one common explanation for a growing interest in theories of justice that look beyond the boundaries of a single nation-state:

> Today we live in a world in which spheres of interaction are constantly expanding, while advanced technology makes it easy to reach the distant needy and vividly broadcast their plight to all. In parallel with the growth of these global relationships, there has been an enormous increase in ethicists' interest in questions regarding the morality of affluence in a world of poverty and the individual's response to

it. In addition to creating new perspectives on individual moral obligation, this discussion is transforming political philosophy. While the initial florescence of interest in theories of justice that began with John Rawls' *A Theory of Justice* (1971) solely concerned relationships among fellow-citizens, theorists of social justice now frequently attend to issues of global inequality and institutional responses to it.[2]

Many, professional ethicists and otherwise, have expressed skepticism about foundational and normative accounts that are not linked closely to social analysis. If an eighteenth-century French philosopher had evoked the plight of the poor in Haiti as an example of "the moral significance of distance," we would immediately argue that he was obscuring historical reality, eliding the fact that his own country created Haiti as a slave colony. Knowledge of the slave trade and related colonial policies would lend necessary context, pointing to the *moral significance of proximity,* not distance. Only the stubborn resolve to desocialize our understanding of Haiti and France would lead us to underline distance and happenstance rather than proximity, causality, and connection.

Notions of distance and proximity are not merely social constructs, but they're social constructs nonetheless. Many discussions of distributive justice across national boundaries reveal a startling naïveté about how political economies work now, and also about how our current social inequalities came to be. To understand that, one must go back to history and other socializing disciplines. Despite talk of globalization as a recent phenomenon, we have long lived in a world in which it was possible, for example, for the Caribbean soil of Haiti to furnish two-thirds of pre-revolutionary France's tropical produce, just as it is possible today for a Haitian housekeeper to tend to our teaching hospitals.

It's a world in which a Ghanaian-born student at Harvard Medical School might return to Ghana to do a summer of Harvard-sponsored research on the causes of the brain drain affecting the country of her birth, and no cognitive dissonance ensues; a world in which recent events and processes are speeding (or slowing) the emergence and retrenchment of social inequalities almost invisible to some who easily traverse national boundaries, while the same social pathologies are glaringly obvious to others who share, however fleetingly, the same social field. It's a world in which HIV and other pathogens spread readily across such boundaries while the fruits of science, including treatment, are blocked at customs. A world in which even discussions of distributive justice erase our historically forged connections with the some of the poorest people in the world, rendering any honest accounting of justice impossible—allowing some to appear generous and others only needy.

It will be my thesis here that we need more, not less, attention to theories of justice. But we need these discussions to be grounded in a sound knowledge of social history, social process, social connection. It is good that ethics should aim to internationalize itself, but it is insufficient. Peter Singer recalls that when he first read *A Theory of Justice*, he "was astonished that a book of nearly 600 pages with that title could fail to tackle the injustice of unequal wealth between different societies."[3] Not to have noticed the existence of that form of inequality is a gross oversight, and Singer is to be commended for wishing to remedy it; but only one philosopher among the thirteen represented in Chatterjee's volume bothers to scold fellow philosophers for their lack of understanding of the *history* of transnational resource flows.[4] Philosopher and political scientist Thomas Pogge enlarges on Singer's astonishment, turning it into something of a rebuke, a rebuke based on a deeper knowledge of facts about our world: "By seeing the problem of poverty merely in terms of assistance, we overlook that our enormous economic advantage is deeply tainted by how it was accumulated over the course of *one* historical process that has devastated the societies and cultures of four continents."[5]

In my view, Pogge is on precisely the right track here. If we want to discuss our obligations to the "distant needy," we need first an honest discussion about how our world got to be the way it is and where it is going. For it's a shared principle, in many discussions of justice, that if we have done harm to someone, we have special obligations to that person, who is more accurately described as our victim and less as a needy but remote citizen of another "society."

Linking social analysis to moral reasoning is a time-honored way of exploring ethical dilemmas, and here I will focus on examples gleaned from working as a physician in Haiti, in Rwanda, and in parts of Boston that aren't even a mile away from Harvard Medical School. I am not about to frame my examples as an "international" comparison or even a transnational one. They point to a *translocal* analysis, certainly, but geography is not the heart of the matter so much as social disparities are.

Although there are many types of social disparity, twenty-first-century poverty deserves particular attention. Poverty is succinctly defined as a lack of money, but twenty-first-century poverty is also about things like access to antiretroviral medications and other fruits of science and progress. Although much work in the social sciences relevant to medicine now "studies up" social gradients, most work, and certainly my own, is conducted in settings of poverty. Sometimes these are settings of extreme poverty, where the major struggle of the day is against hunger and violence and disease; sometimes these are settings of relative poverty, where the struggle is against racism, say, or the lack of basic social entitlements such as medical insurance or affordable housing. Contemporary ethical problems are rooted in these disparities as much as violence and terrorism are. So too are contemporary human rights struggles.

I propose four basic theses:

First, that social inequalities, both local and translocal, can be measured but often are not. However, we still lack the metrics necessary to describe the social cost of such inequalities.

Second, that these inequalities not only are a source of many ethical dilemmas but also constitute in and of themselves our chief, if too little examined, ethical dilemma. The outcome gap and the survival gap—for example, life expectancies that rise in some places even as they fall in others—also constitute our most pressing human rights problem.

Third, that the desocialization of translocal ethical dilemmas is not only a serious epistemological problem but one that further compounds the ethical and human rights dilemmas discussed here.

Fourth, that the engagement of rich-world universities in poor-world research poses ethical problems quite distinct from those identified by institutional review boards. Some of these ethical problems are related to our understanding of what we, as members of universities, owe the destitute sick.

And now, on to the detailed examination.

1. Social inequalities can be measured, but we lack the metrics necessary to describe the true social cost of such inequalities.

There's a brisk debate these days about social inequalities, how to measure them, and whether they're growing or shrinking. It's useful to divide this discussion into smaller components. What do we mean by "social inequalities"? Social categories are an example. For every rigid category imaginable—race is the classic example in this country and in many others, as caste is in India—there exists a significant body of empirical data showing how slippery it is, how thoroughly it depends on processes of social construction and imagination rather than the perception of natural fact. But inequality itself is not so easily argued away. The term "social inequalities," as used here, refers to those stemming from racism, gender bias, or economic deprivation. In worlds both rich and poor, such inequalities are linked together in obvious and less obvious ways. Although you may find gender inequality manifest in the glass ceiling of Fortune 500 companies or in tenure decisions, it is among the poor that it takes its greatest toll. There is, almost everywhere, a noxious synergy between gender- and race-based inequalities and economic inequalities: for example, the majority of poor women in the United States are women of color.

Before turning to metrics, it's worth asking whether social inequalities are growing or shrinking as what is loosely termed the "global economy" grows. Let us turn, in other words, to the globalization debates that serve as the backdrop to the ethical dilemmas mentioned so far. Allow me to quote economist James K. Galbraith, who reviewed this topic a few years ago in a paper for *Daedalus*. "So

what are the facts?" he asks. "Has globalization hurt or helped? Oddly, researchers do not know; mostly they do not ask." Galbraith steers those interested in
measuring the growth or decrease in inequality to the issue of manufacturing
pay, examining global patterns in the years before 1998, the last year for which he
had data. "When the global trend is isolated," he writes, "we find that in the last
two decades, inequality has increased throughout the world in a pattern that cuts
across the effect of national income changes. During the decades that happen
to coincide with the rise of neoliberal ideology, with the breakdown of national
sovereignties, and with the end of Keynesian policies in the global debt crisis of
the early 1980s, inequality rose worldwide."[6]

As might be expected, economists hold widely varying views on this topic,
and even the terms of debate are contested. Some argue that all boats are being
lifted by sharp increases in the volume of global trade; others complain that
years of growth in global trade have meant more suffering for the world's poor;
still others continue to argue, in more Victorian fashion, that inequality spurs
development. These arguments are usually more polemical in character than
based on empirical data, but Galbraith's basic conclusions are acknowledged
by participants on all sides of the globalization debate. In his most recent book,
Jeffrey Sachs, who bemoans facile antiglobalization protests and favors greatly
increased trade, outlines the rising disparity between nations and regions over
the past few centuries.[7] But trade agreements, which are crafted by the powerful,
have long been unfair to the poorer partners.

Thomas Pogge reviews data regarding secular trends in global inequality,
noting that the income gap between the world's richest 20 percent and its poorest
20 percent has increased from a ratio of 30:1 in 1960 to 60:1 in 1990, and then
to 74:1 in 1997. He asks, "If the global economic order plays a major role in the
persistence of severe poverty worldwide and if our governments, acting in our
name, are prominently involved in shaping and upholding this order, then the
deprivation of the distant needy may well engage not merely positive duties to
assist but also more stringent negative duties not to harm."[8]

The causes of increased inequalities are not the only point, nor are their
dimensions or temporal trends: injustice and unfairness are themselves the point.
As Amartya Sen argues in his latest book, *Identity and Violence*,

> Even if the poor who are engaged in the globalized economy were becoming just
> a little richer, this need not imply that the poor are getting a *fair* share of the
> benefits of economic interrelations and of its vast potential. Nor is it adequate to
> ask whether international inequality is getting marginally larger or smaller. To
> rebel against the appalling poverty and staggering inequalities that characterize
> the contemporary world, or to protest against the unfair sharing of the benefits
> of global cooperation, it is not necessary to claim that the inequality not only is
> terribly large, but is also getting marginally *larger*.[9]

What about metrics? Several analysts, including Dan Wikler and Dan Brock, have shown us just what we don't know about measuring health equity. In the first of nine questions posed about metrics, Brock asks, "How should states of health and disability be evaluated?"[10] In 1979, in his Tanner Lecture, Amartya Sen was asking, simply enough, "Equality of what?"[11] When we hear the word "cost," we think of costs in dollars or pounds or euros. But for anyone interested in understanding cost, we have to broaden our analysis substantially, since inequality becomes embodied in strange ways.

Starting in the 1970s, Michael Marmot published a series of papers suggesting that the health of populations was related not only in linear fashion to measures such as GDP but also to indices of social inequality. Specifically, he and his coworkers examined mortality among individuals of different "employment grades" in the British civil service. Whether death was due to coronary artery disease or to other major causes of mortality registered in the dataset, those lower on this middle-class totem pole fared worse than those higher up. What's more, the problem seems to have grown worse in the ensuing thirty years. Citing work published in 1996, Marmot reports that "both for ischaemic heart disease and suicide the social gradient became considerably steeper over the last twenty years."[12]

This line of inquiry was taken up by Richard Wilkinson, who in 1996 published a book called *Unhealthy Societies: The Afflictions of Inequality*. In it, he used associations between indices of social inequality and health outcomes such as life expectancy at birth to argue that unequal societies are noxious to health in ways that are poorly understood. This and similar arguments, using data from more affluent nations, have spawned what is now a cottage industry exploring such concepts as "social capital." Some of that research has been conducted at the Harvard School of Public Health, where Ichiro Kawachi, Norm Daniels, Bruce Kennedy, and others have come to argue that "justice is good for our health."[13]

Justice in what framework of institutions? As we deepen our understanding of social process, administrative and political boundaries become blurred; something that might reasonably be called a global society emerges. Universities are part of it. It's a dizzyingly unequal space, as anyone who makes the short trip from Harvard to Haiti can tell you. In this world, proximity, not distance, is king; connection, not disjuncture, is important. How do we calculate the cost of global inequality? As the rich grow richer, as the poor fail to grow richer, and as the world grows smaller, what sorts of costs might we expect? Amartya Sen's *Identity and Violence,* evaluating the social costs of inequalities of all sorts, takes issue with the tendency, increasingly fashionable among pundits and certain scholars, to divide the world along "civilizational" lines:

In partitioning the population of the world into those belonging to "the Islamic world," "the Western world," "the Hindu world," "the Buddhist world," the divisive power of classificatory priority is implicitly used to place people firmly inside a unique set of rigid boxes. Other divisions (say, between the rich and the poor, between members of different classes and occupations, between people of different politics, between distinct nationalities and residential locations, between language groups, etc.) are all submerged by this allegedly primal way of seeing the differences between people.[14]

Ethicists, sociologists, economists, specialists in public health often think about the social cost of inequalities in a way that subsumes pretty much everything under the rubric "social." But most of the literature on this topic, valuable though it is, has focused on inequalities within a given "society"—a term used, in much ethics literature and in human rights reporting, as a gloss for "nation." In this way of seeing social pathologies, what occurs within the borders of that nation is what counts; connections to other places and other times are hidden. What happens when we insist that both the local and the translocal, the regional and the global, are part of the same question? Sen has long pushed us to address the thorny topic of how we might measure the costs of social inequalities, encouraging us to pay attention to proximity and connections, for the rich world and the poor world are, of course, part of a single world.

How visible translocal social inequalities are, and how noxious or costly they're seen to be, is related to one's relative position in hierarchical social networks. I'd wager that, given changes in telecommunications, our comfort and excess are more readily visible to the world's poor than their suffering is to us. But conspicuous consumption in the face of famine and disease may lead to resentments of which we are only dimly aware. This one-way mirror forms part of the social backdrop for contemporary discussions of medical ethics.

Two thousand years before Rousseau, sages and prophets made inequality a topic of philosophical inquiry. The Greek lyric poet Alcaeus is said to have written the following in the sixth century B.C.:

> The worst of ills, and hardest to endure,
>> Past hope, past cure,
> Is Penury, who, with her sister-mate
> Disorder, soon brings down the loftiest state,
>> And makes it desolate.[15]

Resentment born of indignities is difficult to measure, but it is nonetheless real. It is, apparently, not an exclusively human response, if researchers into primate behavior are to be trusted. The link between inequality and violence is the subject of a large and growing literature. I'll return to this question in considering violence in Rwanda and Haiti.

2. *Social inequalities are a source of many ethical dilemmas, but they also consti-tute our chief ethical dilemma.*

In the previous three decades, much of the literature in medical ethics has focused on issues such as research ethics, organ transplantation, xenotransplantation, brain death, and the quandary ethics of the individual in, for example, an inten-sive care unit. But many people are spared such ethical dilemmas because they never have a chance to become patients at all. Poverty and inequality are tightly linked to access to health care—not that access to care, or to high-quality care, is the only determinant of outcomes. As Fabienne Peter notes, "access to health care is only one social factor among others that influences people's health."[16] Persistent poverty and inequality are thus the hidden source of many of the ethi-cal problems examined at length in the medical ethics literature. I'd argue that they constitute in and of themselves our biggest human rights challenge.

When we enlarge the debate to include not merely access to health care but also access to education, clean water, and other basic economic and social entitle-ments, we move ethics toward the most significant human rights struggles before us today—the social and economic rights of the world's poor, wherever they live.

In my work, I've sought to apply rights language to the problem of who has access to what. Rights language, like moral and ethical reasoning, is used for all manner of purposes, some of them less compelling than others. One disturbing trend has been the use of rights language by powerful governments such as our own to justify military adventures: nothing could more effectively deprive rights language of its moral force. Another persistent problem is a rift in the human rights movement about aims and goals, dividing those who give primary or exclusive attention to guaranteeing political and civil rights from those who advocate the extension of social and economic rights. It was no surprise to me to learn that in settings such as Haiti and Rwanda, many of my patients spoke about substantive entitlements, including the right to health care, clean water, primary education, and food. It was more of a shock to discover the reluctance of mainstream rights organizations in the United States and Western Europe to devote attention to basic social and economic rights: such aspira-tions are regarded as "unrealistic," "difficult to legislate," and even deleterious to more pressing struggles for civil and political rights. The lines were much more sharply drawn than I understood, with the world's largest and most vocal human rights organizations lined up almost exclusively behind civil and politi-cal rights.

In one bizarre example from the field, for years more concern was focused on determining whether HIV testing in Africa or Haiti had been preceded by adequate "pre-test counseling" than on ensuring that those tested would have access to care. Local cultural norms have nothing to do with this obsession; it derives rather from the fact that the voluntary counseling and testing models were exported to these sites from the United States, where civil rights, though not as strong as they should be, have long trumped economic rights, including the right to health care.

The standoff, without concession, between different rights camps is no mere ideological disagreement. Principles have consequences. The choice of civil and political rights over social and economic rights permits the United States to be simultaneously the world's most prominent human rights scold and "an implacable opponent of the right to development."[17] Another consequence is that rights controversies, like the ethical ones to which they're closely linked, are too rarely understood in social context: they easily turn into desocialized debates cast in narrowly legal terms. The failure to understand social context and historical background is, for me (speaking, I fear, for the minority in our profession), the major epistemological problem in medical ethics.

3. The desocialization of ethical dilemmas is not only a serious epistemological problem but one that further compounds ethical dilemmas.

If I've persuaded some of you that social inequalities are noxious and growing, and that poverty and inequality are the leading human rights problems of our time, why are these topics not the focus of more attention in medical ethics? One reason is that growing disciplinary focus and subspecialization lead, often inadvertently, to the evacuation of social dynamics from such inquiry.

The critique of desocialization can take various forms and point to various goals. When anthropologists, for example, talk about desocialization, their point is to reintroduce culture. My teacher and friend Arthur Kleinman got into hot water with some colleagues in medical ethics when he published an overview of the field, taking them to task for failing to ground philosophical debates in social and cultural analysis. He focused less on political economy and more on what he terms the "local social worlds" of those generating or responding to ethical constructs. He wrote, for example, that "medical ethics and human rights concerns must be centered in ethnographically informed evaluations in which local knowledge and local moral processes are made as salient as are the issues in global ethical discourse."[18] Here, I am complaining about something different: a "global ethical discourse" that does not study history and political economy is dishonest.

Kleinman's critique of rights and ethics discourse and the one I am attempting to sketch here are complementary but not identical. Kleinman sought to underline the importance, to ethics, of local moral worlds that did not figure in most normative, foundational, or technocratic accounts.[19] What underpins my critique, in addition to relief that Kleinman and other anthropologists have done the heavy lifting necessary to raise ethicists' awareness of local moral worlds, is the concern that ahistorical foundational accounts of global health equity tell lies about how the world got to be the way it is. Professional rewards come to those who stay within their specialty and wield its tools elegantly. I have nothing against elegance or focus, but it strikes me as artificial to keep history and political economy remote from epidemiology and other ways of measuring health status.

Examples are legion. Research conducted in the midst of great violence doesn't reference it, since there's no room for it in our scholarly journals. I remember one study, published in a pediatric journal in 1999, about AIDS in Rwanda. The article made no mention of violence, even though the research had been conducted between 1988 and 1994, a time of bloody social upheaval, and even though violence and social inequalities were linked to the AIDS epidemic well before the 1994 genocide. Nowhere in the argument, but only in the acknowledgments, does violence deserve a mention: "This article is dedicated to the memory of the mothers, children, and personnel of the project and of the members of the Department of Pediatrics who were murdered in 1994 during the genocide in Rwanda."[20] The authors weren't blind, but they had a narrow—perhaps realistically narrow—idea of what their disciplinary colleagues would consider relevant.

I'm not alone in lamenting the desocialization of ethics and medicine. Although I'm unaware of comprehensive reviews under this rubric, scholars from various disciplines—sociologists of science, anthropologists, psychologists, demographers, epidemiologists, economists, and even philosophers—have signaled the advance of this trend throughout the twentieth century. As specialization proceeds, and new or hardened disciplinary boundaries are erected, there is also a tendency to explore certain social phenomena with little attention to context. For example, fields such as psychology, usually considered a social science, have become focused exclusively on individual, rather than social, psychology. In this way, many social pathologies can be reclassified as personal failings, as Dan Wikler has shown in considering the topic of personal versus social responsibility for health.[21]

This blindness to context amounts to taking sides. It serves the interest of some and not others to keep the social roots of suffering and disease out of view. Most would agree that the sufferers themselves are not well served by any analysis that elides a history of how things came to be the way they are. Do we focus on distance or proximity? On static assessments of disease status at a point in time or on causality and history? When we focus on the social roots of suffering and disease, we return inevitably to the question of justice, but armed, this time, with a better analysis of how things came to be the way they are. This necessarily means disturbing the status quo, as the nineteenth-century Swedish dramatist August Strindberg wryly noted:

What is philosophy?

A seeking of the truth.

Then how can philosophy be the friend of the upper classes?

The upper classes pay the philosopher, in order that he may discover only such truths as are expedient in their eyes.

But suppose uncomfortable truths should be discovered?

They are called lies, and the philosopher gets no pay.

What is history?

The story of the past, presented in a light favorable to the interests of the upper classes.

Suppose the light is unfavorable?

That is scandalous.

What is a scandal?

Anything offending the upper classes.[22]

Strindberg was joking, of course, but his point was serious. Social history, the sociology of science (including social science), and political economy all steer us back toward the social inequality at the root of so many problems in ethics. Strindberg mentioned scandal. Well, what about the scandal of medical research in Africa or India? In the late 1990s, an acrimonious debate was played out in the pages of the *New England Journal of Medicine,* after scholars drew attention to the total lack of care received by the control group in a study of mother-to-child AIDS transmission. What sparked anger was the analogy—in fact, the direct comparison—drawn between the Tuskegee syphilis study and current AIDS research.[23] We like to think that we have learned the lesson of Tuskegee and are now equipped with the necessary moral and institutional safeguards. But in Africa, apparently, sick mothers and children can be used like lab rats. There is no anger like that of an ethicist whose hypocrisy has been unveiled! These debates are not generated by rogue editors in Boston; they are not going away. They are grounded in the history and political economy of our world.

4. The engagement of rich-world universities in research conducted in the poor world poses ethical problems quite distinct from those identified by institutional review boards.

Clinical trials conducted in the poor world are already a subject of discussion for a host of deontological and practical reasons. Leaving aside clinical trials, what about our mere presence in the poor world? What are the effects of this proximity? What about the obligation to do no harm or, to speak honestly, to stop doing harm? Thomas Pogge is brutally honest about the fallacy of theories of justice that magically efface the histories of injustice linking the rich world to the poor world.[24]

Sometimes the best of intentions lead to unintended harm. Peter Uvin's *Aiding Violence: The Development Enterprise in Rwanda* explores how the international aid apparatus helped lay the foundation for genocide in that country. International aid, especially when conducted by governments, quickly turns thuggish, this much we know. But if we ever expected nongovernmental humanitarian aid to Rwanda to be ethically straightforward, consider the experience of the humanitarians who'd come to Rwanda just before, during, or after the genocide.

Most found it nearly impossible to practice medicine there. They could not even be sure in what nation they were practicing, since the boundaries of the struggle to save lives kept shifting and cutting across the lines of military and political struggle. After the cessation of hostilities within Rwandan borders, the humanitarians who'd worked in refugee camps in Zaïre were in an exceptionally difficult position. Many of the camps were in fact run not by the United Nations but by the authors of the genocide, who had fled Rwanda with enormous resources of cash and armaments and set up a parallel government in exile, a government that openly declared its plans to continue the war and complete its genocidal project. More to the point, the *génocidaires* profited directly from the humanitarian aid that poured into Zaïre after the genocide. Fiona Terry, working with Médecins Sans Frontières (MSF) in the camp in Goma, writes searingly about mistakes made in allowing humanitarian aid to be diverted to *génocidaires* and the former Rwandan military, which had regrouped in and around the camps:

> The camps had been used as a base from which the former extremist government, army, and *Interahamwe* militias launched raids on Rwanda to continue the killing they had started in April 1994. The Rwandan government had warned on several occasions that it would break up the camps if nothing was done to control this threat on its border, but no outside state was willing to send armed forces into this dangerous quagmire. Hence those responsible for genocide, the greatest crime against humanity, remained living with impunity in camps run by the United Nations, and the very system established to protect the refugees became the source of their peril.
>
> The history of the Rwandan refugee camps graphically illustrates the paradox of humanitarian action: it can contradict its fundamental purpose by prolonging the suffering it intends to alleviate. Relief agencies rushed to avert immediate disaster among the refugees pouring into Tanzania and Zaïre, but inadvertently

set the scene for the eventual disaster that [one of the camp's residents, a civilian] described. Former leaders manipulated the aid system to entrench their control over the refugees and diverted resources to finance their own activities. In short, humanitarian aid, intended for the victims, strengthened the power of the very people who had caused the tragedy. The consequences were devastating.[25]

The consequences in question included prolonging the conflict in the Congo, where millions have perished over the past several years. But the real cost of such misadventures is not always seen immediately, as Amartya Sen explains in considering the Irish potato famine of the mid-nineteenth century. During the worst years of the famine, there was little in the way of rebellion, even as ships heavily laden with food and other goods left Ireland bound for England. But is it possible to understand the century of conflict that later ensued without reference to grievances registered much earlier? Sen sounds a similar warning in considering Africa today:

> The neglect of the plight of Africa today can have a similarly long-run effect on world peace in the future. What the rest of the world (especially the rich countries) did—or did not do—when at least a quarter of the African population seemed to be threatened with extinction through epidemics, involving AIDS, malaria, and other maladies, might not be forgotten for a very long time to come. We have to understand more clearly how poverty, deprivation, and neglect, and the humiliations associated with asymmetry of power, relate over long periods to a proneness to violence, linked with confrontations that draw on grievances against the top dogs in a world of divided identities.[26]

Top dogs. Not everyone within the university sees himself or herself as a top dog, especially in this society, where money and fame accrue elsewhere. But we are very highly placed dogs, and it behooves us to consider the obligations of the university to the poor world.

CONCLUSIONS

The research university enjoys special prestige in the world today. As First World universities "go global" in various ways, including their newfound enthusiasm for global health, they are caught up in a web of preexisting meanings. Their reputation precedes them, and it's not all favorable. Certainly, universities are part of the rich world, which is often seen skeptically or with warranted envy in settings in which disease is rampant and life expectancy is falling—but aspirations are not. So much of this asymmetry is linked to growing economic inequality, which is shaped in part by rich-world policies that are too rarely the focus of critical scrutiny. Or, rather, the critical evaluation that you might readily hear from poor people, if you were in a position to listen to them, is inaudible on the heights where we seek truth and think of doing good. To quote James Galbraith again, the rise of inequality

> has been, it would appear, a perfect crime. And while statistical forensics can play a small role in pointing this out, no mechanism to reverse the policy exists, still less any that might repair the damage. The developed countries have abandoned the pretense of attempting to foster development in the world at large, preferring to substitute the rhetoric of ungoverned markets for the hard work of stabilizing regulation. The prognosis is grim: a descent into apathy, despair, disease, ecological disaster, and wars of separatism and survival in many of the poorest parts of the world.[27]

Apathy, despair, disease, ecological disaster, and wars of separatism and survival in many of the poorest parts of the world. And, as Galbraith warns us, there exist "no mechanisms to reverse" the policies that have brought us to this point. How, then, do we pursue, with the best of intentions, work in the poorest parts of the world?

Let me be more optimistic than Galbraith and suggest some steps. One first step is to acknowledge the appalling poverty that is the lot of so many; another is to generate knowledge that can be of use in the world today and make sure that it is shared equitably. Imagine if all the discoveries made with public funding— those made under National Institutes of Health sponsorship, for example—were to become freely available to the world's poorest people. This public funding amounts to billions of dollars; what if those expenditures were harnessed to the largest, most direct type of universal public interest?

In 2001, Médecins Sans Frontières requested a license from Yale University to buy generic stavudine, a bedrock of many ARV regimens, from an Indian company that had offered to sell it in South Africa for approximately 3 percent of the price of the branded version. Though Bristol-Myers Squibb had an exclusive license to sell the drug, Yale was the key patent-holder because the drug had been developed at Yale, again with significant public funding. Within three months of receiving the request from MSF, Yale and Bristol-Myers Squibb announced that they would permit the sale of generics in South Africa and that the price of brand-name stavudine would be slashed thirtyfold—from $1,600 to $55—for governments and nongovernmental organizations in sub-Saharan Africa.[28] In contrast, in June 2005, Emory University sold its royalty rights in the antiretroviral Emtriva (emtricitabine) to Gilead for $525 million. While Emory could have used this sale to negotiate conditions for Gilead's licensing, registration, and patenting practices, it has not yet done so. Thus, while Emtriva is recommended by the World Health Organization as a safer and more effective alternative to lamivudine in its first- and second-line antiretroviral therapy guidelines, its prohibitive pricing makes it largely unavailable across the developing world.

I don't think it's too harsh to say that Emory is neglecting its obligations. It becomes easy for Emory to do so in part because in this society, universities belong to the not-for-profit sector and therefore frame the building up of their own endowments and intellectual property portfolios as a virtuous action. This is not entirely wrong: we need universities like Emory and Yale; the whole world benefits from them. But a benefit that is more direct would be a greater benefit. We must not fail to situate the privilege of the rich-world, not-for-profit university in a wider context, one in which, I'm afraid, the cynicism of many a Haitian or Rwandan observer finds its basis.

When Brown University set up a historical commission to look at that famously liberal institution's ties to the slave trade, the purpose was not simply grandstanding, the public display of white guilt, or the achievement of a reputation for purity, but the resocializing of our understanding of privilege and its sources. In this regard, by scrutinizing themselves and their history, universities can join understanding to action and furnish a pattern to actors larger and better organized than themselves—corporations and governments, for example.

A further goal might be to link our research and teaching to service designed to alleviate some of the most devastating problems. Universities must become more involved in the delivery of basic services to—and in the promotion of basic rights for—the poorest citizens of our globalized planet. None of this is to argue that research universities should abandon their focus on generating new knowledge and adopt, instead, a fundamentally humanitarian goal—although a little more generosity in this regard could hardly hurt our standing in the eyes of the world's poor. It's rather to argue that these problems cannot be wished away. We will be faced with hunger, thirst, disease, and violence as long as we venture forth into the world as it is and has long been. Developing new partnerships with groups based on service missions can help universities behave ethically, and less blindly, in Africa, for example.

Although in some universities there is a disdain for all things practical and applied, that could never be the case in a medical school. I believe that every part of the modern university can learn from its medical school's respect for practical applications. I mean, specifically, the establishment of teaching hospitals, often the major purveyor of quality services to the destitute sick of American cities. Over the centuries since their founding, our institutions have grown into islands of privilege and, I believe, decency. Precisely how decent we will appear to posterity remains a question. In order to span the rich world–poor world divide in an ethical way, we need to continue to promote the quest for theories and practices of justice that are honest about proximity and causation. It's less about assisting the distant needy and more about remaking a broken world. As David Hume wrote 250 years ago, in the heyday of the slave ship and the sugar plantation, "the boundaries of justice still grow larger."[29]

NOTES

1. Chatterjee, *The Ethics of Assistance*, p. 1 ("Introduction").
2. Ibid.
3. Singer, "Outsiders," p. 24.
4. "That omission," continues Peter Singer, "cries out for explanation, so I will offer one. Rawls' method is to seek principles of justice by asking what principles persons in the original position would choose, if they were choosing behind a veil of ignorance that concealed from them certain facts about themselves. If we applied this method globally, rather than for a given society, it is obvious that one fact the veil of ignorance should conceal would be whether one is a citizen of a developed nation like the United States, or a less developed nation like Haiti, Bangladesh or Mozambique" (ibid.). Thomas Pogge, in "'Assisting' the Global Poor," his contribution to the Chatterjee volume, offers a rebuttal of the assumption that these are distinct societies. In fact, each of the examples offered—Haiti, Bangladesh, and Mozambique—is embedded in a transnational political economy that has done harm to citizens of those beleaguered and strife-torn countries, all of them born of the violent expansion of colonial empires.
5. Pogge, "'Assisting' the Global Poor," p. 262.
6. Galbraith, "A Perfect Crime," p. 22.
7. Sachs, *The End of Poverty*.
8. Pogge, "'Assisting' the Global Poor," p. 265.
9. Sen, *Identity and Violence*, p. 134.
10. Brock, "Ethical Issues in the Development of Summary Measures of Population Health Status," p. 75.
11. Sen, "Equality of What?"
12. Marmot, "Social Causes for Social Inequalities in Health," p. 41.
13. Daniels, Kennedy, and Kawachi, "Why Justice Is Good for Our Health."
14. Sen, *Identity and Violence*, p. 11.
15. Alcaeus, "Poverty."
16. Peter, "Health Equity and Social Justice," p. 93.
17. Steiner and Alston, *International Human Rights in Context*, p. 1113.
18. Kleinman, "Ethics and Experience," p. 272.
19. Arthur Kleinman puts this in somewhat combative but trenchant terms: "Moral processes differ in a fundamental way from ethical discourse. Whereas moral experience is always about practical engagements in a particular local world, a cultural space that carries political, economic, and psychological specificity—a view from somewhere and actions and reactions that are partisan— ethical discourse is a globally elaborated abstract articulation of and debate over translocal values. It strives for an acontextual universality and objectivity: a view from nowhere" (ibid., p. 270).
20. Spira et al., "Natural History of Human Immunodeficiency Virus Type 1 Infection in Children."
21. Wikler, "Personal and Social Responsibility for Health."
22. Strindberg, "A Catechism for Workers."
23. Lurie and Wolfe, "Unethical Trials of Interventions to Reduce Perinatal Transmission of the Human Immunodeficiency Virus in Developing Countries." See the numerous responses to this article, pro and contra, published in the *New England Journal of Medicine* 338, no. 12 (1998): 836–41.
24. Pogge, "'Assisting' the Global Poor."
25. Terry, *Condemned to Repeat?* pp. 1–2.
26. Sen, *Identity and Violence*, p. 144.
27. Galbraith, "A Perfect Crime," p. 25.
28. Kapczynski et al., "Addressing Global Health Inequities."
29. Hume, *Enquiries concerning Human Understanding and concerning the Principles of Morals*, p. 153.

25

Making Human Rights Substantial

(2008)

Since I've recently been working in Malawi, where maternal mortality is said to be the third highest in the world and where hunger and other afflictions abound, I'll cite a recent essay by an expert on the country: "The tenets of liberalism in both politics and economy are now shared by all the political parties [in Malawi]. . . . Everybody, it seems, is committed to multiparty democracy, human rights, and the market economy."[1]

How are democracy, human rights, and a "market economy" linked together? Are they so linked for the poor in particular? Amartya Sen, among others, has offered compelling evidence that genuinely democratic governance is associated with more development and less poverty.[2] But there is no magic formula that leads from the "shared tenets" of "multiparty democracy, human rights and the market economy" to a reduction in the appalling privations still faced by many Africans and by hundreds of millions elsewhere.

Our ostensible beneficiaries are sometimes called the "voiceless poor." But the epithet is misapplied. They have much to say, and they do so, as any clinician or anthropologist knows. Whether or not we listen to them is a different story. Are human rights and public health groups even prepared to listen? In an essay entitled "Why More Africans Don't Use Human Rights Language," legal scholar Chidi Anselm Odinkalu puts it this way:

In Africa, the realization of human rights is a very serious business indeed. In many cases it is a life and death matter. From the child soldier, the rural dweller deprived of basic health care, the mother unaware that the next pregnancy is not an inexorable fate, the city dweller living in fear of the burglar, the worker owed several months arrears of wages, and the activist organizing against bad government, to the group of rural women seeking access to land so that they may send their children to school with its proceeds, people are acutely aware of the injustices inflicted upon them. Knowledge of the contents of the Universal Declaration [of Human Rights] will hardly advance their condition. What they need is a movement that channels these frustrations into articulate demands that evoke responses from the political process. This the human rights movement is unwilling or unable to provide. In consequence, the real-life struggles for social justice are waged despite human rights groups—not by or because of them—by people who feel that their realities and aspirations are not adequately captured by human rights organizations and their language.[3]

Odinkalu's language is uncompromising. But I don't want to mislead you into thinking that there is little but conflict between human rights groups and the humans desiring to win rights. Despite neoliberal orthodoxy in both international health and human rights, much has changed over the past few years, and some of it for the better.

Allow me to take the example of AIDS. The recent influx of funds designated to treat poor people with AIDS in the spirit of providing a public good, rather than a commodity—the result of efforts on the part of groups led by people living with HIV, student activists, and a small number of organizations serving the destitute with or at risk of AIDS—has challenged modern public health orthodoxy. Pushed by international financial institutions, this orthodoxy has too often sought (and still seeks) to "cap" health expenditures and focus on "cost recovery" in some of the most afflicted places in the world.[4] This is like a call for conserving water just after the house catches fire. But imposing user fees and selling therapy for AIDS did not work in Africa. It was not until diagnosis and care were made rights rather than commodities that people living with AIDS and in poverty had any hope of help. Although many will come to understand that it is ultimately cost-effective to lessen, through the only means possible, the horrific mortality registered among poor people living with HIV, the large-scale efforts I am referring to were not launched on grounds of cost-effectiveness. Instead, they were the result of powerful thinking about ethics and the alleviation of suffering. Human rights and social justice, once staples of public health, are slowly being revived on a grand scale.

How did this come to pass? Could this experience shape rights-based approaches to other problems of poverty? Speaking from our own experience, Partners In Health, which had focused on AIDS prevention for over a decade, launched AIDS treatment for the poor of central Haiti in 1998, an initiative cheered by patients but dismissed by influential international health leaders as neither cost-effective nor sustainable.[5] PIH was then small and without the influence necessary to do more than challenge such orthodoxy. So we turned to the human rights community, launching, in 2001, the Health Action AIDS campaign with Physicians for Human Rights (PHR). To make a long story short, Jim Kim and I went to the PHR board and argued that *this* was what a human rights campaign around AIDS needed to look like: we sought to protect the civil and political rights of people living with HIV at the same time that we protected their right to live. And that goal simply could not be achieved without diagnostic tools, medicines, and even food and water. PHR, it transpired, had never before launched a campaign for social and economic rights. But together we did so energetically, and this effort galvanized many students across the country, echoed and amplified the voices of courageous AIDS activists, and preceded the creation of the Global Fund to Fight AIDS, Tuberculosis, and Malaria as well as major bilateral programs such as the U.S. President's Emergency Plan for AIDS Relief (PEPFAR). These funding mechanisms may have their weaknesses, but at least we're no longer spending all our time arguing about whether or not we should even try to prevent and treat these three major infectious killers.

"FOOD, FOOD, FOOD"

The willingness of the public health community to embrace and promote the right to health is the fulcrum of our ability to address these complexities. Particularly crucial are the responses of global public health leaders. For example, will the inexorable rise of drug-resistant HIV, TB, and malaria lead those who are themselves at no risk of these diseases to argue, whether from Geneva or New York or London, that it is acceptable to use now-inexpensive first-line drugs for AIDS, TB, and malaria, but that it is neither sustainable nor cost-effective to treat more complex forms of these diseases? What if we confess, from Haiti or Rwanda, that many of our patients are hungry and that, last time we checked, the only treatment for hunger is food? What if we tell those who hold the purse strings that we do not really know how to treat diseases, much less how to prevent them, without promoting basic social and economic rights for the poor? Will the next orthodoxy in public health be that it is acceptable to offer medicines but not acceptable to offer access to microcredit, school fees, or food? That it is not "sustainable" to pay community health workers for their labor on behalf of their neighbors, even though we pay ourselves handsomely enough as international health consultants engaged in a network that spans rich world and poor?

Not long ago, in Malawi, I spent time doing home visits to people living with (or dying from) HIV. Most of these patients had not yet received antiretroviral therapy; several also had tuberculosis. They were slated to be enrolled in a treatment program that, though community-based, did not pay community health workers; nor did it include assistance with transportation to and from health centers; nor did it include food or the means to buy it. At the end of the day, over dinner—my colleagues and I enjoyed ready access to food—I mentioned that I had been invited to give a talk to the American Public Health Association and asked what they thought what my message should be. "Food, food, food," intoned one of my colleagues, a former medical student of mine who had completed his training and had spent eighteen months in Malawi working on a research effort. One word, repeated three times. But we all knew just what he meant: that without what some term "wraparound" services (including food), it will not be possible to scale up ambitious programs, because poor people in places like Malawi often don't have enough to eat, nor do they have the resources to go to health centers for a work-up, or the money to pay whatever hidden user fees lurk in ostensibly free AIDS treatment programs.

Over the past few years, we've seen some governments adopt, sometimes reluctantly, treatment programs that are "free" to their poor citizens. The poor show up, only to learn that it costs money to be tested for HIV or that they need an ID card or another laboratory test or a chest film. We've seen programs that claim to prevent transmission of HIV from mother to child but do nothing (or not enough) to provide breast milk substitute, weaning foods, or clean water to women living in poverty. We've even seen programs providing free therapies even as condoms or prophylaxis for opportunistic infections are sold through social marketing schemes funded by resource-rich institutions. These institutions have promoted a public health orthodoxy that leads most people in the richer countries to conclude that it is impossible to sustain public health interventions that do not generate profit or break even.

Food, food, food. How on earth can we make sure that people sick with consumptive diseases like AIDS or tuberculosis recover unless they have access to both medicines and food? That said, even those of us involved in treating such diseases in places like Malawi or Rwanda or Haiti (where food riots recently claimed several lives) know that there is a role for sustainable development. That's why we're involved in efforts to improve seed quality; increase access to fertilizer, water, and microcredit; and implement land reform. These will be difficult programs; "mission creep" will abound. But if we believe in health and human rights, we will need to broaden, very considerably, our efforts to promote social and economic rights for the poor. This, I would argue, is the leading human rights issue now facing public health.

THE CASE OF MATERNAL MORTALITY

Lest this sound too general, allow me to consider maternal mortality. Gender inequality and poverty—together, not apart—are the cause of almost all deaths during childbirth. Half a million women die each year in childbirth, almost exclusively poor women. These deaths can be prevented, but to do so requires that women with obstructed labor have access to modern obstetrics: an operating room, electricity, sutures, blood, clean wards, and good postoperative care.[6] (The major infectious diseases—AIDS, TB, and malaria—also cause a significant share of maternal mortality.)[7] I wish that someone had told me when I first traveled to Haiti, in 1983, that to promote human rights there, we'd need to build operating rooms and procure equipment and supplies; it would have saved us a great deal of time and made us more effective. We did learn that lesson, but only after presiding over the grisly spectacle of young women dying because they were pregnant and poor.

One community-based survey conducted in rural southern Haiti in the early 1980s pegged maternal mortality at 1,400 per 100,000 live births—far and away the highest in the hemisphere.[8] In rural Haiti, rates of cesarean delivery were about zero. Imagine my surprise when I later learned that, elsewhere in Latin America, public health advocates were fighting to *reduce* rates of cesarean delivery. This is the nature of inequality in Latin America: human rights activists could in one setting (Mexico) spend their efforts trying to reduce the number of cesareans, while others, similarly inspired, work in Haiti to increase poor women's access to cesarean delivery. I'd say something here about the ironies of inequality if the story weren't so abominable as to be beyond irony.

I saw the same thing again recently in Malawi. In the largest public maternity ward in the country, in Lilongwe, two obstetricians and a handful of nurses were struggling mightily to deliver twelve thousand babies each year. This is slightly more than the number delivered in Harvard's Brigham and Women's Hospital, where I was trained and still work. The Brigham delivers more babies than any other hospital in New England: we have, in just that one hospital, more than one hundred obstetricians, without counting the dozens of doctors and students training in obstetrics and gynecology. In the Malawian hospital, there is a single operating room; in the Brigham there are more than forty, with four in the women's health center alone. It's almost unheard-of for women to die during childbirth in the United States, though victims of maternal mortality in this country, too, are predominantly poor women of color. Here are some numbers: the maternal mortality ratio in Malawi is pegged at 1,800 per 100,000 live births. In the United States, an estimated 17 women die per 100,000 live births. Twenty-nine other nations, most of them affluent countries with national health insurance, match or beat the U.S. ratio. The figure for Iceland is zero.[9]

In Malawi, I spent some time with Tarek Meguid, one of the two obstetricians tending to the women who deliver their babies, or fail to do so, in the maternity hospital. The day I first visited, Tarek showed me a hospital that was fairly clean but sorely lacked supplies and personnel. The blood bank closed at 5 P.M.; the only way to care for critically ill women or infants was to transfer them to another under-resourced public hospital 2 kilometers away, a difficult procedure since calls had to be made, transport arranged, and so forth. Tarek spoke explicitly in human rights terms even as he detailed the material shortcomings of his facility. Outside the doors of the single operating room was a gurney piled high with surgical drapes in tatters. "This is an abuse of human rights," he said, lifting up one of the rags. "It would never happen if people considered the women we serve as human beings." It pained the doctor that the rate of maternal mortality *within* the hospital was 300 per 100,000 live births. Cold comfort: this appalling figure already represented a sixfold reduction from Malawi's national rate.

Should there be a right to sutures? To sterile drapes? To anesthesia? In 2007, colleagues and friends at PHR took on the issue of maternal mortality in terms that explicitly referred to social and economic rights. In support of their efforts, PIH helped to organize a focus group for PHR's investigation into maternal mortality in Peru. CARE Peru, a local organization with experience providing services to women in remote rural areas, was also instrumental in the project.[10] But to bring down the rate of maternal deaths among poor women in Peru and elsewhere, a wider network of partnerships will be necessary. We will need electricity. We will need gloves. We will need sutures and antihemorrhagics. We will need drapes and hot, clean water. We will need unfettered access to family planning. Making these demands is uncharted territory for human rights organizations, but if we are to move beyond studies, conferences, and exhortations and actually reduce the number of deaths, nothing less is required.

Many groups understand that it's impossible to make rights meaningful without material resources like those I have just mentioned. But human rights orthodoxy has left us weak in this arena. While many who care about rights are prepared to discuss gender inequality, too few of us are ready to buy generators, c-section kits, sutures, or operating-room lamps. Not even contraceptives are given pragmatic consideration. But how on earth will we ever stand in solidarity with women living in poverty if we're unable to move resources, including the fruits of modern science and technology, to them?

Of course, public authorities are the ones who can move such resources most effectively and equitably. A significant part of our work must consist of pressuring political officials to enact redistributive transfers on the scale required—and holding them accountable for performance. Yet even as we grapple collectively with the political challenge, those of us positioned within well-resourced private institutions can and must find short-term strategies to move vital goods quickly from settings where they abound in dizzying excess to places where their utter absence exacts a daily toll of suffering and death.

But many nongovernmental organizations (NGOs), including human rights organizations, regard such pragmatic solidarity as beyond their mandate. Research universities are, by and large, even more oblivious, and rich-world public health authorities are trammeled by the administrative boundaries of county, state, and nation, even as they know that Malawi's nurses, like Malawi's epidemics, transcend borders: nurses move out, epidemics move in. The NGOs that fight for the right to health care by serving the African poor directly frequently do so at the expense of the public sector. Too often, their efforts create a local brain drain by luring nurses, doctors, and other professionals from the public hospitals, like the one in Lilongwe, to "NGOland," where salaries are better and the tools of our trade more plentiful. The chronic dearth of resources that undermines staff retention in the public sector results not only from corruption, a frequent topic of commentary in the international press, but also from the effects of structural adjustment programs, so frequently lauded by the "international community."

How can this sorry human rights situation best be addressed? It's been analyzed exhaustively in survey after survey. And although I confess that PIH, an NGO, has moved into Malawi, I'll add quickly that we do not wish to expand the population of NGOland, nor to repeat our past mistakes. NGOs committed to the rights framework have to learn how to strengthen the public sector, since only governments can guarantee their citizens' rights. No one elected us, the denizens of NGOland, to set things right. We're all self-appointed. Those of us in NGOs and public health will have to learn to move beyond crude notions of cost-effectiveness and sustainability and return to the concept of social justice, which once inspired public health but now seems to embarrass us. First World universities, which are very much in evidence in African capitals, not only have to learn how to challenge public health and rights orthodoxies; they also have to learn how to share their abundant resources if they wish to conduct research across steep grades of inequality. It's fine that there are more American pediatricians than African ones in some of that continent's poorer cities and towns, including Lilongwe, but what are our long-term plans for helping to rebuild health care infrastructure and for training and retaining local professionals in these areas? What are our plans for making certain services, including safe childbirth, a right rather than a commodity?

All this is to say that health and human rights must move beyond the traditional exhortatory role, which stems from insisting on respect for conventions to which most states are signatory, to considering such prosaic issues as supply chains for sutures, generators, magnesium sulfate, and operating-room lights. And, of course, we need to do this at the same time that we continue and expand our struggle for civil and political rights. Enforcing rights is another matter altogether, since it is often the signatory states themselves who are responsible for rights violations, from torture to neglect of the public sector. Even less exposed to human rights activism are the shadow governments above the state: the international financial institutions, the tacit pacts among powerful nations that agree to disagree on Darfur or to ignore genocide in Rwanda until it's too late or to turn a blind eye to the worsening concentration of health and wealth in our inegalitarian world.

But where's the lesion, as we doctors say; what is the source of the problem? Health and human rights must have a legal framework to impose on national governments, true, but who is responsible for spending caps on health and education in the world's poorest countries? Certainly not the hapless medical professionals of those countries, and not the Ministries of Health, either. How can legislation be effective when governments such as Malawi's and Haiti's work with national budgets far less than that of a single Harvard teaching hospital? To understand why there are so few personnel and supplies in Malawi's largest maternity hospital, we'll need more than a local or national frame of analysis; we'll need to lift our eyes to look hard at history, political economy, and the powerful transnational institutions that have determined many policies in postcolonial Africa and in much of Latin America. Where is the support for applying a legal framework to those institutions?

The yield on an expanded and pragmatic view of health and human rights might be greater than we think. Preventing disease, saving lives, eradicating malnutrition, and promoting universal primary education will help to reverse the concentration of power in the hands of a few. It might not be naïve to argue that when people are not facing both destitution and disease, they should be more able to participate in civic processes, both local and national (although, granted, this hopeful hypothesis is not always borne out in affluent democracies). In short, as a public health activist, I advocate challenging the present priorities that place civil and legal rights first and adjourn substantive social and economic rights for another day. It is when people are able to eat and be well that they have the chance to build democratic institutions.

MEASURING THE EFFICACY OF ACCOMPANIMENT

So where does one start in an effort to support "an expanded and pragmatic view of health and human rights"? There is no secret formula, only brute needs. I mentioned food, and also sutures, medications, electricity, water, and other basic goods that may not seem very sexy to most people now commenting on health and human rights. Is this all there is to it—the transfer of ordinary enough material resources, not forgetting money, to the people and places that lack them?[11] We at PIH have found the recruitment and training of community health workers to be a means of working simultaneously on several aspects of the tangle of poverty and disease.

As research shows, under-resourced systems such as public-sector hospitals in places like Haiti and Malawi are unable to retain the nurses and doctors trained there. Here is another cruel paradox: since the local medical personnel were educated, by and large, within publicly financed facilities, their medical training has been supported as much by the local poor, who are taxed indirectly, as by private financing; and yet these doctors and nurses are leaking out of the public system.[12] In order to reverse the brain drain, we will have to invest heavily in institutions such as the maternity hospital in Lilongwe; we will have to make sure not only that health professionals receive salaries that are adequate but also that they have the tools of their trade. One study in urban Kenya shows that, although young physicians are unhappy with their salaries and the way they're treated by their superiors, they are also unhappy because they don't have the diagnostic tools and medications needed in order to treat their patients. "Before training," said one young Kenyan physician, "we thought of doctors as supermen . . . [now] we are only mortuary attendants."[13] How long can African doctors and nurses tolerate being little more than spectators to the grisly parade of suffering and premature death within the walls of that continent's public hospitals? No small amount of that suffering originates within these beleaguered institutions, as witness recent reports of nosocomial outbreaks of tuberculosis, including extensively drug-resistant strains (XDR-TB).[14]

Complementing the hospitals and clinics so desperately in need of renewed investment, community health workers (CHWs) are the pillar of the approach we've devised to deliver high-quality, free health care in settings of extreme poverty. Community health workers are mostly poor people; most have little in the way of formal education; most were unemployed or underemployed prior to becoming CHWs. I insist on the designation "community health *workers*" as distinct from community health *volunteers* (CHVs), the preferred term in NGOland. The word "volunteer" sounds noble but reflects the fact that many NGOs and governments do not pay local people who contribute time and labor to improving the health of their communities. Community health *workers* are paid, however modestly, for their efforts on behalf of their neighbors. Such compensation constitutes, unfortunately, yet another challenge to a regnant orthodoxy—in this case, the assumption that local community members' time and effort need not be valued as highly as those of other partners in health work.

As community members in many settings assume a greater role in health action, a debate simmers over equitable payment for all those who work within the community health arena. Some would have you believe that there's no difference between CHWs and CHVs—that is, between a model in which local people are paid for their work and one in which they are expected to perform similar tasks with no remuneration. This is a fraud perpetuated by our own "community of experts." Those experts who argue that we should encourage volunteerism and not pay the poor for their labor have not imagined themselves in the situation of the vast numbers of rural or urban poor people who would happily become community health workers. The problem with volunteerism is that the people called upon to donate their time are themselves poor (and often sick) and can scarcely afford to spend hours each day checking on their neighbors when they are obligated, NGO fantasies to the contrary, to plant millet and corn in order to feed their own families. That local people are sometimes prepared to accept the nonremunerated CHV role does not mean they don't prefer (and need) the CHW model. If volunteers are poor enough to warrant food assistance, they may declare themselves happy enough to volunteer in order to obtain such support; however, this mutually tolerated fraud is in no way genuinely mutual: the "international health community" promotes it, and the rural and urban poor tolerate it because without this charade, they would receive even less assistance in their efforts to prevent premature death in their beleaguered communities.

We have argued—and argue is the operative word—that community-based care involving CHWs is the very highest standard of care available to the poor who live with chronic disease, whether that disease be AIDS or diabetes or major mental illness. There's a reason that we have taken the model developed in Haiti and applied it not only in rural Rwanda or urban Peru but also in the poorer parts of Boston: in seeking to promote excellent outcomes in treating chronic infectious disease, we've found that doctors and nurses, and even social workers, cannot ensure that our patients are able to adhere to complex regimens unless our patients are offered what we've referred to as "accompaniment."[15] We've come to understand that something far better than supervision emerges when we support CHWs with even modest honoraria or incentives.

Over the past decade, we've sought to present the task of sustaining community-based care in settings of poverty as a human rights challenge. Don't expropriate the labor of the poor; champions of volunteerism within our ranks should feel free to volunteer but should be uncomfortable asking the destitute to do the same. So, although we're embarrassed that the honoraria we provide to our CHWs are so modest, we nonetheless insist on supporting them and seek to promote such remuneration in all the settings in which we work. We've rejected the community volunteer model and its underlying assumption that poor people's work can be had for nothing. We've been rebuked for this stance, but the rebukes have never come from the CHWs or their families or their patients. The rebukes have come from our peers, those obsessed with "sustainability" and "cost-effectiveness." Within international public health circles, we've found ourselves swimming against a strong undercurrent of censorious opinion.

Perhaps if our profession had embraced a rights-based model rather than those now in vogue in public health, we would not be forced to spend so much effort arguing that such care is cost-effective, although it almost certainly is.[16] We have every intention of stooping to the level of our critics in an effort to show that our model is indeed sustainable—we're not proud. But we also argue that the first thing to be sustained is First World commitment to global pandemics and other problems of the world's poor and that this is the way to begin a "virtuous social cycle" that might lift the destitute sick out of extreme poverty.[17]

To bring these disparate themes together in a rights-based framework is, I hope, a useful exercise, as we seek to chart directions for the health and human rights movement. If we believe that health care is a right, we need to address problems such as AIDS and maternal mortality with the highest standard of care possible. If we believe that the treatment for hunger is food, we need to address food insecurity with both short-term and long-term strategies, even if this means that we must learn about improving seed quality and procuring fertilizer and promoting fair trade, which means taking on rich-world agribusiness subsidies. If we believe that it's wrong to appropriate the labor of the poor, we need to insist that community members doing health work be compensated for their labor. If we put even a shred of stock in the notion of solidarity, then we must press for basic social and economic rights for the poor, regardless of whether we term our efforts "wraparound services" or accompaniment.

CONCLUSIONS: A NEW (OLD) RIGHTS PARADIGM

In many senses, nothing I've written here is new. The struggle for social and economic rights has been outlined many times before, the Universal Declaration of Human Rights mentions these rights explicitly, and 155 countries have ratified the International Covenant on Economic, Social and Cultural Rights. My own country is not among them, which will not surprise public health advocates, since we all have a long way to go before we see the right to health care in the United States. But if the basic ideas are hardly novel, the commitment and opportunity to turn them into action mark a fresh departure.

There's much to be done right now if we wish to address orthodoxy in health and human rights. U.S.-based human rights organizations focused on social and economic rights are mostly still small and new. However, their work is gathering momentum, and they are not timid about tackling tough problems. Larger, established organizations that have traditionally focused exclusively on civil and political rights are also coming on board. Amnesty International (AI) now boasts leadership with a clear commitment to social and economic rights and has begun to implement programming in this arena.[18] Indeed, the right to health, and the reduction of maternal mortality in particular, will be a central focus of Amnesty's forthcoming campaign on economic and social rights.

To fully grasp the significance of Amnesty International's recent inclusion of social and economic rights in its proposed programming, it is worth considering not only the importance of the right to health care—including the right to safe motherhood, which is the primary goal of AI's new effort to decrease maternal mortality—but also the cost of erasing the social and economic underpinnings of rights abuses writ large. The narrowly restricted view of rights that has dominated the rights movements based in (and funded by) affluent democracies since the outset of the Cold War has not only erased any serious consideration of social and economic rights but also distorted or at least shaped our understanding of rights abuses as conventionally defined in North America and Western Europe.

It's hard enough, some argue, to understand recent violations of civil and political rights (What, precisely, constitutes such violations? When do they occur? Why? How might they be prevented? What effective legal remedies exist?), not to mention allowing that there are other rights. This elision, this erasure, has not always occurred because of pressure by powerful ideological forces on rights groups, through funding restrictions and within an ethos shaped by the Cold War, to privilege some rights over others. This has certainly happened, as Carol Anderson insists in her magisterial *Eyes Off the Prize*,[19] but more insidious and corrosive erasures also occur. The social constructs now identified as human rights have, in every setting, a history.

Since no social movement is immune from the heavy hand of history, it is important to understand the history of the modern, contested rights movements based in what are termed Western democracies and to see what, during these often bitter struggles, has been brought into relief and what has been erased. Elsewhere and quite recently, discerning observers have written about the sinister ways in which human rights struggles in and regarding Haiti—the very place where French claims to promote "The Rights of Man" were revealed as hypocrisy, since Haiti, not France, was the first to abolish slavery—have been set back in recent years through funding *from* self-declared human rights groups.[20] But, as Odinkalu noted in the blistering critique cited earlier, Amnesty International is not funded by powerful governments; it remains, to this day, an organization funded by individuals objecting to torture and other forms of abuse and to the silencing of the citizenry and the press. (An aside: my first experience as a member of a human rights organization was as a college student, when I joined a group writing letters on behalf of people designated by Amnesty as "prisoners of conscience." I've never regretted it.)

But even groups leery of funding from powerful governments, including Amnesty International, may be "blinkered," as Naomi Klein explains in a new book that every proponent of human rights should read.[21] She reminds us that Amnesty International, in the "loaded context" of the Cold War, developed a "doctrine of strict impartiality: its financing would come exclusively from its members, and it would remain rigorously 'independent of any government, political faction, ideology, economic interest or religious creed.'" This was a reflection of much-needed integrity at a time in which rights were too often defined and supported in order to meet the needs of the powerful. But in its eagerness to eschew any partisan bias, writes Klein, the self-defined independent human rights organization neglected to bring into relief the social and historical backdrop of the rights abuses then occurring in Latin America. Mistakes arose whenever it was deemed unnecessary to explain *why* such abuses occurred, and whenever the sole point was to document and describe abuses. What was really at stake, then as now, Klein argues, was lost in the grim details of detention, torture, and disappearance: "Amnesty's position, emblematic of the human rights movement as a whole at that time, was that since human rights violations were a universal evil, wrong in and of themselves, it was not necessary to determine why abuses were taking place but to document them as meticulously and credibly as possible."[22]

In the 1970s, Latin America was the cauldron of the struggle for human rights in this hemisphere. Tens of thousands of civilians—this is a low estimate—died during efforts to promote basic rights, however they are defined. Almost no one would argue that headway was made during that decade, whether one defined rights primarily as civil, political, economic, or social. Although this death and suffering gave rise to "transnational" rights movements including Amnesty and many others, there remained a fog over those who sought to link, during military dictatorships, gross and obvious violations of rights (torture, murder, the silencing of the press) to the more insidious erosion of the rights of the poor to health care, primary school, water, and employment. The former list of rights generated the lion's share of commentary among the emerging mainstream rights organizations; the latter list of rights generated little commentary among those able to write about what was occurring in so many countries, including Argentina. Klein's assessment of this failure is worth citing at length:

> The narrow scope is most problematic in Amnesty International's 1976 report on Argentina, a breakthrough account of the junta's atrocities and worthy of its Nobel Prize. Yet for all its thoroughness, the report sheds no light on why the abuses were occurring. It asks the questions "to what extent are the violations explicable or necessary" to establish "security"—which was the junta's official rationale for the "dirty war." After the evidence was examined, the report concludes that the threat posed by left-wing guerrillas was in no way commensurate with the level of repression used by the state. . . . But was there some other goal that made the violence "explicable or necessary"? Amnesty made no mention of it. . . . It offered no comment on the deepening poverty or the dramatic reversal of programs to redistribute wealth, though these were the policy centerpieces of junta rule. It carefully lists all the junta laws and decrees that violated civil liberties but named none of the economic decrees that lowered wages and increased prices, thereby violating the right to food and shelter—also enshrined in the UN charter.[23]

Amnesty's selective attention, even at this moment of bold confrontation, shows the effort to forget precisely what we in the public health and human rights movement need most to understand, namely, the ways in which poverty seeps into every aspect of both health and rights. At the grotesque tip of the abuse iceberg, the sorry spectacles of Guantánamo or Abu Ghraib or state-sponsored torture and execution must not command all our outrage; the long and painful processes through which the world's poor meet a premature end deserve it too. When we can discuss solemnly the "right to sutures" even as we discuss gender inequality and torture, we will have succeeded in shifting the agenda in a way that makes sense to the world's poor and marginalized. And that should be the goal of the health and human rights movement in the twenty-first century.

NOTES

1. Englund, *A Democracy of Chameleons,* p. 12.
2. Sen, *Development as Freedom.*
3. Odinkalu, "Why More Africans Don't Use Human Rights Language."
4. Kim and Farmer, "AIDS in 2006—Moving toward One World, One Hope?" (included in this volume as chapter 14).
5. Farmer, Léandre, Mukherjee, Claude, et al., "Community-Based Approaches to HIV Treatment in Resource-Poor Settings."
6. Farmer and Kim, "Surgery and Global Health"; Ivers et al., "Increasing Access to Surgical Services for the Poor in Rural Haiti."
7. Menendez et al., "An Autopsy Study of Maternal Mortality in Mozambique"; Lucas, "Maternal Death, Autopsy Studies, and Lessons from Pathology."
8. Jean-Louis, "Diagnostic de l'état de santé en Haïti."
9. World Health Organization, United Nations Children's Fund, and United Nations Population Fund, *Maternal Mortality in 2000.*
10. Physicians for Human Rights, *Deadly Delays.*
11. Dr. Meguid, the obstetrician who led me through Malawi's largest maternity hospital, wrote that "one does not claim to be in possession of the magic bullet that will solve the problems of health care delivery in rural Africa. On the contrary, I do not believe in bullets, magic or not" (*The Challenge of the Periphery,* p. 5). Since my first visit, Scottish philanthropist Sir Tom Hunter has led an effort to rebuild Malawi's obstetrics infrastructure.
12. In a comprehensive recent report, Physicians for Human Rights summarizes the findings of several studies on the African brain drain: "The vast majority of students in Africa attending health training institutions attend public schools, where tuition is paid for primarily or exclusively by the government. When physicians, nurses, and pharmacists trained in these institutions leave the country, a significant public investment leaves with them. It has been estimated that developing countries spend about $500 million annually on training health professionals who migrate to developed countries. In South Africa, where training a physician costs about $61,000–$97,000 and training a nurse costs about $42,000, the overall loss to that country for all health professionals practicing abroad may top $1 billion" (*An Action Plan to Prevent Brain Drain*).
13. Raviola et al., "HIV, Disease Plague, Demoralization and 'Burnout.'"
14. Centers for Disease Control and Prevention, "Emergence of Mycobacterium Tuberculosis with Extensive Resistance to Second-Line Drugs—Worldwide, 2000–2004." See also Harvard Medical School and Open Society Institute, *The Global Impact of Drug-Resistant Tuberculosis.*
15. Farmer, Nizeye, et al., "Structural Violence and Clinical Medicine" (included in this volume as chapter 18); Shin et al., "Community-Based Treatment of Multidrug-Resistant Tubercu-

losis in Lima, Peru"; Behforouz, Farmer, and Mukherjee, "From Directly Observed Therapy to *Accompagnateurs.*"

16. One recent review addresses, perhaps sympathetically but certainly out of need, the economics of enlisting community health workers; see Walker and Jan, "How Do We Determine Whether Community Health Workers Are Cost-Effective?"

17. Walton et al., "Integrated HIV Prevention and Care Strengthens Primary Health Care" (included in this volume as chapter 13).

18. Amnesty International's latest global survey traces violence and injustice to social and economic inequalities, a new development in the organization's longstanding advocacy of legal and political freedoms: see Amnesty International, *Amnesty International Report 2009.*

19. Anderson, *Eyes Off the Prize.*

20. "Human rights" organizations have in fact often undermined the rights movement in Haiti—and this is true of civil rights as well as of social and economic rights. This sordid tale is only now coming to light: see Hallward, *Damming the Flood;* Robinson, *An Unbroken Agony.* For ongoing coverage of the mechanisms by which the governments of the United States, France, and Canada joined forces with the antidemocratic—and thus anti-rights—elite in Haiti to unseat elected Haitian governments, see the website of the Institute for Justice and Democracy in Haiti (www.ijdh.org [accessed October 12, 2009]), an organization that has sought to document the fate of the democracy and rights movements in Haiti in recent years.

21. Klein, *The Shock Doctrine,* p. 147.

22. Ibid.

23. Ibid., p. 148.

Conclusion

An Interview

(2009)

HAUN SAUSSY: Paul, from a beginning in ethnography, with its emphasis on the local, the specific, and the directly observed, you have gone on to offer accounts of what goes wrong with the whole human species in its many social subdivisions: ideas about "structural violence," inventories of the horrors of war. The categories you operate with on this level seem even broader than the kinds of interactions you were observing at work in the local, specific connections that were the subject of your earliest published writing—namely, the relation between Haiti and its powerful neighbor, the United States, over a long period. Some of your readers have criticized this leap to a global framework as rife with problems: according to them, it's so broad that it disables individual agency; it is driven by moral concerns that may not apply universally; and it has to be justified only "rhetorically," that is, as a ploy for capturing the attention of lay readers. Do you see the shift in the focus of your writing in the same way?

PAUL FARMER: No. For me, it has nothing to do with being a rhetorical ploy. Working with you on this collection forced me—forced us—to think about types of writing and to decide whether to move chronologically or in terms of broad themes. In the end, we broke things down into broad themes rather than following strict chronology.

For an example, I'd like to go back to a paper that I wrote (you read the drafts) in 1987 and published in 1988: "Bad Blood, Spoiled Milk." It's the opening chapter of this book. That paper was trying to stand up to various sorts of demands. One demand was just obvious: what does a graduate student working in Haiti write about? In the 1950s it would have been one thing; in the 1970s it would have been another. For me, having started work in Haiti in 1983, having started a proseminar in anthropology in 1986, I was very much concerned with the fashions of the moment. I remember an essay by George Marcus and Michael Fischer, from *Anthropology as Cultural Critique,* where they said that an anthropology accountable to history and political economy had yet to be written.[1] They had the pulse of the moment. It would be hard to think of a clearer formulation of what was needed in Haiti just then. Haiti has a way of forcing its students to the same combination of interpretation and social process, regardless of academic fashion. What else did Alfred Métraux try to do in the 1950s, what else did Sidney Mintz try to do in the 1970s?

I think that what drove me was not so much the content of anthropology at that moment, or going to medical school, or belonging to a certain school of thought, but really Haiti. The whole idea that we laid out in that article, although it's heavy on symbolic analysis, psychiatric nosology, and other things that I may have been studying at the time, gets back to the very difficult circumstances of life in that place. I was responding not to Marcus and Fischer's demand as such but to the situation in the place where I was doing anthropology.

These days, with a lot of demands on my time, clinical demands, departmental demands (I'm a department chair now, and that takes up time), when I do have a chance to read and write, I still think about that framework. I might, for example, be writing on the life history of a colleague's parent, as in the case of three colleagues: Barbara Rylko-Bauer, whose mother was an enslaved doctor in one of the labor camps in Poland during the Second World War; Philippe Bourgois, whose father was arrested and deported to another camp; and Alisse Waterston, whose immediate family escaped the carnage of that war and went to Cuba—three families whose lives were interrupted by the Nazi regime. The three children have written personal narratives about families whose whole course was transformed by a global war that began in Europe. How do I comment on these biographical narratives, twenty-something years after Madame Gracia told me what she expected from the scholarship I was doing about her village? How would I comment on them in a scholarly journal? The need for an anthropology accountable to history and political economy couldn't be clearer. How would you do a good job by considering these stories as just individual biographies? It's no different with the Haitian village I work in, where people's livelihoods were ruined by a hydroelectric dam in the 1950s, where disease and mortality affect people daily in ways that derive from social conditions. I just don't think the move from small to large is a rhetorical one; I don't think that's true.

Another, more significant trend in the things I write about comes out in your organization of this book. It goes from "Ethnography, History, Political

Economy" to "Anthropology amid Epidemics" and then to "Structural Violence" and to "Human Rights and a Critique of Medical Ethics." Each of these sections is asking, in a similar way, what are the large-scale social forces that determine and drive these local and observable phenomena? For me, that's the same model I apply to the international health bureaucracies, looking at policy; that's the model I apply to human rights, to a critique of human rights rhetoric. And you know, because you originally edited those pieces, that I was trying to write about these questions back in the 1990s. You'll find them all over my first book, *AIDS and Accusation* (1992). I'd like to think that it is not a rhetorical ploy or a change, but an interpretive grid that is useful for understanding a number of very different phenomena.

One thing that is different is my clinical writing, which is not really included in this volume. We talked about including some of it, but I didn't feel that it fit. There, the interpretive framework is set in advance. If I go to rounds, I'll offer an identification of the patient, the chief complaint, past medical history, the physical exam, laboratory studies, and then, for the infectious-disease consultant, an assessment and recommendations. When you write for a clinical journal, you have a methodology piece, a description of the patient, the interventions, the outcomes, and the conclusion. I felt that I couldn't incorporate that kind of writing into this book.

Nonetheless, anthropology and clinical medicine have in common a basis in observation. When you used the phrase "directly observed" in your question, you may have been thinking of ethnography but also of directly observed therapy. As Clifford Geertz said, the chief rhetorical ploy of contemporary anthropology is showing that you were there. I wouldn't make light of showing that you were there. In medicine, being there and directly observing the therapy are critical to good outcomes in chronic disease. This is true of many diseases, not just AIDS but also diabetes, major mental illness, and coronary heart disease. The notion of directly observed therapy—of accompaniment, of accompanying someone over time (that's a theological term, originally, if I'm not mistaken)—comes down to the same thing: what you can see with your own eyes.

If there has been a shift in the writing, it would be a shift in the subject. I'm learning along the way. Could I write *AIDS and Accusation* again today? I couldn't write the Haiti books again for Rwanda or Lesotho; I wouldn't have time to learn those societies from the ground up.

HS: You've been a fairly persistent "agent of change" in the world of medicine and aid. But how does the expert in a region (say, Haiti) and in a problem (say, HIV or multidrug-resistant tuberculosis) gain credibility as a voice addressing worldwide problems like war and inequality?

PF: Do you really think I have credibility in addressing war and inequality? I'm not so sure. I understand that I have credibility on global health, on setting infectious-disease policy globally, on certain pandemics, and I would hope I have some credibility in terms of having put more than twenty-five years, my whole adult life, into implementation and delivery around these topics. I don't think that can be taken away from me or us. We have been there; we've done the work. If you take a head count, Partners In Health currently employs more than eleven thousand people and supports close to fifty institutions, most of them in the public sector, in ten countries. Seventy percent of our workers are community health workers who have never held a job before. This is cumulative—not an argument that's right or wrong. I would imagine that my credibility in this sphere comes from something other than having great writing or theories.

What can I point to? I can say, "We built that hospital." But I can't say, "This work has had great impact in reducing economic inequality or preventing conflict." I don't think I have that credibility. That's one reason I am turning to things like job creation as a way of breaking the cycle of poverty and disease. On areas like Haiti, I think that depth of experience does give you credibility. I would hope I have some about Haiti, more so than on Peru, Rwanda, Lesotho, Russia.

A lot of my credibility comes from being a doctor. Let me tell you a story. A few years back, we were hosting a five-year-old child who had a malignancy called a Wilms tumor invading her kidney, plus metastases in her lungs; it was a lot for a five-year-old to handle. Because she required extensive radiation therapy, which couldn't be done in Haiti, she came to Boston with her mother and stayed in our apartment, a practical solution since I was traveling a lot anyway. I'd come home from the hospital, have dinner with them, hang out, play with the kid, and so on. One evening, some students came to visit the kid—they were great with her—and they said to me that they had been reading one of my books. The girl's mother overheard this and said, "Dr. Paul, you never told me you knew how to read and write."

HS: So your reputation as an infectious-disease specialist didn't automatically transfer into other domains. I might imagine that the broader your reach, the more difficult it is to have an effect; is this so? Is there a difference in the personal efficacy of the specialist with something of a technical approach and that of the generalist addressing moral issues on a global scale?

PF: I never wished to inhabit a public persona. It's still not my wish, and I don't much care for it. The real issue for me is around being an agent of change, and linking humble pragmatism and service to solid analysis and understanding. At Partners In Health, I've been asking: What makes us different? Maybe not a lot; maybe we exaggerate the differences. There are a lot of nongovernmental organizations out there doing impressive and desperately needed work for people's health and well-being. If anything makes us different, it's the feedback loop we've set up, linking service to research and teaching. Most NGOs have no capacity in research or teaching, and most universities have no capacity in service. That's a mistake. To lack the vision to understand that we will not drive forward our work as agents of change without systems analysis, systematic reflection on practice—that's a mistake. Systems thinking, isn't that what history and political economy are? Isn't that what engineering is? Applying it to these stubborn problems, as we can do through our academic tie-ins, is an added level of what the old-school people used to call praxis.

HS: Tracy Kidder's *Mountains Beyond Mountains* was published in 2003. Since then, such organizations as PEPFAR (the U.S. President's Emergency Plan for AIDS Relief) and the Gates and Clinton Foundations have poured billions of dollars into health care in the poor world. (Indeed, Dr. Anthony Fauci, director of the National Institute of Allergies and Infectious Diseases, credited you and PIH with the change in thinking that made these dollars available for AIDS, malaria, and tuberculosis treatment.)[2] How has the landscape changed for you and your coworkers in recent years, and what do you foresee in the near term?

PF: The landscape has changed in enormous ways, most good, some not so good. Anybody who tells you that PEPFAR and the Global Fund to Fight AIDS, Tuberculosis, and Malaria are just fraught with problems and not worth their salt is clearly not involved in humble service. You go from 2002, when there was not a single international financing agency working to treat AIDS, tuberculosis, and malaria, which were taking six million lives a year, no work even to prevent these diseases or develop new diagnostics—you go from that bleak picture to having these fantastic bilateral or multilateral mechanisms focused on integrating prevention and care. (Dr. Fauci, I'd like to add, gets a big piece of the credit for making this happen.) That has changed the landscape irrevocably. Ever since, it has been impossible for anyone to say, "Well, we've never had the experience of treating a chronic, lifelong medical condition among the poor, so it can't be done." Now that these countries and agencies have had that experience, they can't go back. It's irrevocable.

Disbursements began in 2003 for the Global Fund, in 2004 for PEPFAR. This is recent history. What is interesting, after five years, is how quickly people forget. If we cannot seize the moment and strengthen health systems for the poor globally, including in the United States, we're in trouble. We take what in public health terms we call "vertical enthusiasms"—that is, a program only for malaria, safe motherhood, AIDS, breast cancer, or Burkitt's lymphoma—and try to use that exclusive interest to strengthen health systems writ large. That's the landscape now. There's a chapter in the book about this: "Integrated HIV Prevention and Care Strengthens Primary Health Care: Lessons from Rural Haiti," which some colleagues, including a student of mine, and I published in the *Journal of Public Health Policy* in 2004—less than a year after we received the first Global Fund grant in the world.[3]

If you look back at the tempestuous debates over primary health care in 2009, I believe you'll ask yourself, which of the issues being debated now was not already apparent in the first AIDS treatment delivery system in the developing world? Anyone who is trying to work on delivery, and there are millions of us, will see that you can't avoid these questions. In the newspapers, it's always presented as a zero-sum game, as if funds for AIDS are automatically taken away from, say, epilepsy. This mentality of limited resources is so damaging: "If we do AIDS, we can't do epilepsy, or we can't do lymphoma; if we do treatment, we can't do prevention; if we do Comp Lit, we can't do Greek"; and on and on it goes. Yes, resources are scarce. But the resources are less scarce than ever before in human history. (I was saying this back in 1999, if you'll remember, in "Pathologies of Power: Rethinking Health and Human Rights.")[4]

People, never patients, often say to me, "You work on TB, but what about cancer?" I try not to be defensive and I respond, truthfully enough, "Of course I work on cancer!" For me, it was never about this or that disease, but rather about other questions: What about the people we are serving? What ails them? What are their primary problems? Why would we single out one? The answer is, if you can channel these vertical enthusiasms into broader issues, that's good. I've written about cancer, AIDS, surgery, tuberculosis, but always to try to frame specific diseases in the larger context of primary care.[5]

HS: Seen in relation to the Global Fund and PEPFAR, PIH was ahead of the trend, as it had been providing free medical treatment for years to thousands of people abandoned by their existing health systems. What does it mean that the PIH argument is now so widely accepted? Does the PIH model of care translate readily into new areas? Are there hitches in its adoption or adaptation?

PF: Free medical care: it's not thousands now, but millions, who have benefited. What I find startling is how much the term "free medical care" rankles people. Some sociologist should be able to figure it out, but it's puzzling to me. I just did a blurb for a report about health as a human right. Instead of free medical care, I said, the *commodification* of medical care should scandalize us. It startles me to see that people are so irritated by the term "free medical care." When I say "people," of course, I don't mean the poor, who say, "Free medical care? Bring it on!" But policymakers in Africa and Haiti take issue with it. In our publications and materials at PIH, we've learned to be very careful about the words we use. If you say "accessible medical care," it shocks people less than "free medical care," although the meaning can be the same when you're talking about poor people.

The patients were being abandoned because there wasn't a language in which to present their claims and needs. Public health people don't like human rights language very much. They prefer public health language, the language of "public goods for public health." What does that mean? It means free medical care. It means a system where you don't pay more if you're sick and poor, and you're protected from the regressive consequences of a commodity-based financing scheme. I'm a pragmatist; I'm not trying to win a seminar-room argument. We're trying to see health care extended to more and more people, along with basic services such as clean water and primary education.

Let me signal to you another worrisome trend in the language about health interventions: the term "task shifting." It's a phrase used to discuss the resources that have recently become available to treat chronic, serious disease among the poor. But there's a hypocrisy in the term. It makes it sound as if professional A, a doctor, say, was devoting time and effort to treating AIDS and TB, and this work was then shifted to a nurse or other heath worker. That misrepresents the history. In general, nobody was providing care at all. The "shifting" was from providing no care to providing care, but the phrase disguises that fact. However, to point this out annoys health policy people. So why say it? To win an argument? No. But in a book like this, we should say it.

When you ask about how things have changed since our arguments have become "widely accepted," I want to know which arguments of ours have been so widely accepted. Free health care? No—not accepted. The "right to health care" argument? No—not accepted. It's a big struggle; that's why you and I are bringing out this book. The "public goods for public health" argument? We're getting there, somewhat. And, finally, the "breaking the cycle of poverty and disease" argument? This is much more widely accepted, at last.

The arguments have always been multivocal. We've been trying to do several things at once: argue for health care not as a commodity but as a right; advance the use of disease-specific funding and interventions as a way of strengthening health systems; advocate making health care accessible to the poor and those in need; and propose adopting other health care models, such as investment in health care as a way of bringing countries out of poverty. The obscenity of having to pay for medical services, of being unable to, and dying as a consequence; the utility of a rights notion; the limitations of a rights notion; the importance and utility of public health notions—all these have been voiced by us. But as pragmatists, we'll try anything, we'll go anywhere, if it will help the poor majority. In a book like this, we have the space to make deeper, more complex arguments about these issues, something going beyond single solutions for specific contexts.

Hitches in adoption and adaptation? Absolutely. We've covered a number of them in the book.

HS: The initiation of PEPFAR and American involvement in the Global Fund have had the effect of swelling the ranks of NGOs active in the developing world. Has this been an unalloyed benefit to the people these organizations serve? What do you see as the long-term effects of this increase in charitable action? What about the models on which these organizations are built?

PF: It is not an unalloyed benefit. It is an alloyed benefit. In Haiti, we have what we call "the Republic of NGOs." President Clinton asked me to make a list of the various NGOs working in Haiti so that their efforts could be coordinated. This week, for the Clinton Global Initiative and the UN, we've pulled together and are about to publish the list, and we have found over nine thousand NGOs in Haiti. And imagine how many more we may have missed if we had caught up with all the peasant cooperatives and little church initiatives. The Republic of NGOs: it's startling.

Last week, I went directly from Haiti to Rwanda to see my family and give a talk. Another of the speakers at the conference was Dambisa Moyo, who wrote the book *Dead Aid*. She made the argument that no country has ever been pulled out of poverty by aid of that sort. I don't know about this as a general argument; I would like to cast a wider net and, for instance, ask Jim Kim's opinion about the East Asian rebuilding efforts after the war and the emergence of the "tiger economies." But I have to say that the idea that charity is going to substitute for social justice and equity is dangerous. The idea that charity is always bad is also a dangerous idea. I think that swelling the ranks of NGOs can be good, it can bring good consequences. But is it really the long-term strategy for dignity and rights? And the answer is no; the long-term strategy is that people know they have certain rights.

That's what FDR said, not just in 1944 but in the 1920s and 1930s. Cass Sunstein, in his book on Roosevelt's last inaugural, *The Second Bill of Rights*, points out that this is not something Roosevelt started saying just before his death; he was saying it all along. If I'm not mistaken, he couldn't walk for the last twenty-four years of his life. Although he was a rich man, he knew what it was like to be in need. Roosevelt was saying, "I believe in labor rights. I believe in a safety net. I believe in access to education." And I think that's the bottom line for human dignity.

You know, you went to a prep school; I went to a public school. I didn't even know what a prep school was. But we both got into a fancy university, which is where we met at the age of eighteen, in the first week of school, I might add. I got there because from the age of five until I was eighteen, I had the right to go to a public school. Now I'm not claiming that it's the great leveler or equalizer;

we all know it's not. But the important thing is that there was never a question about whether or not I was entitled to a free public education. NGOs are great, but we NGOs are not going to solve the problems of the poor.

HS: According to a 2004 *New England Journal of Medicine* article, "In the United States, as many as 50 percent of patients receiving antiretroviral therapy are infected with viruses that express resistance to at least one of the available antiretroviral drugs."[6] What's the situation with resistant strains of HIV in the world (including the United States)? What's to be done about it? I think I can anticipate your answer: dosages must be adequate and uninterrupted, and for that, they must be free and administered with supervision. But what, if anything, distinguishes drug resistance in the HIV epidemic from that seen with TB?

PF: You did anticipate my response. Therapy must be uninterrupted, which means that it must be accessible or, in many cases, free. There are lots of reasons for that way of administering the drugs, chief among them the need to avoid an epidemic of drug-resistant HIV. But in terms of outcomes, similar arguments could be made for diabetes, hypertension, major mental illness, and so on. If you're interested in the outcome for the patients, the argument that we must be mindful of the potential for developing resistance in the pathogens could be made for other pathologies for which we have a deliverable. It's very expensive to give bad medical care to poor people in a rich country. One reason is the advent of drug resistance. Argentina, a relatively rich country in comparison to the places where we work, spends two-thirds of its public AIDS budget on second-line antiretrovirals because they "burned" the first ones by creating resistance.

About drug resistance in HIV and in TB, I could list you ten differences having to do with modes of transmission, the nature of diagnosis and treatment, and so forth, but for this question I don't think the differences are significant. The main point, the model, is that every infectious pathogen, and even the vectors (think of mosquitoes), over time will acquire resistance to the strategies we've put in place. Be it parasites, viruses, bacteria, microbacteria, over time the pathogens will develop resistance to the strategies we've devised to stop them. Mosquitoes develop resistance to DDT; the malaria parasite develops resistance to the drugs. We, the hosts, adapt, and so do the pathogens and the vectors.

What can be done? The only ethical way to slow the advent of acquired drug resistance is to put in place good programs of prevention and care available to everybody who needs them.

HS: PIH has worked hard to document the health outcomes of its initiatives as part of the process of arguing for the broader adoption of its model. Clearly, when mortality goes down or when people suffering from HIV are able to add years to their lives thanks to free antiretrovirals, the outcomes are positive. But what about the wider effects, economic and other, of providing free high-quality health care to poor people? Or the true costs, again in a wider frame than the patient's individual case, of not providing such health care?

PF: The broad effects of investments in health care are just as visible as the ill effects of leaving things undone. We came to Haiti with a narrow agenda, just to cure the sick, and we found that for systemic reasons we couldn't do that well without getting involved in clean water, in economic projects, in social organization. We're proud to show that the many parts, the many pillars, reinforce one another and make life more livable for people whose times were about as hard as times can be. I'd like to say that PIH has not done this alone. What we've done, we've done through teaching and research, with the help of Harvard University and the Brigham and Women's Hospital. That's how we were able to document what we were doing. If anyone gets the idea that we were doing this alone, that's the wrong message. We had the resources of a university and a teaching hospital behind us. Every university should have that, the University of California, Yale, Duke, and so forth.

HS: What about the argument one sometimes hears that saving the lives of poor people in poor countries only adds to the population and resource burden on the earth and is therefore a soft-hearted approach with untoward consequences?[7]

PF: It's interesting that in twenty-six years I've only heard this a couple of times. Maybe it is often thought. But you know how much public speaking I do to lay audiences—Girl Scout troops, church ladies, graduate schools—and it's really rare that one hears that. The few times I've heard that argument, it came from experts, not laypeople. In all these years of shilling for the poor, that question has come up only a couple of times. People do ask about family planning and other areas, for which we have informed responses. Every other major question, I've been asked thousands of times.

What about it? Well, you know my stock answer: one could argue that unfettered pandemic disease is not the best way to control population size.

HS: Your recent writing identifies the state as the crucial agent in guaranteeing universal access to health care. But your work could not have been done without the support of private foundations and far-seeing individuals. Is there a paradox here? Could a skeptic look at the development of your thinking and say that you came to the state only after the hook had been baited and states were ready to negotiate because of a self-interest created by private charity?

PF: Maybe. I look back to what I was reading and writing in the 1980s. If you were working in Haiti then, what did you want? A decent state that was not a dictatorship. Call me old-fashioned, but I like this idea of one person, one vote. We're not just now tacking on the state as an afterthought. If we start in Haiti under dictatorship, if we start in a federal prison system in Russia, if we start in Rwanda with a government that's trying to break the cycle of poverty, wouldn't you have three different types of state? In graduate school, I read Michel-Rolph Trouillot's *Haiti, State against Nation*. This problem of the state, of resistance and private initiative, is one I've been struggling with my whole adult life. I've heard this cynical narrative about NGOs trying to make a claim on state resources too, but it's not the way it worked for us. There are a lot of private charities that get in too deep and then want to be bailed out. But we—all of us NGOs together—should not do that.

HS: In "Getting There from Here," published in the *New Yorker*, Atul Gawande observes that "every industrialized nation in the world except the United States has a national system that guarantees affordable health care for all its citizens. . . . But each has taken a drastically different form, and the reason has rarely been ideology. Rather, each country has built on its own history, however imperfect, unusual, and untidy."[8] In contrast to this argument for historical specificity and path-dependency, the PIH model is designed to be extensible and generalizable. Does the PIH experience indicate a path for creating universal health care systems where none have yet been implemented, including, perhaps, in the United States?

PF: I've been asked a lot for my view on American health care. Well, "it would be a good idea," to quote Gandhi. I've seen the very best in American health care and the very worst. If someone has a complex medical emergency and they can be schlepped from rural Maine or Jordan or Haiti and end up at a place like the Brigham, that's good for them. But the expenditure of 16 to 20 percent of GDP that we currently have is not sustainable with an aging population. I get that. It's too expensive. So at what points can a layperson like me who doesn't know the American health system make an inroad? Universal access is important. Bringing Americans into the network. I feel the same way about the Guatemalans or the Bolivians. It doesn't matter to me who the patients are. I do know that giving poor people bad medical care in a rich country is a bad idea.

Looking at this as an American, a doctor, but no expert on health care in the United States, the debate seems to me entirely ideological, not driven by data or evidence. If it were an evidence-driven debate, we would have a public option already enshrined as law. And so I'm watching, just as an American, and saying, I hope we do a good job.

Atul is a friend and colleague; we trained together. Back in medical school, we would see the same patients, and I would read his notes: they were both concise and elegantly written, and I always said, "There's only one surgeon I know at the Brigham whose notes on a chart are worthy of the *New Yorker*."

We gave a talk together at the American Surgical Association, and he said something about my work, our work, that disturbed me a little bit. He said, "I'm not a humanitarian or a generous person like Paul; I'm just trying to use the data to improve surgical services for a wide number of patients." I said, "Atul, (a) I find you perfectly humanitarian in your clinical work; and (b) we're also trying to use these data to move forward better delivery systems." So I'm not sure where he got that. But in his article, the thing that must be intriguing to Americans and especially to those in political power is this: in the same country, even the same county, you can have clinical results that are all over the map, radical differences in quality and outcome.[9]

So does PIH indicate a path? I'll say one thing. On chronic disease, the highest standard of care is community-based care, with community health workers. Whether we have lots of doctors per capita or very few, community-based care is still the highest standard of care for chronic disease. The model of accompaniment that we developed in Haiti in the 1980s—we ended up bringing it to Boston to improve the management of chronic disease where people were falling through the cracks.[10]

There's one more thing about the model we developed out of our Haitian experience. The United States now has high unemployment and a financial crisis. Wouldn't it be good to create a half-million jobs in America to do something generative and decent? Train five hundred thousand or a million community health workers; they would enjoy the work, build social capital, and use this as a springboard for getting into college or another degree program and finding other jobs that might be even more rewarding. Or some might like to remain health workers forever. I think it's a good plan for lots of reasons. One, outcomes; two, it's a dignified job, taking care of other people; three, we need some quick wins. You don't think you could get people in an area with crushing unemployment like New Haven or Hartford to accept an offer of training and payment? It's not rocket science.

HS: What do you see as having been accomplished by slogans like "Three by Five," the push declared by the World Health Organization to start 3 million poor patients on antiretrovirals by 2005? Do such initiatives deliberately set impossible targets, counting on failure to have an educational effect? Do they perhaps contribute to cynicism about the effectiveness of multinational health bureaucracies?

PF: I was involved in that one, so I can tell you: it was aspirational, always, but it was never intended to set up conditions for failure. I don't know if Jim Kim invented the slogan, but in his time at the WHO he was the force behind "Three by Five." We fought hard to meet the target and got to 1.9 or 2 million in 2005, and I could hardly believe we did so well. At the time, Jim said, "I'll take the rap for failing." Well, if that's failure, then what about every other global health initiative?

The smallpox eradication initiative: there's an example of success. I've been teaching about the smallpox campaign, using an article by Paul Greenough that's a critique of the heavy-handed approaches applied in the service of an end that I think we would all agree was noble.[11] What I want the students to grapple with is that this was a huge public health victory, the big victory of the twentieth century, but what are the costs? How do we calculate them? I'm not trying to have students agree with what I think about it; I want them to struggle with it as I have. The goal was to eradicate smallpox—and guess what, it worked. It was the perfect vertical program: there was no nonhuman host to serve as a reservoir; we had a Cold War truce to work on this; no one's interests were served by smallpox continuing to be a threat. The counterargument for the class, just last week at Harvard College, was an article by Ciro de Quadros, the man credited with the successful eradication of polio.[12] It's really about the struggle between the vertical and the horizontal, in medical terms; but Greenough, as a social scientist, comes in to show the high political cost of enforcing vaccination practically at gunpoint. Eradication programs are possible only if there's universality. They went in and they were tough. It worked, but now there will be decades of discussion about the cost. Yet the benefit, to use crass terms, the return on investment for that intervention, is huge.

"Three by Five" was a great idea. There was so much resistance to it, but the idea was to set a goal and try to meet it. By the way, the 3 million target was far exceeded as of mid-2006. As for contributing to cynicism, I just don't believe it. A lot of bureaucracies, according to Max Weber, are cynical whether we will or not.

HS: What are the implications of the current financial crisis for the objectives of PIH and similar organizations? Is the news simply bad, or does the imminence of recession or depression change public attitudes about spending and investment in a constructive way?

PF: If you're trying to raise money for eleven thousand employees serving some millions of patients, it feels very burdensome and daunting. In December 2008, Ophelia Dahl and I wrote a memo to our donors, where we made the argument that in times of financial crisis it is imperative that we find more resources, not fewer, to protect human lives—a very Rooseveltian sort of argument.[13] It was difficult, as you know, but our donations were up something like 18 percent over the past two years. How was that done? By daily efforts. At the same time, our expenditures were planned to be up 22 percent. Our reasonable, optimistic, engaged objectives—for building new hospitals, accommodating new patients—could not be met. Not because we shrank, but because we couldn't grow fast enough to meet need and capacity.

The imminence of depression hasn't changed Americans' attitude about the need to be generous toward those less fortunate. It may have even made for better attitudes. I was worried that people would say we can't feed our own, but that hasn't happened. Public attitudes toward supporting our work have never been better. The problem is that the public doesn't have the resources it used to have. The contraction of the world economy has been real, cutting into the savings of generous individuals. So we have been trying to double the size of our donor base rather than double the size of the gifts. A broader appeal has a lot going for it. I think that this crisis will force us to reexamine our dependency on carbon fuels, for example. With fifty hospitals, we have a lot of energy needs.

The most important thing for a group like PIH is not to get stuck in paradigms and models that we mastered years ago, ideas that worked before. You have to keep innovating. The "learning institution" is not a goofy corporate idea. According to Weber, any institution can get stuck. If we are to be a nimble institution, we have to respond to new conditions, whether financial, environmental, epidemiological, or social. All those things are fundamentally social. Berger and Luckmann were right.[14]

NOTES

1. Marcus and Fischer, *Anthropology as Cultural Critique*, p. 86. This idea is also discussed in the introduction to part 1 of this book and in the concluding pages of Farmer, "Bad Blood, Spoiled Milk" (chapter 1 of this volume).

2. Waring, "PIH's Farmer Speaks on Antibiotic Resistance."

3. Walton et al., "Integrated HIV Prevention and Care Strengthens Primary Health Care" (included in this volume as chapter 13).

4. Farmer, "Pathologies of Power"; this argument was further developed in the 2003 book *Pathologies of Power*, chap. 9 (included in this volume as chapter 21).

5. On the right to surgery, see Farmer and Kim, "Surgery and Global Health."

6. Clavel and Hance, "HIV Drug Resistance," p. 1023.

7. On May 4, 2008, CBS's *60 Minutes* broadcast a feature segment on PIH's activities (Pitts, "Dr. Farmer's Remedy for World Health"). Comments posted online by viewers included the following:

Call me cold hearted but I think his program should include a sterilization program. The 45 year old woman with eleven kids with complications during her delivery infuriated me. No reason on God's green earth for anyone much less an impoverished person to have that many children. [Comment by TheRock107, May 4 and 5, 2008]

I think this is bunk! He should be doing this in the United States of AMERICA! He's turning his back on his own! [Comment by ladyharley05, May 5, 2008]

I find it quite unnerving whenever I come across any article praising someone for giving away (free) medical care to any outside the USA when so much help is needed here . . . especially when that same physician was educated here.

Just now offering "help" in the way of knowledge rather than personal assistance to Americans is insulting. What about the millions here that are in need of medical care? Why aren't physicians willing to do for those who helped them acquire that knowledge that they so freely give away to third world countries now? Was it any of them who gave this man his scholarships? No!

Where's his compassion for those less fortunate—where he spent his youth? Praise should be given to those who deserve it and charity begins at home . . . or should! [Comment by feya1, May 5, 2008]

While I am impressed with Dr. Farmers altruism I find it amazing that with all of those sick and starving people the words "birth control" never came up. Without birth control how can he ever hope to get ahead, obviously he can't. As he is one of eight children himself is it possible his religion is clouding his judgement, he is a phony saint. [Comment by hahnse, May 6, 2008]

8. Gawande, "Getting There from Here," p. 30.

9. Dr. Farmer's answer refers to a second article by Gawande, "The Cost Conundrum."

10. Behforouz, Farmer, and Mukherjee, "From Directly Observed Therapy to *Accompagnateurs*."

11. Paul Greenough, "Intimidation, Coercion, and Resistance in the Final Stages of the South Asian Smallpox Eradication Campaign, 1973–1975."

12. Ciro A. de Quadros, "The Whole Is Greater."

13. Partners In Health, "Holiday Message from Ophelia Dahl and Paul Farmer," December 17, 2008; link available at www.pih.org/inforesources/newsletters/PIH_e-bulletin_1208.pdf (accessed October 10, 2009).

14. Berger and Luckmann, *The Social Construction of Reality.*

ACKNOWLEDGMENTS

A round decade ago, I dedicated a book to Haun Saussy. I was lucky enough to have met him during my first week of college—a sunny fall day in 1978. It was clear, even then, that Haun was an editing marvel (he was seeking contributions, from a group of eighteen-year-old creative writing students, for a literary magazine), but little did I know then how important our friendship would prove to my own intellectual development. Haun scrutinizes everything I write. This holds as true for my first papers, published in the late eighties, as it does for those published in the past couple of years—and even for those never before seen in print. For three decades of friendship and wise counsel, my greatest debt as a physician-anthropologist who seeks to put pen to paper is to Haun.

My debts to others are many and no less heartfelt. I have received steadfast encouragement from Fritz and Yolande Lafontant, Ophelia Dahl, Jim Yong Kim, Didi Bertrand, Thomas J. White, and the staff of Partners In Health.

For indispensable academic advice and guidance over the years, I am indebted to Arthur Kleinman, Leon Eisenberg, Byron Good, Mary-Jo DelVecchio Good, and Barbara Rylko-Bauer.

The work described here has been supported by numerous private donors as well as the Charles A. Dana Foundation; Project Bread; the MacArthur Foundation; the World AIDS Foundation; Family Planning International Assistance; the Global Fund to Fight AIDS, Tuberculosis, and Malaria; the Haitian Ministry of Health; the Harvard Medical School's Division of AIDS; and the Clinton Foundation.

The editors and anonymous reviewers of many journals are to be thanked for their collegial critique over the years; the journals and edited volumes in which earlier versions of my essays were published are noted in the Credits section of this book.

My work has been enriched by the collaboration, advice, and input of many friends, students, and colleagues, among them Zoe Agoos, Greg Bates, Mercedes Becerra, Agnes Binagwaho, Jennie Weiss Block, Allan Brandt, Wayne Cavalier, Rose-Marie Chierici, Marie-

Flore Chipps, Noam Chomsky, Beth Collins, Veena Das, Marie-Marcelle Deschamps, Nancy Dorsinville, Linda Garro, Nicole Gastineau Campos, Melissa Gillooly, the members of the Groupe d'Etude sur le Sida et la Classe Paysanne (especially Maxi Raymonville), Isabella Harty-Hugues, Marcia Inhorn, the participants in the Institute for Health and Social Justice seminar "Women, Poverty, and AIDS," François Jean, Yolande Jean and her son "Joe," Lernéus Joseph, Thérèse and Poteau Joseph, Arthur Kleinman, Sarah LeVine, Jamie Maguire, Sally Falk Moore, Mariette Murphy, Ed Nardell, Deogratias Niyizonkiza, Jeffrey Parsonnet, Maral Poladian, the members of Proje Sante Fanm, Simon Robin, Naomi Rosenberg, Ricardo Sanchez, Gino Strada, Loïc Wacquant, David Walton, Alisse Waterston, Sarah Widmer, Paul Willis, Alice Yang, and Howard Zinn.

Paul Farmer

My gratitude and admiration go to the leaders and members of Partners In Health: Ophelia Dahl, Jim Yong Kim, Thomas J. White, Yolande Lafontant, Father Fritz Lafontant, Loune Viaud, and many others. For help and encouragement in bringing this book to completion, I thank Zoe Agoos, Dore Brown, Cordt Byrne, Jonathan K. Cohen, Tracy Kidder, Sophia Kostelanetz, Dominick LaCapra, Emily Morell, Tej Nuthulaganti, Mary Renaud, Naomi Schneider, Cathy Shufro, Olga Solovieva, and Alice Yang.

Haun Saussy

Aalen, O.O., V.T. Farewell, D. De Angelis, N.E. Day, and O.N. Gill. "New Therapy Explains the Fall in AIDS Incidence with a Substantial Rise in Number of Persons on Treatment Expected." *AIDS* 13, no. 1 (1999): 103–8.

Abbott, Elizabeth. *Haiti: The Duvaliers and Their Legacy.* New York: McGraw-Hill, 1988.

——— (as Elizabeth Abbott Namphy). *Tropical Obsession: A Universal Tragedy in Four Acts Set in Haiti.* Port-au-Prince: Éditions H. Deschamps, 1986.

Abbott, Karen. "Parolee with Tuberculosis Sues County Jail, State Prison." *Rocky Mountain News (Colo.),* April 2, 1998, p. 31A.

Abdool Karim, Quarraisha, and Salim S. Abdool Karim. "South Africa: Host to a New and Emerging HIV Epidemic." *Sexually Transmitted Infections* 75, no. 3 (1999): 139–40.

Ackerknecht, Erwin Heinz. *Rudolf Virchow: Doctor, Statesman, Anthropologist.* Madison: University of Wisconsin Press, 1953.

Addington, W.W. "Patient Compliance: The Most Serious Remaining Problem in the Control of Tuberculosis in the United States." *Chest* 76, no. 6 Suppl. (1979): 741–43.

Agamben, Giorgio. *Homo Sacer: Sovereign Power and Bare Life.* Translated by Daniel Heller-Roazen. Stanford, Calif.: Stanford University Press, 1998.

———. *Remnants of Auschwitz: The Witness and the Archive.* New York: Zone Books, 1999.

Aïach, P., R. Carr-Hill, S. Curtis, and R. Illsey. *Les inégalités sociales de santé en France et en Grande-Bretagne.* Paris: INSERM, 1987.

Akinbami, Lara J., and Kenneth C. Schoendorf. "Trends in Childhood Asthma: Prevalence, Health Care Utilization, and Mortality." *Pediatrics* 110, no. 2 (2002): 315–22.

Alcaeus. "Poverty." In *The Cry for Justice: An Anthology of the Literature of Social Protest,* edited by Upton Sinclair, Edward Sagarin, and Albert Teichner, p. 440. New York: L. Stuart, 1963.

Alden, Edward, Guy Dinmore, and Christopher Swann. "Wolfowitz Nomination a Shock for Europe." *Financial Times,* March 17, 2005, p. 39.

Alegría, Claribel. "Nocturnal Visits." In *Poetry Like Bread: Poets of the Political Imagination,* edited by Martin Espada, pp. 18–19. Willimantic, Conn.: Curbstone Press, 2000.

Alexander, A. "Money Isn't the Issue; It's (Still) Political Will." *TB Monitor* 5, no. 5 (1998): 53.

Alexander, Priscilla. *Prostitutes Prevent AIDS: A Manual for Health Educators.* San Francisco: California Prostitutes Education Project (CAL-PEP), 1988.

———. "Sex Workers Fight against AIDS: An International Perspective." In *Women Resisting AIDS: Feminist Strategies of Empowerment,* edited by Beth Schneider and Nancy E. Stoller, pp. 99–123. Philadelphia: Temple University Press, 1995.

Al-Rubeyi, B. I. "Mortality before and after the Invasion of Iraq in 2003." *Lancet* 364, no. 9448 (2004): 1834–35.

Alston, Philip. "Conjuring Up New Human Rights: A Proposal for Quality Control." *American Journal of International Law* 78, no. 3 (1984): 607–21.

Alvarez, Maria, and Gerald Murray. "Socialization for Scarcity: Child Feeding Beliefs and Practices in a Haitian Village." Port-au-Prince: USAID/Haiti, 1981.

Aly, Götz, Peter Chroust, and Christian Pross. *Cleansing the Fatherland: Nazi Medicine and Racial Hygiene.* Baltimore: Johns Hopkins University Press, 1994.

Ambinder, R. F., C. Newman, G. S. Hayward, R. Biggar, M. Melbye, L. Kestens, E. Van Marck, P. Piot, P. Gigase, and P. B. Wright. "Lack of Association of Cytomegalovirus with Endemic African Kaposi's Sarcoma." *Journal of Infectious Diseases* 156, no. 1 (1987): 193–97.

American Psychiatric Association. *Diagnostic and Statistical Manual of Mental Disorders.* 3rd ed. Washington, D.C.: American Psychiatric Association, 1980.

Americas Watch and National Coalition for Haitian Refugees. *Silencing a People: The Destruction of Civil Society in Haiti.* New York: Human Rights Watch, 1993.

Amnesty International. *Amnesty International Report 2009: The State of the World's Human Rights.* London: Amnesty International Press, 2009. http://thereport.amnesty.org/sites/report2009.amnesty.org/files/documents/air09-en.pdf (accessed October 9, 2009).

———. *Carnage and Despair: Iraq Five Years On.* London: Amnesty International, 2008.

———. *Torture in Russia: "This Man-Made Hell."* New York: Amnesty International, 1997.

Anand, Sudhir, Fabienne Peter, and Amartya Kumar Sen, eds. *Public Health, Ethics, and Equity.* New York: Oxford University Press, 2004.

Andersen, Martin Edwin. *Dossier secreto: Argentina's Desaparecidos and the Myth of the "Dirty War."* Boulder, Colo.: Westview Press, 1993.

Anderson, Carol. *Eyes Off the Prize: The United Nations and the African American Struggle for Human Rights, 1944–1955.* Cambridge: Cambridge University Press, 2003.

Angell, Marcia. "The Ethics of Clinical Research in the Third World." *New England Journal of Medicine* 337, no. 12 (1997): 847–49.

———. "Investigators' Responsibilities for Human Subjects in Developing Countries." *New England Journal of Medicine* 342, no. 13 (2000): 967–69.

———. "Tuskegee Revisited." *Wall Street Journal,* October 18, 1997, pp. A1, A22.

Anjos, Marcio Fabri dos. "Medical Ethics in the Developing World: A Liberation Theology Perspective." *Journal of Medicine and Philosophy* 21, no. 6 (1996): 629–37.

Annas, G. J. "Detention of HIV-Positive Haitians at Guantánamo: Human Rights and Medical Care." *New England Journal of Medicine* 329, no. 8 (1993): 589–92.

Anton, Donna. "Mother Courage: Musings of a Marine Mother." www.donna-anton.com/ wordpress (accessed July 9, 2009).

Appadurai, Arjun, ed. *The Social Life of Things: Commodities in Cultural Perspective.* Cambridge: Cambridge University Press, 1986.

Aral, S., and K. Holmes. "Sexually Transmitted Diseases in the AIDS Era." *Scientific American* 264, no. 2 (1991): 62–69.

Arendt, Hannah. *Eichmann in Jerusalem; A Report on the Banality of Evil.* New York: Viking, 1963.

Asad, Talal, ed. *Anthropology and the Colonial Encounter.* New York: Humanities Press, 1973.

———. "On Torture, or Cruel, Inhuman, and Degrading Treatment." In *Social Suffering,* edited by Arthur Kleinman, Veena Das, and Margaret M. Lock, pp. 285–308. Berkeley: University of California Press, 1997.

Associated Press. "Experimental Drug Gives Researchers Optimism for New Treatment for TB." *St. Louis Post-Dispatch,* June 22, 2000, p. A9.

Bachman, Ronet, and Linda E. Saltzman. *Violence against Women: Estimates from the Redesigned National Crime Victimization Survey.* Special report, Bureau of Justice Statistics, U.S. Department of Justice, NCJ-154348, August 1995. www.ojp.usdoj.gov/ bjs/abstract/femvied.htm (accessed July 9, 2009).

Bangsberg, D., J. P. Tulsky, F. M. Hecht, and A. R. Moss. "Protease Inhibitors in the Home-less." *Journal of the American Medical Association* 278, no. 1 (1997): 63–65.

Barnhoorn, Florie, and Hans Adriaanse. "In Search of Factors Responsible for Noncom-pliance among Tuberculosis Patients in Wardha District, India." *Social Science and Medicine* 34, no. 3 (1992): 291–306.

Barros, Jacques. *Haïti, de 1804 à nos jours.* Paris: Éditions L'Harmattan, 1984.

Bartholomew, C., W. C. Saxinger, J. W. Clark, M. Gail, A. Dudgeon, B. Mahabir, B. Hull-Drysdale, F. Cleghorn, R. C. Gallo, and W. A. Blattner. "Transmission of HTLV-I and HIV among Homosexual Men in Trinidad." *Journal of the American Medical Associa-tion* 257, no. 19 (1987): 2604–8.

Basaglia, Franco. *Psychiatry Inside-Out: Selected Writings of Franco Basaglia.* Edited by Nancy Scheper-Hughes and Anne Lovell. New York: Columbia University Press, 1987.

Bastien, Rémy. *Le paysan haïtien et sa famille: Vallée de Marbial.* Paris: Karthala, 1985.

Bateson, Mary Catherine, and Richard A. Goldsby. *Thinking AIDS.* Reading, Mass.: Addison-Wesley, 1988.

Bauman, Zygmunt. *Globalization: The Human Consequences.* New York: Columbia Uni-versity Press, 1998.

Bayer, R. "Does Anything Work? Public Health and the Nihilist Thesis." Paper presented at the annual meeting of the American Public Health Association, New York, Novem-ber 1996.

Bayer, R., C. Stayton, M. Desvarieux, C. Healton, S. Landesman, and W. Y. Tsai. "Directly Observed Therapy and Treatment Completion for Tuberculosis in the United States: Is Universal Supervised Therapy Necessary?" *American Journal of Public Health* 88, no. 7 (1998): 1052–58.

Beach, R. S., and P. F. Laura. "Nutrition and the Acquired Immunodeficiency Syndrome." *Annals of Internal Medicine* 99, no. 4 (1983): 565–66.

Becerra, M. C., J. Freeman, J. Bayona, S. S. Shin, J. Y. Kim, J. J. Furin, B. Werner, A. Sloutsky, R. Timperi, P. E. Farmer, et al. "Using Treatment Failure under Effective Directly Observed Short-Course Chemotherapy Programs to Identify Patients with Multidrug-Resistant Tuberculosis." *International Journal of Tuberculosis and Lung Disease* 4, no. 2 (2000): 108–14.

Becerra-Valdivia, Mercedes C. "Epidemiology of Tuberculosis in the Northern Shanty-towns of Lima, Peru." Sc.D. diss., Harvard University, 1999.

Behforouz, Heidi L., Paul E. Farmer, and Joia S. Mukherjee. "From Directly Observed Therapy to *Accompagnateurs*: Enhancing AIDS Treatment Outcomes in Haiti and in Boston." *Clinical Infectious Diseases* 38, no. 5 Suppl. (2004): S429–S436.

Bell, Beverly. *Walking on Fire: Haitian Women's Stories of Survival and Resistance*. Ithaca, N.Y.: Cornell University Press, 2001.

Benkimoun, Paul. "Contre le sida, 'on peut soulever des montagnes.'" *Le Monde,* November 29, 2008.

Berger, Peter L., and Thomas Luckmann. *The Social Construction of Reality: A Treatise in the Sociology of Knowledge*. Garden City, N.Y.: Anchor Books, 1967.

Berkelman, R. L., and J. M. Hughes. "The Conquest of Infectious Diseases: Who Are We Kidding?" *Annals of Internal Medicine* 119, no. 5 (1993): 426–28.

Bernier, Olivier. *Pleasure and Privilege: Life in France, Naples, and America, 1770–1790*. Garden City, N.Y.: Doubleday, 1981.

Berreman, Gerald D. "'Bringing It All Back Home': Malaise in Anthropology." In *Reinventing Anthropology,* edited by Dell H. Hymes, pp. 83–98. New York: Vintage Books, 1974.

Bifani, P. J., B. B. Plikaytis, V. Kapur, K. Stockbauer, X. Pan, M. L. Lutfey, S. L. Moghazeh, W. Eisner, T. M. Daniel, M. H. Kaplan, et al. "Origin and Interstate Spread of a New York City Multidrug-Resistant Mycobacterium Tuberculosis Clone Family." *Journal of the American Medical Association* 275, no. 6 (1996): 452–57.

Bilmes, Linda J., and Joseph E. Stiglitz. "The Iraq War Will Cost Us $3 Trillion, and Much More." *Washington Post,* March 9, 2008, p. B1.

Binford, Leigh. *The El Mozote Massacre: Anthropology and Human Rights*. Tucson: University of Arizona Press, 1996.

Birns, Larry, and Michael Marx McCarthy. "Haiti Needs U.S. Aid, Not Ineffective Manipulation." *Miami Herald,* December 21, 2001.

Bland, R. M., N. C. Rollins, A. Coutsoudis, and H. M. Coovadia. "Breastfeeding Practices in an Area of High HIV Prevalence in Rural South Africa." *Acta Paediatrica* 91, no. 6 (2002): 704–11.

Bloom, Barry R., and Christopher J. L. Murray. "Tuberculosis: Commentary on a Reemergent Killer." *Science* 257, no. 5073 (1992): 1055–64.

Blower, Sally, and Paul E. Farmer. "Predicting the Public Health Impact of Antiretrovirals: Preventing HIV in Developing Countries." *AIDScience,* no. 11 (2003). www.aidscience.org/Articles/AIDScience033.asp (accessed July 10, 2009).

Blower, Sally, Li Ma, Paul E. Farmer, and Serena Koenig. "Predicting the Impact of Antiretrovirals in Resource-Poor Settings: Preventing HIV Infections Whilst Controlling Drug Resistance." *Current Drug Targets—Infectious Disorders* 3, no. 4 (2003): 345–53.

Bobat, Raziya, Dhayendree Moodley, Anna Coutsoudis, and Hoosen Coovadia. "Breast-feeding by HIV-1-Infected Women and Outcome in Their Infants: A Cohort Study from Durban, South Africa." *AIDS* 11, no. 13 (1997): 1627–33.

Boff, Leonardo. *Faith on the Edge: Religion and Marginalized Existence.* Translated by Robert R. Barr. San Francisco: Harper and Row, 1989.

Boff, Leonardo, and Clodovis Boff. *Introducing Liberation Theology.* Translated by Paul Burns. Maryknoll, N.Y.: Orbis Books, 1987.

Bogdanich, Walt, and Jenny Nordberg. "Mixed U.S. Signals Helped Tilt Haiti toward Chaos." *New York Times,* January 29, 2006.

Boodhoo, Kenneth. "The Economic Dimension of U.S.-Caribbean Policy." In *The Caribbean Challenge: U.S. Policy in a Volatile Region,* edited by H. Michael Erisman, pp. 72–91. Boulder, Colo.: Westview Press, 1984.

Börjesson, Kristina. *Feet to the Fire: The Media after 9/11. Top Journalists Speak Out.* Amherst, N.Y.: Prometheus Books, 2005.

Boseley, Sarah. "13.4M Children Are AIDS Orphans, Says Report." *Guardian* (U.K.), July 11, 2002. www.guardian.co.uk/aids/story/0,,753051,00.html (accessed July 10, 2009).

Bourdieu, Pierre. *Acts of Resistance: Against the Tyranny of the Market.* Translated by Richard Nice. New York: The New Press, 1998.

———. *Contre-feux: Propos pour servir à la résistance contre l'invasion néo-libérale.* Paris: Liber-Raisons D'Agir, 1998.

———. *In Other Words: Essays towards a Reflexive Sociology.* Translated by Matthew Adamson. Cambridge: Polity Press, 1990.

———. *Interventions, 1961–2001: Science sociale et action politique.* Edited by Franck Poupeau and Thierry Discepolo. Montreal: Comeau and Nadeau, 2002.

———. *Pascalian Meditations.* Translated by Richard Nice. Cambridge: Polity Press, 2000.

Bourdieu, Pierre, et al. *La misère du monde.* Paris: Éditions du Seuil, 1993.

———. *The Weight of the World: Social Suffering in Contemporary Society.* Translated by Priscilla Parkhurst Ferguson et al. Stanford, Calif.: Stanford University Press, 1999.

Bourgois, Philippe I. "Confronting Anthropology, Education, and Inner-City Apartheid." *American Anthropologist* 98, no. 2 (1996): 249–58.

———. "Families and Children in the U.S. Inner City." In *Small Wars: The Cultural Politics of Childhood,* edited by Nancy Scheper-Hughes and Carolyn Fishel Sargent, pp. 331–51. Berkeley: University of California Press, 1998.

———. *In Search of Respect: Selling Crack in El Barrio.* 2nd ed. Cambridge: Cambridge University Press, 2003.

———. "Missing the Holocaust: My Father's Account of Auschwitz from August 1943 to June 1944." *Anthropological Quarterly* 78, no. 1 (2005): 89–123.

Bourgois, Philippe I., Nancy Scheper-Hughes, Didier Fassin, Linda Green, H. K. Heggenhougen, Laurence Kirmayer, and Loïc Wacquant. "Commentary on Farmer, Paul, 'An Anthropology of Structural Violence.'" *Current Anthropology* 45, no. 3 (2004): 317–22.

Bowser, Diana, Sarthak Das, Renee Szostek, and Shelly Toussi. *Domestic Violence and Disability.* New Haven: n.p., 1997.

Brandt, Allan M. "AIDS: From Social History to Social Policy." In *AIDS: The Burdens of History,* edited by Elizabeth Fee and Daniel M. Fox, pp. 147–71. Berkeley: University of California Press, 1988.

———. *No Magic Bullet: A Social History of Venereal Disease in the United States since 1880.* New York: Oxford University Press, 1987.

Brauman, Rony. "L'assistance humanitaire internationale." In *Dictionnaire d'éthique et de philosophie morale,* edited by Monique Canto-Sperber, pp. 96–101. Paris: Presses Universitaires de France, 1997.

———. "Refugee Camps, Population Transfers, and NGOs." In *Hard Choices: Moral Dilemmas in Humanitarian Intervention,* edited by Jonathan Moore, pp. 177–94. Lanham, Md.: Rowman and Littlefield, 1998.

Braun, M. M., B. I. Truman, B. Maguire, G. T. DiFerdinando Jr., G. Wormser, R. Broaddus, and D. L. Morse. "Increasing Incidence of Tuberculosis in a Prison Inmate Population: Association with HIV Infection." *Journal of the American Medical Association* 261, no. 3 (1989): 393–97.

Brecht, Bertolt. *Mother Courage and Her Children: A Chronicle of the Thirty Years' War.* Translated by Eric Bentley. New York: Grove Weidenfeld, 1991.

Bretton Woods Commission and Bretton Woods Committee. *Bretton Woods: Looking to the Future. Conference Proceedings, Washington, D.C., July 20–22, 1994.* Washington, D.C.: Bretton Woods Committee, 1994.

Briggs, Charles L., Paul E. Farmer, and Catherine A. Christen. *Infectious Diseases and Social Inequality in Latin America: From Hemispheric Insecurity to Global Cooperation.* Washington, D.C.: Woodrow Wilson International Center for Scholars, 1999. www.wilsoncenter.org/topics/docs/ACF35C.pdf (accessed July 11, 2009).

Brock, Dan W. "Broadening the Bioethics Agenda." *Kennedy Institute of Ethics Journal* 10, no. 1 (2000): 21–38.

———. "Ethical Issues in the Development of Summary Measures of Population Health Status." In *Summarizing Population Health: Directions for the Development and Application of Population Metrics,* edited by Marilyn J. Field and Marthe R. Gold, pp. 74–81. Washington, D.C.: National Academies Press, 1998.

Brody, Howard. *The Healer's Power.* New Haven: Yale University Press, 1992.

Brown, Peter. "Introduction: Anthropology and Disease Control." *Medical Anthropology* 7, no. 1 (1983): 1–8.

Brown, Robert McAfee. *Liberation Theology: An Introductory Guide.* Louisville, Ky.: Westminster/John Knox Press, 1993.

Brudney, K., and J. Dobkin. "Resurgent Tuberculosis in New York City: Human Immunodeficiency Virus, Homelessness, and the Decline of Tuberculosis Control Programs." *American Review of Respiratory Disease* 144, no. 4 (1991): 745–49.

———. "A Tale of Two Cities: Tuberculosis Control in Nicaragua and New York City." *Seminars in Respiratory Infections* 6, no. 4 (1991): 261–72.

Brutus, Jean-Robert. "Problèmes d'éthique liés au dépistage du virus HIV-1." Paper presented at the Congrès des Médecins Francophones d'Amérique, Fort-de-France, Martinique, June 12–16, 1989.

———. "Séroprevalence de HIV parmi les femmes enceintes à Cité Soleil, Haïti." Paper presented at the Fifth International Conference on AIDS, Montreal, June 5–7, 1989.

Bukhman, Gene. "Reform and Resistance in Post-Soviet Tuberculosis Control." PhD diss., University of Arizona, Tucson, 2001.

Buncombe, Andrew. "UN Admits Haiti Force Is Not Up to the Job It Faces." *Independent (U.K.)*, July 30, 2005, p. 31.

Burdick, John. *Looking for God in Brazil: The Progressive Catholic Church in Urban Brazil's Religious Arena*. Berkeley: University of California Press, 1993.

Burgard, S. A., and D. J. Treiman. "Trends and Racial Differences in Infant Mortality in South Africa." *Social Science and Medicine* 62, no. 5 (2006): 1126–37.

Burnham, G., R. Lafta, S. Doocy, and L. Roberts. "Mortality after the 2003 Invasion of Iraq: A Cross-Sectional Cluster Sample Survey." *Lancet* 368, no. 9545 (2006): 1421–28.

Burns, John F. "U.S. Envoy Sees Her Role Reverse." *International Herald Tribune*, November 26, 2001.

Byrd, W. Michael, and Linda A. Clayton. *An American Health Dilemma: Race, Medicine, and Health Care in the United States, 1900–2000*. 2 vols. New York: Routledge, 2000.

Calhoun, Craig. "U.S. and Multilateral Efforts to Fight HIV/AIDS: Are We Making Progress?" Address to the Bretton Woods Committee, December 17, 2003.

Campbell, Donald T. "Herskovits, Cultural Relativism, and Metascience." In *Cultural Relativism: Perspectives in Cultural Pluralism*, edited by Melville J. Herskovits, pp. v–xxiii. New York: Random House, 1972.

Caputo, John D. *Against Ethics: Contributions to a Poetics of Obligation with Constant Reference to Deconstruction*. Bloomington: Indiana University Press, 1993.

Carovano, K. "More Than Mothers and Whores: Redefining the AIDS Prevention Needs of Women." *International Journal of Health Services* 21, no. 1 (1991): 131–42.

Carpenter, Frank G. *Lands of the Caribbean: The Canal Zone, Panama, Costa Rica, Nicaragua, Salvador, Honduras, Guatemala, Cuba, Jamaica, Haiti, Santo Domingo, Porto Rico, and the Virgin Islands*. Garden City, N.Y.: Doubleday, Page, 1925.

Castiglione, Baldassare. *The Book of the Courtier*. Translated by John Singleton. Garden City, N.Y.: Doubleday, 1959.

Castillo, Otto René. "Apolitical Intellectuals." In *Against Forgetting: Twentieth Century Poetry of Witness*, edited by Carolyn Forché, pp. 607–8. New York: Norton, 1993.

Centers for Disease Control and Prevention. "Current Trends: Acquired Immunodeficiency Syndrome (AIDS) Update—United States." *Morbidity and Mortality Weekly Report* 32, no. 24 (1983): 309–11. www.aegis.org/pubs/mmwr/1983/MM3224.html (accessed September 13, 2009).

———. "Current Trends: AIDS in Women—United States." *Morbidity and Mortality Weekly Report* 39, no. 47 (1990): 845–46.

———. "Diphtheria Outbreak—Russian Federation, 1990–1993." *Morbidity and Mortality Weekly Report* 42, no. 43 (1993): 840–41, 847.

———. "Emergence of Mycobacterium Tuberculosis with Extensive Resistance to Second-Line Drugs—Worldwide, 2000–2004." *Morbidity and Mortality Weekly Report* 55, no. 11 (2006): 301–5.

———. "Opportunistic Infections and Kaposi's Sarcoma among Haitians in the United States." *Morbidity and Mortality Weekly Report* 31, no. 26 (1982): 353–54, 360–61.

———. "Outbreak of Multidrug-Resistant Tuberculosis—Texas, California, and Pennsylvania." *Morbidity and Mortality Weekly Report* 39, no. 22 (1990): 369–72.

———. "*Pneumocystis* Pneumonia—Los Angeles." *Morbidity and Mortality Weekly Report* 30, no. 21 (1981): 250–52.

———. "Prevention and Control of Tuberculosis in Correctional Institutions: Recommendations of the Advisory Committee for the Elimination of Tuberculosis." *Morbidity and Mortality Weekly Report* 38, no. 18 (1989): 313–20, 325.

———. "Primary Multidrug-Resistant Tuberculosis—Ivanovo Oblast, Russia, 1999." *Morbidity and Mortality Weekly Report* 48, no. 30 (1999): 661–64.

———. *Reported Tuberculosis in the United States, 1999.* Atlanta: Centers for Disease Control and Prevention, 2000.

———. "Update: AIDS among Women—United States, 1994." *Morbidity and Mortality Weekly Report* 44, no. 5 (1995): 81–84.

———. "Update on Kaposi's Sarcoma and Opportunistic Infections in Previously Healthy Persons—United States." *Morbidity and Mortality Weekly Report* 31, no. 22 (1982): 294, 300–301.

———. "U.S. HIV and AIDS Cases Reported through June 1995." *HIV/AIDS Surveillance Report* 7, no. 1 (1995). www.cdc.gov/hiv/topics/surveillance/resources/reports/pdf/hivsur71.pdf (accessed July 11, 2009).

Chaisson, Richard E., Jeanne C. Keruly, and Richard D. Moore. "Race, Sex, Drug Use, and Progression of Human Immunodeficiency Virus Disease." *New England Journal of Medicine* 333, no. 12 (1995): 751–56.

Chambers, Veronica. "Betrayal Feminism." In *Listen Up: Voices from the Next Feminist Generation,* edited by Barbara Findlen, pp. 21–28. Seattle: Seal Press, 1995.

Chan-Tack, Kirk M., José F. Díaz, Wya A. Geerligs, Richard van Altena, Tjip S. van der Werf, Ariel Pablos-Méndez, Mario C. Raviglione, and Paul Nunn. "Antituberculosis-Drug Resistance." *New England Journal of Medicine* 339, no. 15 (1998): 1079–80.

Chapman, Audrey R., and Leonard S. Rubenstein, eds. *Human Rights and Health: The Legacy of Apartheid.* Prepared by the American Association for the Advancement of Science and Physicians for Human Rights (U.S.). Washington, D.C.: American Association for the Advancement of Science, 1998.

Charlemagne, Manno. *Manno Charlemagne.* Recording. Miami: Mini Records, 1988.

Charles, Claude. "Brief Comments on the Occurrence, Etiology, and Treatment of Indisposition." *Social Science and Medicine. Part B: Medical Anthropology* 13, no. 2 (1979): 135–36.

Chatterjee, Deen K., ed. *The Ethics of Assistance: Morality and the Distant Needy.* Cambridge: Cambridge University Press, 2004.

Chaulet, Pierre. "Compliance with Anti-Tuberculosis Chemotherapy in Developing Countries." *Tubercle* 68, no. 2 Suppl. (1987): 19–24.

———. "Les nouveaux tuberculeux." *Journal de la tuberculose et du SIDA* 6, no. 4 (1996): 6–8.

Chaze, William. "In Haiti, a View of Life at the Bottom." *U.S. News and World Report* 95, no. 18 (1983): 41–42.

Chen, Kwan-Hwa, and Gerald Murray. "Truths and Untruths in Village Haiti: An Experiment in Third-World Survey Research." In *Culture, Natality, and Family Planning,* edited by John F. Marshall and Steven Polgar, pp. 241–62. Chapel Hill: Carolina Population Center, University of North Carolina, 1976.

Chien, Arnold, Margaret Connors, and Kenneth Fox. "The Drug War in Perspective." In *Dying for Growth: Global Inequality and the Health of the Poor,* edited by Jim Yong Kim, Joyce V. Millen, Alec Irwin, and John Gershman, pp. 293–327. Monroe, Maine: Common Courage Press, 2000.

Chomsky, Noam. *Turning the Tide: U.S. Intervention in Central America and the Struggle for Peace.* Boston: South End Press, 1985.

Chomsky, Noam, and Edward S. Herman. *After the Cataclysm: Postwar Indochina and the Construction of Imperial Ideology.* Boston: South End Press, 1979.

———. *The Political Economy of Human Rights.* 2 vols. Boston: South End Press, 1979.

———. *The Washington Connection and Third World Fascism.* Boston: South End Press, 1979.

Chopp, Rebecca S. *The Praxis of Suffering: An Interpretation of Liberation and Political Theologies.* Maryknoll, N.Y.: Orbis Books, 1986.

Chossudovsky, Michel. *The Globalization of Poverty and the New World Order.* 2nd ed. Shanty Bay, Ontario: Global Outlook, 2003.

Chrétien, Jean-Pierre. *The Great Lakes of Africa: Two Thousand Years of History.* New York: Zone Books, 2003.

Churchill, Larry R. "Are We Professionals? A Critical Look at the Social Role of Bioethics." *Daedalus* 128, no. 4 (1999): 253–74.

Ciancaglini, Sergio, and Martin Granovsky. *Nada más que la verdad: El juicio a las juntas.* Buenos Aires: Planeta, 1995.

Clatts, Michael C. "All the King's Horses and All the King's Men: Some Personal Reflections on Ten Years of AIDS Ethnography." *Human Organization* 53, no. 1 (1994): 93–95.

———. "Disembodied Acts: On the Perverse Use of Sexual Categories in the Study of High-Risk Behavior." In *Culture and Sexual Risk: Anthropological Perspectives on AIDS,* edited by Han ten Brummelhuis and Gilbert H. Herdt, pp. 241–56. Amsterdam: Gordon and Breach, 1995.

Clavel, François, and Allan F. Hance. "HIV Drug Resistance." *New England Journal of Medicine* 350, no. 10 (2004): 1023–35.

Clinton, Bill, and Al Gore. *Putting People First: How We Can All Change America.* New York: Times Books, 1992.

Cohen, Lawrence. *No Aging in India: Alzheimer's, the Bad Family, and Other Modern Things.* Berkeley: University of California Press, 1998.

Cohn, D. L., B. J. Catlin, K. L. Peterson, F. N. Judson, and J. A. Sbarbaro. "A 62-Dose, 6-Month Therapy for Pulmonary and Extrapulmonary Tuberculosis: A Twice-Weekly, Directly Observed, and Cost-Effective Regimen." *Annals of Internal Medicine* 112, no. 6 (1990): 407–15.

Coker, Richard. "'Extrapolitis': A Disease More Threatening Than TB in Russia?" *European Journal of Public Health* 10, no. 2 (2000): 148–50.

Cole, S. T., and A. Telenti. "Drug Resistance in Mycobacterium Tuberculosis." *European Respiratory Journal* 20, Suppl. (1995): 701S–713S.

Collaborative Study Group of AIDS in Haitian-Americans. "Risk Factors for AIDS among Haitians Residing in the United States: Evidence of Heterosexual Transmission." *Journal of the American Medical Association* 257, no. 5 (1987): 635–39.

Collins, Patricia Hill. *Black Feminist Thought: Knowledge, Consciousness, and the Politics of Empowerment.* Boston: Unwin Hyman, 1990.

Comandancia General del EZLN. "Primera declaración de la Selva Lacandona." Chiapas, Mexico, 1993. www.bibliotecas.tv/chiapas/ene94/dic93a.html (accessed July 10, 2009).

Comisión de la Verdad para El Salvador. "De la locura a la esperanza: La guerra de doce años en El Salvador; Informe de la Comisión de la Verdad para El Salvador." *ECA: Estudios Centroamericanos* 48, no. 533 (1993): 161–326.

Comisión Nacional Sobre la Desaparición de Personas. *Nunca más: The Report of the Argentine National Commission on the Disappeared.* New York: Farrar, Straus and Giroux, 1986.

Concannon, Brian, Jr. "Beyond Complementarity: The International Criminal Court and National Prosecutions—A View from Haiti." *Columbia Human Rights Law Review* 32, no. 1 (2000): 201–50.

Connolly, Ceci. "Study: Uninsured Don't Get Needed Health Care; Delayed Diagnoses, Premature Deaths Result." *Washington Post,* May 22, 2002.

Connors, M. M. "The Politics of Marginalization: The Appropriation of AIDS Prevention Messages among Injection Drug Users." *Culture, Medicine, and Psychiatry* 19, no. 4 (1995): 425–52.

Conrad, Joseph. *Heart of Darkness.* New York: Penguin, 1999.

Conrad, P. "The Meaning of Medications: Another Look at Compliance." *Social Science and Medicine* 20, no. 1 (1985): 29–37.

Coreil, Jeannine. "Parallel Structures in Professional and Folk Health Care: A Model Applied to Rural Haiti." *Culture, Medicine, and Psychiatry* 7, no. 2 (1983): 131–51.

———. "Traditional and Western Responses to an Anthrax Epidemic in Rural Haiti." *Medical Anthropology* 4 (1980): 79–105.

Coutsoudis, Anna. "Infant Feeding Dilemmas Created by HIV: South African Experiences." *Journal of Nutrition* 135, no. 4 (2005): 956–59.

Crofton, J. "The Contribution of Treatment to the Prevention of Tuberculosis." *Bulletin of the International Union against Tuberculosis and Lung Disease* 32 (1962): 643–53.

Csordas, Thomas J. *Embodiment and Experience: The Existential Ground of Culture and Self.* Cambridge: Cambridge University Press, 1994.

———. "Embodiment as a Paradigm for Anthropology." *Ethos* 18, no. 1 (1990): 5–47.

Cueto, Marcos. "Sanitation from Above: Yellow Fever and Foreign Intervention in Peru, 1919–1922." *Hispanic American Historical Review* 72, no. 1 (1992): 1–22.

Cufino Svitone, E., R. Garfield, M. I. Vasconcelos, and V. Araujo Craveiro. "Primary Health Care Lessons from the Northeast of Brazil: The Agentes de Saude Program." *Revista Panamericana de Salud Publica* 7, no. 5 (2000): 293–302.

Curry, F. J. "Neighborhood Clinics for More Effective Outpatient Treatment of Tuberculosis." *New England Journal of Medicine* 279, no. 23 (1968): 1262–67.

d'Adesky, Anne-Christine. *Moving Mountains: The Race to Treat Global AIDS.* London: Verso, 2004.

———. "Silence = Death, AIDS in Haiti." *Advocate* 577, May 21, 1991, p. 30.

Dallaire, Roméo, and Brent Beardsley. *Shake Hands with the Devil: The Failure of Humanity in Rwanda.* New York: Carroll and Graf, 2004.

Daly, Christopher T., John Doody, and Kim Paffenroth, eds. *Augustine and History.* Lanham, Md.: Lexington Books, 2008.

Daniels, Norman. "Justice, Health, and Health Care." In *Medicine and Social Justice: Essays on the Distribution of Health Care,* edited by Rosamond Rhodes, M. Pabst Battin, and Anita Silvers, pp. 6–23. New York: Oxford University Press, 2002.

Daniels, Norman, Bruce P. Kennedy, and Ichiro Kawachi. "Why Justice Is Good for Our Health: The Social Determinants of Health Inequalities." *Daedalus* 128, no. 4 (1999): 215–51.

Danner, Mark. *The Massacre at El Mozote: A Parable of the Cold War.* New York: Vintage Books, 1994.

———. *The Secret Way to War: The Downing Street Memo and the Iraq War's Buried History.* Preface by Frank Rich. New York: New York Review of Books, 2006.

———. "The Truth at El Mozote." *New Yorker,* December 6, 1993, pp. 50–133.

Das, A., S. Jana, A. K. Chakraborty, L. Khodakevich, M. S. Chakraborty, and N. K. Pal. "Community Based Survey of STD/HIV Infection among Commercial Sex-Workers in Calcutta (India). Part-III: Clinical Findings of Sexually Transmitted Diseases (STD)." *Journal of Communicable Diseases* 26, no. 4 (1994): 192–96.

Das, Sarthak. "AIDS in India: An Ethnography of HIV/AIDS amongst Bombay's Commercial Sex Workers." A.B. thesis, Harvard University, 1995.

———. "Prostitution and AIDS: HIV and Bombay's Commercial Sex Workers." M.P.H. thesis, Yale University, 2000.

Das, Veena. *Life and Words: Violence and the Descent into the Ordinary.* Berkeley: University of California Press, 2007.

———. *Violence and Subjectivity.* Berkeley: University of California Press, 2000.

Davis, David Brion. *The Problem of Slavery in the Age of Revolution, 1770–1823.* Ithaca, N.Y.: Cornell University Press, 1975.

Davis, Mike. *Late Victorian Holocausts: El Niño, Famines, and the Making of the Third World.* London: Verso, 2001.

de Bruyn, Maria. "Women and AIDS in Developing Countries: The XIIth International Conference on the Social Sciences and Medicine." *Social Science and Medicine* 34, no. 3 (1992): 249–62.

"Declaration of Alma-Ata." Adopted at the International Conference on Primary Health Care, Alma-Ata, USSR, September 6–12, 1978. www.who.int/hpr/NPH/docs/declaration_almaata.pdf (accessed July 2, 2009).

del Rio, C., S. Green, C. Abrams, and J. Lennox. "From Diagnosis to Undetectable: The Reality of HIV/AIDS Care in the Inner City." Paper presented at the eighth annual

Conference on Retroviruses and Opportunistic Infections, Chicago, February 4–8, 2001.

Denison, Rebecca. "Call Us Survivors! Women Organized to Respond to Life-Threatening Diseases (WORLD)." In *Women Resisting AIDS: Feminist Strategies of Empowerment*, edited by Beth Schneider and Nancy E. Stoller, pp. 195–207. Philadelphia: Temple University Press, 1995.

de Quadros, Ciro A. "The Whole Is Greater: How Polio Was Eradicated from the Western Hemisphere." In *The Practice of International Health: A Case-Based Orientation*, edited by Daniel Perlman and Ananya Roy, pp. 54–69. New York: Oxford University Press, 2008.

Deschamps, M. M., J. W. Pape, M. Desvarieux, P. Williams-Russo, S. Madhavan, J. L. Ho, and W. D. Johnson Jr. "A Prospective Study of HIV-Seropositive Asymptomatic Women of Childbearing Age in a Developing Country." *JAIDS: Journal of Acquired Immune Deficiency Syndromes* 6, no. 5 (1993): 446–51.

Des Jarlais, D. C. "AIDS and the Use of Injected Drugs." *Scientific American* 270, no. 2 (1994): 82–87.

Des Jarlais, D. C., K. Choopanya, S. Vanichseni, K. Plangsringarm, W. Sonchai, M. Carballo, P. Friedmann, and S. R. Friedman. "AIDS Risk Reduction and Reduced HIV Seroconversion among Injection Drug Users in Bangkok." *American Journal of Public Health* 84, no. 3 (1994): 452–55.

Des Jarlais, D. C., and S. R. Friedman. "Needle Sharing among IVDUs at Risk for AIDS." *American Journal of Public Health* 78, no. 11 (1988): 1498–99.

Des Jarlais, D. C., S. R. Friedman, and C. Casriel. "Target Groups for Preventing AIDS among Intravenous Drug Users: 2. The 'Hard' Data Studies." *Journal of Consulting and Clinical Psychology* 58, no. 1 (1990): 50–56.

Des Jarlais, D. C., S. R. Friedman, K. Choopanya, S. Vanichseni, and T. P. Ward. "International Epidemiology of HIV and AIDS among Injecting Drug Users." *AIDS* 6, no. 10 (1992): 1053–68.

Des Jarlais, D. C., S. R. Friedman, and J. L. Sotheran. "The First City: HIV among Intravenous Drug Users in New York City." In *AIDS: The Making of a Chronic Disease*, edited by Elizabeth Fee and Daniel M. Fox, pp. 279–98. Berkeley: University of California Press, 1992.

Des Jarlais, D. C., S. R. Friedman, and T. P. Ward. "Harm Reduction: A Public Health Response to the AIDS Epidemic among Injecting Drug Users." *Annual Review of Public Health* 14 (1993): 413–50.

Des Jarlais, D. C., H. Hagan, S. R. Friedman, P. Friedmann, D. Goldberg, M. Frischer, S. Green, K. Tunving, B. Ljungberg, and A. Wodak. "Maintaining Low HIV Seroprevalence in Populations of Injecting Drug Users." *Journal of the American Medical Association* 274, no. 15 (1995): 1226–31.

Des Jarlais, D. C., N. S. Padian, and W. Winkelstein Jr. "Targeted HIV-Prevention Programs." *New England Journal of Medicine* 331, no. 21 (1994): 1451–53.

Des Jarlais, D. C., J. Wenston, S. R. Friedman, J. L. Sotheran, R. Maslansky, M. Marmor, S. Yancovitz, and S. Beatrice. "Implications of the Revised Surveillance Definition:

AIDS among New York City Drug Users." *American Journal of Public Health* 82, no. 11 (1992): 1531–33.

Desormeaux, J., M. P. Johnson, J. S. Coberly, P. Losikoff, E. Johnson, R. Huebner, L. Geiter, H. Davis, J. Atkinson, R. E. Chaisson, et al. "Widespread HIV Counseling and Testing Linked to a Community-Based Tuberculosis Control Program in a High-Risk Population." *Bulletin of the Pan American Health Organization* 30, no. 1 (1996): 1–8.

Desvarieux, M., and J. W. Pape. "HIV and AIDS in Haiti: Recent Developments." *AIDS Care* 3, no. 3 (1991): 271–79.

de Villiers, S. "Tuberculosis in Anthropological Perspective." *South African Journal of Ethnology* 14 (1991): 69–72.

DeWitt, Karen. "Many Americans Back Singapore's Decision to Flog Teen." *Fort Worth Star-Telegram,* April 10, 1994, p. 4.

Diamond, Jared M. *Collapse: How Societies Choose to Fail or Succeed.* New York: Viking, 2005.

Diamond, Stanley. *In Search of the Primitive: A Critique of Civilization.* New Brunswick, N.J.: Transaction Books, 1974.

DiBacco, Thomas V. "Tuberculosis on the Rebound—A Disease Thought Tamed Is Again Causing Concern." *Washington Post,* January 27, 1998.

"Did He Go or Was He Pushed?" *Economist* 370, no. 8365 (2004): 24.

Dlugy, Yana. "The Prisoners' Plague—Overcrowded Jails Are Fueling a Frightening New Epidemic of Drug-Resistant Tuberculosis." *Newsweek,* July 5, 1999, pp. 18–20.

Donnelly, John. "Prevention Urged in AIDS Fight: Natsios Says Fund Should Spend Less on HIV Treatment." *Boston Globe,* June 7, 2001, p. A8.

Dos Reis, A. R. "Norplant in Brazil: Implantation Strategy in the Guise of Scientific Research." *Issues in Reproductive and Genetic Engineering: Journal of International Feminist Analysis* 3 (1990): 111–18.

Dostoevsky, Fyodor. *Crime and Punishment.* Translated by Richard Pevear and Larissa Volokhonsky. New York: Vintage Books, 1993.

———. *A Writer's Diary.* Translated by Kenneth Lantz. 3 vols. Evanston, Ill.: Northwestern University Press, 1993–94.

Dozon, Jean-Pierre, and Didier Fassin. *Critique de la santé publique: Une approche anthropologique.* Paris: Balland, 2001.

———. *The White Plague: Tuberculosis, Man, and Society.* 2nd ed. New Brunswick, N.J.: Rutgers University Press, 1992.

Dubos, René J., and Jean Dubos, eds. *The White Plague: Tuberculosis, Man, and Society.* New Brunswick, N.J.: Rutgers University Press, 1992.

Dubrac, Ferdinand. *Traité de jurisprudence médicale et pharmaceutique.* Paris: Baillière, 1822.

Dugger, Celia. "Rural Haitians Are Vanguard in AIDS Battle." *New York Times,* November 30, 2004, p. A1.

Dunn, Frederick L. "Social Determinants in Tropical Disease." In *Tropical and Geographic Medicine,* edited by Kenneth S. Warren and Adel A. F. Mahmoud, pp. 1086–96. New York: McGraw-Hill, 1984.

Dunn, Frederick L., and Craig R. Janes. "Introduction: Medical Anthropology and Epidemiology." In *Anthropology and Epidemiology: Interdisciplinary Approaches to the Study of Health and Disease,* edited by Craig R. Janes, Ron Stall, and Sandra M. Gifford, pp. 3–34. Dordrecht: Reidel, 1986.

Duranton, Alexandre. *Cours de droit français, suivant le code civil.* 21 vols. 6th ed. Paris: G. Thorel, E. Guilbert, 1844.

"Durban Declaration and Programme of Action." Adopted at the World Conference against Racism, Racial Discrimination, Xenophobia, and Related Intolerance, Durban, South Africa, August 31–September 8, 2001. Final version at www.un.org/WCAR/durban.pdf (accessed September 13, 2009).

Dussel, Inés, Silvia Finocchio, and Silvia Gojman. *Haciendo memoria en el país de nunca más.* Buenos Aires: Eudeba, 1997.

Easterbrook, P. J., J. C. Keruly, T. Creagh-Kirk, D. D. Richman, R. E. Chaisson, and R. D. Moore. "Racial and Ethnic Differences in Outcome in Zidovudine-Treated Patients with Advanced HIV Disease: Zidovudine Epidemiology Study Group." *Journal of the American Medical Association* 266, no. 19 (1991): 2713–18.

Eckardt, Irina. "Challenging Complexity: Conceptual Issues in an Approach to New Disease." *Annals of the New York Academy of Sciences* 740 (1994): 408–17.

Einstein, Albert, and Bertrand Russell. "The Russell-Einstein Manifesto." In *The Manhattan Project: The Birth of the Atomic Bomb in the Words of Its Creators, Eyewitnesses, and Historians,* edited by Cynthia Kelly, pp. 444–47. New York: Black Dog and Leventhal, 2007.

Eisenberg, Leon. "Rudolf Ludwig Karl Virchow, Where Are You Now That We Need You?" *American Journal of Medicine* 77, no. 3 (1984): 524–32.

Eisenberg, Leon, and Arthur Kleinman. *The Relevance of Social Science for Medicine.* Dordrecht: Reidel, 1981.

Eisenhower, Dwight David. "The Chance for Peace." Speech to the American Society of Newspaper Editors, April 16, 1953. www.eisenhowermemorial.org/speeches/19530416%20Chance%20for%20Peace.htm (accessed July 2, 2009).

Ellerbrock, T. V., S. Chamblee, T. J. Bush, J. W. Johnson, B. J. Marsh, P. Lowell, R. J. Trenschel, C. F. Von Reyn, L. S. Johnson, and C. R. Horsburgh Jr. "Human Immunodeficiency Virus Infection in a Rural Community in the United States." *American Journal of Epidemiology* 160, no. 6 (2004): 582–88.

Ellerbrock, T. V., S. Lieb, P. E. Harrington, T. J. Bush, S. A. Schoenfisch, M. J. Oxtoby, J. T. Howell, M. F. Rogers, and J. J. Witte. "Heterosexually Transmitted Human Immunodeficiency Virus Infection among Pregnant Women in a Rural Florida Community." *New England Journal of Medicine* 327, no. 24 (1992): 1704–9.

Emanuel, Ezekiel J., David Wendler, and Christine Grady. "What Makes Clinical Research Ethical?" *Journal of the American Medical Association* 283, no. 20 (2000): 2701–11.

Englund, Harri, ed. *A Democracy of Chameleons: Politics and Culture in the New Malawi.* Uppsala: Nordic Africa Institute, 2002.

"Enquête: Projet de marketing social." Port-au-Prince: Centre de Recherche Appliquée, 1998.

Epstein, Helen. "God and the Fight against AIDS." *New York Review of Books* 52, no. 7 (2005): 47–51.

———. "The Lost Children of AIDS." *New York Review of Books* 52, no. 17 (2005): 41–46.

Espinal, M. A., S. J. Kim, P. G. Suarez, K. M. Kam, A. G. Khomenko, G. B. Migliori, J. Baez, A. Kochi, C. Dye, and M. C. Raviglione. "Standard Short-Course Chemotherapy for Drug-Resistant Tuberculosis: Treatment Outcomes in 6 Countries." *Journal of the American Medical Association* 283, no. 19 (2000): 2537–45.

Espinal, M. A., A. Laszlo, L. Simonsen, F. Boulahbal, S. J. Kim, A. Reniero, S. Hoffner, H. L. Rieder, N. Binkin, C. Dye, et al. (for the World Health Organization–International Union against Tuberculosis and Lung Disease Working Group on Anti-Tuberculosis Drug Resistance Surveillance). "Global Trends in Resistance to Antituberculosis Drugs." *New England Journal of Medicine* 344, no. 17 (2001): 1294–1303.

Fabian, Johannes. *Time and the Other: How Anthropology Makes Its Object.* 2nd ed. New York: Columbia University Press, 2002. Originally published in 1983.

Fairchild, A. L., and G. M. Oppenheimer. "Public Health Nihilism vs. Pragmatism: History, Politics, and the Control of Tuberculosis." *American Journal of Public Health* 88, no. 7 (1998): 1105–17.

Fanon, Frantz. *Toward the African Revolution: Political Essays.* New York: Monthly Review Press, 1967.

———. *The Wretched of the Earth.* New York: Grove Press, 1965.

Farmer, Paul E. "AIDS: A Biosocial Problem with Social Solutions." *Anthropology News* 44 (2003): 5–7.

———. *AIDS and Accusation: Haiti and the Geography of Blame.* Updated with a new preface. Berkeley: University of California Press, 2006. Originally published in 1992.

———. "AIDS and Accusation: Haiti, Haitians, and the Geography of Blame." In *Culture and AIDS: The Human Factor,* edited by Douglas A. Feldman, pp. 67–91. New York: Praeger, 1990.

———. "AIDS-Talk and the Constitution of Cultural Models." *Social Science and Medicine* 38, no. 6 (1994): 801–9.

———. "An Anthropology of Structural Violence (Sidney W. Mintz Lecture for 2001)." *Current Anthropology* 45, no. 3 (2004): 305–25.

———. "Bad Blood, Spoiled Milk: Bodily Fluids as Moral Barometers in Rural Haiti." *American Ethnologist* 15, no. 1 (1988): 62–83.

———. "The Banality of Agency: Bridging Personal Narrative and Political Economy." *Anthropological Quarterly* 78, no. 1 (2005): 125–35.

———. "Blood, Sweat, and Baseballs: Haiti in the West Atlantic System." *Dialectical Anthropology* 13, no. 1 (1988): 83–99.

———. "Challenging Orthodoxies: The Road Ahead for Health and Human Rights." *Health and Human Rights: An International Journal* 10, no. 1 (2008): 5–19.

———. "The Consumption of the Poor: Tuberculosis in the Twenty-First Century." *Ethnography* 1, no. 2 (2000): 183–216.

———. "Cruel and Unusual: Drug-Resistant Tuberculosis as Punishment." In *Sentenced to Die? The Problem of TB in Prisons in Eastern Europe and Central Asia,* edited by Vivien Stern, pp. 70–88. London: International Centre for Prison Studies, King's College, 1999.

———. "Culture, Society, and the Dynamics of HIV Transmission in Rural Haiti." In *Cul-*

ture and Sexual Risk: Anthropological Perspectives on AIDS, edited by Han ten Brummelhuis and Gilbert H. Herdt, pp. 3–28. Amsterdam: Gordon and Breach, 1995.

———. "Douze points en faveur de la restitution à Haïti de la dette française." *L'Union,* November 11, 2003.

———. "Ethnography, Social Analysis, and the Prevention of Sexually Transmitted HIV Infection among Poor Women in Haiti." In *The Anthropology of Infectious Disease: International Health Perspectives,* edited by Marcia C. Inhorn and Peter J. Brown, pp. 413–38. Amsterdam: Gordon and Breach, 1997.

———. "The Exotic and the Mundane: Human Immunodeficiency Virus in Haiti." *Human Nature* 1 (1990): 415–46.

———. "Haiti's Lost Years: Lessons for the Americas." *Current Issues in Public Health* 2 (1996): 143–51.

———. *Infections and Inequalities: The Modern Plagues.* Berkeley: University of California Press, 1999.

———. "'Landmine Boy' and the Tomorrow of Violence." In *Global Health in Times of Violence,* edited by Barbara Rylko-Bauer, Linda Whiteford, and Paul Farmer, pp. 41–62. Santa Fe: SAR Press, 2009.

———. "Letter from Haiti." *AIDS Clinical Care* 9, no. 11 (1997): 83–85.

———. "Listening for Prophetic Voices in Medicine." *America (NY)* 177, no. 1 (1997): 8–10, 12–13.

———. "The Major Infectious Diseases in the World—To Treat or Not to Treat?" *New England Journal of Medicine* 345, no. 3 (2001): 208–10.

———. "Managerial Successes, Clinical Failures." *International Journal of Tuberculosis and Lung Disease* 3, no. 5 (1999): 365–67.

———. "Mother Courage and the Future of War." *Social Analysis* 52, no. 2 (2008): 165–84.

———. "Never Again? Reflections on Human Values and Human Rights." Tanner Lecture on Human Values, March 30, 2005. In *The Tanner Lectures on Human Values, Vol. 26,* edited by Grethe B. Peterson, pp. 139–88. Salt Lake City: University of Utah Press, 2006. www.tannerlectures.utah.edu/lectures/documents/Farmer_2006.pdf (accessed July 15, 2009).

———. "New Disorder, Old Dilemmas: AIDS and Anthropology in Haiti." In *The Time of AIDS: Social Analysis, Theory, and Method,* edited by Gilbert H. Herdt and Shirley Lindenbaum, pp. 287–318. Newbury Park, Calif.: Sage, 1992.

———. "On Suffering and Structural Violence: A View from Below." *Daedalus* 125, no. 1 (1996): 261–83.

———. *Pathologies of Power: Health, Human Rights, and the New War on the Poor.* Reprinted with a new preface by the author. Foreword by Amartya Sen. Berkeley: University of California Press, 2004. Originally published in 2003.

———. "Pathologies of Power: Rethinking Health and Human Rights." *American Journal of Public Health* 89, no. 10 (1999): 1486–96.

———. "Political Violence and Public Health in Haiti." *New England Journal of Medicine* 350, no. 15 (2004): 1483–86.

———. "Prevention without Treatment Is Not Sustainable." *National AIDS Bulletin (Australia)* 13 (2000): 6–9, 40.

———. "Sending Sickness: Sorcery, Politics, and Changing Concepts of AIDS in Rural Haiti." *Medical Anthropology Quarterly* 4, no. 1 (1990): 6–27.

———. "The Significance of Haiti." In *Haiti: Dangerous Crossroads,* edited by North American Congress on Latin America (NACLA), pp. 217–30. Boston: South End Press, 1995.

———. "Social Inequalities and Emerging Infectious Diseases." *Emerging Infectious Diseases* 2, no. 4 (1996): 259–69.

———. "Social Medicine and the Challenge of Biosocial Research." In *Innovative Structures in Basic Research: Ringberg Symposium, 4–7 October 2000,* pp. 55–73. Munich: Generalverwaltung der Max-Planck-Gesellschaft, Referat Press- und Öffentlichkeitsarbeit, 2002.

———. "Social Scientists and the New Tuberculosis." *Social Science and Medicine* 44, no. 3 (1997): 347–58.

———. "TB Superbugs: The Coming Plague on All Our Houses." *Natural History* 108, no. 3 (1999): 46–53.

———. *The Uses of Haiti.* 3rd ed. Monroe, Maine: Common Courage Press, 2006. Originally published in 1994; 2nd ed. published in 2003.

———. "La violence structurelle et la matérialité du social." Leçon inaugurale, Chaire internationale, November 9, 2001. Collège de France, Paris.

———. "La violence structurelle et la matérialité du social." *Lettre du Collège de France,* no. 4 (2002).

———. "Who Removed Aristide?" *London Review of Books* 26, no. 8 (2004): 28–31.

———. "Women, Poverty, and AIDS." In *Women, Poverty, and AIDS: Sex, Drugs, and Structural Violence,* edited by Paul Farmer, Margaret Connors, and Janie Simmons, pp. 3–38. Monroe, Maine: Common Courage Press, 1996.

Farmer, Paul E., Jaime Bayona, and Mercedes Becerra. "Multidrug-Resistant Tuberculosis and the Need for Biosocial Perspectives." *International Journal of Tuberculosis and Lung Disease* 5, no. 10 (2001): 885–86.

Farmer, Paul E., Jaime Bayona, Mercedes Becerra, et al. "Poverty, Inequality, and Drug Resistance: Meeting Community Needs in the Global Era." In *Proceedings of the International Union against Tuberculosis and Lung Disease, North American Region Conference,* February 27–March 2, Chicago, pp. 88–101.

Farmer, Paul E., Jaime Bayona, Mercedes Becerra, Jennifer Furin, Cassis Henry, Howard Hiatt, Jim Yong Kim, Carole Mitnick, Edward Nardell, and Sonya Shin. "The Dilemma of MDR-TB in the Global Era." *International Journal of Tuberculosis and Lung Disease* 2, no. 11 (1998): 869–76.

Farmer, Paul E., Jaime Bayona, Sonya Shin, Lourdes Alvarez, Mercedes Becerra, Edward Nardell, Carlos Núñez, Epifanio Sánchez, Ralph Timperi, and Jim Yong Kim. "Preliminary Outcomes of Community-Based MDRTB Treatment in Lima, Peru." Paper presented at the Conference on Global Lung Health and the annual meeting of the International Union against Tuberculosis and Lung Disease, Bangkok, November 23–26, 1998.

Farmer, Paul E., and Mercedes Becerra. "Biosocial Research and the TDR Agenda." *TDR News,* no. 66 (2001): 5–7. Special Programme for Research and Training in Tropical

Diseases. www.who.int/tdrold/publications/tdrnews/news66/biosocial.htm (accessed October 10, 2009).

Farmer, Paul E., and Didi Bertrand. "Hypocrisies of Development and the Health of the Haitian Poor." In *Dying for Growth: Global Inequality and the Health of the Poor,* edited by Jim Yong Kim, Joyce V. Millen, Alec Irwin, and John Gershman, pp. 65–89. Monroe, Maine: Common Courage Press, 2000.

Farmer, Paul E., and Nicole Gastineau Campos. "Rethinking Medical Ethics: A View from Below." *Developing World Bioethics* 4, no. 1 (2004): 17–41.

Farmer, Paul E., Margaret Connors, and Janie Simmons, eds. *Women, Poverty, and AIDS: Sex, Drugs, and Structural Violence.* Monroe, Maine: Common Courage Press, 1996.

Farmer, Paul E., Jennifer J. Furin, Jaime Bayona, Mercedes Becerra, Cassis Henry, Howard Hiatt, Jim Yong Kim, Carole D. Mitnick, Edward Nardell, and Sonya Shin. "Management of MDR-TB in Resource-Poor Countries." *International Journal of Tuberculosis and Lung Disease* 3, no. 8 (1999): 643–45.

Farmer, Paul E., Jennifer J. Furin, and Sonya Shin. "Managing Multidrug-Resistant Tuberculosis." *Journal of Respiratory Diseases* 21, no. 1 (2000): 53–56.

Farmer, Paul E., and Nicole Gastineau. "Rethinking Health and Human Rights: Time for a Paradigm Shift." *Journal of Law, Medicine, and Ethics* 30, no. 4 (2002): 655–66.

Farmer, Paul E., and Jim Yong Kim. "Community-Based Approaches to the Control of Multidrug-Resistant Tuberculosis: Introducing 'DOTS-Plus.'" *British Medical Journal* 317, no. 7159 (1998): 671–74.

———. "Resurgent TB in Russia: Do We Know Enough to Act?" *European Journal of Public Health* 10, no. 2 (2000): 150–53.

———. "Surgery and Global Health: A View from beyond the OR." *World Journal of Surgery* 32, no. 4 (2008): 533–36.

Farmer, Paul E., Jim Yong Kim, Carole D. Mitnick, and Ralph Timperi. "Responding to Outbreaks of Multidrug-Resistant Tuberculosis: Introducing DOTS-Plus." In *Tuberculosis: A Comprehensive International Approach,* edited by Lee B. Reichman and Earl S. Hershfield, pp. 447–69. New York: Dekker, 2000.

Farmer, Paul E., and Arthur Kleinman. "AIDS as Human Suffering." *Daedalus* 118, no. 2 (1989): 135–60.

Farmer, Paul E., Alexander S. Kononets, Sergei E. Borisov, Alex Goldfarb, Timothy Healing, and Martin McKee. "Recrudescent Tuberculosis in the Russian Federation." In *The Global Impact of Drug-Resistant Tuberculosis,* by Harvard Medical School and Open Society Institute, pp. 39–83. Boston: Program in Infectious Disease and Social Change, Department of Social Medicine, Harvard Medical School, 1999.

Farmer, Paul E., Fernet Léandre, Jaime Bayona, and Myrtha Louissant. "DOTS-Plus for the Poorest of the Poor: The Partners In Health Experience." Abstract. *International Journal of Tuberculosis and Lung Disease* 5, no. 11, Suppl. 1 (2001): S257.

Farmer, Paul E., Fernet Léandre, Joia S. Mukherjee, Marie Sidonise Claude, Patrice Nevil, Mary C. Smith Fawzi, Serena P. Koenig, Arachu Castro, Mercedes C. Becerra, Jeffrey Sachs, et al. "Community-Based Approaches to HIV Treatment in Resource-Poor Settings." *Lancet* 358, no. 9279 (2001): 404–9.

Farmer, Paul E., Fernet Léandre, Joia S. Mukherjee, Rajesh Gupta, Laura Tarter, and

Jim Yong Kim. "Community-Based Treatment of Advanced HIV Disease: Introducing DOT-HAART (Directly Observed Therapy with Highly Active Antiretroviral Therapy)." *Bulletin of the World Health Organization* 79, no. 12 (2001): 1145–51.

Farmer, Paul E., and Edward A. Nardell. "Nihilism and Pragmatism in Tuberculosis Control." *American Journal of Public Health* 88, no. 7 (1998): 1014–15.

Farmer, Paul E., Bruce Nizeye, Sara Stulac, and Salmaan Keshavjee. "Structural Violence and Clinical Medicine." *PLoS Medicine* 3, no. 10 (2006): e449.

Farmer, Paul E., Simon Robin, St. Luc Ramilus, and Jim Yong Kim. "Tuberculosis, Poverty, and 'Compliance': Lessons from Rural Haiti." *Seminars in Respiratory Infections* 6, no. 4 (1991): 254–60.

Farmer, Paul E., and Mary C. Smith Fawzi. "Unjust Embargo Deepens Haiti's Health Crisis." *Boston Globe,* December 30, 2002, p. A15.

Farmer, Paul E., Mary C. Smith Fawzi, and Patrice Nevil. "Unjust Embargo of Aid for Haiti." *Lancet* 361, no. 9355 (2003): 420–23.

Farmer, Paul E., and David A. Walton. "Condoms, Coups, and Ideology of Prevention: Facing Failure in Rural Haiti." In *Catholic Ethicists on HIV/AIDS Prevention,* edited by James F. Keenan, Jon Fuller, Lisa Sowle Cahill, and Kevin T. Kelly, pp. 108–19. New York: Continuum, 2000.

Farmer, Paul E., David A. Walton, and Jennifer J. Furin. "The Changing Face of AIDS: Implications for Policy and Practice." In *The Emergence of AIDS: The Impact on Immunology, Microbiology, and Public Health,* edited by Kenneth H. Mayer and Hank Pizer, pp. 139–61. Washington, D.C.: American Public Health Association, 2000.

Fassin, Didier. "The Embodiment of Inequality: AIDS as a Social Condition and the Historical Experience in South Africa." *EMBO Reports* 4 (2003): S1–S9.

———. *L'espace politique de la santé: Essai de généalogie.* Paris: Presses Universitaires de France, 1996.

———. "Exclusion, Underclass, Marginalidad: Figures contemporaines de la pauvreté urbaine en France, aux États-Unis, et en Amérique Latine." *Revue Française de Sociologie* 37, no. 1 (1996): 37–75.

Fauci, A.S. "The AIDS Epidemic—Considerations for the 21st Century." *New England Journal of Medicine* 341, no. 14 (1999): 1046–50.

Feachem, Richard. "HAART—The Need for Strategically Focused Investments." *Bulletin of the World Health Organization* 79, no. 12 (2001): 1152–53.

"Federal Poverty Level Not Realistic." *Omaha World-Herald,* October 18, 1994, p. A9.

Feilden, R., J. Allman, J. Montague, and J. Rohde. "Health, Population, and Nutrition in Haiti: A Report Prepared for the World Bank." Boston: Management Sciences for Health, 1981.

Feldberg, Georgina D. *Disease and Class: Tuberculosis and the Shaping of Modern North American Society.* New Brunswick, N.J.: Rutgers University Press, 1995.

Ferguson, James. *Papa Doc, Baby Doc: Haiti and the Duvaliers.* Oxford: Blackwell, 1988.

Field, M.G. "The Health Crisis in the Former Soviet Union: A Report from the 'Post-War' Zone." *Social Science and Medicine* 41, no. 11 (1995): 1469–78.

Fife, D., and C. Mode. "AIDS Incidence and Income." *JAIDS: Journal of Acquired Immune Deficiency Syndromes* 5, no. 11 (1992): 1105–10.

Fischer-Homberger, Esther. *Medezin vor Gericht: Gerichtsmedizin von der Renaissance bis zur Aufklärung.* Bern: Huber, 1983.

Forster, E. M. *Maurice: A Novel.* New York: Norton, 1971.

Foucault, Michel. *The History of Sexuality.* New York: Pantheon Books, 1978.

——. *Surveiller et punir: Naissance de la prison.* Paris: Gallimard, 1971.

Frain, Sébastien. *Arrests du Parlement de Bretagne, pris des mémoires et plaidoyers de feu M. Sébastien Frain.* Edited by Pierre Hevin. 3rd ed. 2 vols. Rennes: P. Garnier, 1684.

Francisque, Edouard. *La structure économique et sociale de Haïti.* Port-au-Prince: Imprimerie Henri Deschamps, 1986.

French, Howard W. "AIDS Research in Africa: Juggling Risks and Hopes." *New York Times,* October 9, 1997, pp. A1, A14.

Frenk, J., and F. Chacon. "Bases conceptuales de la nueva salud internacional." *Salud Publica de Mexico* 33 (1991): 307–13.

Fridkin, Scott K., Jeffrey C. Hageman, Melissa Morrison, Laurie Thomson Sanza, Kathryn Como-Sabetti, John A. Jernigan, Kathleen Harriman, Lee H. Harrison, Ruth Lynfield, Monica M. Farley, et al. "Methicillin-Resistant Staphylococcus Aureus Disease in Three Communities." *New England Journal of Medicine* 352, no. 14 (2005): 1436–44.

Fried, Edward R., and Philip H. Trezise, eds. *Third World Debt: The Next Phase.* Washington, D.C.: Brookings Institution, 1989.

Frieden, T. R., P. I. Fujiwara, R. M. Washko, and M. A. Hamburg. "Tuberculosis in New York City—Turning the Tide." *New England Journal of Medicine* 333, no. 4 (1995): 229–33.

Friedman, Lloyd N., Michael T. Williams, Tejinder P. Singh, and Thomas R. Frieden. "Tuberculosis, AIDS, and Death among Substance Abusers on Welfare in New York City." *New England Journal of Medicine* 334, no. 13 (1996): 828–33.

Friedman, Samuel R., and Don C. Des Jarlais. "HIV among Drug Injectors: The Epidemic and the Response." *AIDS Care* 3, no. 3 (1991): 239–50.

Friedman, Samuel R., Don C. Des Jarlais, and Jo L. Sotheran. "AIDS Health Education for Intravenous Drug Users." *Health Education Quarterly* 13, no. 4 (1986): 383–93.

Friedman, Thomas L. "U.S. to Release 158 Haitian Detainees." *New York Times,* June 10, 1993, p. A12.

Friedrich, Ernst. *Krieg dem Kriege! Guerre à la Guerre! War against War! Oorlog aan den Oorlog!* Berlin: "Freie Jugend," 1924.

Frimodt-Möller, J. "Domiciliary Drug Therapy of Pulmonary Tuberculosis in a Rural Population in India." *Tubercle* 49, Suppl. (1968): 22–23.

Fuchs, Victor R. *Who Shall Live? Health, Economics, and Social Choice.* New York: Basic Books, 1974.

Fuller, R. Buckminster. *Operating Manual for Spaceship Earth.* Carbondale: Southern Illinois University Press, 1969.

Fullilove, Mindy Thompson, Robert E. Fullilove III, Katherine Haynes, and Shirley Gross. "Black Women and AIDS Prevention: A View towards Understanding the Gender Rules." *Journal of Sex Research* 27, no. 1 (1990): 47–64.

Fullilove, Mindy Thompson, Robert Fullilove III, Gail Kennedy, and Michael Smith.

"Trauma, Crack, and HIV Risk." Paper presented at the Eighth International Conference on AIDS, Amsterdam, July 19–24, 1992.

Fullilove, Mindy Thompson, E. Anne Lown, and Robert E. Fullilove III. "Crack 'Hos and Skeezers: Traumatic Experiences of Women Crack Users." *Journal of Sex Research* 29, no. 2 (1992): 275–87.

Fullilove, Robert E. "Community Disintegration and Public Health: A Case Study of New York City." In Institute of Medicine, *Assessing the Social and Behavioral Science Base for HIV/AIDS Prevention and Intervention,* pp. 93–116. Washington, D.C.: National Academies Press, 1995.

Fumento, Michael. *The Myth of Heterosexual AIDS.* Washington, D.C.: Regnery, 1993. Originally published in 1990.

Furin, Jennifer J. "The Clinical Management of Drug-Resistant Tuberculosis." *Current Opinion in Pulmonary Medicine* 13, no. 3 (2007): 212–17.

Furin, Jennifer J., Mercedes C. Becerra, Sonya S. Shin, Jim Yong Kim, Jaime Bayona, and Paul E. Farmer. "Effect of Administering Short-Course, Standardized Regimens in Individuals Infected with Drug-Resistant Mycobacterium Tuberculosis Strains." *European Journal of Clinical Microbiology and Infectious Diseases* 19, no. 2 (2000): 132–36.

Gail, Mitchell H., Philip S. Rosenberg, and James J. Goedert. "Therapy May Explain Recent Deficits in AIDS Incidence." *JAIDS: Journal of Acquired Immune Deficiency Syndromes* 3, no. 4 (1990): 296–306.

Gaines, Atwood D., and Paul E. Farmer. "Visible Saints: Social Cynosures and Dysphoria in the Mediterranean Tradition." *Culture, Medicine, and Psychiatry* 10, no. 4 (1986): 295–330.

Gakidou, Emmanuela, and Gary King. "Measuring Total Health Inequality: Adding Individual Variation to Group-Level Differences." *International Journal for Equity in Health* 1, no. 1 (2002). www.pubmedcentral.nih.gov/articlerender.fcgi?artid=140140 (accessed September 14, 2009).

Galbraith, James K. "A Perfect Crime: Inequality in the Age of Globalization." *Daedalus* 131, no. 1 (2002): 11–25.

Galeano, Eduardo H. *Open Veins of Latin America: Five Centuries of the Pillage of a Continent.* New York: Monthly Review Press, 1997.

———. "Those Little Numbers and People." In *The Book of Embraces,* translated by Cedric Belfrage, p. 81. New York: Norton, 1992.

Galtung, Johan. "Cultural Violence." *Journal of Peace Research* 27, no. 3 (1990): 291–305.

———. "Violence, Peace, and Peace Research." *Journal of Peace Research* 6, no. 3 (1969): 167–91.

Garrett, Laurie. "Bragging in Bangkok." *New York Times,* July 16, 2004, p. A21.

———. *The Coming Plague: Newly Emerging Diseases in a World Out of Balance.* New York: Farrar, Straus and Giroux, 1994.

———. "Public Health and the Mass Media." *Current Issues in Public Health* 1 (1995): 147–50.

———. "TB Surge in Former East Bloc." *Newsday,* March 25 1998, p. A21.

Garro, Linda C. "Explaining High Blood Pressure: Variation in Knowledge about Illness." *American Ethnologist* 15, no. 1 (1988): 98–119.

Gawande, Atul. "The Cost Conundrum: What a Texas Town Can Teach Us about Health Care." *New Yorker*, June 1, 2009. www.newyorker.com/reporting/2009/06/01/090601fa _fact_gawande (accessed October 10, 2009).

———. "Getting There from Here: How Should Obama Reform Health Care?" *New Yorker*, January 26, 2009. www.newyorker.com/reporting/2009/01/26/090126fa_fact _gawande (accessed October 10, 2009).

Geertz, Clifford. "Anti Anti-Relativism: Distinguished Lecture." *American Anthropologist* 86, no. 2 (1984): 263–78.

———. *Works and Lives: The Anthropologist as Author.* Stanford, Calif.: Stanford University Press, 1988.

Gellner, Ernest. *Relativism and the Social Sciences.* Cambridge: Cambridge University Press, 1985.

Gerstoft, J., J. O. Nielsen, E. Dickmeiss, T. Ronne, P. Platz, and L. Mathiesen. "The Acquired Immunodeficiency Syndrome (AIDS) in Denmark: A Report from the Copenhagen Study Group of AIDS on the First 20 Danish Patients." *Acta Medica Scandinavica* 217, no. 2 (1985): 213–24.

Gervais, Myriam. "Étude de la pratique des ajustements au Niger et au Rwanda." *Labor, Capital, and Society* 26, no. 1 (1993): 20–41.

Gifford, Sandra M. "The Meaning of Lumps: A Case Study of the Ambiguities of Risk." In *Anthropology and Epidemiology: Interdisciplinary Approaches to the Study of Health and Disease*, edited by Craig R. Janes, Ron Stall, and Sandra M. Gifford, pp. 213–48. Dordrecht: Reidel, 1986.

Gilks, Charles, Carla AbouZahr, and Tomris Türmen. "HAART in Haiti—Evidence Needed." *Bulletin of the World Health Organization* 79, no. 12 (2001): 1154–55.

Gilligan, James. *Violence: Reflections on a National Epidemic.* New York: Vintage Books, 1997.

Gilman, Sander. "AIDS and Syphilis: The Iconography of Disease." In *AIDS: Cultural Analysis, Cultural Activism*, edited by Douglas Crimp, pp. 87–107. Cambridge, Mass.: MIT Press, 1988.

Gilson, L., R. Mkanje, H. Grosskurth, F. Mosha, J. Picard, A. Gavyole, J. Todd, P. Mayaud, R. Swai, L. Fransen, et al. "Cost-Effectiveness of Improved Treatment Services for Sexually Transmitted Diseases in Preventing HIV-1 Infection in Mwanza Region, Tanzania." *Lancet* 350, no. 9094 (1997): 1805–9.

Gitlin, Todd. *The Twilight of Common Dreams: Why America Is Wracked by Culture Wars.* New York: Henry Holt, 1995.

Glendon, Mary Ann. *Rights Talk: The Impoverishment of Political Discourse.* New York: Free Press, 1991.

Global AIDS Policy Coalition. *Status and Trends of the HIV/AIDS Pandemic as of January 1, 1995.* Cambridge, Mass.: Harvard School of Public Health/François-Xavier Bagnoud Center for Health and Human Rights, 1995.

———. *Status and Trends of the HIV/AIDS Pandemic as of January 1, 1996.* Cambridge,

Mass.: Harvard School of Public Health/François-Xavier Bagnoud Center for Health and Human Rights, 1996.

Global Fund to Fight AIDS, Tuberculosis, and Malaria. "Haiti's Response to HIV/AIDS." Grant proposal and agreement. www.theglobalfund.org/programs/grant/?compid=483&grantid=29&lang=en&CountryId=HTI (accessed October 12, 2009).

Glover, Jonathan. *Humanity: A Moral History of the Twentieth Century.* New Haven: Yale University Press, 2000.

Goble, M., M. D. Iseman, L. A. Madsen, D. Waite, L. Ackerson, and C. R. Horsburgh Jr. "Treatment of 171 Patients with Pulmonary Tuberculosis Resistant to Isoniazid and Rifampin." *New England Journal of Medicine* 328, no. 8 (1993): 527–32.

Goeman, J., A. Meheus, and P. Piot. "Epidemiology of Sexually Transmissible Diseases in Developing Countries in the Era of AIDS." *Annales de la Société Belge de la Médecine Tropicale* 71, no. 2 (1991): 81–113.

Goldberger, Joseph, G. A. Wheeler, and Edgar Sydenstricker. "A Study of the Relation of Family Income and Other Economic Factors to Pellagra Incidence in Seven Cotton-Mill Villages of South Carolina in 1916." *Public Health Reports* 35, no. 46 (1920): 2673–2714.

Goma Epidemiology Group. "Public Health Impact of Rwandan Refugee Crisis: What Happened in Goma, Zaïre, in July, 1994?" *Lancet* 345, no. 8946 (1995): 339–44.

Good, Byron J. "The Heart of What's the Matter: The Semantics of Illness in Iran." *Culture, Medicine, and Psychiatry* 1, no. 1 (1977): 25–58.

Good, Byron J., and Mary-Jo DelVecchio Good. "Towards a Meaning-Centered Analysis of Popular Illness Categories: 'Fright Illness' and 'Heart Distress' in Iran." In *Cultural Conceptions of Mental Health and Therapy,* edited by Anthony J. Marsella and Geoffrey M. White, pp. 141–66. Dordrecht: Reidel, 1982

Goodman, Alan H., and Thomas L. Leatherman. *Building a New Biocultural Synthesis: Political-Economic Perspectives on Human Biology.* Ann Arbor: University of Michigan Press, 1998.

Goose, Stephen D., and Frank Smyth. "Arming Genocide in Rwanda—The High Cost of Small Arms Transfers." *Foreign Affairs* 73, no. 5 (1994): 86–96.

Gordon, Michael R. "Fateful Choice on Iraq Army Bypassed Debate." *New York Times,* March 17, 2008, p. A1.

Gorman, M. "The AIDS Epidemic in San Francisco: Epidemiological and Anthropological Perspectives." In *Anthropology and Epidemiology: Interdisciplinary Approaches to the Study of Health and Disease,* edited by Craig R. Janes, Ron Stall, and Sandra M. Gifford, pp. 157–74. Dordrecht: Reidel, 1986.

Gottlieb, Daniel J., Alexa S. Beiser, and George T. O'Connor. "Poverty, Race, and Medication Use Are Correlates of Asthma Hospitalization Rates." *Chest* 108, no. 1 (1995): 28–35.

Gottlieb, Sami L., John M. Douglas Jr., D. Scott Schmid, Gail Bolan, Michael Iatesta, C. Kevin Malotte, Jonathan Zenilman, Mark Foster, Anna E. Barón, John F. Steiner, et al. "Seroprevalence and Correlates of Herpes Simplex Virus Type 2 Infection in Five Sexually-Transmitted-Disease Clinics." *Journal of Infectious Diseases* 186, no. 10 (2002): 1381–89.

Goudsmit, J. "Malnutrition and Concomitant Herpesvirus Infection as a Possible Cause of Immunodeficiency Syndrome in Haitian Infants." *New England Journal of Medicine* 309, no. 9 (1983): 554–55.

Gourevitch, Philip. *We Wish to Inform You That Tomorrow We Will Be Killed with Our Families: Stories from Rwanda.* New York: Farrar, Straus and Giroux, 1998.

Grange, J. M., and F. Festenstein. "The Human Dimension of Tuberculosis Control." *Tubercle and Lung Disease* 74, no. 4 (1993): 219–22.

Gray, R. H., T. C. Quinn, D. Serwadda, N. K. Sewankambo, F. Wabwire-Mangen, and M. J. Wawer. "The Ethics of Research in Developing Countries." *New England Journal of Medicine* 343, no. 5 (2000): 361–63.

Green, Edward C. "New Challenges to the AIDS Prevention Paradigm." *Anthropology News* 44 (2003): 5–7.

Green, Linda. *Fear as a Way of Life: Mayan Widows in Rural Guatemala.* New York: Columbia University Press, 1999.

Green, Reginald Herbold. "Politics, Power, and Poverty: Health for All in 2000 in the Third World?" *Social Science and Medicine* 32, no. 7 (1991): 745–55.

Greene, Graham. *The Comedians.* London: Bodley Head, 1966.

Greenfield, W. R. "Night of the Living Dead II: Slow Virus Encephalopathies and AIDS: Do Necromantic Zombiists Transmit HTLV-III/LAV during Voodooistic Rituals?" *Journal of the American Medical Association* 256, no. 16 (1986): 2199–2200.

Greenough, Paul. "Intimidation, Coercion, and Resistance in the Final Stages of the South Asian Smallpox Eradication Campaign, 1973–1975." *Social Science and Medicine* 41, no. 5 (1995): 633–45.

Greifinger, Robert B., Nancy J. Heywood, and Jordan B. Glaser. "Tuberculosis in Prison: Balancing Justice and Public Health." *Journal of Law, Medicine, and Ethics* 21, no. 3–4 (1993): 332–41.

Griffin, Thomas M. *Haiti Human Rights Investigation, November 11–21, 2004.* Center for the Study of Human Rights, University of Miami Law School. Washington, D.C.: Ecumenical Program on Central America and the Caribbean, 2005. www.law.miami .edu/cfshr/pdf/CSHR_Report_1111–21_2004.pdf (accessed October 8, 2009).

Groopman, J. E. "Viruses and Human Neoplasia: Approaching Etiology." *American Journal of Medicine* 75, no. 3 (1983): 377–80.

Grove, Robert D., and Alice M. Hetzel. *Vital Statistics Rates in the United States, 1940–1960.* Washington, D.C.: U.S. Department of Health, Education, and Welfare, 1968.

Grover, Jan Zita. "AIDS: Keywords." In *AIDS: Cultural Analysis, Cultural Activism,* edited by Douglas Crimp, pp. 17–31. Cambridge, Mass.: MIT Press, 1988.

Grunwald, Joseph, Leslie Delatour, and Karl Voltaire. "Offshore Assembly in Haiti." In *Haiti—Today and Tomorrow: An Interdisciplinary Study,* edited by Charles Robert Foster and Albert Valdman, pp. 231–52. Lanham, Md.: University Press of America, 1984.

Guérin, J. M., R. Malebranche, R. Elie, A. C. Laroche, G. D. Pierre, E. Arnoux, T. J. Spira, J. M. Dupuy, T. A. Seemayer, and C. Pean-Guichard. "Acquired Immune Deficiency Syndrome: Specific Aspects of the Disease in Haiti." *Annals of the New York Academy of Sciences* 437 (1984): 254–63.

Guillermoprieto, Alma. *The Heart That Bleeds: Latin America Now.* New York: Knopf, 1994.

Gupta, Rajesh, Jim Y. Kim, Marcos A. Espinal, Jean-Michel Caudron, Bernard Pecoul, Paul E. Farmer, and Mario C. Raviglione. "Responding to Market Failures in Tuberculosis Control." *Science* 293, no. 5532 (2001): 1049–51.

Gutiérrez, Gustavo. *The Power of the Poor in History: Selected Writings.* Maryknoll, N.Y.: Orbis Books, 1983.

———. *A Theology of Liberation: History, Politics, and Salvation.* Maryknoll, N.Y.: Orbis Books, 1973.

Gwatkin, D. R., and P. Heuveline. "Improving the Health of the World's Poor." *British Medical Journal* 315, no. 7107 (1997): 497–98.

Gwinn, M., M. Pappaioanou, J. R. George, W. H. Hannon, S. C. Wasser, M. A. Redus, R. Hoff, G. F. Grady, A. Willoughby, and A. C. Novello. "Prevalence of HIV Infection in Childbearing Women in the United States: Surveillance Using Newborn Blood Samples." *Journal of the American Medical Association* 265, no. 13 (1991): 1704–8.

Haggett, P. "Geographical Aspects of the Emergence of Infectious Diseases." *Geographic Annals* 76 (1994): 91–104.

Haitian Ministry of Health and Population. "AIDS: An Epidemic That Threatens Haitian Development." Presented by the Haitian delegation at the Special United Nations Assembly on HIV/AIDS, New York, June 25–27, 2001.

Hallward, Peter. *Damming the Flood: Haiti, Aristide, and the Politics of Containment.* London: Verso, 2007.

———. "Option Zero in Haiti." *New Left Review* 27 (2004): 23–47.

Halsey, N., R. Boulos, and J. Brutus. "HIV Antibody Prevalence in Pregnant Haitian Women." *Abstracts of the Third International Conference on AIDS,* Washington, D.C., June 1987, p. 174.

Hancock, Graham. *Lords of Poverty: The Power, Prestige, and Corruption of the International Aid Business.* New York: Atlantic Monthly Press, 1989.

Hansen, Jonathan M. "Guantánamo Bay: An American Story." Cambridge, Mass.: David Rockefeller Center for Latin American Studies, Harvard University, 2007.

Hardt, Michael, and Antonio Negri. *Empire.* Cambridge, Mass.: Harvard University Press, 2000.

Harries, Anthony D., and Dermot Maher. *TB/HIV: A Clinical Manual.* Geneva: World Health Organization, 1996.

Harrison, Lawrence E. "Voodoo Politics." *Atlantic Monthly* 271, no. 6 (1993): 101–8.

Hartog, François. *Régimes d'historicité: Présentisme et expériences du temps.* Paris: Seuil, 2003.

Harvard AIDS Institute. "HAI Forum Panelists Debate the True Numbers of the AIDS Epidemic." *Harvard AIDS Institute Monthly Report,* May 1990, pp. 2–6.

Harvard Medical School and Open Society Institute. *The Global Impact of Drug-Resistant Tuberculosis.* Boston: Program in Infectious Disease and Social Change, Department of Social Medicine, Harvard Medical School, 1999.

Hatch, Elvin. *Culture and Morality: The Relativity of Values in Anthropology.* New York: Columbia University Press, 1983.

Hatzfeld, Jean. *The Antelope's Strategy: Living in Rwanda after the Genocide.* New York: Farrar, Straus and Giroux, 2009.

———. *Dans le nu de la vie: Récits des marais rwandais.* Paris: Seuil, 2000.

———. *Life Laid Bare: The Survivors in Rwanda Speak.* New York: Other Press, 2006.

———. *Machete Season: The Killers in Rwanda Speak. A Report.* New York: Farrar, Straus and Giroux, 2005.

———. *Une saison de machettes: Récits.* Paris: Seuil, 2003.

Hayner, Priscilla B. *Unspeakable Truths: Confronting State Terror and Atrocity.* New York: Routledge, 2001.

Heggenhougen, H. K. "Are the Marginalized the Slag-Heap of Globalization? Disparity, Health, and Human Rights." *Health and Human Rights* 4, no. 1 (1999): 205–13.

———. "Therapeutic Anthropology: Response to Shiloh's Proposal." *American Anthropologist* 81, no. 3 (1979): 647–51.

———. "Will Primary Health Care Efforts Be Allowed to Succeed?" *Social Science and Medicine* 19, no. 3 (1984): 217–24.

Heinlein, Peter. "UN Peacekeeping Chief: Haiti Worse than Darfur." *Voice of America,* June 28, 2005. www.voanews.com/english/archive/2005-06/2005-06-28-voa63.cfm (accessed September 14, 2009).

Henkin, Louis. *International Law, Politics, Values, and Functions. General Course on Public International Law.* Dordrecht: M. Nijhoff, 1990.

Herbert, Bob. "Refusing to Save Africans." *New York Times,* June 11, 2001. www.nytimes.com/2001/06/11/opinion/11HERB.html (accessed September 4, 2009).

Hersh, Seymour M. *Chain of Command: The Road from 9/11 to Abu Ghraib.* New York: HarperCollins, 2004.

Hilts, Philip J. "7 Haitians Held at Guantanamo Unconscious in a Hunger Strike." *New York Times,* February 15, 1993.

Hinman, Alan R., James M. Hughes, Dixie E. Snider, and Mitchell L. Cohen. "Meeting the Challenge of Multidrug-Resistant Tuberculosis: Summary of a Conference." *Morbidity and Mortality Weekly Report* 41, RR-11 (1992): 49–57.

Hochschild, Adam. *Bury the Chains: Prophets and Rebels in the Fight to Free an Empire's Slaves.* Boston: Houghton Mifflin, 2005.

———. *King Leopold's Ghost: A Story of Greed, Terror, and Heroism in Colonial Africa.* Boston: Houghton Mifflin, 1998.

Hollibaugh, Amber. "Lesbian Denial and Lesbian Leadership in the AIDS Epidemic: Bravery and Fear in the Construction of a Lesbian Geography of Risk." In *Women Resisting AIDS: Feminist Strategies of Empowerment,* edited by Beth Schneider and Nancy E. Stoller, pp. 219–30. Philadelphia: Temple University Press, 1995.

Holmes, King K., and Sevgi O. Aral. "Behavioral Interventions in Developing Countries." In *Research Issues in Human Behavior and Sexually Transmitted Diseases in the AIDS Era,* edited by Judith N. Wasserheit, Sevgi O. Aral, and King K. Holmes, pp. 318–44. Washington, D.C.: American Society for Microbiology, 1991.

Hong Kong Chest Service/British Medical Research Council. "Controlled Trial of 4 Three-Times-Weekly Regimens and a Daily Regimen All Given for 6 Months for Pulmonary Tuberculosis. Second Report: The Results up to 24 Months." *Tubercle* 63, no. 2 (1982): 89–98.

Horton, Richard. "Iraq: Time to Signal a New Era for Health in Foreign Policy." *Lancet* 368, no. 9545 (2006): 1395–97.

———. "Towards the Elimination of Tuberculosis." *Lancet* 346, no. 8978 (1995): 790.

Hughes, Robert. *Culture of Complaint: The Fraying of America.* New York: Oxford University Press, 1993.

Human Rights Watch. "Exposing the Source: U.S. Companies and the Production of Antipersonnel Mines." *Human Rights Watch Arms Project,* April 1997, vol. 9, no. 2 (G). www.hrw.org/reports/pdfs/g/general/general2974.pdf (accessed July 2, 2009).

Human Rights Watch/Americas, Jesuit Refugee Service, and National Coalition for Haitian Refugees. *Fugitives from Injustice: The Crisis of Internal Displacement in Haiti.* Washington, D.C.: Human Rights Watch/Americas, August 1994. www.hrw.org/reports/pdfs/h/haiti/haiti948.pdf (accessed July 2, 2009).

Human Rights Watch/Americas and National Coalition for Haitian Refugees. *Terror Prevails in Haiti: Human Rights Violations and Failed Diplomacy.* Written and edited by Anne Fuller, Kathie Klarreich, Allyson Collins, and Robert Kimzey. New York: Human Rights Watch/Americas, April 1994. www.hrw.org/reports/pdfs/h/haiti/haiti 944.pdf (accessed July 2, 2009).

Human Rights Watch/The Arms Project and Physicians for Human Rights. *Landmines: A Deadly Legacy.* New York: Human Rights Watch, 1993.

Hume, David. *Enquiries concerning Human Understanding and concerning the Principles of Morals.* Edited by L. A. Selby-Bigge and P. H. Nidditch. 3rd ed. Oxford: Clarendon Press, 1975.

Hunter, Nan D. "Complications of Gender: Women, AIDS, and the Law." In *Women Resisting AIDS: Feminist Strategies of Empowerment,* edited by Beth Schneider and Nancy E. Stoller, pp. 32–56. Philadelphia: Temple University Press, 1995.

Hurbon, Laënnec. *Le barbare imaginaire.* Paris: Éditions du Cerf, 1988.

Hymes, Dell H. "The Uses of Anthropology: Critical, Political, Personal." In *Reinventing Anthropology,* edited by Dell H. Hymes, pp. 3–79. New York: Vintage Books, 1974.

Ignatieff, Michael. *Human Rights as Politics and Idolatry.* Edited and with an introduction by Amy Gutmann. Princeton, N.J.: Princeton University Press, 2001.

Immerman, Richard H. *The CIA in Guatemala: The Foreign Policy of Intervention.* Austin: University of Texas Press, 1982.

"Improved STD Treatment: A Message of Hope." *AIDS Analysis Africa* 5, no. 5 (1994): 10–11.

Inhorn, Marcia C. "Medical Anthropology and Epidemiology: Divergences or Convergences?" *Social Science and Medicine* 40, no. 3 (1995): 285–90.

Inhorn, Marcia C., and Peter J. Brown. "Anthropology of Infectious Disease." *Annual Review of Anthropology* 19 (1990): 89–117.

———, eds. *The Anthropology of Infectious Disease: International Health Perspectives.* Amsterdam: Gordon and Breach, 1997.

Institute of Medicine. Board on Health Care Services, Committee on the Consequences of Uninsurance. *Care without Coverage: Too Little, Too Late.* Washington, D.C.: National

Academies Press, 2002. www.nap.edu/openbook.php?isbn=0309083435 (accessed July 11, 2009).

Integrated Regional Information Network (IRIN). "Rwanda: Funding Shortage Retards Mine Action Efforts." *Laying Landmines to Rest? IRIN Web Special on Humanitarian Mine Action,* November 2004, pp. 37–38. www.irinnews.org/pdf/in-depth/Humanitarian -Mine-Action-IRIN-In-Depth.pdf (accessed July 11, 2009).

Inter-American Commission on Human Rights. *Report on the Situation of Human Rights in Haiti, 1995.* Washington, D.C.: Organization of American States, 1995. www.cidh .oas.org/countryrep/EnHa95/eh95int.htm (accessed July 12, 2009).

International Campaign to Ban Landmines (ICBL). *Landmine Monitor Report 1999: Toward a Mine-Free World.* www.icbl.org/lm/1999 (accessed July 12, 2009).

———. *Landmine Monitor Report 2007: Toward a Mine-Free World.* www.icbl.org/lm/ 2007 (accessed July 12, 2009).

———. "Rwanda." *Landmine Monitor Report 1999: Toward a Mine-Free World.* www.icbl .org/lm/1999/rwanda.html (accessed July 12, 2009).

———. "Rwanda." *Landmine Monitor Report 2007: Toward a Mine-Free World.* www.icbl .org/lm/2007/rwanda.html (accessed July 12, 2009).

International Military Tribunal (Nuremberg). "Judgment and Sentences." *American Journal of International Law* 41, no. 1 (1947): 172–333.

Iraq Family Health Survey Study Group (A. H. Alkhuzai, I. J. Ahmad, M. J. Hweel, T. W. Ismail, H. H. Hasan, A. R. Younis, O. Shawani, V. M. Al-Jaf, M. M. Al-Alak, L. H. Rasheed, S. M. Hamid, N. Al-Gasseer, F. A. Majeed, N. A. Al Awqati, M. M. Ali, J. T. Boerma, and C. Mathers). "Violence-Related Mortality in Iraq from 2002 to 2006." *New England Journal of Medicine* 358, no. 5 (2008): 484–93.

Iseman, Michael D. "Tailoring a Time-Bomb: Inadvertent Genetic Engineering." *American Review of Respiratory Disease* 132, no. 4 (1985): 735–36.

———. "Treatment of Multidrug-Resistant Tuberculosis." *New England Journal of Medicine* 329, no. 11 (1993): 784–91.

Ivers, Louise, Evan Garfein, Josué Augustin, Maxi Raymonville, Alice Yang, David Sugarbaker, and Paul Farmer. "Increasing Access to Surgical Services for the Poor in Rural Haiti: Surgery as a Public Good for Public Health." *World Journal of Surgery* 32, no. 4 (2008): 537–42.

Jacoby, Russell. *Dogmatic Wisdom: How the Culture Wars Divert Education and Distract America.* New York: Doubleday, 1994.

James, C. L. R. *The Black Jacobins; Toussaint L'Ouverture and the San Domingo Revolution.* 2nd ed. New York: Vintage Books, 1963.

Jameton, A., and J. Pierce. "Environment and Health: 8. Sustainable Health Care and Emerging Ethical Responsibilities." *Canadian Medical Association Journal* 164, no. 3 (2001): 365–69.

Janes, Craig R. "Migration and Hypertension: An Ethnography of Disease Risk in an Urban Samoan Community." In *Anthropology and Epidemiology: Interdisciplinary Approaches to the Study of Health and Diseases,* edited by Craig R. Janes, Ron Stall, and Sandra M. Gifford, pp. 175–212. Dordrecht: Reidel, 1986.

Janes, Craig R., Ron Stall, and Sandra M. Gifford, eds. *Anthropology and Epidemiology:*

Interdisciplinary Approaches to the Study of Health and Disease. Dordrecht: Reidel, 1986.

Janzen, John M. "Therapy Management: Concept, Reality, Process." *Medical Anthropology Quarterly* 1, no. 1 (1987): 68–84.

Jean-Louis, R. "Diagnostic de l'état de santé en Haïti." *Forum Libre (Santé, Médicine et Democratie en Haïti)* 1 (1989): 11–20.

Jereb, J. A., G. D. Kelly, S. W. Dooley Jr., G. M. Cauthen, and D. E. Snider Jr. "Tuberculosis Morbidity in the United States: Final Data, 1990." *Morbidity and Mortality Weekly Report, CDC Surveillance Summaries* 40, no. 3 (1991): 23–27.

Jha, P., B. Stirling, and A. S. Slutsky. "Weapons of Mass Salvation: Canada's Role in Improving the Health of the Global Poor." *Canadian Medical Association Journal* 170, no. 1 (2004): 66–67.

Johnson, K. M., J. V. Lange, P. A. Webb, and F. A. Murphy. "Isolation and Partial Characterisation of a New Virus Causing Acute Haemorrhagic Fever in Zaire." *Lancet* 1, no. 8011 (1977): 569–71.

Johnson, Warren, and Jean Pape. "AIDS in Haiti." In *AIDS: Pathogenesis and Treatment*, edited by Jay A. Levy, pp. 65–78. New York: Dekker, 1989.

Joint United Nations Programme on HIV/AIDS. *AIDS in Africa: Three Scenarios to 2025.* Geneva: UNAIDS, 2005. www.unaids.org/unaids_resources/images/AIDSScenarios/ AIDS-scenarios-2025_report_en.pdf (accessed July 12, 2009).

———. "Selected Issues: Prevention, Care, and Funding [Part II]." *UNAIDS Questions and Answers,* 2006. http://data.unaids.org/pub/GlobalReport/2006/20060530-Q-A_Part2 _en.pdf (accessed September 14, 2009).

Kahn, Joseph. "Rich Nations Consider Fund of Billions to Fight AIDS." *New York Times,* April 28, 2001, p. A10.

Kaiser Commission on Medicaid and the Uninsured. "Health Insurance Coverage in America: 2004 Data Update." www.kff.org/uninsured/upload/Health-Coverage-in -America-2004-Data-Update-Report.pdf (accessed June 15, 2009).

Kajiyama, W., S. Kashiwagi, H. Ikematsu, J. Hayashi, H. Nomura, and K. Okochi. "Intrafamilial Transmission of Adult T-Cell Leukemia Virus." *Journal of Infectious Diseases* 154, no. 5 (1986): 851–57.

Kapczynski, Amy, Samantha Chaifetz, Zachary Katz, and Yochai Benkler. "Addressing Global Health Inequities: An Open Licensing Approach for University Innovations." *Berkeley Technology Law Journal* 20, no. 2 (2005): 1031–1114.

Katon, Wayne, Arthur Kleinman, and Gary Rosen. "Depression and Somatization: A Review. Part I." *American Journal of Medicine* 72, no. 1 (1982): 127–35.

———. "Depression and Somatization: A Review. Part II." *American Journal of Medicine* 72, no. 2 (1982): 241–47.

Kauffman, L. A. "The Diversity Game." *Village Voice,* August 31, 1993, pp. 29, 32.

Kaufman, Carol E. "Contraceptive Use in South Africa under Apartheid." *Demography* 35, no. 4 (1998): 421–34.

Kawachi, Ichiro, and Bruce P. Kennedy. *The Health of Nations: Why Inequality Is Harmful to Your Health.* New York: The New Press, 2002.

Kawachi, Ichiro, Bruce P. Kennedy, Kimberly Lochner, and Deborah Prothrow-Stith.

"Social Capital, Income Inequality, and Mortality." *American Journal of Public Health* 87, no. 9 (1997): 1491–98.

Keane, Fergal. *Season of Blood: A Rwandan Journey.* New York: Viking, 1995.

———. "Why 'Never Again' Keeps Happening." *BBC News,* July 2005. http://news.bbc.co .uk/2/hi/programmes/from_our_own_correspondent/4641773.stm (accessed July 12, 2009).

Keane, John. *Reflections on Violence.* London: Verso, 1996.

Keegan, Victor. "Second Front: Highway Robbery by the Super-Rich." *Guardian* (U.K.), July 22, 1996, p. T2.

Kernaghan, Charles. *Haiti after the Coup: Sweatshop or Real Development?* New York: U.S. National Labor Committee, 1993.

Kidder, Tracy. *Mountains Beyond Mountains: The Quest of Dr. Paul Farmer, a Man Who Would Cure the World.* New York: Random House, 2003.

———. "The Trials of Haiti." *Nation* 277, no. 13 (2003): 26–30.

Kiev, Ari. *Transcultural Psychiatry.* New York: Free Press, 1972.

Kim, Jim Yong, and Paul E. Farmer. "AIDS in 2006—Moving toward One World, One Hope?" *New England Journal of Medicine* 355, no. 7 (2006): 645–47.

Kim, Jim Yong, Jennifer J. Furin, Aaron D. Shakow, Joyce V. Millen, Joel G. Brenner, Marshall W. Fordyce, Evan Lyon, Jaime Bayona, and Paul E. Farmer. "Treatment of Multidrug-Resistant Tuberculosis (MDR-TB): New Strategies for Procuring Second- and Third-Line Drugs." Abstract. *International Journal of Tuberculosis and Lung Disease* 3, no. 9, Suppl. 1 (1999): S81.

Kim, Jim Yong, and Charlie Gilks. "Scaling Up Treatment—Why We Can't Wait." *New England Journal of Medicine* 353, no. 22 (2005): 2392–94.

Kim, Jim Yong, Joyce V. Millen, Alec Irwin, and John Gershman, eds. *Dying for Growth: Global Inequality and the Health of the Poor.* Monroe, Maine: Common Courage Press, 2000.

Kim, Jim Yong, Aaron Shakow, Jaime Bayona, Joe Rhatigan, and Emma L. Rubín de Celis. "Sickness amidst Recovery: Public Debt and Private Suffering in Peru." In *Dying for Growth: Global Inequality and the Health of the Poor,* edited by Jim Yong Kim, Joyce V. Millen, Alec Irwin, and John Gershman, pp. 127–53. Monroe, Maine: Common Courage Press, 2000.

Kim, Jim Yong, Aaron Shakow, Arachu Castro, Chris Vanderwarker, and Paul E. Farmer. "Tuberculosis Control." In *Global Public Goods for Health: Health Economic and Public Health Perspectives,* edited by Richard Smith, Robert Beaglehole, David Woodward, and Nick Drager, pp. 54–72. Oxford: Oxford University Press, 2003.

Kimerling, M. E., H. Kluge, N. Vezhnina, T. Iacovazzi, T. Demeulenaere, F. Portaels, and F. Matthys. "Inadequacy of the Current WHO Re-Treatment Regimen in a Central Siberian Prison: Treatment Failure and MDR-TB." *International Journal of Tuberculosis and Lung Disease* 3, no. 5 (1999): 451–53.

Kinney, Eleanor D. "The International Human Right to Health: What Does This Mean for Our Nation and World?" *Indiana Law Review* 34 (2001): 1457–75.

Kirmayer, Laurence J. "Failures of Imagination: The Refugee's Narrative in Psychiatry." *Anthropology and Medicine* 10, no. 2 (2003): 167–85.

———. "Reflections on Embodiment." In *Social and Cultural Lives of Immune Systems,* edited by James MacLynn Wilce, pp. 282–302. London: Routledge, 2003.

Klein, D. E., G. Sullivan, D. L. Wolcott, J. Landsverk, S. Namir, and F. I. Fawzy. "Changes in AIDS Risk Behaviors among Homosexual Male Physicians and University Students." *American Journal of Psychiatry* 144, no. 6 (1987): 742–47.

Klein, Herbert S. *African Slavery in Latin America and the Caribbean.* New York: Oxford University Press, 1986.

Klein, Naomi. *No Logo: Taking Aim at the Brand Bullies.* New York: Picador, 2000.

———. *The Shock Doctrine: The Rise of Disaster Capitalism.* New York: Henry Holt, 2007.

Kleinman, Arthur. "Ethics and Experience: An Anthropological Approach to Health Equity." In *Public Health, Ethics, and Equity,* edited by Sudhir Anand, Fabienne Peter, and Amartya Kumar Sen, pp. 269–82. New York: Oxford University Press, 2004.

———. "Experience and Its Moral Modes: Culture, Human Conditions, and Disorder." Tanner Lecture on Human Values, April 1998. In *Tanner Lectures on Human Values, Vol. 20,* edited by Grethe B. Peterson, pp. 357–420. Salt Lake City: University of Utah Press, 1999. www.tannerlectures.utah.edu/lectures/documents/Kleinman99.pdf (accessed July 15, 2009).

———. "Neurasthenia and Depression: A Study of Somatization and Culture in China." *Culture, Medicine, and Psychiatry* 6, no. 2 (1982): 117–90.

———. *Patients and Healers in the Context of Culture: An Exploration of the Borderland between Anthropology, Medicine, and Psychiatry.* Berkeley: University of California Press, 1980.

———. *Social Origins of Distress and Disease: Depression, Neurasthenia, and Pain in Modern China.* New Haven: Yale University Press, 1986.

———. *What Really Matters: Living a Moral Life amidst Uncertainty and Danger.* New York: Oxford University Press, 2006.

———. *Writing at the Margin: Discourse between Anthropology and Medicine.* Berkeley: University of California Press, 1995.

Kleinman, Arthur, Veena Das, and Margaret M. Lock, eds. *Social Suffering.* Berkeley: University of California Press, 1997.

Kleinman, Arthur, Leon Eisenberg, and Byron Good. "Culture, Illness, and Care: Clinical Lessons from Anthropologic and Cross-Cultural Research." *Annals of Internal Medicine* 88, no. 2 (1978): 251–58.

Kleinman, Arthur, and Byron Good, eds. *Culture and Depression: Studies in the Anthropology and Cross-Cultural Psychiatry of Affect and Disorder.* Berkeley: University of California Press, 1985.

Kleinman, Arthur, and Joan Kleinman. "The Appeal of Experience; the Dismay of Images: Cultural Appropriations of Suffering in Our Times." In *Social Suffering,* edited by Arthur Kleinman, Veena Das, and Margaret M. Lock, pp. 1–24. Berkeley: University of California Press, 1997.

———. "Suffering and Its Professional Transformation: Towards an Ethnography of Experience." Paper presented at the First Conference of the Society for Psychological Anthropology, October 6–8, 1989, San Diego, Calif.

Kochi, Arata. "Tuberculosis Control—Is DOTS the Health Breakthrough of the 1990s?" *World Health Forum* 18, nos. 3–4 (1997): 225–32.

Koenig, R. E., J. Pittaluga, M. Bogart, M. Castro, F. Nunez, I. Vilorio, L. Delvillar, M. Calzada, and J. A. Levy. "Prevalence of Antibodies to the Human Immunodeficiency Virus in Dominicans and Haitians in the Dominican Republic." *Journal of the American Medical Association* 257, no. 5 (1987): 631–34.

Koselleck, Reinhart. *L'expérience de l'histoire.* Edited and with a preface by Michaël Werner. Paris: Gallimard/Seuil, 1997.

Koss, Mary, Paul Koss, and Joy Woodruff. "Deleterious Effects of Criminal Victimization on Women's Health and Medical Utilization." *Archives of Internal Medicine* 151, no. 2 (1991): 342–47.

Kraut, Alan M. *Silent Travelers: Germs, Genes, and the "Immigrant Menace."* New York: Basic Books, 1994.

Krieger, Nancy. "Embodying Inequality: A Review of Concepts, Measures, and Methods for Studying Health Consequences of Discrimination." *International Journal of Health Services* 29, no. 2 (1999): 295–352.

———. "Proximal, Distal, and the Politics of Causation: What's Level Got to Do with It?" *American Journal of Public Health* 98, no. 2 (2008): 221–30.

Krieger, Nancy, and Elizabeth Fee. "Social Class: The Missing Link in U.S. Health Data." *International Journal of Health Services* 24, no. 1 (1994): 25–44.

Krieger, Nancy, Diane Rowley, Allen Herman, Byllye Avery, and Mona Phillips. "Racism, Sexism, and Social Class: Implications for Studies of Health, Disease, and Well-Being." *American Journal of Preventive Medicine* 9, no. 6, Suppl. (1993): 82–122.

Krieger, Nancy, and Sally Zierler. "Accounting for Health of Women." *Current Issues in Public Health* 1 (1995): 251–56.

Kristof, Nicholas. "All Ears for Tom Cruise, All Eyes on Brad Pitt." *New York Times,* February 23, 2005, p. A19.

———. "The Secret Genocide Archive." *New York Times,* July 26, 2005, p. A19.

Kroeber, Alfred L. *Anthropology: Culture, Patterns, and Processes.* New York: Harcourt, 1963.

Krueger, Leigh E., Robert W. Wood, Paula H. Diehr, and Clare L. Maxwell. "Poverty and HIV Seropositivity: The Poor Are More Likely to Be Infected." *AIDS* 4, no. 8 (1990): 811–14.

Kuhn, Thomas S. *The Structure of Scientific Revolutions.* 2nd ed. Chicago: University of Chicago Press, 1970.

Kundera, Milan. *The Book of Laughter and Forgetting.* Translated by Aaron Asher. New York: HarperCollins, 1996.

Kwiatkowski, Lynn M. *Struggling with Development: The Politics of Hunger and Gender in the Philippines.* Boulder, Colo.: Westview Press, 1998.

Lacey, Marc. "Women's Voices Rise as Rwanda Reinvents Itself." *New York Times,* February 26, 2005, p. A3.

LaFeber, Walter. *Inevitable Revolutions: The United States in Central America.* New York: Norton, 1984.

Laga, M., A. Manoka, M. Kivuvu, B. Malele, M. Tuliza, N. Nzila, J. Goeman, F. Behets,

V. Batter, and M. Alary. "Non-Ulcerative Sexually Transmitted Diseases as Risk Factors for HIV-1 Transmission in Women: Results from a Cohort Study." *AIDS* 7, no. 1 (1993): 95–102.

Laguerre, Michel S. *Afro-Caribbean Folk Medicine.* South Hadley, Mass.: Bergin and Garvey, 1987.

Lambert, Bruce. "Now, No Haitians Can Donate Blood." *New York Times,* March 14, 1990.

Lancaster, Roger N. *Thanks to God and the Revolution: Popular Religion and Class Consciousness in the New Nicaragua.* New York: Columbia University Press, 1988.

Landmine Action. *Explosive Remnants of War: Unexploded Ordnance and Post-Conflict Communities.* March 2002. www.landmineaction.org/resources/ERW%20-%20UXO%20and%20post-conflict%20communities.pdf (accessed July 12, 2009).

Lange, W. R., and J. H. Jaffe. "AIDS in Haiti." *New England Journal of Medicine* 316, no. 22 (1987): 1409–10.

Langley, Lester D. *The United States and the Caribbean in the Twentieth Century.* Athens: University of Georgia Press, 1989.

Langone, John. "AIDS: The Latest Scientific Facts." *Discover,* December 1985, pp. 40–56.

Larson, A. "Social Context of Human Immunodeficiency Virus Transmission in Africa: Historical and Cultural Bases of East and Central African Sexual Relations." *Reviews of Infectious Diseases* 11, no. 5 (1989): 716–31.

Latour, Bruno. *The Pasteurization of France.* Cambridge, Mass.: Harvard University Press, 1988.

Latour, Bruno, and Steve Woolgar. *Laboratory Life: The Social Construction of Scientific Facts.* London: Sage, 1979.

Lawless, Robert. *Haiti's Bad Press.* Rochester, Vt.: Schenkman Books, 1992.

Leacock, Eleanor Burke. *Myths of Male Dominance: Collected Papers on Women Cross Culturally.* New York: Monthly Review Press, 1981.

le Carré, John. "A War We Cannot Win." *Nation* 273, no. 16 (2001): 15–17.

Leclerc, Annette, Didier Fassin, Hélène Grandjean, and Monique Kaminski, eds. *Les inégalités sociales de santé.* Paris: Éditions la Découverte, 2000.

Lederberg, Joshua, Robert E. Shope, and Stanley C. Oaks Jr., eds. *Emerging Infections: Microbial Threats to Health in the United States.* Institute of Medicine, Committee on Emerging Microbial Threats to Health. Washington, D.C.: National Academies Press, 1992.

Lee, JeeYeun. "Beyond Bean Counting." In *Listen Up: Voices from the Next Feminist Generation,* edited by Barbara Findlen, pp. 205–11. Seattle: Seal Press, 1995.

Leibowitch, Jacques. *A Strange Virus of Unknown Origin.* New York: Ballantine, 1985.

Lemarchand, René. "The Rwanda Genocide." In *Century of Genocide: Critical Essays and Eyewitness Accounts,* 2nd ed., edited by Samuel Totten, William S. Parsons, and Israel W. Charny, pp. 395–414. New York: Routledge, 2004.

Lemp, G. F., A. M. Hirozawa, J. B. Cohen, P. A. Derish, K. C. McKinney, and S. R. Hernandez. "Survival for Women and Men with AIDS." *Journal of Infectious Diseases* 166, no. 1 (1992): 74–79.

Levi, Primo. *Survival in Auschwitz: The Nazi Assault on Humanity.* New York: Collier, 1961.

Levinas, Emmanuel. *Totality and Infinity: An Essay on Exteriority.* Translated by Alphonso Lingis. Pittsburgh: Duquesne University Press, 1969.

Levine, Norman D. "Editor's Preface." In *Malaria in the Interior Valley of North America,* edited by Norman D. Levine. Urbana: University of Illinois Press, 1964.

Levins, Richard. "Preparing for Uncertainty." *Ecosystem Health* 1, no. 1 (1995): 47–57.

Lewis, Diane K. "African-American Women at Risk: Notes on the Sociocultural Context of AIDS Infection." In *Women Resisting AIDS: Feminist Strategies of Empowerment,* edited by Beth Schneider and Nancy E. Stoller, pp. 57–73. Philadelphia: Temple University Press, 1995.

Leyburn, James Graham. *The Haitian People.* Introduction by Sidney W. Mintz. New Haven: Yale University Press, 1966.

Liautaud, B., C. Laroche, J. Duvivier, and C. Pean-Guichard. "Le sarcôme de Kaposi en Haïti: Foyer méconnu ou récemment apparu?" *Annals of Dermatological Venereology* 110 (1983): 213–19.

Liautaud, B., J. W. Pape, and M. Pamphile. "Le sida dans les Caraïbes." *Médecine et Maladies Infectieuses* 18, no. 5 Suppl. (1988): 687–97.

Lieban, R. W. "Traditional Medical Beliefs and the Choice of Practitioners in a Philippine City." *Social Science and Medicine* 10, no. 6 (1976): 289–96.

Liebow, Elliot. *Tally's Corner: A Study of Negro Streetcorner Men.* Boston: Back Bay Books, 1968.

Lindenbaum, Shirley. *Kuru Sorcery: Disease and Danger in the New Guinea Highlands.* Palo Alto, Calif.: Mayfield, 1979.

Lipovetsky, Gilles. *L'ère du vide: Essais sur l'individualisme contemporain.* Paris: Gallimard, 1983.

Little, Susan J., Sarah Holte, Jean-Pierre Routy, Eric S. Daar, Marty Markowitz, Ann C. Collier, Richard A. Koup, John W. Mellors, Elizabeth Connick, Brian Conway, et al. "Antiretroviral-Drug Resistance among Patients Recently Infected with HIV." *New England Journal of Medicine* 347, no. 6 (2002): 385–94.

Lock, Margaret M. *Encounters with Aging: Mythologies of Menopause in Japan and North America.* Berkeley: University of California Press, 1995.

———. "Protests of a Good Wife and Wise Mother: The Medicalization of Distress in Japan." In *Health, Illness, and Medical Care in Japan: Cultural and Social Dimensions,* edited by Edward Norbeck and Margaret Lock, pp. 130–57. Honolulu: University of Hawaii Press, 1987.

Lockett, Gloria. "CAL-PEP: The Struggle to Survive." In *Women Resisting AIDS: Feminist Strategies of Empowerment,* edited by Beth Schneider and Nancy E. Stoller, pp. 208–18. Philadelphia: Temple University Press, 1995.

Long, R., M. Scalcini, J. Manfreda, G. Carre, E. Philippe, E. Hershfield, L. Sekla, and W. Stackiw. "Impact of Human Immunodeficiency Virus Type 1 on Tuberculosis in Rural Haiti." *American Review of Respiratory Disease* 143, no. 1 (1991): 69–73.

Lorch, Donatella. "F.D.A. Policy to Limit Blood Is Protested." *New York Times,* April 21, 1990.

Lowenthal, I. "Labor, Sexuality, and the Conjugal Contract in Rural Haiti." In *Haiti— Today and Tomorrow: An Interdisciplinary Study,* edited by Charles Robert Foster and Albert Valdman, pp. 15–33. Lanham, Md.: University Press of America, 1984.

Lucas, S. "Maternal Death, Autopsy Studies, and Lessons from Pathology." *PLoS Medicine* 5, no. 2 (2008): e48.

Lucas, S. B., A. Hounnou, C. Peacock, A. Beaumel, and G. Djomand. "The Mortality and Pathology of HIV Infection in a West African City." *AIDS* 7, no. 12 (1993): 1569–79.

Lundahl, Mats. *The Haitian Economy: Man, Land, and Markets.* London: Croom, 1987.

Lurie, M., A. Harrison, D. Wilkinson, and S. Abdool Karim. "Circular Migration and Sexual Networking in Rural Kwazulu/Natal: Implications for the Spread of HIV and Other Sexually Transmitted Diseases." *Health Transition Review* 7, no. 3 (1997): 17–27.

Lurie, P., P. Hintzen, and R. A. Lowe. "Socioeconomic Obstacles to HIV Prevention and Treatment in Developing Countries: The Roles of the International Monetary Fund and the World Bank." *AIDS* 9, no. 6 (1995): 539–46.

Lurie, P., and S. M. Wolfe. "Unethical Trials of Interventions to Reduce Perinatal Transmission of the Human Immunodeficiency Virus in Developing Countries." *New England Journal of Medicine* 337, no. 12 (1997): 853–56.

MacArthur, John R. *Second Front: Censorship and Propaganda in the 1991 Gulf War.* Berkeley: University of California Press, 2004.

MacKenzie, William R., Neil J. Hoxie, Mary E. Proctor, M. Stephen Gradus, Kathleen A. Blair, Dan E. Peterson, James J. Kazmierczak, David G. Addiss, Kim R. Fox, Joan B. Rose, et al. "A Massive Outbreak in Milwaukee of Cryptosporidium Infection Transmitted through the Public Water Supply." *New England Journal of Medicine* 331, no. 3 (1994): 161–67.

Macklin, Ruth. *Against Relativism: Cultural Diversity and the Search for Ethical Universals in Medicine.* New York: Oxford University Press, 1999.

Mahmoudi, Artin, and Michael D. Iseman. "Pitfalls in the Care of Patients with Tuberculosis: Common Errors and Their Association with the Acquisition of Drug Resistance." *Journal of the American Medical Association* 270, no. 1 (1993): 65–68.

Mamdani, Mahmood. *When Victims Become Killers: Colonialism, Nativism, and the Genocide in Rwanda.* Princeton, N.J.: Princeton University Press, 2001.

Mann, Jonathan M. "AIDS and Human Rights: Where Do We Go from Here?" *Health and Human Rights* 3, no. 1 (1998): 143–49.

———. "Global AIDS: Critical Issues for Prevention in the 1990s." *International Journal of Health Services* 21, no. 3 (1991): 553–59.

Mann, Jonathan M., Sofia Gruskin, Michael A. Grodin, and George J. Annas. *Health and Human Rights: A Reader.* New York: Routledge, 1999.

Mann, Jonathan M., and Daniel Tarantola, eds. *AIDS in the World II: Global Dimensions, Social Roots, and Responses.* New York: Oxford University Press, 1996.

———. "Responding to HIV/AIDS: A Historical Perspective." *Health and Human Rights* 2, no. 4 (1998): 5–8.

Mann, Jonathan M., Daniel Tarantola, and Thomas W. Netter, eds. *AIDS in the World: The Global AIDS Policy Coalition.* Cambridge, Mass.: Harvard University Press, 1992.

Manz, Beatriz. *Paradise in Ashes: A Guatemalan Journey of Courage, Terror, and Hope.* Berkeley: University of California Press, 2004.

Marcus, George E., and Michael M. J. Fischer. *Anthropology as Cultural Critique: An Experimental Moment in the Human Sciences.* Chicago: University of Chicago Press, 1986.

Margalit, Avishai. *The Ethics of Memory*. Cambridge, Mass.: Harvard University Press, 2002.

Margono, F., A. Garely, J. Mroueh, and H. Minkoff. "Tuberculosis among Pregnant Women—New York City, 1985–1992." *Morbidity and Mortality Weekly Report* 42, no. 31 (1993): 605, 611–12.

Marmot, Michael G. "Social Causes for Social Inequalities in Health." In *Public Health, Ethics, and Equity,* edited by Sudhir Anand, Fabienne Peter, and Amartya Kumar Sen, pp. 37–62. New York: Oxford University Press, 2004.

———. "Social Differentials in Health within and between Populations." *Daedalus* 123, no. 4 (1994): 197–216.

Marseille, E., P. B. Hofmann, and J. G. Kahn. "HIV Prevention before HAART in Sub-Saharan Africa." *Lancet* 359, no. 9320 (2002): 1851–56.

Marsella, Anthony J. "Thoughts on Cross-Cultural Studies on the Epidemiology of Depression." *Culture, Medicine, and Psychiatry* 2, no. 4 (1978): 343–57.

Martin, Emily. *The Woman in the Body: A Cultural Analysis of Reproduction*. Boston: Beacon, 1987.

Mason, Alpheus Thomas. *Harlan Fiske Stone: Pillar of the Law*. New York: Viking, 1956.

Massing, Michael. *Now They Tell Us: The American Press and Iraq*. New York: New York Review of Books, 2004.

Mata, J. I. "Integrating the Client's Perspective in Planning a Tuberculosis Education and Treatment Program in Honduras." *Medical Anthropology* 9, no. 1 (1985): 57–64.

Mathai, R., P. V. Prasad, M. Jacob, P. G. Babu, and T. J. John. "HIV Seropositivity among Patients with Sexually Transmitted Diseases in Vellore." *Indian Journal of Medical Research* 91 (1990): 239–41.

Mayaud, Philippe, Sarah Hawkes, and David Mabey. "Advances in Control of Sexually Transmitted Diseases in Developing Countries." *Lancet* 351 Suppl. 3 (1998): 29–32.

Mbewu, Anthony. "Antiretroviral Therapy Is Only Part of It." *Bulletin of the World Health Organization* 79, no. 12 (2001): 1152.

McBarnett, L. "Women and Poverty: The Effects on Reproductive Status." In *Too Little, Too Late: Dealing with the Health Needs of Women in Poverty,* edited by Cesar A. Perales and Lauren S. Young, pp. 55–81. New York: Harrington Park Press, 1988.

McBride, David. *From TB to AIDS: Epidemics among Urban Blacks since 1900*. Albany: SUNY Press, 1991.

McCarthy, Susan A., R. Merrill McPhearson, Anthony M. Guarino, and Jack L. Gaines. "Toxigenic Vibrio Cholerae O1 and Cargo Ships Entering Gulf of Mexico." *Lancet* 339, no. 8793 (1992): 624–25.

McConnochie, Kenneth M., Mark J. Russo, John T. McBride, Peter G. Szilagyi, Ann-Marie Brooks, and Klaus J. Roghmann. "Socioeconomic Variation in Asthma Hospitalization: Excess Utilization or Greater Need?" *Pediatrics* 103, no. 6 (1999): e75.

McCord, C., and H. P. Freeman. "Excess Mortality in Harlem." *New England Journal of Medicine* 322, no. 3 (1990): 173–77.

McKenna, Matthew T., Eugene McCray, and Ida Onorato. "The Epidemiology of Tuberculosis among Foreign-Born Persons in the United States, 1986 to 1993." *New England Journal of Medicine* 332, no. 16 (1995): 1071–76.

McKeown, Thomas, and R.G. Record. "Reasons for the Decline of Mortality in England and Wales during the Nineteenth Century." *Population Studies* 16, no. 2 (1962): 94–122.

McMichael, Anthony J. "The Health of Persons, Populations, and Planets: Epidemiology Comes Full Circle." *Epidemiology* 6, no. 6 (1995): 633–36.

Médecins Sans Frontières. "MSF Ends Tuberculosis Treatment in Kemerovo Region, Russia." Press release, September 30, 2003. www.msf.org/msfinternational/invoke.cfm ?component=pressrelease&objectid=D657393B-C8E6-4CD7-9835259FD4F8AFEF &method=full_html (accessed July 14, 2009).

Meguid, Tarek. *The Challenge of the Periphery.* Capetown, South Africa: HARPS Publishers, 2001.

Meja, Volker, and Nico Stehr, eds. *Knowledge and Politics: The Sociology of Knowledge Dispute.* London: Routledge, 1990.

——, eds. *The Sociology of Knowledge.* 2 vols. Cheltenham: Elgar, 1999.

Mellors, J.W., and M. Barry. "Malnutrition or AIDS in Haiti?" *New England Journal of Medicine* 310, no. 17 (1984): 1119–20.

Menendez, C., C. Romagosa, M.R. Ismail, C. Carrilho, F. Saute, N. Osman, F. Machungo, A. Bardaji, L. Quinto, A. Mayor, et al. "An Autopsy Study of Maternal Mortality in Mozambique: The Contribution of Infectious Diseases." *PLoS Medicine* 5, no. 2 (2008): e44.

Menzies, R., I. Rocher, and B. Vissandjee. "Factors Associated with Compliance in Treatment of Tuberculosis." *Tubercle and Lung Disease* 74, no. 1 (1993): 32–37.

Meredith, Martin. *The Fate of Africa: From the Hopes of Freedom to the Heart of Despair— A History of Fifty Years of Independence.* New York: Public Affairs, 2005.

Merino, N., R.L. Sanchez, A. Muñoz, G. Prada, C.F. Garcia, and B.F. Polk. "HIV-1, Sexual Practices, and Contact with Foreigners in Homosexual Men in Colombia, South America." *JAIDS: Journal of Acquired Immune Deficiency Syndromes* 3, no. 4 (1990): 330–34.

Merleau-Ponty, Maurice. *Phénoménologie de la perception.* Paris: Gallimard, 1945.

Merton, Robert K. "The Unanticipated Consequences of Purposive Social Action." *American Sociological Review* 1, no. 6 (December 1936): 894–904.

Métellus, Jean. *Haïti: Une nation pathétique.* Paris: Denoël, 1987.

Métraux, Alfred. "Médecine et vodou en Haïti." *Acta Tropica* 10, no. 1 (1953): 28–68.

——. *Voodoo in Haiti.* Translated by Hugo Charteris. New York: Schocken Books, 1972.

Michael, J.M., and M.A. Michael. "Health Status of the Australian Aboriginal People and the Native Americans—A Summary Comparison." *Asia-Pacific Journal of Public Health* 7, no. 2 (1994): 132–36.

Michaels, Jim. "Behind Success in Ramadi: An Army Colonel's Gamble." *USA Today,* May 1, 2007, p. A1.

Millen, Joyce V., and Timothy H. Holtz. "Dying for Growth, Part I: Transnational Corporations and the Health of the Poor." In *Dying for Growth: Global Inequality and the Health of the Poor,* edited by Jim Yong Kim, Joyce V. Millen, Alec Irwin, and John Gershman, pp. 177–223. Monroe, Maine: Common Courage Press, 2000.

Miller, J. "'Your Life Is on the Line Every Night You're on the Streets': Victimization and Resistance among Street Prostitutes." *Humanity and Society* 17 (1993): 422–46.

Mintz, Sidney Wilfred. "The Caribbean Region." In *Slavery, Colonialism, and Racism: Essays,* edited by Sidney Wilfred Mintz, pp. 45–71. New York: Norton, 1974.

———. *Caribbean Transformations.* New York: Columbia University Press, 1989.

———. "Introduction." In *Voodoo in Haiti,* by Alfred Métraux, pp. 1–14. New York: Schocken Books, 1972.

———. "The Localization of Anthropological Practice: From Area Studies to Transnationalism." *Critique of Anthropology* 18, no. 2 (1998): 117–33.

———. "The So-Called World System: Local Initiative and Local Response." *Dialectical Anthropology* 2, no. 1 (1977): 253–70.

———. *Sweetness and Power: The Place of Sugar in Modern History.* New York: Viking, 1985.

Mitchell, J. L., J. Tucker, P. O. Loftman, and S. B. Williams. "HIV and Women: Current Controversies and Clinical Relevance." *Journal of Women's Health* 1, no. 1 (1992): 35–39.

Mitnick, C., J. Bayona, E. Palacios, S. Shin, J. Furin, F. Alcantara, E. Sanchez, M. Sarria, M. Becerra, M. C. Smith Fawzi, S. Kapiga, J. Y. Kim, P. E. Farmer, et al. "Community-Based Therapy for Multidrug-Resistant Tuberculosis in Lima, Peru." *New England Journal of Medicine* 348, no. 2 (2003): 119–28.

Mitty, Jennifer A., Grace E. Macalino, Lauri B. Bazerman, Helen G. Loewenthal, Joseph W. Hogan, Cynthia J. MacLeod, and Timothy P. Flanigan. "The Use of Community-Based Modified Directly Observed Therapy for the Treatment of HIV-Infected Persons." *JAIDS: Journal of Acquired Immune Deficiency Syndromes* 39, no. 5 (2005): 545–50.

Montesquiou, Alfred de. "Missionaries, Schoolkids, and Bystanders—No One Is Safe from Haiti's Kidnappers." Associated Press, December 26, 2005.

Moore, Alexander, and Ronald LeBaron. "The Case for a Haitian Origin of the AIDS Epidemic." In *The Social Dimensions of AIDS: Method and Theory,* edited by Douglas A. Feldman and Thomas M. Johnson, pp. 77–93. New York: Praeger, 1986.

Moore, Richard D., David Stanton, Ramana Gopalan, and Richard E. Chaisson. "Racial Differences in the Use of Drug Therapy for HIV Disease in an Urban Community." *New England Journal of Medicine* 330, no. 11 (1994): 763–68.

Moore, Sally Falk. "Explaining the Present: Theoretical Dilemmas in Processual Ethnography." *American Ethnologist* 14, no. 4 (1987): 727–36.

Moreau de Saint-Méry, Médéric Louis Élie. *Description topographique, physique, civile, politique et historique de la partie française de l'isle Saint-Domingue ... à l'époque du 18 Octobre 1789. . . .* Saint-Denis, France: Société française d'histoire d'outre-mer, 2004. Originally published in 1797.

Morse, S. S. "Factors in the Emergence of Infectious Diseases." *Emerging Infectious Diseases* 1, no. 1 (1995): 7–15.

Moses, Peter, and John Moses. "Haiti and the Acquired Immune Deficiency Syndrome." *Annals of Internal Medicine* 99, no. 4 (1983): 565.

Moyo, Dambisa. *Dead Aid: Why Aid Is Not Working and How There Is a Better Way for Africa.* New York: Farrar, Straus and Giroux, 2009.

Muir, D. G., and M. A. Belsey. "Pelvic Inflammatory Disease and Its Consequences in the Developing World." *American Journal of Obstetrics and Gynecology* 138, no. 7, pt. 2 (1980): 913–28.

Mukherjee, Joia S. "HIV-1 Care in Resource-Poor Settings: A View from Haiti." *Lancet* 362, no. 9388 (2003): 994–95.

———, ed. *The PIH Guide to the Community-Based Treatment of HIV in Resource-Poor Settings.* 2nd ed. Boston: Partners In Health, 2008.

Mukherjee, Joia S., Margaly Colas, Paul E. Farmer, Fernet Léandre, Wesler Lambert, Maxi Raymonville, Serena Koenig, David Walton, Patrice Nevil, Nirlande Louissant, et al. *Access to Antiretroviral Treatment and Care: Experience of the HIV Equity Initiative, Cange, Haiti: Case Study.* Geneva: World Health Organization, 2003.

Muldoon, Mark. *Tricks of Time: Bergson, Merleau-Ponty, and Ricoeur in Search of Time, Self, and Meaning.* Pittsburgh: Duquesne University Press, 2006.

Murphy, E. L., J. P. Figueroa, W. N. Gibbs, A. Brathwaite, M. Holding-Cobham, D. Waters, B. Cranston, B. Hanchard, and W. A. Blattner. "Sexual Transmission of Human T-Lymphotropic Virus Type I (HTLV-I)." *Annals of Internal Medicine* 111, no. 7 (1989): 555–60.

Murray, Christopher J. L. "Social, Economic, and Operational Research on Tuberculosis: Recent Studies and Some Priority Questions." *Bulletin of the International Union against Tuberculosis and Lung Disease* 66, no. 4 (1991): 149–56.

Murray, Christopher J. L., and Alan D. Lopez, eds. *The Global Burden of Disease: A Comprehensive Assessment of Mortality and Disability from Diseases, Injuries, and Risk Factors in 1990 and Projected to 2020; Summary.* On behalf of the World Health Organization and the World Bank. Cambridge, Mass.: Harvard School of Public Health, 1996.

Murray, Christopher J. L., Karel Styblo, and Annik Rouillon. "Tuberculosis in Developing Countries: Burden, Intervention, and Cost." *Bulletin of the International Union against Tuberculosis and Lung Disease* 65, no. 1 (1990): 6–24.

Murray, Gerald. "Women in Perdition: Ritual Fertility Control in Haiti." In *Culture, Natality, and Family Planning,* edited by John F. Marshall and Steven Polgar, pp. 59–78. Chapel Hill: Carolina Population Center, University of North Carolina, 1976.

Murray, Stephen O. "A Note on Haitian Tolerance of Homosexuality." In *Male Homosexuality in Central and South America,* edited by Stephen O. Murray, pp. 92–100. San Francisco: Instituto Obregón, 1987.

Murray, Stephen O., and Kenneth Payne. "Medical Policy without Scientific Evidence: The Promiscuity Paradigm and AIDS." *California Sociologist* 11, no. 1–2 (1988): 13–54.

Mushikiwabo, Louise, and Jack Kramer. *Rwanda Means the Universe: A Native's Memoir of Blood and Bloodlines.* New York: St. Martin's Press, 2006.

Nachman, Steven R. "Wasted Lives: Tuberculosis and Other Health Risks of Being Haitian in a U.S. Detention Camp." *Medical Anthropology Quarterly* 7, no. 3 (1993): 227–59.

Nachman, Steven R., and Ginette Dreyfuss. "Haitians and AIDS in South Florida." *Medical Anthropology Quarterly* 17, no. 2 (1986): 32–33.

Naik, T. N., S. Sarkar, H. L. Singh, S. C. Bhunia, Y. I. Singh, P. K. Singh, and S. C. Pal. "Intravenous Drug Users—A New High-Risk Group for HIV Infection in India." *AIDS* 5, no. 1 (1991): 117–18.

Nairn, Allan. "Behind Haiti's Paramilitaries." *Nation* 259, no. 13 (1994): 458–61.

———. "The Eagle Is Landing." *Nation* 259, no. 10 (1994): 344–48.

Nardell, E. A. "Beyond Four Drugs: Public Health Policy and the Treatment of the Individual Patient with Tuberculosis." *American Review of Respiratory Disease* 148, no. 1 (1993): 2–5.

Nataraj, Shyamala. "Indian Prostitutes Highlight AIDS Dilemmas." *Development Forum* 18 (November–December 1990): 1–16.

National Center for Health Statistics. "Annual Summary of Births, Marriages, Divorces, and Deaths: United States, 1993." *Monthly Vital Statistics Report* 42, no. 13, October 11, 1994. Hyattsville, Md.: Centers for Disease Control and Prevention, Public Health Service. www.cdc.gov/nchs/data/mvsr/supp/mv42_13acc.pdf (accessed September 14, 2009).

———. *Health, United States, 1998, with Socioeconomic Status and Health Chartbook.* Hyattsville, Md.: Centers for Disease Control and Prevention, National Center for Health Statistics, 1998. www.cdc.gov/nchs/data/hus/hus98.pdf (accessed July 14, 2009).

———. *Health, United States, 2000, with Adolescent Health Chartbook.* Hyattsville, Md.: Centers for Disease Control and Prevention, National Center for Health Statistics, 2000. www.cdc.gov/nchs/data/hus/hus00.pdf (accessed September 14, 2009).

National Center for Infectious Diseases. *Addressing Emerging Infectious Disease Threats: A Prevention Strategy for the United States.* Atlanta: Centers for Disease Control and Prevention, 1994.

National Priorities Project. "Bringing the Federal Budget Home: Costs of War." www.nationalpriorities.org/costofwar_home (accessed July 14, 2009).

National Research Council, Panel on Monitoring the Social Impact of the AIDS Epidemic. *The Social Impact of AIDS in the United States.* Edited by Albert R. Jonsen and Jeff Stryker. Washington, D.C.: National Academies Press, 1993.

Nations, M. "Epidemiological Research on Infectious Disease: Quantitative Rigor or Rigor Mortis? Insights from Ethnomedicine." In *Anthropology and Epidemiology: Interdisciplinary Approaches to the Study of Health and Diseases,* edited by Craig R. Janes, Ron Stall, and Sandra M. Gifford, pp. 97–124. Dordrecht: Reidel, 1986.

Navarro, Vicente. "Race or Class versus Race and Class: Mortality Differentials in the United States." *Lancet* 336, no. 8725 (1990): 1238–40.

Neier, Aryeh. *War Crimes: Brutality, Genocide, Terror, and the Struggle for Justice.* New York: Times Books, 1998.

———. "What Should Be Done about the Guilty?" *New York Review of Books* 37, no. 1 (1990): 32–35.

Nelson-Pallmeyer, Jack. *Brave New World Order: Must We Pledge Allegiance?* Maryknoll, N.Y.: Orbis Books, 1992.

Neptune-Anglade, Mireille. *L'autre moitié du développement: À propos du travail des femmes en Haïti.* Montreal: Éditions des Alizés—ERCE, 1986.

Neu, Harold C. "The Crisis in Antibiotic Resistance." *Science* 257, no. 5073 (1992): 1064–73.

Neuffer, Elizabeth. *The Key to My Neighbor's House: Seeking Justice in Bosnia and Rwanda.* New York: Picador, 2001.

Neugebauer, R. "Research on Violence in Developing Countries: Benefits and Perils." *American Journal of Public Health* 89, no. 10 (1999): 1473–74.

Newbury, Catharine. *The Cohesion of Oppression: Clientship and Ethnicity in Rwanda, 1860–1960*. New York: Columbia University Press, 1988.

Newsholme, A. "The Present Position of the Tuberculosis Problem." *Proceedings of the Institute of Medicine of Chicago* 35, no. 3 (1982): 102–4.

Nguyen, Vinh-Kim. "The Shape of Things to Come? Give Drugs to Africa and Help Rebuild Its Health Care, Says a Canadian Doctor, Because We're All at Risk." *Globe and Mail,* July 11, 2000, p. A15.

Nguyen, Vinh-Kim, and Karine Peschard. "Anthropology, Inequality, and Disease: A Review." *Review of Anthropology* 32 (2003): 447–74.

Nightingale, E. O., K. Hannibal, H. J. Geiger, L. Hartmann, R. Lawrence, and J. Spurlock. "Apartheid Medicine: Health and Human Rights in South Africa." *Journal of the American Medical Association* 264, no. 16 (1990): 2097–2102.

Norbeck, Edward, and Margaret Lock, eds. *Health, Illness, and Medical Care in Japan: Cultural and Social Dimensions*. Honolulu: University of Hawaii Press, 1987.

Nordstrom, Carolyn. *Global Outlaws: Crime, Money, and Power in the Contemporary World*. Berkeley: University of California Press, 2007.

———. *Shadows of War: Violence, Power, and International Profiteering in the Twenty-First Century*. Berkeley: University of California Press, 2004.

———. "The Tomorrow of Violence." In *Violence*, edited by Neil L. Whitehead, pp. 223–42. Santa Fe: School of American Research Press, 2004.

Nyamathi, A., C. Bennett, B. Leake, C. Lewis, and J. Flaskerud. "AIDS-Related Knowledge, Perceptions, and Behaviors among Impoverished Minority Women." *American Journal of Public Health* 83, no. 1 (1993): 65–71.

Nyhan, David. "Murder in Haiti." *Boston Globe,* March 19, 1992.

Obeyesekere, Gananath. "Depression, Buddhism, and the Work of Culture in Sri Lanka." In *Culture and Depression: Studies in the Anthropology and Cross-Cultural Psychiatry of Affect and Disorder,* edited by Arthur Kleinman and Byron Good, pp. 134–52. Berkeley: University of California Press, 1985.

Obiora, L. Amede. "Bridges and Barricades: Rethinking Polemics and Intransigence in the Campaign against Female Circumcision." *Case Western Reserve Law Review* 47, no. 2 (1997): 275–379.

Odinkalu, Chidi Anselm. "Why More Africans Don't Use Human Rights Language." *Human Rights Dialogue* 2, no. 1 (1999): 3–4. www.cceia.org/resources/publications/dialogue/2_01/articles/602.html (accessed October 10, 2009).

Oldstone, Michael B. A. *Viruses, Plagues, and History.* New York: Oxford University Press, 1998.

Olliaro, P., J. Cattani, and D. Wirth. "Malaria, the Submerged Disease." *Journal of the American Medical Association* 275, no. 3 (1996): 230–33.

O'Neill, William G. "The Roots of Human Rights Violations in Haiti." *Georgetown Immigration Law Journal* 7, no. 1 (1993): 87–117.

Onoge, O. "Capitalism and Public Health: A Neglected Theme in the Medical Anthropology of Africa." In *Topias and Utopias in Health: Policy Studies,* edited by Stanley R. Ingman and Anthony E. Thomas, pp. 219–32. The Hague: Mouton, 1975.

Oppenheimer, Gerald. "In the Eye of the Storm: The Epidemiological Construction of

AIDS." In *AIDS: The Burdens of History,* edited by Elizabeth Fee and Daniel M. Fox, pp. 267–300. Berkeley: University of California Press, 1988.

Orwell, George. *The Collected Essays, Journalism, and Letters of George Orwell.* 4 vols. Edited by Sonia Brownell Orwell and Ian Angus. New York: Harcourt Brace Jovanovich, 1968.

Osborn, June E. "Public Health and the Politics of AIDS Prevention." *Daedalus* 118, no. 3 (1989): 123–44.

Osmond, D.H., K. Page, J. Wiley, K. Garrett, H.W. Sheppard, A.R. Moss, L. Schrager, and W. Winkelstein. "HIV Infection in Homosexual and Bisexual Men 18 to 29 Years of Age: The San Francisco Young Men's Health Study." *American Journal of Public Health* 84, no. 12 (1994): 1933–37.

Oster, Emily. "Treating HIV Doesn't Pay." *Forbes* 176, no. 2 (2005): 44.

Osterberg, Lars, and Terrence Blaschke. "Adherence to Medication." *New England Journal of Medicine* 353, no. 5 (2005): 487–97.

Ott, Katherine. *Fevered Lives: Tuberculosis in American Culture since 1870.* Cambridge, Mass.: Harvard University Press, 1996.

Paavonen, J., L. Koutsky, and N. Kiviat. "Cervical Neoplasia and Other STD-Related Genital and Anal Neoplasias." In *Sexually Transmitted Diseases,* edited by King K. Holmes, pp. 561–62. New York: McGraw-Hill, 1990.

Pablos-Méndez, A., M.C. Raviglione, A. Laszlo, N. Binkin, H.L. Rieder, F. Bustreo, D.L. Cohn, C.S. Lambregts-van Weezenbeek, S.J. Kim, P. Chaulet, and P. Nunn. "Global Surveillance for Anti-Tuberculosis Drug Resistance, 1994–1997; World Health Organization–International Union against Tuberculosis and Lung Disease Working Group on Anti-Tuberculosis Drug Resistance Surveillance." *New England Journal of Medicine* 338, no. 23 (1998): 1641–49. [Erratum published in *New England Journal of Medicine* 339, no. 2 (1998): 139a.]

Packard, Randall M. *White Plague, Black Labor: Tuberculosis and the Political Economy of Health and Disease in South Africa.* Berkeley: University of California Press, 1989.

Packard, Randall M., and Paul Epstein. "Epidemiologists, Social Scientists, and the Structure of Medical Research on AIDS in Africa." *Social Science and Medicine* 33, no. 7 (1991): 771–83; discussion 783–94.

Pan American Health Organization. "Country Health Profile: Haiti, 2001." www.paho.org/English/SHA/prflHAI.htm (accessed July 6, 2009).

———. "The Haiti Crisis: Health Risks." 2004. www.paho.org/english/dd/ped/HaitiHealthImpact.htm (accessed July 14, 2009).

———. *Reported Cases of Notifiable Diseases in the Americas.* Washington, D.C.: Pan American Health Organization, 1967.

Pape, Jean W. "Tuberculosis and HIV in the Caribbean: Approaches to Diagnosis, Treatment, and Prophylaxis." *Topics in HIV Medicine* 12, no. 5 (2004): 144–49.

Pape, Jean W., and Warren D. Johnson Jr. "AIDS in Haiti: 1982–1992." *Clinical Infectious Diseases* 17 Suppl. 2 (1993): S341–S345.

———. "Epidemiology of AIDS in the Caribbean." In *AIDS and HIV Infection in the Tropics (Baillière's Clinical Tropical Medicine and Communicable Diseases),* edited by Peter Piot and Jonathan M. Mann, pp. 31–42. London: Baillière Tindall, 1988.

Pape, J. W., B. Liautaud, F. Thomas, J. R. Mathurin, M. M. St. Amand, M. Boncy, V. Péan, M. Pamphile, A. C. Laroche, and J. Dehovitz. "The Acquired Immunodeficiency Syndrome in Haiti." *Annals of Internal Medicine* 103, no. 5 (1985): 674–78.

Pape, J. W., B. Liautaud, F. Thomas, J. R. Mathurin, M. M. St Amand, M. Boncy, V. Péan, M. Pamphile, A. C. Laroche, and W. D. Johnson Jr. "Characteristics of the Acquired Immunodeficiency Syndrome (AIDS) in Haiti." *New England Journal of Medicine* 309, no. 16 (1983): 945–50.

———. "Risk Factors Associated with AIDS in Haiti." *American Journal of the Medical Sciences* 291, no. 1 (1986): 4–7.

Patel, Mahesh S. "Problems in the Evaluation of Alternative Medicine." *Social Science and Medicine* 25, no. 6 (1987): 669–78.

Paton, N. I., S. Sangeetha, A. Earnest, and R. Bellamy. "The Impact of Malnutrition on Survival and the CD4 Count Response in HIV-Infected Patients Starting Antiretroviral Therapy." *HIV Medicine* 7, no. 5 (2006): 323–30.

Patterson, Orlando. *Slavery and Social Death: A Comparative Study.* Cambridge, Mass.: Harvard University Press, 1982.

Patz, J. A., P. R. Epstein, T. A. Burke, and J. M. Balbus. "Global Climate Change and Emerging Infectious Diseases." *Journal of the American Medical Association* 275, no. 3 (1996): 217–23.

Paul, Emmanuel. "La première enfance: Maternité et techniques populaires." *Bulletin du Bureau d'Ethnologie* 4, no. 31 (1965): 19–63.

Pax Christi International. *Pax Christi Newsletter* 13, 1992.

Peter, Fabienne. "Health Equity and Social Justice." In *Public Health, Ethics, and Equity,* edited by Sudhir Anand, Fabienne Peter, and Amartya Kumar Sen, pp. 93–106. New York: Oxford University Press, 2004.

Pfeifer, Sylvia. "Public-Private Partnership Attacks Tuberculosis—Aim Is to Spur Development of New Drugs." *Chicago Tribune,* October 20, 2000, p. 7.

Philippe, Jeanne, and Jean Baptiste Romain. "Indisposition in Haiti." *Social Science and Medicine. Part B: Medical Anthropology* 13, no. 2 (1979): 129–33.

Physicians for Human Rights. *An Action Plan to Prevent Brain Drain: Building Equitable Health Systems in Africa.* July 1, 2004. http://physiciansforhumanrights.org/library/report-2004-july.html (accessed July 14, 2009).

———. *Deadly Delays: Maternal Mortality in Peru. A Rights-Based Approach to Safe Motherhood.* http://physiciansforhumanrights.org/library/report-2007-11-28.html (accessed July 14, 2009).

———. "Health Action AIDS Campaign." http://physiciansforhumanrights.org/hiv-aids (accessed July 14, 2009).

———. *Health Care Held Hostage: Human Rights Violations and Violations of Medical Neutrality in Chiapas, Mexico.* Report submitted by Alicia Ely Yamin, Victor B. Penchaszadeh, and Thomas S. Crane. Boston: Physicians for Human Rights, 1999.

Pitts, Byron. "Dr. Farmer's Remedy for Global Health." *60 Minutes,* CBS, May 4, 2008. www.cbsnews.com/stories/2008/05/01/60minutes/main4063191.shtml (accessed October 9, 2009).

Pivnick, Anitra. "HIV Infection and the Meaning of Condoms." *Culture, Medicine, and Psychiatry* 17, no. 4 (1993): 431–53.

———. "Loss and Regeneration: Influences on the Reproductive Decisions of HIV Positive, Drug-Using Women." *Medical Anthropology* 16, no. 1 (1994): 39–62.

Pivnick, Anitra, Audrey Jacobson, Kathleen Eric, Lynda Doll, and Ernest Drucker. "AIDS, HIV Infection, and Illicit Drug Use within Inner-City Families and Social Networks." *American Journal of Public Health* 84, no. 2 (1994): 271–74.

Pivnick, Anitra, Audrey Jacobson, Kathleen Eric, Michael Mulvihill, Ming Ann Hsu, and Ernest Drucker. "Reproductive Decisions among HIV-Infected, Drug-Using Women: The Importance of Mother-Child Coresidence." *Medical Anthropology Quarterly* 5, no. 2 (1991): 153–69.

Pogge, Thomas. "'Assisting' the Global Poor." In *The Ethics of Assistance: Morality and the Distant Needy,* edited by Deen K. Chatterjee, pp. 260–88. Cambridge: Cambridge University Press, 2004.

Poinsignon, Y., Z. Marjanovic, and D. Farge. "Maladies infectieuses nouvelles et résurgentes liées à la pauvreté." *Revue du Praticien* 46, no. 15 (1996): 1827–38.

Polakow, Valerie. "Lives of Welfare Mothers: On a Tightrope without a Net." *Nation* 260, no. 17 (1995): 590–92.

———. *Lives on the Edge: Single Mothers and Their Children in the Other America.* Chicago: University of Chicago Press, 1993.

Pollak, Michael. *Les homosexuels et le SIDA: Sociologie d'une épidémie.* Paris: A.M. Métailié, 1988.

Porter, J.D., and K.P. McAdam. "The Re-Emergence of Tuberculosis." *Annual Review of Public Health* 15 (1994): 303–23.

Pottier, Johan. *Re-Imagining Rwanda: Conflict, Survival, and Disinformation in the Late Twentieth Century.* Cambridge: Cambridge University Press, 2002.

Powell, Cathy. "'Life' at Guantánamo: The Wrongful Detention of Haitian Refugees." *Reconstruction* 2, no. 2 (1993): 58–68

Preston, Richard. *The Hot Zone.* New York: Random House, 1994.

Price, Laurie. "Ecuadorian Illness Stories: Cultural Knowledge in Natural Discourse." In *Cultural Models in Language and Thought,* edited by Dorothy C. Holland and Naomi Quinn, pp. 313–42. Cambridge: Cambridge University Press, 1987.

Price-Mars, Jean. *La République d'Haïti et la République Dominicaine; les aspects divers d'un problème d'histoire, de géographie et d'ethnologie, depuis les origines du peuplement de l'île antiléenne en 1492, jusqu'à l'évolution des deux états qui en partagent la souveraineté en 1953.* Port-au-Prince: Collection du Tricinquantenaire de l'Indépendance d'Haïti, 1953.

Prime Minister's Office, United Kingdom. "Prime Minister's Official Spokesperson Morning Briefing: Iraq." October 29, 2004. www.number10.gov.uk/Page6496 (accessed July 14, 2009).

Prince, Rod. *Haiti: Family Business.* Latin America Bureau Special Brief. London: Latin America Bureau, 1985.

Prunier, Gérard. *The Rwanda Crisis: History of a Genocide.* New York: Columbia University Press, 1997.

Quigley, Fran. *Walking Together, Walking Far: How a U.S. and African Medical School Partnership Is Winning the Fight against HIV/AIDS*. Foreword by Paul Farmer. Bloomington: Indiana University Press, 2009.

Quinn, Naomi, and Dorothy Holland. "Culture and Cognition." In *Cultural Models in Language and Thought*, edited by Dorothy C. Holland and Naomi Quinn, pp. 3–42. Cambridge: Cambridge University Press, 1987.

Quinn, T.C., M.J. Wawer, N. Sewankambo, D. Serwadda, C. Li, F. Wabwire-Mangen, M.O. Meehan, T. Lutalo, and R.H. Gray. "Viral Load and Heterosexual Transmission of Human Immunodeficiency Virus Type 1: Rakai Project Study Group." *New England Journal of Medicine* 342, no. 13 (2000): 921–29.

Racine, Marie M.B., and Kathy Ogle. *Like the Dew That Waters the Grass: Words from Haitian Women*. Washington, D.C.: Ecumenical Program on Central America and the Caribbean (EPICA), 1999.

Rajaduraipandi, K., K. Mani, K. Panneerselvam, M. Mani, M. Bhaskar, and P. Manikandan. "Prevalence and Antimicrobial Susceptibility Pattern of Methicillin Resistant Staphylococcus Aureus: A Multicentre Study." *Indian Journal of Medical Microbiology* 24, no. 1 (2006): 34–38.

Ramachandran, P., and R. Prabhakar. "Defaults, Defaulter Action, and Retrieval of Patients during Studies on Tuberculous Meningitis in Children." *Tubercle and Lung Disease* 73, no. 3 (1992): 170–73.

Raviola, Giuseppe, M'Imunya Machoki, Esther Mwaikambo, and Mary-Jo DelVecchio Good. "HIV, Disease Plague, Demoralization and 'Burnout': Resident Experience of the Medical Profession in Nairobi, Kenya." *Culture, Medicine, and Psychiatry* 26, no. 1 (2002): 55–86.

Rawls, John. *A Theory of Justice*. Cambridge, Mass.: Harvard University Press, 1999.

Raymonville, M., F. Léandre, R. Saintard, M. Colas, and M. Louissaint. "Prevention of Mother-to-Child Transmission of HIV in Rural Haiti: The Partners In Health Experience [Poster]." Paper presented at Multicultural Caribbean United against HIV/AIDS conference, Santo Domingo, Dominican Republic, March 5–7, 2004.

Reeves, W.C., W.E. Rawls, and L.A. Brinton. "Epidemiology of Genital Papillomaviruses and Cervical Cancer." *Reviews of Infectious Diseases* 11, no. 3 (1989): 426–39.

Reichman, Lee B. "Tuberculosis Elimination—What's to Stop Us?" *International Journal of Tuberculosis and Lung Disease* 1, no. 1 (1997): 3–11.

Renteln, Alison Dundes. "Relativism and the Search for Human Rights." *American Anthropologist* 90, no. 1 (1988): 56–72.

Republic of South Africa, Department of National Health. *Health Trends in South Africa, 1994*. Pretoria: Department of National Health, 1994.

Reverby, Susan. *Tuskegee's Truths: Rethinking the Tuskegee Syphilis Study*. Chapel Hill: University of North Carolina Press, 2000.

Rey, Terry. "Junta, Rape, and Religion in Haiti." *Journal of Feminist Studies in Religion* 15, no. 2 (1999): 73–100.

Reyes, Hernán, and Rudi Coninx. "Pitfalls of Tuberculosis Programmes in Prisons." *British Medical Journal* 315, no. 7120 (1997): 1447–50.

Ricoeur, Paul. *Time and Narrative*. 3 vols. Translated by Kathleen Blamey and David Pellauer. Chicago: University of Chicago Press, 1984.

Ridgeway, James. *The Haiti Files: Decoding the Crisis*. Washington, D.C.: Essential Books/ Azul Editions, 1994.

Rieder, H. L. "Tuberculosis among American Indians of the Contiguous United States." *Public Health Reports* 104, no. 6 (1989): 653–57.

Rieff, David. "No Exit Strategy." *Nation* 281, no. 4 (2005): 31–36.

Roberts, L., R. Lafta, R. Garfield, J. Khudhairi, and G. Burnham. "Mortality before and after the 2003 Invasion of Iraq: Cluster Sample Survey." *Lancet* 364, no. 9448 (2004): 1857–64.

Robinson, Randall. *An Unbroken Agony: Haiti, from Revolution to the Kidnapping of a President*. New York: Basic Civitas Books, 2007.

Rohde, David. "Musharraf Redraws Constitution, Blocking Prospects for Democracy." *New York Times*, August 22, 2002.

Roizman, Bernard, ed. *Infectious Diseases in an Age of Change: The Impact of Human Ecology and Behavior on Disease Transmission*. National Academy of Sciences. Washington, D.C.: National Academies Press, 1995.

Rosaldo, Michelle Zimbalist, and Louise Lamphere, eds. *Woman, Culture, and Society*. Stanford, Calif.: Stanford University Press, 1974.

Rosaldo, Renato. "From the Door of His Tent: The Fieldworker and the Inquisitor." In *Writing Culture: The Poetics and Politics of Ethnography*, edited by James Clifford and George E. Marcus, pp. 77–97. Berkeley: University of California Press, 1986.

Roseberry, William. "Political Economy." *Annual Review of Anthropology* 17 (1988): 161–85.

———. "The Unbearable Lightness of Anthropology." *Radical History Review* 65 (1996): 5–25.

Rosenkrantz, Barbara Gutmann. "Preface." In *The White Plague: Tuberculosis, Man, and Society*, edited by René J. Dubos and Jean Dubos, pp. xiii–xxxiv. New Brunswick, N.J.: Rutgers University Press, 1992.

Rousseau, Jean-Jacques. *Discourse on the Origin of Inequality*. Translated by Franklin Philip. Edited with an introduction and notes by Patrick Coleman. Oxford: Oxford University Press, 1999. First published in 1755.

Rubel, Arthur J., and Linda C. Garro. "Social and Cultural Factors in the Successful Control of Tuberculosis." *Public Health Reports* 107, no. 6 (1992): 626–36.

Ryan, Frank. *The Forgotten Plague: How the Battle against Tuberculosis Was Won—and Lost*. Boston: Little, Brown, 1993.

Ryan, William. *Blaming the Victim*. New York: Pantheon, 1971.

Rylko-Bauer, Barbara. "Lessons about Humanity and Survival from My Mother and from the Holocaust." *Anthropological Quarterly* 78, no. 1 (2005): 11–41.

Rylko-Bauer, Barbara, and Paul E. Farmer. "Managed Care or Managed Inequality? A Call for Critiques of Market-Based Medicine." *Medical Anthropology Quarterly* 16 (2002): 476–502.

Sabatier, Renée. *Blaming Others: Prejudice, Race, and Worldwide AIDS*. Edited by John Tinker. Washington: Panos Institute, 1988.

Sachs, Jeffrey. *The End of Poverty: Economic Possibilities for Our Time*. New York: Penguin, 2005.

Sadat, Leila Nadya. "Ghost Prisoners and Black Sites: Extraordinary Rendition under International Law." *Case Western Reserve Journal of International Law* 37, no. 2/3 (2006): 309–42.

Saltus, Richard. "Journal Departures Reflect AIDS Dispute." *Boston Globe*, October 16, 1997, p. A11.

Sampson, J.H., and J. Neaton. "On Being Poor with HIV." *Lancet* 344, no. 8930 (1994): 1100–1101.

Sanchez, Thomas. *Mile Zero*. New York: Vintage Books, 1990.

Satcher, David. "Emerging Infections: Getting Ahead of the Curve." *Emerging Infectious Diseases* 1, no. 1 (1995): 1–6.

Scalcini, M., G. Carré, M. Jean-Baptiste, E. Hershfield, S. Parker, J. Wolfe, K. Nelz, and R. Long. "Antituberculous Drug Resistance in Central Haiti." *American Review of Respiratory Disease* 142, no. 3 (1990): 508–11.

Schachter, Oscar. *International Law in Theory and Practice*. Dordrecht: M. Nijhoff, 1991.

Scheper-Hughes, Nancy. "Culture, Scarcity, and Maternal Thinking: Maternal Detachment and Infant Survival in a Brazilian Shantytown." *Ethos* 13, no. 4 (1985): 291–317.

———. *Death without Weeping: The Violence of Everyday Life in Brazil*. Berkeley: University of California Press, 1992.

———. "An Essay: 'AIDS and the Social Body.'" *Social Science and Medicine* 39, no. 7 (1994): 991–1003.

———. "The Global Traffic in Human Organs." *Current Anthropology* 41, no. 2 (2000): 191–224.

———. "The Primacy of the Ethical: Propositions for a Militant Anthropology." *Current Anthropology* 36, no. 3 (1995): 409–40.

———. "Small Wars and Invisible Genocides." *Social Science and Medicine* 43, no. 5 (1996): 889–900.

———. "Three Propositions for a Critically Applied Medical Anthropology." *Social Science and Medicine* 30, no. 2 (1990): 189–97.

———. *A World Cut in Two: The Global Traffic in Organs*. Berkeley: University of California Press, forthcoming.

Scheper-Hughes, Nancy, and Philippe I. Bourgois, eds. *Violence in War and Peace: An Anthology*. Malden, Mass.: Blackwell, 2004.

Scheper-Hughes, Nancy, and Margaret M. Lock. "The Mindful Body: A Prolegomenon to Future Work in Medical Anthropology." *Medical Anthropology Quarterly* 1, no. 1 (1987): 6–41.

Schiff, Eugene. "Deadly Bureaucracy: Dominican Republic Retreats from '3x5' Commitments, Lowers ARV Access Goals." Agua Buena Human Rights Organization, September 13, 2004. www.aguabuena.org/ingles/articules/dominicanburocracy.html (accessed July 16, 2009).

Schiller, Nina Glick. "The Invisible Women: Caregiving and the Construction of AIDS Health Services." *Culture, Medicine, and Psychiatry* 17, no. 4 (1993): 487–512.

Schmidt, Hans. *The United States Occupation of Haiti, 1915–1934.* New Brunswick, N.J.: Rutgers University Press, 1995. Originally published in 1971.

Schmidt, Paul F. "Some Criticisms of Cultural Relativism." *Journal of Philosophy* 52, no. 25 (1955): 780–91.

Schneider, Beth, and Nancy E. Stoller, eds. *Women Resisting AIDS: Feminist Strategies of Empowerment.* Philadelphia: Temple University Press, 1995.

Schoenbaum, E. E., and M. P. Webber. "The Underrecognition of HIV Infection in Women in an Inner-City Emergency Room." *American Journal of Public Health* 83, no. 3 (1993): 363–68.

Schoenholtz, Andrew I. "Aiding and Abetting Persecutors: The Seizure and Return of Haitian Refugees in Violation of the U.N. Refugee Convention and Protocol." *Georgetown Immigration Law Journal* 7, no. 1 (1993): 67–85.

Schoepf, Brooke Grundfest. "AIDS Action-Research with Women in Kinshasa, Zaire." *Social Science and Medicine* 37, no. 11 (1993): 1401–13.

———. "Gender, Development, and AIDS: A Political Economy and Cultural Framework." In *Women and International Development Annual,* edited by Rita S. Gallin, Anne Ferguson, and Janice Harper, pp. 53–85. Boulder, Colo.: Westview Press, 1993.

———. "Women, AIDS, and Economic Crisis in Central Africa." *Canadian Journal of African Studies/Revue Canadienne des Études Africaines* 22, no. 3 (1988): 625–44.

Schwab, Peter. *Cuba: Confronting the U.S. Embargo.* New York: St. Martin's Press, 1999.

Scott, Clarissa. "Haitian Blood Beliefs and Practices in Miami, Florida." Paper presented at the annual meeting of the American Anthropological Association, New Orleans, November 1973.

Scott, James C. *Domination and the Arts of Resistance: Hidden Transcripts.* New Haven: Yale University Press, 1990.

———. *The Moral Economy of the Peasant: Rebellion and Subsistence in Southeast Asia.* New Haven: Yale University Press, 1976.

———. *Weapons of the Weak: Everyday Forms of Peasant Resistance.* New Haven: Yale University Press, 1985.

Selik, R. M., S. Y. Chu, and J. W. Buehler. "HIV Infection as Leading Cause of Death among Young Adults in U.S. Cities and States." *Journal of the American Medical Association* 269, no. 23 (1993): 2991–94.

Sen, Amartya Kumar. *Development as Freedom.* New York: Knopf, 1999.

———. "Equality of What?" Tanner Lecture on Human Values, May 22, 1979. In *Equal Freedom: Selected Tanner Lectures in Human Values,* edited by Stephen Darwall, pp. 307–31. Ann Arbor: University of Michigan Press, 1995. www.tannerlectures.utah .edu/lectures/documents/sen80.pdf (accessed July 15, 2009).

———. *Identity and Violence: The Illusion of Destiny.* New York: Norton, 2006.

———. "Missing Women." *British Medical Journal* 304, no. 6287 (1992): 587–88.

———. "Mortality as an Indicator of Economic Success and Failure." *Economic Journal* 108, no. 446 (1998): 1–25.

Sengupta, Sarthak. *Tribes of the Eastern Himalayas.* New Delhi: Mittal, 2001.

Shacochis, Bob. *The Immaculate Invasion.* New York: Viking, 1999.

Shadid, Anthony. "Fighting Scourges with Funds: Once Almost Ignored, Malaria, TB Research See Flood of Cash." *Boston Globe,* May 30, 2001, p. C4.

Shattuck, John H. F. *Freedom on Fire: Human Rights Wars and America's Response.* Cambridge, Mass.: Harvard University Press, 2003.

Shears, Paul. *Tuberculosis Control Programmes in Developing Countries.* 2nd ed. Oxford: Oxfam, 1988.

Shiloh, Ailon. "Therapeutic Anthropology: The Anthropologist as Private Practitioner." *American Anthropologist* 79, no. 2 (1977): 443–45.

Shin, Sonya, Jennifer J. Furin, Jaime Bayona, Kedar Mate, Jim Yong Kim, and Paul E. Farmer. "Community-Based Treatment of Multidrug-Resistant Tuberculosis in Lima, Peru: 7 Years of Experience." *Social Science and Medicine* 59, no. 7 (2004): 1529–39.

Shkilnyk, Anastasia M. *A Poison Stronger Than Love: The Destruction of an Ojibwa Community.* New Haven: Yale University Press, 1985.

Shuger, Scott. "Supreme Court Cover-Up." *Slate,* March 30, 2000. www.slate.com/id/1004976/ (accessed July 15, 2009).

Sibeko, Lindiwe, Mohammed Ali Dhansay, Karen E. Charlton, Timothy Johns, and Katherine Gray-Donald. "Beliefs, Attitudes, and Practices of Breastfeeding Mothers from a Periurban Community in South Africa." *Journal of Human Lactation* 21, no. 1 (2005): 31–38.

Simpson, Christopher. *The Splendid Blond Beast: Money, Law, and Genocide in the Twentieth Century.* New York: Grove Press, 1993.

Sinclair, Upton, Edward Sagarin, and Alfred Teichner, eds. *The Cry for Justice: An Anthology of the Literature of Social Protest.* New York: L. Stuart, 1963.

Singapore Tuberculosis Service/British Medical Research Council. "Five-Year Follow-Up of a Clinical Trial of Three 6-Month Regimens of Chemotherapy Given Intermittently in the Continuation Phase in the Treatment of Pulmonary Tuberculosis." *American Review of Respiratory Disease* 137 (1988): 1147–50.

Singer, M. "AIDS and the Health Crisis of the U.S. Urban Poor: The Perspective of Critical Medical Anthropology." *Social Science and Medicine* 39, no. 7 (1994): 931–48.

———. "Beyond the Ivory Tower: Critical Praxis in Medical Anthropology." In *Understanding and Applying Medical Anthropology,* edited by Peter J. Brown, pp. 225–39. Mountain View, Calif.: Mayfield, 1998.

Singer, M., F. Valentin, H. Baer, and Z. Jia. "Why Does Juan Garcia Have a Drinking Problem? The Perspective of Critical Medical Anthropology." *Medical Anthropology* 14, no. 1 (1992): 77–108.

Singer, Peter. "Outsiders: Our Obligations to Those Beyond Our Borders." In *The Ethics of Assistance: Morality and the Distant Needy,* edited by Deen K. Chatterjee, pp. 11–32. Cambridge: Cambridge University Press, 2004.

Singler, Jennifer, and Paul E. Farmer. "Treating HIV in Resource-Poor Settings." *Journal of the American Medical Association* 288, no. 13 (2002): 1652–53.

Skogly, Sigrun I. "Structural Adjustment and Development: Human Rights—An Agenda for Change." *Human Rights Quarterly* 15, no. 4 (1993): 751–78.

Skolnick, A. A. "Some Experts Suggest the Nation's 'War on Drugs' Is Helping Tuberculosis Stage a Deadly Comeback." *Journal of the American Medical Association* 268, no. 22 (1992): 3177–78.

Slutzker, Laurence, Jean-Baptiste Brunet, John Karon, and James Curran. "Trends in the United States and Europe." In *AIDS in the World: The Global Aids Policy Coalition,* edited by Jonathan M. Mann, Daniel Tarantola, and Thomas W. Netter, pp. 605–16. Cambridge, Mass.: Harvard University Press, 1992.

Small, P. M., and A. Moss. "Molecular Epidemiology and the New Tuberculosis." *Infectious Agents and Disease* 2, no. 3 (1993): 132–38.

Small, P. M., R. W. Shafer, P. C. Hopewell, S. P. Singh, M. J. Murphy, E. Desmond, M. F. Sierra, and G. K. Schoolnik. "Exogenous Reinfection with Multidrug-Resistant *Mycobacterium tuberculosis* in Patients with Advanced HIV Infection." *New England Journal of Medicine* 328, no. 16 (1993): 1137–44.

Smillie, W. G., and D. L. Augustine. "Vital Capacity of the Negro Race." *Journal of the American Medical Association* 87, no. 25 (1926): 2055–58.

Smith Fawzi, Mary C., W. Lambert, J. M. Singler, S. P. Koenig, F. Léandre, P. Nevil, D. Bertrand, M. S. Claude, J. Bertrand, J. J. Salazar, et al. "Prevalence and Risk Factors of STDs in Rural Haiti: Implications for Policy and Programming in Resource-Poor Settings." *International Journal of STD and AIDS* 14 (2003): 848–53.

Snider, D. E., Jr. "The Impact of Tuberculosis on Women, Children, and Minorities in the United States." Paper presented at the World Congress on Tuberculosis, Bethesda, Md., November 1992.

Snider, D. E., Jr., J. Graczyk, E. Bek, and J. Rogowski. "Supervised Six-Months Treatment of Newly Diagnosed Pulmonary Tuberculosis Using Isoniazid, Rifampin, and Pyrazinamide with and without Streptomycin." *American Review of Respiratory Disease* 130, no. 6 (1984): 1091–94.

Snider, D. E., Jr., and W. L. Roper. "The New Tuberculosis." *New England Journal of Medicine* 326, no. 10 (1992): 703–5.

Snider, D. E., Jr., L. Salinas, and G. D. Kelly. "Tuberculosis: An Increasing Problem among Minorities in the United States." *Public Health Reports* 104, no. 6 (1989): 646–53.

Sobrino, Jon. *Spirituality of Liberation: Toward Political Holiness.* Maryknoll, N.Y.: Orbis Books, 1988.

Solórzano, A. "Sowing the Seeds of Neo-Imperialism: The Rockefeller Foundation's Yellow Fever Campaign in Mexico." *International Journal of Health Services* 22, no. 3 (1992): 529–54.

Sontag, Susan. *Regarding the Pain of Others.* New York: Farrar, Straus and Giroux, 2003.

"South Florida Braces for Haitian Time Bomb." *Orlando Sentinel,* January 11, 1993, p. A1.

Spence, D. P., J. Hotchkiss, C. S. Williams, and P. D. Davies. "Tuberculosis and Poverty." *British Medical Journal* 307, no. 6907 (1993): 759–61.

Spira, R., P. Lepage, P. Msellati, P. Van De Perre, V. Leroy, A. Simonon, E. Karita, and F. Dabis. "Natural History of Human Immunodeficiency Virus Type 1 Infection in Children: A Five-Year Prospective Study in Rwanda. Mother-to-Child HIV-1 Transmission Study Group." *Pediatrics* 104, no. 5 (1999): e56.

Spitzer, Robert, and Janet Williams. "Proposed Revisions in the DSM-III Classification of Anxiety Disorders Based on Research and Clinical Experience." In *Anxiety and the Anxiety Disorders,* edited by A. Hussain Tuma and Jack D. Maser, pp. 297–323. Hillsdale, N.J.: Erlbaum, 1985.

Sprinkle, Robert H. Review: "Pathologies of Power: Health, Human Rights, and the New War on the Poor." *Journal of the American Medical Association* 292, no. 5 (2004): 631–32.

Standaert, B., and A. Meheus. "Le cancer de col utérin en Afrique." *Médecine d'Afrique Noire* 32 (1985): 406–15.

Stanley, Alessandra. "Russians Lament the Crime of Punishment." *New York Times,* January 8, 1988, p. A1.

Starn, Orin. "Missing the Revolution: Anthropologists and the War in Peru." In *Rereading Cultural Anthropology,* edited by George E. Marcus, pp. 152–80. Durham, N.C.: Duke University Press, 1992.

Steadman, Kimberly Jill. "Struggling for a 'Never Again': A Comparison of the Human Rights Reports in Post-Authoritarian Argentina and Chile." A.B. thesis, Harvard University, 1997.

Stein, Z. "What Was New at Yokohama—Women's Voices at the 1994 International HIV/AIDS Conference." *American Journal of Public Health* 84, no. 12 (1994): 1887–88.

Steiner, Henry J., and Philip Alston. *International Human Rights in Context: Law, Politics, Morals. Text and Materials.* New York: Oxford University Press, 1996.

Stern, Vivien, ed. *Sentenced to Die? The Problem of TB in Prisons in Eastern Europe and Central Asia.* London: International Centre for Prison Studies, 1999.

———. *A Sin against the Future: Imprisonment in the World.* Boston: Northeastern University Press, 1998.

Stiglitz, Joseph, and Linda Bilmes. "The Three Trillion Dollar War: The Costs of the Iraq and Afghanistan Conflicts Have Grown to Staggering Proportions." *Times (U.K.),* February 23, 2008. www.timesonline.co.uk/tol/comment/columnists/guest_contributors/article3419840.ece (accessed July 15, 2009).

St. Louis, M. E., G. A. Conway, C. R. Hayman, C. Miller, L. R. Petersen, and T. J. Dondero. "Human Immunodeficiency Virus Infection in Disadvantaged Adolescents: Findings from the U.S. Job Corps." *Journal of the American Medical Association* 266, no. 17 (1991): 2387–91.

Stockman, Farah, and Susan Milligan. "Before Fall of Aristide, Haiti Hit by Aid Cutoff." *Boston Globe,* March 7, 2004.

Stoller, Nancy E. "Lesbian Involvement in the AIDS Epidemic: Changing Roles and Generational Differences." In *Women Resisting AIDS: Feminist Strategies of Empowerment,* edited by Beth Schneider and Nancy E. Stoller, pp. 270–85. Philadelphia: Temple University Press, 1995.

Stop TB Initiative. *Tuberculosis and Sustainable Development: The Stop TB Initiative 2000 Report.* Geneva: World Health Organization, 2000. www.stoptb.org/stop_tb_initiative/assets/documents/rap-lit.pdf (accessed June 10, 2009).

Strada, Gino. *Green Parrots: A War Surgeon's Diary.* Foreword by Howard Zinn. Milan: Charta, 2004.

Strathern, Marilyn, ed. *Audit Cultures: Anthropological Studies in Ethics, Accountability, and the Academy.* London: Routledge, 2000.

Straus, Scott. *The Order of Genocide: Race, Power, and War in Rwanda*. Ithaca. N.Y.: Cornell University Press, 2006.

Strindberg, A. "A Catechism for Workers." In *The Cry for Justice: An Anthology of the Literature of Social Protest*, edited by Upton Sinclair, Edward Sagarin and Albert Teichner, pp. 729–30. New York: L. Stuart, 1963.

Styblo, K. "Overview and Epidemiological Assessment of the Current Global Tuberculosis Situation: With an Emphasis on Tuberculosis Control in Developing Countries." *Zeitschrift für Erkrankungen der Atmungsorgane* 173, no. 1 (1989): 6–17.

Sumartojo, Esther. "When Tuberculosis Treatment Fails: A Social Behavioral Account of Patient Adherence." *American Review of Respiratory Disease* 147 (1993): 1311–20.

Sunstein, Cass R. *The Second Bill of Rights: FDR's Unfinished Revolution and Why We Need It More Than Ever*. New York: Basic Books, 2004.

Swoboda, Frank, and Martha McNeil Hamilton. "Congress Passes $15 Billion Airline Bailout." *Washington Post*, September 22, 2001.

Szymborska, Wisława. *Poems, New and Collected, 1957–1997*. Translated by Stanislaw Baranczak and Clare Cavanagh. New York: Harcourt Brace, 1998.

———. *View with a Grain of Sand: Selected Poems*. Translated by Stanislaw Baranczak and Clare Cavanagh. New York: Harcourt Brace, 1995.

Tacitus. "Agricola." In *"Agricola" and "Germany,"* edited and translated by Anthony R. Birley. Oxford: Oxford University Press, 1999.

Tahaoğlu, K., T. Törün, T. Sevim, G. Ataç, A. Kir, L. Karasulu, I. Özmen, and N. Kapakli. "The Treatment of Multidrug-Resistant Tuberculosis in Turkey." *New England Journal of Medicine* 345, no. 3 (2001): 170–74.

Talbot, E. A., M. Moore, E. McCray, and N. J. Binkin. "Tuberculosis among Foreign-Born Persons in the United States, 1993–1998." *Journal of the American Medical Association* 284, no. 22 (2000): 2894–2900.

Talisuna, A. O., P. Bloland, and U. D'Alessandro. "History, Dynamics, and Public Health Importance of Malaria Parasite Resistance." *Clinical Microbiology Reviews* 17, no. 1 (2004): 235–54.

Taussig, Michael T. *The Nervous System*. New York: Routledge, 1992.

———. "Reification and the Consciousness of the Patient." *Social Science and Medicine* 148 (1980): 3–13.

———. *Shamanism, Colonialism, and the Wild Man: A Study in Terror and Healing*. Chicago: University of Chicago Press, 1986.

Tayler, E., C. P. Besse, and T. Healing. "Tuberculosis in Siberia." *Lancet* 343, no. 8903 (1994): 968.

Taylor, Christopher C. "King Sacrifice, President Habyarimana, and the Iconography of Pregenocidal Rwandan Political Literature." In *Violence*, edited by Neil L. Whitehead, pp. 79–105. Santa Fe: School of American Research Press, 2004.

"TB Returns with a Vengeance." *Washington Post*, August 3, 1996, p. A19.

Telzak, E. E., K. Sepkowitz, P. Alpert, S. Mannheimer, F. Medard, W. el-Sadr, S. Blum, A. Gagliardi, N. Salomon, and G. Turett. "Multidrug-Resistant Tuberculosis in Patients without HIV Infection." *New England Journal of Medicine* 333, no. 14 (1995): 907–11.

Terry, Fiona. *Condemned to Repeat? The Paradox of Humanitarian Action.* Ithaca, N.Y.: Cornell University Press, 2002.

Third East African/British Medical Research Council Study. "Controlled Clinical Trial of Four Short-Course Regimens of Chemotherapy for Two Durations in the Treatment of Pulmonary Tuberculosis: Second Report." *Tubercle* 61, no. 2 (1980): 59–69.

Thomas, Lewis. *The Youngest Science: Notes of a Medicine-Watcher.* New York: Viking, 1983.

Tjaden, Patricia Godeke, and Nancy Thoennes. *Prevalence, Incidence, and Consequences of Violence against Women: Findings from the National Violence against Women Survey.* Washington, D.C.: U.S. Department of Justice, National Institute of Justice, and Centers for Disease Control and Prevention, 1998.

Toltzis, Philip, Richard C. Stephens, Ina Adkins, Emilia Lombardi, Shobhana Swami, Andrea Snell, and Victoria Cargill. "Human Immunodeficiency Virus (HIV)-Related Risk-Taking Behaviors in Women Attending Inner-City Prenatal Clinics in the Mid-West." *Journal of Perinatology* 19, no. 7 (1999): 483–87.

Totten, Samuel, William S. Parsons, and Israel W. Charny, eds. *Century of Genocide: Critical Essays and Eyewitness Accounts.* 2nd ed. New York: Routledge, 2004.

Treichler, Paula A. "AIDS, Gender, and Biomedical Discourse: Current Contests for Meaning." In *AIDS: The Burdens of History,* edited by Elizabeth Fee and Daniel M. Fox, pp. 190–266. Berkeley: University of California Press, 1988.

———. "AIDS, Homophobia, and Biomedical Discourse: An Epidemic of Signification." In *AIDS: Cultural Analysis, Cultural Activism,* edited by Douglas Crimp, pp. 31–37. Cambridge, Mass.: MIT Press, 1988.

Trouillot, Michel-Rolph. *Haiti, State against Nation: The Origins and Legacy of Duvalierism.* New York: Monthly Review Press, 1990.

———. *Les racines historiques de l'état duvaliérien.* Port-au-Prince: Deschamps, 1986.

Tully, Julia, and Kathryn Dewey. "Private Fears, Global Loss: A Cross-Cultural Study of the Insufficient Milk Syndrome." *Medical Anthropology* 9, no. 3 (1985): 225–44.

Turett, G. S., E. E. Telzak, L. V. Torian, S. Blum, D. Alland, I. Weisfuse, and B. A. Fazal. "Improved Outcomes for Patients with Multidrug-Resistant Tuberculosis." *Clinical Infectious Diseases* 21, no. 5 (1995): 1238–44.

Turner, Jonathan H. "Analytical Theorizing." In *Social Theory Today,* edited by Anthony Giddens and Jonathan H. Turner, pp. 156–94. Stanford, Calif.: Stanford University Press, 1987.

Turner, Victor Witter. *The Forest of Symbols: Aspects of Ndembu Ritual.* Ithaca, N.Y.: Cornell University Press, 1967.

Turshen, Meredeth. *The Political Ecology of Disease in Tanzania.* New Brunswick, N.J.: Rutgers University Press, 1984.

"Uganda: HIV Project Runs Out of Infant Milk." *The New Vision,* August 12, 2003. http://allafrica.com/stories/200308120677.html (accessed September 12, 2009).

UNAIDS. "2002 Report on the Global HIV Epidemic." Geneva: UNAIDS, 2002.

UNICEF. *HIV and Infant Feeding.* New York: United Nations Children's Fund, 2002.

———. "Saving Children from the Tragedy of Landmines." Press release, April 4, 2006. www.unicef.org/media/media_32034.html (accessed July 16, 2009).

United Nations. *Mission of Technical Assistance to the Republic of Haiti*. Lake Success, N.Y.: United Nations, 1949.

———. *Our Common Future: Report of the World Commission on Environment and Development*. 1987. www.un-documents.net/wced-ocf.htm (accessed July 16, 2009).

———. *Report on the Situation of Human Rights in Haiti*. Submitted to the General Assembly, Fiftieth Session, by Adama Dieng, independent expert, in accordance with Commission on Human Rights resolution 1995/70. Agenda item 112(b), A/50/714, November 1, 1995. www.unhchr.ch/Huridocda/Huridoca.nsf/TestFrame/ad4f1980704bc90d80256723005e32e4?Opendocument (accessed September 13, 2009).

———. "Universal Declaration of Human Rights." Adopted by the United Nations General Assembly on December 10, 1948. www.un.org/Overview/rights.html (accessed July 16, 2009).

United Nations Commission on Human Rights. *Situation of Human Rights in Haiti*. Submitted by Marco Tulio Bruni Celli, Special Rapporteur. Geneva: United Nations Economic and Social Council, 1995.

United Nations Development Programme. *Human Development Report 1990: Concept and Measurement of Human Development*. New York: Oxford University Press for UNDP, 1990. http://hdr.undp.org/en/reports/global/hdr1990 (accessed May 14, 2009).

———. *Human Development Report 1998: Consumption for Human Development*. New York: Oxford University Press for UNDP, 1998. http://hdr.undp.org/en/reports/global/hdr1998 (accessed May 14, 2009).

———. *Human Development Report 1999: Globalization with a Human Face*. Background Papers. 2 vols. New York: Oxford University Press for UNDP, 1999. http://hdr.undp.org/en/reports/global/hdr1999 (accessed May 14, 2009).

———. *Young Women: Silence, Susceptibility, and the HIV Epidemic*. New York: UNDP, 1992.

United Nations Food and Agriculture Organization. "The State of Food Insecurity in the World." Rome: United Nations Food and Agriculture Organization, 2000. www.fao.org/DOCREP/X8200E/X8200E00.htm (accessed July 16, 2009).

U.S. Bureau of the Census. *1990 Census of Population and Housing*. Washington, D.C.: Government Printing Office, 1993. www.census.gov/prod/www/abs/decennial/1990.htm (accessed July 16, 2009).

U.S. Central Intelligence Agency. "Haiti: Country Profile." *The World Factbook 2001*. Washington, D.C.: Central Intelligence Agency, 2001. Available through EBSCO Publishing, Academic Search Premier, Ipswich, Mass. (accessed September 11, 2009).

———. "Haiti: Country Profile." *The World Factbook 2007*. Washington, D.C.: Central Intelligence Agency, 2007. Available through EBSCO Publishing, Academic Search Premier, Ipswich, Mass. (accessed September 11, 2009).

U.S. Department of Health and Human Services. "The Surgeon General's Call to Action to Prevent and Decrease Overweight and Obesity." December 13, 2001. www.surgeongeneral.gov/topics/obesity (accessed July 16, 2009).

Uvin, Peter. *Aiding Violence: The Development Enterprise in Rwanda*. West Hartford, Conn.: Kumarian Press, 1998.

Varmus, Harold, and David Satcher. "Ethical Complexities of Conducting Research in Developing Countries." *New England Journal of Medicine* 337, no. 14 (1997): 1003–5.

Vastey, Pompée-Valentin. *Notes à M. le Baron de V. P. Malouet, ministre de la marine et des colonies, de Sa Majesté Louis XVIII, et ancien administrateur des colonies et de la marine, ex-colon de Saint-Domingue* . . . Cap-Haïtien: P. Roux, 1814.

Victora, C. G., J. P. Vaughan, F. C. Barros, A. C. Silva, and E. Tomasi. "Explaining Trends in Inequities: Evidence from Brazilian Child Health Studies." *Lancet* 356, no. 9235 (2000): 1093–98.

Vieux, Serge-Henri. *Le plaçage: Droit coutumier et famille en Haïti.* Paris: Publisud, 1989.

Virchow, Rudolf Ludwig Karl. *Die Einheitsbestrebungen in der Wissenschaftlichen Medicin.* Berlin: G. Reimer, 1849.

———. "Was die 'medizinische Reform' will." *Die Medizinische Reform* 1 (1848). www .uni-heidelberg.de/institute/fak5/igm/g47/bauerz15.htm (accessed July 16, 2009).

Vissière, Isabelle, and Jean Louis Vissière. *La traite des noirs au siècle des Lumières: Témoignages de négriers.* Paris: A. M. Métailié, 1982.

Wacquant, Loïc J. D. *Body and Soul: Notebooks of an Apprentice Boxer.* Oxford: Oxford University Press, 2004.

Wagner, Roy. *The Invention of Culture.* Englewood Cliffs, N.J.: Prentice-Hall, 1975.

Waldholz, Michael. "Precious Pills: New AIDS Treatment Raises Tough Question of Who Will Get It—For the Poor, High Costs, Rigid Regimens Dim Drug Cocktails' Promise. A Major Issue for Medicaid." *Wall Street Journal,* July 3, 1996.

Walensky, R. P., A. D. Paltiel, E. Losina, L. M. Mercincavage, B. R. Schackman, P. E. Sax, M. C. Weinstein, and K. A. Freedberg. "The Survival Benefits of AIDS Treatment in the United States." *Journal of Infectious Diseases* 194, no. 1 (2006): 11–19.

Walker, Damian G., and Stephen Jan. "How Do We Determine Whether Community Health Workers Are Cost-Effective? Some Core Methodological Issues." *Journal of Community Health* 30, no. 3 (2005): 221–29.

Wallace, Rodrick. "Social Disintegration and the Spread of AIDS: Thresholds for Propagation along 'Sociogeographic' Networks." *Social Science and Medicine* 33, no. 10 (1991): 1155–62.

———. "Social Disintegration and the Spread of AIDS—II. Meltdown of Sociogeographic Structure in Urban Minority Neighborhoods." *Social Science and Medicine* 37, no. 7 (1993): 887–96.

———. "A Synergism of Plagues: 'Planned Shrinkage,' Contagious Housing Destruction, and AIDS in the Bronx." *Environmental Research* 47 (1988): 1–33.

———. "Urban Desertification, Public Health, and Public Order: 'Planned Shrinkage,' Violent Death, Substance Abuse, and AIDS in the Bronx." *Social Science and Medicine* 31, no. 7 (1990): 801–13.

Wallace, Rodrick, Mindy Fullilove, Robert Fullilove, Peter Gould, and Deborah Wallace. "Will AIDS Be Contained within U.S. Minority Urban Populations?" *Social Science and Medicine* 39, no. 8 (1994): 1051–62.

Wallerstein, Immanuel Maurice. *After Liberalism.* New York: The New Press, 1995.

———. "The Insurmountable Contradictions of Liberalism: Human Rights and the Rights of Peoples in the Geoculture of the Modern World-System." *South Atlantic Quarterly* 46 (1995): 1161–78.

———. *The Modern World-System: Capitalist Agriculture and the Origins of the European World-Economy in the Sixteenth Century.* New York: Academic Press, 1974.

———. "World-Systems Analysis." In *Social Theory Today,* edited by Anthony Giddens and Jonathan H. Turner, pp. 309–24. Stanford, Calif.: Stanford University Press, 1987.

Walton, David A., Paul E. Farmer, and R. Dillingham. "Social and Cultural Factors in Tropical Medicine: Reframing Our Understanding of Disease." In *Tropical Infectious Diseases: Principles, Pathogens, and Practice,* edited by Richard L. Guerrant, David H. Walker, and Peter F. Weller, pp. 26–35. Philadelphia: Elsevier Churchill Livingstone, 2005.

Walton, David A., Paul E. Farmer, Wesler Lambert, Fernet Léandre, Serena P. Koenig, and Joia S. Mukherjee. "Integrated HIV Prevention and Care Strengthens Primary Health Care: Lessons from Rural Haiti." *Journal of Public Health Policy* 25, no. 2 (2004): 137–58.

Ward, Martha C. "A Different Disease: HIV/AIDS and Health Care for Women in Poverty." *Culture, Medicine, and Psychiatry* 17, no. 4 (1993): 413–30.

———. "Poor and Positive: Two Contrasting Views from inside the HIV/AIDS Epidemic." *Practicing Anthropology* 15, no. 4 (1993): 59–61.

———. "Women's Health, Women's Lives." *Medical Anthropology Quarterly* 12, no. 3 (1998): 384–90.

Waring, Belle. "PIH's Farmer Speaks on Antibiotic Resistance." *NIH Record* 61, no. 3, February 6, 2006, p. 1. http://nihrecord.od.nih.gov/newsletters/2009/02_06_2009/story1.htm (accessed October 9, 2009).

Warner, David C. "Health Issues at the U.S.–Mexican Border." *Journal of the American Medical Association* 265, no. 2 (1991): 242–47.

Warren, Kenneth S., and Adel A. F. Mahmoud. *Geographic Medicine for the Practitioner.* New York: Springer-Verlag, 1985.

Wasser, S. C., M. Gwinn, and P. Fleming. "Urban-Nonurban Distribution of HIV Infection in Childbearing Women in the United States." *JAIDS: Journal of Acquired Immune Deficiency Syndromes* 6, no. 9 (1993): 1035–42.

Waterston, Alisse. *Street Addicts in the Political Economy.* Philadelphia: Temple University Press, 1993.

Waterston, Alisse, and Barbara Rylko-Bauer. "Out of the Shadows of History and Memory: Personal Family Narratives in Ethnographies of Rediscovery." *American Ethnologist* 33, no. 3 (2006): 397–412.

Watts, Sheldon J. *Epidemics and History: Disease, Power, and Imperialism.* New Haven: Yale University Press, 1997.

Wedel, Janine R. *Collision and Collusion: The Strange Case of Western Aid to Eastern Europe, 1989–1998.* New York: St. Martin's Press, 1998.

Weidman, Hazel. *Miami Health Ecology Project Report: A Statement on Ethnicity and Health.* Miami: University of Miami, 1978.

Weisman, Jonathan. "Projected Iraq War Costs Soar—Total Spending Is Likely to More Than Double, Analysis Finds." *Washington Post,* April 27, 2006, p. A16.

Whitehead, M., A. Scott-Samuel, and G. Dahlgren. "Setting Targets to Address Inequalities in Health." *Lancet* 351, no. 9111 (1998): 1279–82.

Whitehead, Neil L. *Violence*. Santa Fe: School of American Research Press, 2004.

Whitmore, George. *Someone Was Here: Profiles in the AIDS Epidemic.* New York: New American Library, 1988.

Wiese, Helen Jean Coleman. "The Interaction of Western and Indigenous Medicine in Haiti in Regard to Tuberculosis." Ph.D. diss., University of North Carolina at Chapel Hill, 1971.

———. "Tuberculosis in Rural Haiti." *Social Science and Medicine* 8, no. 6 (1974): 359–62.

Wikan, Unni. "Illness from Fright or Soul Loss: A North Balinese Culture-Bound Syndrome?" *Culture, Medicine, and Psychiatry* 13, no. 1 (1989): 25–50.

Wikler, Daniel. "Personal and Social Responsibility for Health." In *Public Health, Ethics, and Equity,* edited by Sudhir Anand, Fabienne Peter, and Amartya Kumar Sen, pp. 109–34. Oxford: Oxford University Press, 2004.

Wiktor, Stefan Z., Madeleine Sassan-Morokro, Alison D. Grant, Lucien Abouya, John M. Karon, Chantal Maurice, Gaston Djomand, Alain Ackah, Kouao Domoua, Auguste Kadio, et al. "Efficacy of Trimethoprim-Sulphamethoxazole Prophylaxis to Decrease Morbidity and Mortality in HIV-1-Infected Patients with Tuberculosis in Abidjan, Côte d'Ivoire: A Randomised Controlled Trial." *Lancet* 353, no. 9163 (1999): 1469–75.

Wilentz, Amy. *The Rainy Season: Haiti since Duvalier.* New York: Simon and Schuster, 1989.

Wilkinson, Richard G. "The Epidemiological Transition: From Material Scarcity to Social Disadvantage?" *Daedalus* 123, no. 4 (1994): 61–77.

———. *Unhealthy Societies: The Afflictions of Inequality.* London: Routledge, 1996.

Williams, Juan. "Powell Defends U.S. Stance on Haiti: U.S. Wasn't Prepared to 'Prop Up' a 'Failing' Aristide." Extended interview with Colin Powell, *Morning Edition,* National Public Radio, March 9, 2004. Audio available at www.npr.org/templates/story/story .php?storyId=1752713 (accessed October 10, 2009).

Willis, Paul E. *Learning to Labor: How Working Class Kids Get Working Class Jobs.* New York: Columbia University Press, 1981.

Wilson, Carter. *Hidden in the Blood: A Personal Investigation of AIDS in the Yucatán.* New York: Columbia University Press, 1995.

Wilson, Mary E. "Travel and the Emergence of Infectious Diseases." *Emerging Infectious Diseases* 1, no. 2 (1995): 39–46.

Wilson, Ruth P., and Moses Pounds. "AIDS in African-American Communities and the Public Health Response: An Overview." *Transforming Anthropology* 4, no. 1–2 (1993): 9–16.

Wilson, William J. *The Declining Significance of Race: Blacks and Changing American Institutions.* 2nd ed. Chicago: University of Chicago Press, 1980.

Winter, Deborah DuNann, and Dana C. Leighton. "Structural Violence, Introduction." In *Peace, Conflict, and Violence: Peace Psychology for the Twenty-First Century,* edited by Daniel Christie, Richard Wagner, and Deborah DuNann Winter, pp. 99–101. Upper Saddle River, N.J.: Prentice Hall, 2001.

Wise, P. H. "Confronting Racial Disparities in Infant Mortality: Reconciling Science and Politics." *American Journal of Preventive Medicine* 9 (1993): 7–16.

Wolf, Eric R. *Europe and the People without History.* Berkeley: University of California Press, 1997.

Wolf, Eric R., Joel S. Kahn, William Roseberry, and Immanuel Maurice Wallerstein. "Perilous Ideas: Race, Culture, People." With Comments and Reply. *Current Anthropology* 35, no. 1 (1994): 1–12.

Woloch, Alex. *The One vs. the Many: Minor Characters and the Space of the Protagonist in the Novel.* Princeton, N.J.: Princeton University Press, 2003.

World Bank. *Social Indicators of Development, 1994.* Baltimore: Johns Hopkins University Press, 1994.

——. *World Development Indicators 1999.* Washington, D.C.: World Bank, 1999.

World Health Organization. "Cholera in the Americas." *Weekly Epidemiological Record* 67, no. 6 (1992): 33–39.

——. "Constitution of the World Health Organization." Adopted July 22, 1946, New York. http://avalon.law.yale.edu/20th_century/decad051.asp (accessed July 16, 2009).

——. "Coordination of DOTS-Plus Pilot Projects for the Management of MDR-TB: Proceedings of a Meeting, Geneva, 29 January 1999." Edited by Marcos A. Espinal. Geneva: World Health Organization, 1999.

——. "Ebola Haemorrhagic Fever in Zaïre, 1976. Report of an International Commission." *Bulletin of the World Health Organization* 56, no. 2 (1978): 271–93.

——. *Global Health Situation and Projections: Estimates.* Division of Epidemiological Surveillance and Health Situation and Trend Assessment. Geneva: World Health Organization, 1992.

——. *Global Tuberculosis Control: WHO Report 2001.* Geneva: World Health Organization, 2001.

——. "Maternal Mortality: Helping Women Off the Road to Death." *WHO Chronicle* 40 (1985): 175–83.

——. *Report, Multidrug Resistant Tuberculosis (MDR TB): Basis for the Development of an Evidence-Based Case-Management Strategy for MDR TB within the WHO's DOTS Strategy. Proceedings of 1998 Meetings and Protocol Recommendations.* Edited by Marcos A. Espinal. WHO/TB, 99.260. Geneva: World Health Organization, 1999. http://whqlibdoc.who.int/hq/1999/WHO_TB_99.260.pdf (accessed July 11, 2009).

——. *Scaling Up Antiretroviral Therapy in Resource-Limited Settings: Treatment Guidelines for a Public Health Approach.* Geneva: World Health Organization, 2004. www.who.int/hiv/pub/prev_care/en/arvrevision2003en.pdf (accessed July 16, 2009).

——. *Towards Universal Access: Scaling Up Priority HIV/AIDS Interventions in the Health Sector. Progress Report 2008.* Geneva: World Health Organization, 2008. www.who.int/hiv/pub/towards_universal_access_report_2008.pdf (accessed July 16, 2009).

——. *Treatment of Tuberculosis: Guidelines for National Programmes.* Geneva: World Health Organization, 1991.

——. *WHO Tuberculosis Programme: Framework for Effective Tuberculosis Control.* Geneva: World Health Organization, 1994.

———. *The World Health Report, 1995: Bridging the Gaps.* Geneva: World Health Organization, 1995.

———. *The World Health Report, 2003: Shaping the Future.* Geneva: World Health Organization, 2003.

World Health Organization Global Tuberculosis Programme. *Anti-Tuberculosis Drug Resistance in the World.* WHO/IUATLD Global Project on Anti-Tuberculosis Drug Resistance Surveillance. Geneva: World Health Organization Global Tuberculosis Programme, 1997. http://whqlibdoc.who.int/HQ/1997/WHO_TB_97.229.pdf (accessed July 16, 2009).

———. *Anti-Tuberculosis Drug Resistance in the World, Third Global Report.* WHO/IUATLD Global Project on Anti-Tuberculosis Drug Resistance Surveillance. Geneva: World Health Organization, 2004. www.who.int/tb/publications/who_htm_tb_2004_343/en (accessed July 16, 2009).

———. *Groups at Risk: WHO Report on the Tuberculosis Epidemic, 1996.* Geneva: World Health Organization, 1996. http://whqlibdoc.who.int/hq/1996/WHO_TB_96.198.pdf (accessed July 16, 2009).

———. *TB Treatment Observer,* no. 2 (1997).

———. *TB: WHO Report on the Tuberculosis Epidemic 1997.* Geneva: World Health Organization, 1997.

———. *WHO Report on the Tuberculosis Epidemic, 1995: Stop TB at the Source.* Geneva: World Health Organization, 1995.

World Health Organization and UNAIDS. "UNAIDS/WHO AIDS Epidemic Update 2005." Geneva: World Health Organization, 2005.

———. "UNAIDS/WHO Epidemiological Fact Sheets on HIV/AIDS and Sexually Transmitted Infections, 2004 Update." Directory. http://data.unaids.org/Publications/Fact-Sheets01 (accessed September 12, 2009).

World Health Organization, United Nations Children's Fund, and United Nations Population Fund. *Maternal Mortality in 1995: Estimates Developed by WHO, UNICEF, UNFPA.* Report prepared by Carla AbouZahr and Tessa M. Wardlaw. Geneva: World Health Organization, 2001.

———. *Maternal Mortality in 2000: Estimates Developed by WHO, UNICEF, UNFPA.* Report prepared by Carla AbouZahr and Tessa M. Wardlaw. Geneva: World Health Organization, 2004. http://whqlibdoc.who.int/publications/2004/9241562706.pdf (accessed July 16, 2009).

Worth, Dooley. "Minority Women and AIDS: Culture, Race, and Gender." In *Culture and AIDS: The Human Factor,* edited by D. A. Feldman, pp. 111–36. New York: Praeger, 1990.

———. "Sexual Decision-Making and AIDS: Why Condom Promotion among Vulnerable Women Is Likely to Fail." *Studies in Family Planning* 20, no. 6 (1989): 297–307.

Wyatt, G. E. "Transaction Sex and HIV Risks: A Woman's Choice?" Paper presented at the conference HIV Infection in Women: Setting a New Agenda, Washington, D.C., February 22–24, 1995.

Yerushalmy, J. "The Increase in Tuberculosis Proportionate Mortality among Non-White Young Adults." *Public Health Reports* 61, no. 8 (1946): 251–58.

Zacchia, Paolo. *Quaestiones medico-legales.* 9 vols. Loudun, Belgium: Anisson, 1621–1635.

Zanmi Lasante. "Rapport trimestriel des données de base." Cange, Haiti: Zanmi Lasante, 1993.

Zierler, Sally. "Hitting Hard: HIV and Violence." In *The Gender Politics of HIV/AIDS in Women: Perspectives on the Pandemic in the United States,* edited by Nancy Goldstein and Jennifer L. Manlowe, pp. 207–21. New York: New York University Press, 1997.

Zinsser, Hans. *Rats, Lice, and History; Being a Study in Biography, Which, after Twelve Preliminary Chapters Indispensable for the Preparation of the Lay Reader, Deals with the Life History of Typhus Fever.* Boston: Little, Brown, 1935.

Zwi, Anthony B. "How Should the Health Community Respond to Violent Political Conflict?" *PLoS Medicine* 1, no. 1 (2004): e14.

EDITORIAL NOTE AND CREDITS

EDITORIAL NOTE

The essays in this book were chosen to reflect the main interests of Paul Farmer's writing; to show the interconnectedness of his contributions in anthropology, medicine, health policy, and political advocacy; and to give a sense of the development of his ideas over more than a quarter-century of activity. The order in which they are presented is roughly chronological, but also by field: the reader can observe Farmer solidifying his grasp of issues in Haiti, then extending the insights to other places and other issues. Some of the pieces are chapters excerpted from Farmer's books; a number were written in collaboration with colleagues. Each chapter shows, I feel, a turning point in his work: a concern discovered, a claim documented, a challenge announced. The original contexts in which these essays appeared are highly dissimilar. Some of the chapters were research papers submitted to specialized journals for anthropologists or medical practitioners; others were editorials invited by the same journals; still others began as lectures for a broad public or addresses to professional associations. All have been edited in order to make them freestanding essays and, in some cases, to bring their content up to date. (The first three pieces, however, have not been extensively updated. Their arguments are inseparable from their historical context, namely, an early stage in the understanding of AIDS.) Notes have sometimes been added to allow cross-referencing among the various essays. Digressions and repetitions have been trimmed, as have a number of illustrations. I am grateful to Paul for discussing these changes with me on many occasions and giving them his approval and for helping me, a philologist, understand his area of endeavor.

Haun Saussy

CREDITS

Chapter 1, "Bad Blood, Spoiled Milk: Bodily Fluids as Moral Barometers in Rural Haiti," was first published in *American Ethnologist* 15, no. 1 (1988): 62–83. Reproduced by permission of the American Anthropological Association. Not for sale or further reproduction.

Chapter 2, "Sending Sickness: Sorcery, Politics, and Changing Concepts of AIDS in Rural Haiti," was first published in *Medical Anthropology Quarterly* 4, no. 1 (1990): 6–27. Reproduced by permission of the American Anthropological Association. Not for sale or further reproduction. Additional passages are derived from "AIDS and Accusation: Haiti, Haitians, and the Geography of Blame," in Douglas A. Feldman, ed., *Culture and AIDS: The Human Factor* (New York: Praeger, 1990), pp. 67–91; and from "AIDS-Talk and the Constitution of Cultural Models," *Social Science and Medicine* 38, no. 6 (1994): 801–9.

Chapter 3, "The Exotic and the Mundane: Human Immunodeficiency Virus in Haiti," was originally published in *Human Nature* 1 (1990): 415–46, copyright © 1990 by Walter de Gruyter Inc., New York. It is reprinted with the kind permission of Springer Science+Business Media.

Chapter 4, "Ethnography, Social Analysis, and the Prevention of Sexually Transmitted HIV Infection among Poor Women in Haiti," was originally published in Marcia C. Inhorn and Peter J. Brown, eds., *The Anthropology of Infectious Disease: International Health Perspectives* (Amsterdam: Gordon and Breach, 1997), pp. 413–38.

Chapter 5, "From Haiti to Rwanda: AIDS and Accusations," was first published as the afterword to the second edition of *Aids and Accusation* (Berkeley: University of California Press, 2006).

Chapter 6, "Rethinking 'Emerging Infectious Diseases,'" is taken from chapter 2 of *Infections and Inequalities: The Modern Plagues* (Berkeley: University of California Press, 1999), pp. 37–58. An earlier version was published as "Social Inequalities and Emerging Infectious Diseases," *Emerging Infectious Diseases* 2, no. 4 (1996): 259–69.

Chapter 7, "Social Scientists and the New Tuberculosis," was first published in *Social Science and Medicine* 44, no. 3 (1997): 347–58.

Chapter 8, "Optimism and Pessimism in Tuberculosis Control: Lessons from Rural Haiti," is a shortened version of chapter 8 of Farmer, *Infections and Inequalities: The Modern Plagues* (Berkeley: University of California Press, 1999), pp. 211–27.

Chapter 9, "Cruel and Unusual: Drug-Resistant Tuberculosis as Punishment," was first published in Vivien Stern, ed., *Sentenced to Die? The Problem of TB in Prisons in Eastern Europe and Central Asia* (London: International Centre for Prison Studies, King's College, 1999), pp. 70–88.

Chapter 10, "The Consumption of the Poor: Tuberculosis in the Twenty-First Century," was originally published in *Ethnography* 1, no. 2 (2000): 183–216. A still earlier version appeared as chapter 7 of *Infections and Inequalities: The Modern Plagues* (Berkeley: University of California Press, 1999), pp. 184–210.

Chapter 11, "Social Medicine and the Challenge of Biosocial Research," was first published in *Innovative Structures in Basic Research: Ringberg Symposium, 4–7 October 2000* (Munich: Generalverwaltung der Max-Planck-Gesellschaft, Referat Press- und Öffentlichkeitsarbeit, 2002), pp. 55–73.

Chapter 12, "The Major Infectious Diseases in the World—To Treat or Not to Treat?" first appeared in the *New England Journal of Medicine* 345, no. 3 (2001): 208–10.

Chapter 13, "Integrated HIV Prevention and Care Strengthens Primary Health Care: Lessons from Rural Haiti," written by David A. Walton, Paul Farmer, Wesler Lambert, Fernet Léandre, Serena P. Koenig, and Joia S. Mukherjee, was first published in the *Journal of Public Health Policy* 25, no. 2 (2004): 137–58.

Chapter 14, "AIDS in 2006—Moving toward One World, One Hope?" written by Jim Yong Kim and Paul Farmer, was first published in the *New England Journal of Medicine* 355, no. 7 (2006): 645–47.

Chapter 15, "Women, Poverty, and AIDS," from Paul Farmer, Margaret Connors, and Janie Simmons, eds., *Women, Poverty, and AIDS: Sex, Drugs, and Structural Violence* (Monroe, Maine: Common Courage Press, 1996), pp. 3–38, is reprinted with the generous permission of Greg Bates and Common Courage Press.

A preliminary version of chapter 16, "On Suffering and Structural Violence: Social and Economic Rights in the Global Era," was published as "On Suffering and Structural Violence: A View from Below," *Daedalus* 125, no. 1 (1996): 261–83; and then, with revisions, as chapter 1 of *Pathologies of Power: Health, Human Rights, and the New War on the Poor* (Berkeley: University of California Press, 2003), pp. 29–50.

Chapter 17, "An Anthropology of Structural Violence," delivered as the 2001 Sidney W. Mintz Lecture in Anthropology on November 27, 2001, at Johns Hopkins University, was originally published in *Current Anthropology* 45, no. 3 (2004): 305–25, including commentary (pp. 317–22) by Philippe Bourgois, Nancy Scheper-Hughes, Didier Fassin, Linda Green, H. K. Heggenhougen, Laurence Kirmayer, and Loïc Wacquant. Copyright © 2004 by The Wenner-Gren Foundation for Anthropological Research.

An earlier version of chapter 18, "Structural Violence and Clinical Medicine," written by Paul Farmer, Bruce Nizeye, Sara Stulac, and Salmaan Keshavjee, was published in the online scientific journal *PLoS Medicine* 3, no. 10 (2006): e449.

Chapter 19, "Mother Courage and the Costs of War," was first published as "Mother Courage and the Future of War," in *An Anthropology of War*, ed. Alisse Waterston (New York: Berghahn Books, 2009), pp. 165–184.

Chapter 20, "'Landmine Boy' and Stupid Deaths," is a recasting of an article which previously appeared as "'Landmine Boy' and the Tomorrow of Violence," in Barbara Rylko-Bauer, Linda Whiteford, and Paul Farmer, eds., *Global Health in Times of Violence* (Santa Fe: SAR Press, 2009), pp. 41–62. Copyright © 2009 by the School for Advanced Research, Santa Fe, New Mexico.

Chapter 21, "Rethinking Health and Human Rights: Time for a Paradigm Shift," was originally published in the *American Journal of Public Health* 89, no. 10 (1999): 1486–96, as "Pathologies of Power: Rethinking Health and Human Rights." The version published here is revised from chapter 9 of *Pathologies of Power: Health, Human Rights, and the New War on the Poor* (Berkeley: University of California Press, 2003), pp. 213–46.

A version of chapter 22, "Rethinking Medical Ethics: A View from Below," written by Paul Farmer and Nicole Gastineau Campos, was previously published in *Developing World Bioethics* 4, no. 1 (2004): 17–41.

Chapter 23, "Never Again? Reflections on Human Values and Human Rights," was a lecture delivered at the University of Utah, March 30, 2005, as part of the series of Tanner Lectures on Human Values. It is reprinted by courtesy of the Tanner Foundation and the University of Utah Press.

Chapter 24, "Rich World, Poor World: Medical Ethics and Global Inequality," was delivered as the George Gay Lecture in the Harvard Medical School, May 2, 2006.

An earlier version of chapter 25, "Making Human Rights Substantial," was published as "Challenging Orthodoxies: The Road Ahead for Health and Human Rights," *Health and Human Rights: An International Journal* 10, no. 1 (2008): 5–19. That essay was based in part on Paul Farmer's keynote address to the 134th annual meeting of the American Public Health Association, Boston, November 5, 2006.

CALIFORNIA SERIES IN PUBLIC ANTHROPOLOGY

The California Series in Public Anthropology emphasizes the anthropologist's role as an engaged intellectual. It continues anthropology's commitment to being an ethnographic witness, to describing, in human terms, how life is lived beyond the borders of many readers' experiences. But it also adds a commitment, through ethnography, to reframing the terms of public debate—transforming received, accepted understandings of social issues with new insights, new framings.

Series Editor: Robert Borofsky (Hawaii Pacific University)

Contributing Editors: Philippe Bourgois (University of Pennsylvania), Paul Farmer (Partners in Health), Alex Hinton (Rutgers University), Carolyn Nordstrom (University of Notre Dame), and Nancy Scheper-Hughes (UC Berkeley)

University of California Press Editor: Naomi Schneider

TEXT
10/12.5 Minion Pro

DISPLAY
Minion Pro

COMPOSITOR
BookMatters, Berkeley

ILLUSTRATOR
Bill Nelson

INDEXER
Marcia Carlson

PRINTER/BINDER
Sheridan Books